Clinical Laboratory
Urinalysis and Body Fluids

Robert L. Sunheimer MSMT (ASCP) SC, SLS

Professor Emeritus

Dep...   ...Science

...University

...cuse, NY

Linda Graves, Ed.D., MT (ASCP)

Program Director, Medical Laboratory Technology Program

University of Maine at Presque Isle

Presque Isle, Maine

Wendy Stockwin, BS, MT (ASCP) SBB

Clinical Instructor

Department of Clinical Laboratory Science

SUNY Upstate Medical University

Syracuse, NY

PEARSON

Boston   Columbus   Indianapolis   New York   San Francisco   Upper Saddle River
Amsterdam   Cape Town   Dubai   London   Madrid   Milan   Munich   Paris   Montreal   Toronto
Delhi   Mexico City   Sao Paulo   Sydney   Hong Kong   Seoul   Singapore   Taipei   Tokyo

Publisher: Julie Levin Alexander
Publisher's Assistant: Regina Bruno
Editor in Chief: Marlene McHugh Pratt
Executive Editor: John Goucher
Editorial Project Manager: Jonathan Cheung
Editorial Assistant: Ericia Vivani
Development Editor: Anne Seitz/Learning and Performance
    Improvement Group
Director of Marketing: David Gesell
Marketing Manager: Brittany Hammond
Marketing Specialist: Michael Sirinides
Project Management Lead: Cynthia Zonneveld
Project Manager: Patricia Gutierrez

Operations Specialist: Nancy Maneri-Miller
Art Director: Mary Siener
Text Designer: Candace Rowley
Cover Designer: Carly Schnur
Media Director: Amy Peltier
Lead Media Project Manager: Lorena Cerisano
Full-Service Project Management: Patty Donovan, Laserwords
    Private Limited
Composition: Laserwords Private Limited
Printer/Binder: R.R. Donnelley/Willard
Cover Printer: Phoenix Color/Hagerstown
Text Font: Minion Pro Display 10/12

Credits and acknowledgments for content borrowed from other sources and reproduced, with permission, in this textbook appear on appropriate page within text.

Notice: The author and the publisher of this book have taken care to make certain that the information given is correct and compatible with the standards generally accepted at the time of publication. Nevertheless, as new information becomes available, changes in treatment and in the use of equipment and procedures become necessary. The reader is advised to carefully consult the instruction and information material included in each piece of equipment or device before administration. Students are warned that the use of any techniques must be authorized by their medical advisor, where appropriate, in accordance with local laws and regulations. The publisher disclaims any liability, loss, injury, or damage incurred as a consequence, directly or indirectly, of the use and application of any of the contents of this book.

Many of the designations by manufacturers and seller to distinguish their products are claimed as trademarks. Where those designations appear in this book, and the publisher was aware of a trademark claim, the designations have been printed in initial caps or all caps.

Library of Congress Cataloging-in-Publication Data
Sunheimer, Robert L., author.
  Clinical laboratory urinalysis and body fluids / Robert L. Sunheimer, Linda Graves, Wendy Stockwin.
     p. ; cm.
  Includes bibliographical references and index.
  ISBN 978-0-13-278404-7 — ISBN 0-13-278404-1
  I. Graves, Linda, author. II. Stockwin, Wendy, author. III. Title.
  [DNLM: 1. Urinalysis—methods. 2. Bodily Secretions—chemistry. 3. Body Fluids—chemistry. 4. Clinical Laboratory Techniques—methods. 5. Safety Management. QY 185]
RB53
616.07'566—dc23

2014021174

10 9 8 7 6 5 4 3 2 1

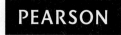

ISBN 10: 0-13-278404-1
ISBN 13: 978-0-13-278404-7

To my wife, Bonny; my daughter, Kristin; and my son Mark. —*Robert L. Sunheimer*

To the current students and graduates of the MLT program of the University of Maine at Presque Isle and the MLT Program of Maine. I continue to be extremely proud of the laboratory professionals who are graduates of the program. To my husband, Bill, who always provides support and encouragement.

—*Linda Graves*

Those who teach are lifelong learners. I dedicate this work to all my students who continue to teach me every day. —*Wendy Stockwin*

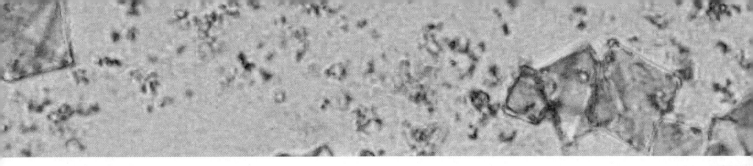

Contents

APPENDICES

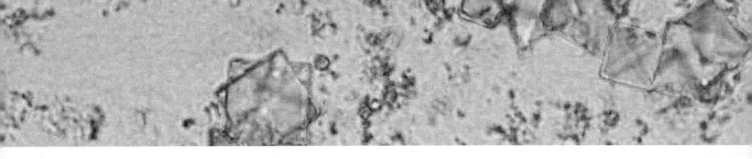

Acknowledgments

Clinical Laboratory Urinalysis and Body Fluids is a massive project and the product of many individuals. The editors guided us through the various steps in the process and offered encouragement when we needed a little push to keep going. Reviewers gave us extremely valuable feedback and suggestions on our various chapters.

Special thanks are extended to the staff of Pearson Health Science: John Goucher, Executive Editor, who kept in touch throughout the long process; Associate Editors Jonathan Cheung, Melissa Kerian, and Monica Moosang kept us on track and provided support: Anne Seitz and Laura Horowitz were invaluable support during the assembling of the manuscript. We couldn't have done it without their help!

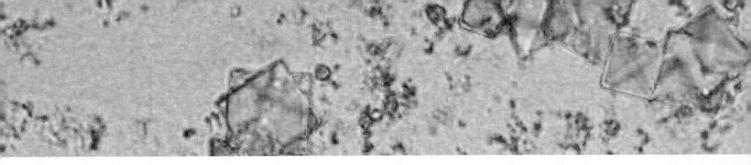

Reviewers

Jimmy Boyd, MLS (ASCP)
Arkansas State University – Beebe
Beebe, Arkansas

Karen Chandler, M.A.MLS (ASCP)
University of Texas Pan American
Edinburg, TX

Lee Danielson, PhD, MLS (ASCP)
University of New Mexico-School of Medicine
Albuquerque, NM

Kathryn Dugan, MEd, MT(ASCP)
Auburn University — Montogomery
Montgomery, AL

Amy Gatautis. MBA, MT(ASCP)SC
Cuyahoga College – Metro Campus
Cleveland, Ohio

Risa Grimme, MA, BS, MT(ASCP)
Calhoun Community College
Decatur, Alabama

Nancy Heldt, MT(ASCP)
Oakton Community College
Des Plaines, Illinois

Lori Howard, MLFSC, BSMT(ASCP)SM
Halifax Community College
Weldon, North Carolina

Cheryl Jackson-Harris, MSMT(ASCP)SHCM
California State University – Dominguez Hills
Carson, California

Steve Johnson, MS, MT(ASCP)
Saint Vincent Health Center School of Med Technology
Erie, Pennsylvania

Rhoda Jost, MSH, MT(ASCP)
Florida State College at Jacksonville
Jacksonville, Florida

Amy Kapanka, MS, MT(ASCP)SC
Hawkeye Community College
Waterloo, Iowa

Janis Livingston, MLT, MT(ASCP)
Midlands Technical College
Columbia, South Carolina

Sonja Nehr-kanet, MS, MLS (ASCP)
Idaho State University
Pocatello, Idaho

Amanda Reed, BA, M.Ed., BS, CLS(ASCP)CM
Saint Louis University
Saint Louis, Missouri

Diane Schmaus, MA, MT(ASCP)
McLennan Community College
Waco, Texas

Tonya Shearin-Patterson, MT(ASCP)MCH
York College, CUNY
Jamaica, New York

Rosalyn Singleton, MT(ASCP)
Northeast Mississippi Community College
Booneville, Mississippi

Jean Sparks, MLS(ASCP), PhD Molecular Biology
Texas A&M University — Corpus Christi
College Station, TX

Dawn Williamson, MS
Southeastern Community College
Whiteville, North Carolina

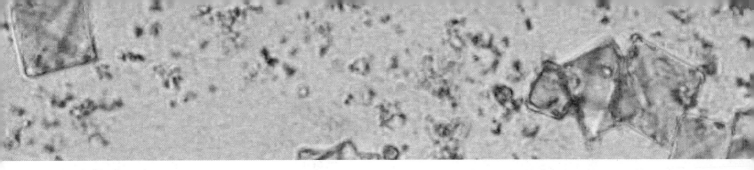

Safety

Objectives

LEVEL I

Following successful completion of this chapter, the learner will be able to:

1. Identify elements of an exposure control plan.
2. List five examples of personal protective equipment (PPE) and engineered controls used to protect laboratory staff and indicate when they should be used.
3. List five examples of potentially infectious body fluids and provide examples of what contaminants may be present.
4. Describe the purpose of a chemical hygiene plan.
5. Identify equipment in a laboratory and administrative areas that may emit harmful radiation.
6. List five important safety procedures to follow when handling electrical equipment.
7. Identify the classes of fires and the appropriate type of fire extinguisher to use.
8. Define the acronyms RACE and PASS.
9. Explain the proper way to store compressed gas cylinders and what may happen if the cylinders fall to the floor.
10. Identify three types of waste generated by a clinical laboratory and identify an agency that may provide information on safe disposal.
11. List five examples of risk factors for cumulative trauma disorders and state a method to mitigate them.
12. Discuss the significant aspects of selected workplace safety issues.

LEVEL II

Following successful completion of this chapter, the learner will be able to:

1. Select the appropriate Codes of Federal Register (CFR) to review for a specific safety issue.
2. Identify elements of an exposure control plan and discuss measures to reduce the possibility of accidental exposure.

Chapter Outline

(continued)

Objectives *(continued)*

3. Identify elements of a chemical hygiene plan and indicate the importance of such a plan.
4. Provide specific examples of information available in an SDS and explain why this information is important to laboratory workers.
5. Interpret a selected NFPA 704-M warning label and discuss the proper procedure for handling the substance.
6. Compare and contrast ionizing radiation and nonionizing radiation and identify four sources of nonionizing radiation.

7. Recognize all the potential electrical hazards found in a clinical laboratory.
8. Discuss the reason why compressed gas cylinders must be stored in an upright position and secured to the wall or bench.
9. Identify issues that should be included in the development of a waste management policy and discuss their impact on the laboratory.
10. Explain the importance of ergonomics in the workplace.
11. Identify several workplace safety issues and explain their role in clinical laboratories.

Key Terms

Bloodborne pathogens
Carcinogen
Chemical hygiene plan
Codes of Federal Regulations
Cumulative trauma disorders

Engineered control
Ergonomics
Exposure control plan
Hazard Identification System
Incident command system

Nonionizing radiation
Occupational Safety and
  Health Administration
Personal protective equipment
Safety Data Sheets

Teratogen
Universal precautions
Xenobiotic

A CASE IN POINT

A member of the laboratory staff was asked to clean out a closet storage area where chemicals had been stored and came upon a bottle of concentrated hydrochloric acid.

Questions to Consider

1. What is the NFPA704-M placard designations for health hazard, fire/flammability, reactivity, and special hazard?

2. What is the physical appearance of the chemical?
3. Where can you look for information regarding the safety issues for this chemical?
4. What important information about the chemical should be the focus for this laboratory worker?
5. What specific steps should be taken to properly handle, use, and dispose of this chemical?

Safe laboratory practices are the responsibility of everyone who enters the facility. Knowledge and common sense are the keys to ensure that accidents are kept to a minimum. All laboratory staff should develop an appreciation for safety because working safely is as much an attitude as it is a practice.

LABORATORY SAFETY

A substantial number of organizations are actively involved in providing a safe environment for laboratory personnel, including state, federal, professional, and accrediting agencies. Some examples are listed in Table 1-1 ★, and we will discuss one organization specifically in the section following.

OCCUPATIONAL SAFETY AND HEALTH ADMINISTRATION

The U.S. **Occupational Safety and Health Administration** (OSHA) is a federal agency within the Department of Labor that was created by Congress through public law 91-596 in 1970 to

★ **TABLE 1-1** Organizations Involved in Providing Safety Standards, Guidelines, Education, and Procedures for Clinical Laboratories

Abbreviation	Organization
CAP	College of American Pathologists
ASCP	American Society for Clinical Pathology
AACC	American Association for Clinical Chemistry
CDC	Centers for Disease Control and Prevention
DNV	Det Norske Veritas (hospital accreditation)
EPA	Environmental Protection Agency
OSHA	Occupational Safety and Health Administration
JC (JCAHO)	The Joint Commission (formerly JCAHO, Joint Commission on Accreditation of Healthcare Organizations)
CLIS (NCCLS)	Clinical and Laboratory Standards Institute (formerly National Committee for Clinical Laboratory Standards)
NIOSH	National Institute for Occupational Safety and Health
NFPA	National Fire Protection Agency

provide standards of safety for all men and women in workplace facilities. OSHA standards are found in the **Codes of Federal Regulations** (CFR). The standard most associated with clinical laboratories is Standard 29 CFR, which is divided into several sections identified using part numbers and standard numbers (e.g., 1910.1450, titled "Occupational Exposure to Hazardous Chemicals in the Laboratories").[1] A list of parts and standards relevant to clinical laboratories is shown in Table 1-2 ★. Detailed information for each part may be found in the Federal Register, document 29 CFR.

Four major OSHA programs have made a significant impact upon the safety practices in clinical laboratories:

- Occupational exposure to hazardous chemicals in laboratories (29CFR 1910.1450).

- Hazard Communication (29 CFR1910.1200), which includes Right to Know, OSHA poster 2203, and SDS. In 1988, OSHA expanded this regulation to include hospital workers.

- Occupational exposure to bloodborne pathogens (29 CFR 1910.1030). In 1991 OSHA issued the Bloodborne Pathogens Standard to protect workers from this risk.

- In 2001, in response to the Needlestick Safety and Prevention Act, OSHA revised the occupational exposure to bloodborne pathogens (29 CFR 1910.1030) to include needlestick safety.

☑ CHECKPOINT 1-1

Which Codes of Federal Regulations (CFR) may assist a laboratory supervisor in developing a policy for the proper handling of patient specimens?

★ **TABLE 1-2** Relevant OSHA Standards, Including the Respective Titles for Clinical Laboratories

1910.94	Ventilation	
1910.97	Nonionizing radiation	
1910.101	Compressed gases (General requirements)	
1910.120	Hazardous waste operations and emergency response	
1910.134	Respiratory protection	
1910.155	Fire protection	
	1910 Subpart L	Portable fire extinguishers
	1910 Subpart S	Electrical
	1910 Subpart Z	Toxic and hazardous substances
1910.1030	Bloodborne pathogens	
1910.1048	Formaldehyde	
1910.1096	Ionizing radiation	
1910.1200	Hazard communications	
1910.1450	Occupational exposure to hazardous chemicals in laboratories	

BIOHAZARDS/UNIVERSAL PRECAUTION

Exposure Control Plan

OSHA requires all laboratories to develop and implement an **exposure control plan**,[2] which is designed to help prevent accidental exposure of laboratory personnel to bloodborne pathogens. **Bloodborne pathogens** are pathogenic microorganisms that are present in human blood and can cause disease in humans. These pathogens include, but are not limited to, hepatitis B virus (HBV) and human immunodeficiency virus (HIV). The exposure control plan also includes procedures for the proper handling and disposal of all medical waste produced by the laboratory as well as sections on (1) purpose, (2) scope, (3) references, (4) definition of terms, (5) delineation of responsibilities, and (6) detailed procedural steps.

Biological Hazards

Laboratory personnel must be aware of potential sources of exposure to infectious agents such as HBV and HIV from

- Centrifuge accidents.
- Needle punctures.
- Spilling infectious material on bench surfaces.
- Cuts and scratches from contaminated glassware.
- Removing stoppers from blood drawing tubes.

Universal precautions* is a practice described by National Institute for Occupational Safety and Health (NIOSH) in which every clinical laboratory should treat all human blood and other potentially infectious material as if it was known to contain infectious agents such a HBV, HIV, and other bloodborne pathogens.[3] Examples of infectious materials include all human blood, vaginal secretions, semen, tissue, and the following fluids: pleural, peritoneal, pericardial, amniotic, cerebrospinal, and synovial. Universal precautions do not applied to feces, nasal secretion, saliva (except in dental settings), sputum, sweat, tears, urine, and vomit unless it contains visible blood. Hands and other skin surfaces should be washed immediately and thoroughly if contaminated with blood or other body fluids. Hands should also be washed immediately after gloves are removed.[4]

Mouthpieces, resuscitation bags, and other ventilation devices should be available for use in areas in which the need for resuscitation is predictable to minimize the need for emergency mouth-to-mouth resuscitation, although saliva has not been implicated in HIV transmission. Healthcare workers who have exudative lesions or weeping dermatitis should refrain from all direct patient care and from handling patient-care equipment until the condition resolves.

Pregnant healthcare workers are not known to be at greater risk of contracting HIV infection than healthcare workers who are not pregnant; however, if a healthcare worker develops an HIV infection

---

*The CDC has replaced the term *Universal Precautions* with the terms *standard precautions* and *transmission-based precautions* for healthcare workers. The difference between the three is shown below:

Universal precautions—for fluids liable to have blood or are visibly bloody

Standard precautions—for all body substances except sweat

Transmission-based precautions—specific for new microbes

during pregnancy, the infant is at risk of infection resulting from perinatal transmission. Because of this risk, pregnant healthcare workers should be especially familiar with and strictly adhere to precautions to minimize the risk of HIV transmission.[5]

Hand Hygiene Practices

Transmission of pathogens most often occurs via the contaminated hands of healthcare workers. Accordingly, hand hygiene (i.e., hand washing with soap and water or use of a waterless, alcohol-based hand rub) has long been considered one of the most important infection control measures for preventing the transmission of infectious agents.

The CDC recommends vigorous rubbing together of all lathered surfaces for at least 15 seconds followed by rinsing in a flowing stream of water as shown in Box 1-1.[6] If hands are visibly soiled, more time may be required. Hand hygiene is still necessary after gloves are removed because gloves may become perforated and bacteria can multiply rapidly on gloved hands.

- Individuals will wash their hands immediately or as soon as possible after removal of gloves or other PPE and after hand contact with blood or other potentially infectious materials.

- Hands are to be washed between all patient contacts, before eating, drinking, smoking, applying cosmetics or lip balm, manipulating contact lenses, handling of personal devices (e.g., book bags and cell phones), and after using the restroom.

Needlestick Regulations

OSHA updated 29 CFR 1910.1030 to include the Needlestick Safety and Preventions Act,[7,8] which requires that needles used for withdrawing blood must have a "built-in safety feature or mechanism that effectively reduces the risk of an exposure incident." All laboratories must provide the appropriate devices and monitor their use as part of a quality assurance program.

The Centers for Disease Control and Prevention (CDC) reported that implementing the following measures may prevent needlestick injuries:[9]

- Use safe and effective alternatives to needles.
- Participate in the selection and evaluation of needle safety devices.
- Use only devices equipped with safety mechanisms.
- Do not recap needles.
- Implement a plan that will ensure safe handling and disposal of needles.
- Immediately dispose of used needles in the proper sharps disposal containers.
- Communicate needlestick hazards to employees.
- Participate in infection control training.

☑ CHECKPOINT 1-2

What is the term that describes the following? Every clinical laboratory should treat all human blood and other potentially infectious material as if they were known to contain infectious agents such a HBV, HIV, and other bloodborne pathogens.

Personal Protective Equipment

Personal protective equipment (PPE) is specialized clothing or equipment worn by an employee for protection against a hazard. General work clothes (e.g., uniforms, pants, shirts, or blouses) not intended to function as protection against a hazard are not considered PPE. Several examples of PPE are shown in Figure 1-1 ■.

BOX 1-1   Hand Hygiene Procedure

Hand wash procedure	Comments
1. Turn on water faucet to a cool temperature.	Water that is too hot can affect skin integrity.
2. Place hands under water.	To aid soap activation.
3. Dispense one pump action volume of soap.	Excessive volume of soap product may cause drying of hands, and dry cracked hands may harbor bacteria, viruses, and fungi.
4. Rubbing briskly, wash all surfaces of hands, including between fingers, for at least 15 seconds.	The focus of good hand washing technique is to initiate mechanical removal of dirt and microorganisms, using friction and rinsing under running water.
5. Rinse thoroughly under running water.	To reduce skin irritation from soap residue.
6. Pat hands dry with paper towels, discarding the paper towels in a waste container.	
7. If using a hand-operated faucet, use a dry paper towel to turn off faucet.	All faucet handles are considered contaminated.

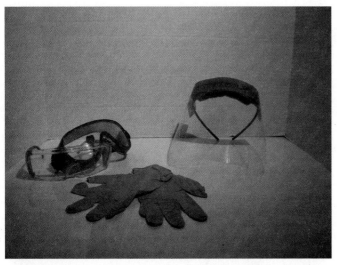

FIGURE 1-1 Personal Protective Equipment (PPE) Including Gloves, Face Shield, Safety Goggles with Side Shield

Gloves

The routine use of gloves to protect laboratory staff against exposure to bloodborne pathogens was included in 29 CFR 1910.1030. As laboratory staff began wearing gloves on a daily basis for a prolonged time, reports of skin sensitivities traceable to the plastic gloves increased. Skin sensitivities may be due to either protein from the rubber tree or to the chemicals used in the production of latex. NIOSH has recommended that employers provide gloves with reduced protein content (e.g., latex free and powder- or cornstarch-free gloves). In addition, every employee should be provided with continuing education and training materials about latex allergies, and high-risk employees should be screened periodically for allergy symptoms.

Gloves are also available to protect employees from exposure to chemicals (e.g., acids, bases, and solvents). Glove materials highly rated for handling acids and bases include nitrile, neoprene, and natural rubber. Nitrile- and neoprene-based gloves are also acceptable for handling organic solvents. For guidance on proper selection of gloves, refer to the MAPA® Spontex, Inc. (Columbia, TN) chemical resistance guide.

Eyewear

Laboratory staff occasionally chooses not to properly protect their eyes while handling hazardous materials. Workers who wear glasses often feel "safe" and do not believe that additional eyewear is necessary. Conventional or prescription eyeglasses are not impervious to chemicals, and therefore they are not considered to be safety glasses. Proper eyewear is described as glasses or goggles that provide protection to the sides of the face as well as the front. The lenses must also be impervious to chemicals. Another acceptable face-eye protection device is the face shield.

Respirators

Respirators are required for selected laboratory procedures. Most notable is the handling of pathogenic microorganisms such as strains of *Mycobacterium tuberculosis*.[10] Respirators should contain high-efficiency particulate air (HEPA) filters if no other engineering controls are available. Handling of certain chemicals may require the use of a respirator. The Safety Data Sheet (SDS) explained later in the section on chemical safety, accompanying the chemical should indicate whether a respirator is required. Filtration respirators will require the use of one or two cartridges designed to filter out hazardous chemical vapors. Strict adherence to all safety recommendations is necessary when handling hazardous materials requiring the use of any type of respirator.

Laboratory Coats and Footwear

Laboratory coats should be provided to employees by the employer. Laboratory coats should be designed with the following features:

- They must have cuffed sleeves and be full length.
- The material should be resistant to liquids.
- The construction of lab coats resistant to liquids includes layers of polypropylene, spun bonded filaments, and melt-blown polypropylene microfibers.

A spun bonded filament refers to the process of producing filaments or webs from polypropylene and other organic substances that will restrict fluids from passing through. Melt-blown polypropylene is a thermally bonded ultrafine fiber that has been self-bonded, forming a three-dimensional random microporous structure. This material is impervious to the passage of liquids through the fibers. Laboratory staff should keep their laboratory coats buttoned to avoid contaminating their street clothes.

Laboratory staff should also wear footwear that is comfortable and safe. The shoe material should be nonporous. No open toed shoes, sandals, or flip-flops should be worn in the laboratory.

Engineered Controls

An **engineered control** is defined as safety equipment that isolates or removes the bloodborne pathogen hazard from the workplace and represents the preferred method for controlling hazards. Several examples of engineered controls are listed in Box 1-2 and shown in Figure 1-2 ■.

BOX 1-2 Examples of Several Safety-Engineered Controls

Splash shields
Biosafety cabinets
Secondary containers
Impervious needle boxes
Automatic pipettes
Centrifuge caps
Self-sheathing needles

Glass versus Plastic

Exposure to broken glass in the laboratory poses a similar risk to that posed by a needlestick. Therefore, clinical laboratories should use products that reduce the risk of exposure to broken glass. Many glass products, including specimen collection tubes, capillary tubes, pipettes, and slides, can be replaced by their plastic counterparts. Benefits of converting to plasticware are (1) reduced cost in biohazard waste disposal because plastic is lighter than glass and (2) that plastics can be incinerated, thus reducing waste "downstream." Laboratory staff must remember that when switching to plasticware, especially blood collection tubes, they must review the manufacturer's data and verify method performance characteristics (e.g., accuracy, precision, and interference) related to the plasticware.

Biosafety Levels

The CDC and National Institutes of Health (NIH) have developed criteria for handling infectious materials. These criteria are classified into four biosafety levels: biosafety levels 1 (BSL1) through 4 (BSL4).[11] Table 1-3 ★ provides a portion of the information contained in the reference cited. Knowledge of BSLs is required when questions arise regarding proper use and functional parameters of laboratory hoods.

☑ CHECKPOINT 1-3

True or False: It is acceptable to wear comfortable sandals with exposed toes in a clinical laboratory.

★ **TABLE 1-3** Biosafety Levels 1-4 with Associated Agents

BSL	Agents
BSL1	Not known to cause diseases in healthy adults consistently
BSL2	Associated with human disease; hazard by percutaneous injury, ingestion, and mucous membrane exposure
BSL3	Indigenous or exotic agents with potential for aerosol transmission; disease may have serious or lethal consequences
BSL4	Dangerous/exotic agents, which pose high risk of life-threatening disease; aerosol-transmitted lab infections; or related agents with unknown risk of transmission

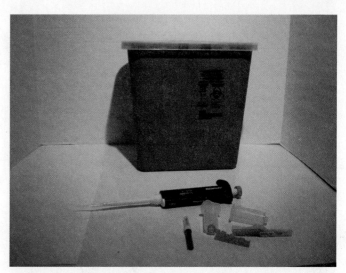

■ **FIGURE 1-2** Engineered Controls. Puncture-Resistant Sharps Container, Pipet, and Safety Needle Cover

Toxic Substances

Toxic substances pose a potentially significant and long-lasting risk to all laboratory personnel. Chemicals in this group have the potential to affect the offspring of female workers. The term **xenobiotic** refers to a substance that is foreign to a living organism and usually harmful. The routes of entry for xenobiotic substances include the following:

- Pulmonary
- Oral
- Transcutaneous absorption
- Percutaneous (ocular contact)

Once a xenobiotic enters the body, it circulates until a suitable cellular receptor is located. Examples of receptors include the following:

- Membranes
- Antibodies
- Circulating carrier proteins
- Water-soluble intracellular proteins
- Intracellular cytoskeletal proteins

A xenobiotic substance that results in the production of a cancer-producing tumor is termed a **carcinogen**. Examples of compounds currently classified as carcinogens that may be found in laboratories are

- Asbestos
- Arsenic
- Benzene
- Benzidine
- Nickel

Teratogens

A **teratogen** is a substance that acts preferentially on an embryo at precise stages of its development, thereby leading to possible anomalies and malformations. *Organogenesis* is a term that describes the process that can occur in the 15th through 60th day of fetal development, where the embryo is most sensitive to the action of a teratogenic substance. Examples of teratogens include thalidomide, polyaromatic hydrocarbons, dimethylmercury, diethylstilbestrol (DES), and vinyl chloride.

☑ CHECKPOINT 1-4

A laboratory staff member complains that she develops allergy-like symptoms when donning a particular type of glove. What type of glove would you recommend that she use to prevent these symptoms?

CHEMICAL SAFETY

Chemical safety awareness is of paramount importance in the clinical laboratory. The staff technologist may handle several different types of chemicals in a working day. Therefore, knowledge of the compounds, their associated hazards, and proper handling is very important in reducing the extent of injury in case of an accidental exposure.

Chemical Hygiene Plan

OSHA recommends that each laboratory establish a **chemical hygiene plan**.[12] This plan is designed to provide laboratory staff with information necessary to handle chemicals. Several specific elements included in the hygiene plan are listed in Box 1-3.

Operating Procedures

Specific operating protocols should be developed for proper disposition of accidents in the laboratories involving chemical spills. After accidents that involve chemicals splashed into the eyes, they must be flushed immediately with copious amounts of water from an eyewash station (Figure 1-3 ■). The eyewash station should be plumbed to a continuous source of water (60–100°F) and be handicapped accessible. Maintenance of eyewash devices should include periodic flushing to ensure sufficient flow of water and to minimize bacterial growth in the lines that could lead to eye infections. When chemicals, especially corrosives, are splashed into the eyes, they should be rinsed for 15 minutes continuously and without interruption in an eyewash or under a faucet if an eyewash is unavailable. Chemical exposure to other body tissues also requires that the affected body tissue be flushed with water using a faucet or shower, after which a physician should evaluate the victim. Flushing should last for at least 15 minutes.

Chemical spills occur in laboratories and should be approached with care. Laboratory staff should be properly trained to respond in a safe manner. Every laboratory staff should have knowledge of the chemicals being used, available resources, first aid procedures, and the proper steps to assess the impact of a spill.

Appropriate response to a chemical spill is dictated by the size of the spill. A small spill is typically described as a spill of less than 20 to 30 cc, or one ounce of toxic material, or up to one gallon of low-toxicity chemical. Large chemical spills are defined as spills greater than one gallon or 20 to 30 cc of a chemical that is highly hazardous. Once the size of a spill is determined, the appropriate response must be initiated.

Small chemical spills can be managed by laboratory staff. The SDSs should be available and knowledge of chemical NFPA 704-M labels may be helpful. All laboratories should have a chemical spill kit available. A commercial kit for most types of spills is available and is shown in Figure 1-4 ■. All-purpose absorbents—for example, kitty litter, vermiculite, and sand—can also be used. These materials are useful to form a dike to contain the spill. Before cleaning up the spill, remember to wear appropriate PPE. As a minimum, this includes gloves and protective eyewear.

Depending on the size and type of spill, protective clothing, protective foot covering, and a respirator may be needed. Pick up any broken glass with tongs or some other mechanical device. Do not use your hands. Place absorbent material over the spill, making sure not to spread the liquid. Transfer all contaminated material into a plastic bag.

BOX 1-3 Specific Elements Included in the OSHA Chemical Hygiene Plan

Glossary of terms

A description of standard operating procedures

An inventory of all chemicals

Safety Data Sheets (SDS)

Proper labeling and storage of chemicals

An inventory of personal protective equipment

A description of engineering controls

Procedures for waste removal and disposal

Requirements for employees' physical and medical consultations

Training requirements

Procedures for proper record keeping

Designation of a chemical hygiene officer and safety committee

---

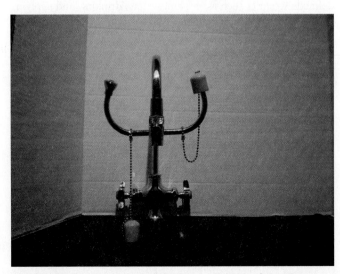

■ **FIGURE 1-3** Eyewash Station with Dual Jet Eye Washers

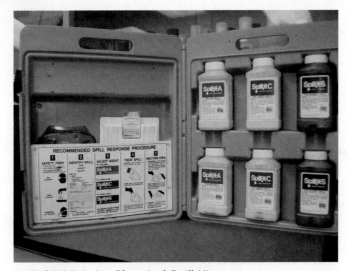

■ **FIGURE 1-4** Chemical Spill Kit

Label the bag with the name of the hazardous material. Finally, contact the appropriate hazardous spill team or emergency health team. The incident should be documented, first aid issues addressed, and an analysis of the incident should be initiated to assess the appropriateness of the response and measures to prevent reoccurrence.

The response for a large chemical spill requires a higher level of expertise and coordination of the departments within an institution. A large chemical spill typically requires evacuation of the area. The doors to the affected room should be closed to contain the vapors or gases. Appropriate notification of external response crews depends on the nature and size of the chemical spill. For example, a spill may dictate the need for fire department, HAZMAT crew, or an institutional safety department. Be prepared to provide the responding crews with the necessary information about the spill (e.g., name of chemical(s) and approximate quantity of material spilled). Finally, do not reenter the area until advised by an appropriate authority that it is safe to do so.

Policies for avoiding unnecessary chemical exposure must be defined. Activities such as smoking, eating, drinking, and applying cosmetics must be prohibited in all workstations. Wearing of proper footwear must be enforced. No sandals, canvas shoes, or any open-toed footware should be allowed. Staff with long hair or loose clothing and jewelry should be reminded that these items must be secured. Contact lenses should not be worn in the laboratory because they prevent proper washing of the eyes in the case of a chemical splash. In addition, plastic lenses may be damaged by organic vapors, which may lead to chronic eye infections. Hand washing after handling chemicals and before leaving the laboratory should be emphasized.

Safety Data Sheets (SDSs) are documents that provide information about the chemical substances. Each sheet consists of 16 sections, including identification, composition, hazards, first aid, firefighting concerns, and safe handling, that are relevant to the chemical being used. SDSs must be obtained for all chemicals and must be located in an area available to all laboratory personnel at any time. The format of the SDS has been standardized by the American National Standards Institute (ANSI), which makes the document easier to interpret.[13]

Identifying and Labeling Chemicals

Proper labeling of chemicals is described in OSHA standard 29 CFR 1910.1450. The actual labeling system has been adopted from the **Hazard Identification System** developed by the National Fire Protection Agency (NFPA).[14] This identification system, referred to as the 704-M Identification System, categorizes chemicals into nine classes of hazardous materials:

- Explosives
- Compressed gases
- Flammable liquids
- Flammable solids
- Oxidizer materials
- Toxic materials
- Radioactive materials
- Corrosive materials
- Miscellaneous materials not classified by any other means

Materials are identified using four small, diamond-shaped symbols grouped into a large diamond shape, as shown in Figure 1-5 ■. The smaller diamonds are colored coded to represent a specific health hazard as shown in Table 1-4 ★. The degree of hazard is rated using a scale of 0 to 4, with 4 indicating the most serious risk. Chemical labels on the original containers must not be removed or defaced. For chemicals not in their original containers, the labeling information must include at least the following information:

- Identification of the hazardous chemical
- Route of body entry
- Health hazard
- Physical hazard
- Target organ(s) affected

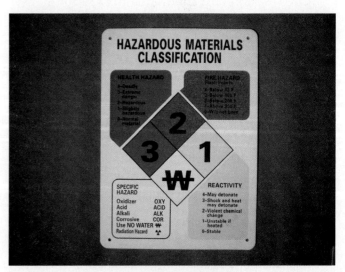

■ **FIGURE 1-5** NFPA 704-M. Identification System Using Diamond-Shaped Symbol

★ **TABLE 1-4** NFPA 704–M Identification System of Warning Labels for Chemical Hazards

Color-codes	Interpretations	
Blue–Health Hazard	4-Deadly	
	3-Extreme danger	
	2-Hazardous	
	1-Slightly hazardous	
	0-Normal material	
Red–Fire Hazard		
Flash points	4-Below 73°F	
	3-Below 100°F	
	2-Below 200°F	
	1-Above 200°F	
	0-Will not burn	
Yellow–Reactivity	4-May detonate	
	3-Shock and heat may detonate	
	2-Violent chemical change	
	1-Unstable if heated	
	0-Stable	
White–Specific Hazards	Oxidizer	OXY
	Corrosive	COR
	Acid	ACID
	Alkali	ALK
	Use no water	W̶
	Radiation	☢

☑ CHECKPOINT 1-5

The container for a chemical received in the clinical laboratory reveals a symbol with a capital letter W with a line drawn through it (W̶) in the white diamond of the NFPA 704-M identification designation. What information does this disclose to the laboratory staff?

Storage and Inventory of Chemicals

A chemical inventory should be conducted on an annual basis. An accurate listing of all chemicals and their hazards should be made available at all times. During the inventory process, the technologist should focus on the following:

- Keep only the amount of chemicals that is needed. Less is better.
- If possible, purchase chemicals in plastic containers to avoid breaking glass.
- Rotate the chemical inventory and note expiration dates.
- Dispose of chemicals if not used within a year—especially peroxide-forming compounds.
- Make sure all secondary containers are properly labeled.
- If possible, relocate corrosive, flammable, and reactive chemicals to below eye level.

BOX 1-4 Examples of Poor Chemical Storage Practices

Chemicals stored in random order

Chemicals stored in alphabetical order

Chemicals stored by poorly chosen categories

Chemicals stored in a hood while the hood is in use for other purposes

Flammables stored in domestic (household-type) refrigerators

Food stored beside chemicals in refrigerator

Chemicals stored on shelves above eye level

Stacking chemicals on top of each other

Overcrowded shelves

Shelving on which chemicals are stored is not strong enough to support chemicals

Shelves not securely fastened to a permanent structure

Poor or nonexistent inventory control

Containers with no labels or inappropriate labels

Containers stored on the floor

Caps on containers are missing, not secured, or badly deteriorated

Proper storage of hazardous materials in the laboratory is very important. Several examples of poor storage practices are shown in Box 1-4. Examples of problems with storing chemicals alphabetically are shown in Table 1-5 ★.[15]

Categorical storage of chemicals is a safe approach for separating potentially reactive chemicals. Each chemical must be stored in its respective hazardous category. For example, inorganic acids such as hydrochloric acid (HCL) and sulfuric acid (H_2SO_4) should be stored as a group and should not be stored with caustic bases, such as sodium hydroxide (NaOH) and ammonium hydroxide (NH_4OH). Chemicals classified as oxidizing compounds, such as potassium dichromate and silver nitrate, can be stored together, but away from

★ **TABLE 1-5** Problems Associated with Storing Chemicals Alphabetically

Chemical Combinations	Problems
Acetic acid + acetaldehyde	Small amounts of acetic acid will cause the acetaldehyde to polymerize, releasing a large amount of heat.
Ammonium nitrate + acetic acid	Mixture will ignite, especially with concentrated acids
Hydrogen peroxide + ferrous sulfide	Vigorous reaction, highly exothermic
Lead perchlorate + methanol	Explosive mixture if agitated
Potassium cyanide + potassium nitrite	Potentially explosive mixture if heated

other compounds. Chemical compatibility charts are available that outline general classes of incompatible chemical.[16]

Flammable chemicals must be stored in an appropriate safety cabinet (see section entitled "Safety Cabinets") and should not be mixed in with other classes of compounds. Volatile or flammable liquids should never be stored in refrigerators that are not designed to accommodate hazards the solvents may create. If the laboratory has corrosive or flammable chemicals that require refrigeration, there are several manufacturers that distribute explosion-proof and corrosion-proof refrigerators. These units are designed to comply with NFPA and OSHA specifications.

Transferring chemicals from one container to another can result in an accident or overexposure. Therefore, care must be taken to avoid these situations. A bottle should never be held by its neck, but instead should be gripped firmly around its body with one or both hands, depending on the size of the bottle. Acids must be diluted slowly by adding them to water while mixing. Never add water to a concentrated acid. Transferring volatile or flammable chemicals should be conducted in an OSHA-approved fume hood. In addition, safety glasses should be worn whenever transferring chemicals from one container to another. Acids, caustic materials, and strong oxidizing agents should be mixed in the sink. This provides water for cooling and confinement of the reagent in case of a spill.

Transporting chemicals throughout the laboratory can be hazardous. For safe transport of any chemical, place it in an approved secondary container. Chemicals in glass bottles should be transported in rubber or plastic containers that protect them from breakage and, in the event of breakage, help to contain the spill. To move heavy containers or multiple numbers of containers from one area of the laboratory to another, use a cart.

Potentially Explosive Compounds

Laboratory staff must be aware of any chemicals that have the potential to explode or detonate. An *explosive* chemical is described as a chemical that causes a sudden release of pressure, gas, or heat when subjected to shock, pressure, or high temperatures. Dried picric acid may explode if the container is dropped (Figure 1-6 ■). Azides, specifically lead azide, are explosives that may detonate when heated or shaken. Heavy-metal azides are formed when solutions or reagents containing sodium azide are exposed to heavy metals or their salts. Heavy-metal azides can accumulate under certain circumstances, for example, in metal pipelines, and thus lead to violent explosions. Anhydrous and monohydrate perchloric acid are explosive, but the usual aqueous solutions are stable in the absence of organic compounds. The crystalline form of the acid, which is explosive and shock sensitive, can precipitate on a hood surface. Information regarding the explosive nature of chemicals may be found in their accompanying SDSs.

Cryogenic Material

Cryogenic liquids (cryogens) are liquefied gases that are kept in their liquid state at very low temperatures. The word *cryogenic* means "producing, or related to, low temperatures," and all cryogenic liquids are extremely cold. Cryogenic liquids have boiling points below $-150°C$ ($-238°F$). Carbon dioxide and nitrous oxide, which have slightly higher boiling points, are sometimes included in this category. All cryogenic liquids are gases at normal temperatures and pressures. These gases must be cooled below room temperature before an increase in pressure can liquefy them. Various cryogens become liquids under different conditions of temperature and pressure, but all have two properties in common: (1) They are extremely cold and (2) small amounts of liquid can expand into very large volumes of gas.

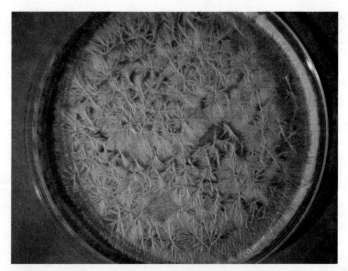

■ **FIGURE 1-6** Dried Picric Acid May Explode If the Container is Dropped

The vapors and gases released from cryogenic liquids also remain very cold. They often condense the moisture in air, creating a highly visible fog. In poorly insulated containers, some cryogenic liquids actually condense the surrounding air, forming a liquid air mixture. Cryogenic liquids are classified as "compressed gases" according to North American Industrial Classification System (NAICS) 325120, which replaced the Standard Industrial Classification Code 2813. Everyone who works with cryogenic liquids must be aware of their hazards and know how to work with them safely.

Cryogenic liquids such as liquid nitrogen, helium, and oxygen are, by definition, extremely cold. Contact of exposed skin to cryogenic liquids and can produce a painful burn. A splash of cryogenic liquid in the eye can cause loss of vision. Whenever handling cryogenic liquids, always wear proper personal protective equipment, including a lab coat that is buttoned, heavy gloves, and a face shield or safety goggles. Hazards associated with cryogens include the following:

- Fire or explosion
- Asphyxiation
- Pressure buildup
- Embrittlement of material
- Tissue damage

Formaldehyde

Formaldehyde (formalin) is a colorless liquid with a characteristic pungent odor that is routinely used in laboratories for tissue processing. Deleterious health effects of formaldehyde exposure include respiratory cancer, dermatitis, sensory irritation (eye, nose, and throat), and sensitization. In addition to inhalation hazards, solutions of formaldehyde can damage skin and eye tissue immediately upon contact. OSHA and specific state guidelines have been established to assist laboratories in handling and disposing of this chemical.

Safety Cabinets

Limit the amount of flammable materials required for storage in the laboratory. OSHA defines the maximum amount of flammable and combustible liquids that can be stored in laboratories using approved flammable storage cabinets. The safety regulations pertinent to these limits are defined by the solvent's classification. The classification of flammable solvents is determined by their flash points, with Class IA and IB solvents being the most combustible. Large amounts of volatile solvents must be stored in a safety cabinet approved by NFPA to meet OSHA standards. The cabinet should be properly vented, and the use of self-closing doors is encouraged.

Chemical Waste

Disposal of chemical waste is the responsibility of the individual laboratories. The responsibility and liability start at the time the chemical is brought into or made in the laboratory and continues through the time that the waste has been rendered harmless. The 1976 Resource Conservation and Recovery Act (RCRA) dictate this "cradle-to-grave" responsibility and liability. The RCRA established a system for managing nonhazardous and hazardous solid waste in an environmentally sound manner. Specifically, it provides for the management of hazardous wastes from the point of origin to the point of final disposal. RCRA also promotes resource recovery and waste minimization.[17] In addition, each laboratory must comply with all local, state Department of Environmental Conservation (DEC), and U.S. Environmental Protection Agency (EPA) mandates.[18]

Laboratories are identified by RCRA as "waste generators," and they require a permit for proper waste disposal. Laboratories are considered small-quantity waste generators and are therefore governed by the policies and procedures appropriate to the corresponding permit. Pouring chemicals down the sink drain should not be done without authorization from the laboratories' environmental health and safety officer. Examples of chemicals that must not be disposed of by pouring down sink drains include:

- Organic solvents with boiling point of less than 50°C
- Hydrocarbons
- Halogenated hydrocarbons
- Nitro compounds
- Mercaptan
- Freon
- Azides and peroxides
- Concentrated acids and bases

☑ CHECKPOINT 1-6

A staff technologist was organizing the chemical storage area and was placing the chemicals in alphabetical order. The technologist placed a container of acetic acid next to a container of ammonium nitrate.

1. What recommendation would you make to the technologist for a safer method to store these chemicals?
2. What reason would you provide as a rationale for not storing acetic acid next to ammonium nitrate?

MINI-CASE 1-3

Sam was transferring a serum sample using a 5.0 ml volumetric glass pipet to a 250 mL glass volumetric flask containing 6M hydrochloric acid. When Sam was finished, he inadvertently left the glass pipet in the flask. A few minutes later as he turned and reached for another flask, he struck the glass pipet and tipped the flask over, spilling the solution onto the bench, floor, his shoes, lab coat, and pants. Sam was wearing a lab coat, unbuttoned, no eyewear, and he was using a pipetting bulb to aspirate the serum sample.

1. Identify safety practices Sam chose to ignore.
2. What is the appropriate course of action for Sam to follow in response to the chemical spill?

RADIATION SAFETY

Clinical laboratory personnel may be exposed to two types of radiation sources: *nonionizing* and *ionizing*. Both types can pose a considerable health risk to exposed workers if not properly controlled. **Nonionizing radiation** sources emit electromagnetic radiation that does not possess sufficient energy per quantum to ionize atoms or molecules by removing an electron from an atom or molecule. This type of radiation ranges from extremely low frequency (ELF) to ultraviolet (UV). Ionizing radiation sources emit particles (alpha, beta, neutrons) and electromagnetic (x-rays, gamma rays) radiation.

Sources of nonionizing radiation commonly found in clinical laboratories include the following:

- Microwaves
- Infrared lamps and lasers
- Visible lamps (tungsten-halogen)
- Ultraviolet lamps (xenon and deuterium)

Protective measures usually include some type of shielding and/or containment devices that will protect the user from direct exposure. The tissues of the eyes are the most vulnerable, therefore appropriate eyewear is recommended.[19]

Laser light is used in several commercial brands of office copiers and printers. Lasers typically emit radiation in the infrared, visible, and ultraviolet regions of the electromagnetic spectrum; they are primarily an eye and skin hazard. Common lasers used in clinical and research laboratories include CO_2 IR laser, helium-neon, neodymium, yttrium aluminum garnet (YAG), ruby visible lasers, and the nitrogen UV laser. Special precautions must be followed when maintaining these light sources, and it is critical that the user avoid direct exposure to laser beams.

ELECTRICAL SAFETY

Working with electricity can be dangerous. Laboratory technologists work with electricity directly (e.g., when troubleshooting electrical components) and indirectly (e.g., by operating the analyzers). Technologists are often exposed to electrical hazards (e.g., overloaded circuits, frayed wires, electrically charged equipment near a water source).

Handling "live" or charged electrical devices requires the user to be completely focused on his or her task and be aware of any possible hazards. Several examples of proper safety recommendations while working with electrical equipment are listed in Box 1-5.

BOX 1-5 Electrical Safety Recommendations

- Use properly grounded electrical circuits and devices.
- Electrical wires and cords should have no frayed edges, cuts, or exposed wiring.
- Use of extension cords should be discouraged.
- Multi-plug adapters and "cheater" plugs (two prongs to three-prong adapters) should not be used.
- Use only Underwriters Laboratory (UL)–approved fuse-protected multiple socket surge protectors.
- Use ground fault interrupter (GFI) receptacles (plugs) in areas where there is a source of water, for example, sink faucets and water filtration systems.
- Keep heat sources and liquids away from outlets.
- Do not handle any electrical devices with damp or wet hands.
- Train employees emergency response procedures for electrical shock injuries.
- Electrical panels should be clear of obstacles for easy access (clear an area of materials at least 3 feet from the panel).
- Never work on exposed electrical devices alone.
- All shocks should be reported immediately, including small "tingles."
- Do not work on or attempt to repair any instrument while the power is still on.
- Unplug equipment when not in use.

FIRE SAFETY

OSHA and the NFPA have combined their resources to provide policies, procedures, and standards for fire safety. State and local government agencies have adopted these standards for laboratories and businesses with the ability to fine laboratories for non-compliance. Visit http://www.NFPA.org and http://www.osha.gov to see the latest standards.

Laboratories should have available the means to extinguish a small fire in a room, confine fire, and extinguish clothing that has caught on fire. Common sense, personal safety, and the safety of others must be considered before attempting to extinguish a fire. Examples of fire safety devices that are used for extinguishing in the laboratory include (1) a fire blanket that can be used to smother fires, especially effective for a situation where a person's clothes catch fire; (2) safety showers designed to provide several gallons of water that can be used for extinguishing; and (3) fire extinguishers.

Several types of extinguishers are available for fire suppression and include a dry chemical type displayed in Figure 1-7 ■. Laboratories should have an extinguisher available near each door and on opposite sides of the laboratory. Laboratory staff should know the location of these extinguishers and be trained on the proper operation of each type of extinguisher available in the laboratory.

Fire extinguishers are designed to suppress and extinguish different classes of fires. The fire suppression agents within the extinguishers characterize the different types of extinguishers. The classes of fires are designated by capital letters A, B, C, and D. The classes of fires, recommended extinguishing agents, and types of hazards suitable for each type of extinguisher are shown in Table 1-6 ★. Many laboratories have opted to use a fire extinguisher rated A, B, C (also referred to as all purpose). This type of extinguisher uses a dry chemical substance to smother an active fire.

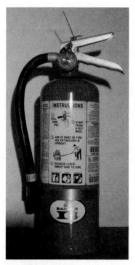

■ **FIGURE 1-7** Dry Chemical Fire Extinguisher

The appropriate extinguishing agent to use for computer fires is Halon 1301 (bromotrifluoromethane) or Halon 1211 (bromo-chlorodifluoromethane), which is currently being replaced with Halotron® (American Pacific AMPAC™ Halotron®, Las Vegas, Nevada USA 89109).

Sprinkler systems are located in most buildings according to local fire code regulations and OSHA standards.[20] NFPA 13 discusses the policies and procedures relevant to sprinkler systems. Another important safety issue involves the storage of materials near sprinkler heads. NFPA guidelines state "the minimum vertical clearance between sprinkler and material below shall be 18 inches."[21]

Two commonly used acronyms relevant to fire-related emergencies are defined in Box 1-6. Individuals in a situation to initiate RACE should exercise extreme caution and common sense before commencing this procedure.

Every hospital, outpatient clinic, and other medical-related facility has instituted procedures for alerting occupants of a fire-related emergency. Some facilities use a public announcement system of codes (e.g., *code Elmer* or *code red*) to alert staff that there is a fire emergency. Automatic alarm systems use flashing lights and loud sounds to warn the staff that there may be a fire emergency. Larger institutions may have a fire brigade of employees who will respond immediately to fire-related emergencies. Whatever alarm method is used, every laboratory staff member should know what to do when the alarm sounds.

HAZARDOUS MATERIALS

Compressed Gases

The Department of Transportation (DOT) regulates the labeling of gas cylinders that are transported by interstate carriers. NFPA diamond-shaped labels, discussed previously, are used on all large cylinders and boxes containing small cylinders. The OSHA standards regarding compressed gases are based on information from the Compressed Gas Association, Inc.[22]

Gases may be

• Flammable or combustible

• Corrosive

• Explosive

• Poisonous

• Inert

• A combination of the aforementioned hazards

The laboratory staff should be aware of two important aspects of compressed gases. First, the staff should know the dangers, if any, associated with the gases they are using. Second, staff must know the proper procedure for securing gas cylinders (see last paragraph of this section).

The contents of the cylinder must be clearly identified. Such identification is stamped or stenciled onto the container or label. Never

★ **TABLE 1-6** Lists of Classes of Fires, Associated Hazards, and Proper Types of Extinguishers to Use

Fire Class	Hazard	Extinguisher Type
A	Ordinary combustible material (e.g., paper, wood, cloth, and some rubber and plastic material)	Water or dry chemical
B	Flammable combustible liquids, gasses, grease, and similar materials	Drug chemical or carbon dioxide
C	Energized electrical equipment	Carbon dioxide, dry chemical, or Halotron (Halon)
D	Combustible metals such as magnesium, titanium, sodium, and potassium	Specific for the type of metal in question

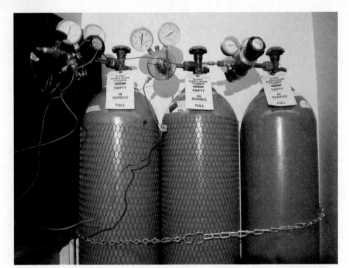

■ **FIGURE 1-8** Proper Storage of Compressed Gas Cylinders

rely on the color of a cylinder for identification. Color-coding is not reliable because the same color may be used for different types of gases. Always read the label.

Signs should be conspicuously posted in the area where flammable gases are used. These signs must identify the gas and appropriate precautions to take if a problem arises. For example, if a laboratory has a cylinder of hydrogen gas, a sign should be posted that indicates that it is a flammable gas and no smoking or open flames are allowed.

Because gases are contained in highly pressurized metal containers, the large amount of potential energy resulting from compression of the gas makes the cylinder a potential rocket or fragmentation bomb. Cylinders must be kept in an upright position and secured to the wall using a chain that will prevent the cylinder from tipping. Proper storage of compressed gas cylinders is shown in Figure 1-8 ■. Cylinders may also be attached to bench tops, placed in a holding cage, or have a non-tip base attached. If a gas cylinder does fall, the immediate concern is that the on-off valve or regulator located on the top of the cylinder may break off. If the value breaks off, the gas may be released at a very high velocity, causing the cylinder to propel like a rocket.

WASTE MANAGEMENT ISSUES

The three types of waste generated in most laboratories are chemical, radioactive, and biohazardous. OSHA and the CDC provide specific guidelines on proper disposal of all types of waste materials. In addition, each state defines specific procedures to follow that are appropriate for the state's resources (e.g., some states may have a radioactive dumpsite or large landfill sites whereas other states may not). A few procedures for laboratories to consider if they are creating waste materials are the following:

- Create a recycling program.
- Dispose of the waste according to guidelines provided by federal, state, and local authorities.
- Create a waste management plan.

- Instruct employees on the types of liquids that can be discharged into the sewers.
- Obtain a discharge permit for the laboratory.
- Monitor sewer discharge.
- Properly label waste containers.
- Separate incompatible waste and/or materials.

WORKPLACE SAFETY ISSUES

Ergonomics

Ergonomics is described as the study of problems related to people adjusting to their environment. Employers and employees must work together to adapt working conditions to suit the worker. Laboratory work involves a myriad of tasks that are challenging to the mind and body. Over time, serious complications can develop from performing some tasks that may render the staff member nonfunctional and perhaps cause the worker to leave the work force. Every effort must be made to seek better ways to perform daily laboratory work and thus ensure a long and healthy work life for the employee.

Cumulative Trauma Disorders

One way to identify tasks that may place employees at risk of developing problems is to perform a cumulative trauma disorders (CTD) risk factor survey. **Cumulative trauma disorders**, also "cumulative trauma syndrome," "repetitive motion disorder," and "overuse syndrome," refer to disorders associated with overloading of particular muscle groups from repeated use or maintaining a constrained posture (Figure 1-9 ■). The disorders typically develop over periods of weeks, months, or years and may involve tendons, as in de Quervain's disease; nerve entrapment, as in carpal tunnel syndrome; muscles, as in tension neck syndrome; or blood vessels, as in vibration white-finger disease or occupational Raynaud's phenomenon.[23,24] Risk factors that are associated with CTD are shown in Box 1-7.

Noise and Hearing Conservation

Clinical laboratories—especially highly automated, heavily populated facilities—generate a substantial amount of low-level noise due to the high amount of activity and communications. Low-level noise, or "white noise," can result in fatigue, irritation, and headaches. OSHA standard 1910.95 Subpart app G allows a *time weighted average* (TWA) of up to 85 decibels/8 hours.[25] This revised amendment requires that employees be placed in a hearing conservation program if they are exposed to noise levels that exceed this TWA.

Ventilation Devices

Laboratory Hoods

Laboratory hoods, also called fume hoods, are used to ventilate unwanted fumes from chemical reagents. According to OSHA guidelines outlined in 1910.1450 App A, a laboratory hood with 2.5 linear feet of hood space per person should be provided for every two workers if they spend most of their time working with chemicals.[26] Each hood should have a continuous monitoring device to allow convenient confirmation of adequate hood performance.

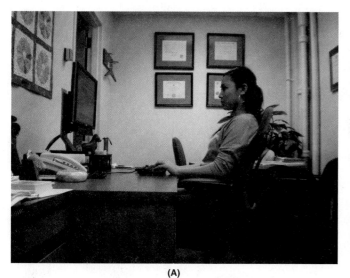

(A)

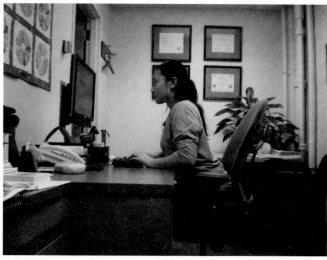

(B)

■ **FIGURE 1-9** Sitting Position for Using a Computer.
(A) Proper position while sitting in an ergonomically correct chair includes a monitor screen slightly below eye level, eyes 20 to 40 inches away from monitor with head vertical, posture is upright and straight with arms resting comfortably on armrest. (B) Improper position includes slouching posture, head bent and to close to monitor screen, and arms raised above armrest.

Biosafety Cabinets

More sophisticated biohazard hoods or biological safety cabinets that can remove particulates are available depending on the needs of the laboratory. A typical BSL II hood is shown in Figure 1-10 ■. An abbreviated listing of specifications for Class I-III biosafety cabinets is provided in Table 1-7 ★. Class I and II biosafety cabinets are appropriate for BSL II and III, whereas class III cabinets must be used for BSL III and IV.[27]

All ventilation devices should be checked periodically for proper flow rates, and HEPA filters should be changed according

---

BOX 1-7 List of Cumulative Trauma Disorder (CTD) Risk Factors

Repetitive and prolonged activity

Forceful exertions, usually with the hands

Prolonged static postures

Awkward postures of the upper body, for example, reaching above the shoulders or behind the back

Continued physical contact with work surfaces, such as contact with edges

Excessive vibration from equipment

Working in a cold temperature

Poor body mechanics, for example, continued bending at the waist, lifting from below the knuckles or above the shoulder, or twisting at the waist.

Lifting or moving objects of excessive weight or asymmetric sizes

Prolonged sitting, especially with poor posture

Lack of adjustable chairs, footrest, body supports, and adjustable work surfaces at workstation

Slippery footing

Noise

Lifting

Repetitive stress issues

Standing for long periods of time

☑ CHECKPOINT 1-8

One of the staff technologists reported to her supervisor that she had been more tired than usual, somewhat irritable, and experiencing several headaches within the past several weeks. The laboratory facility contains four large chemistry analyzers, two hematology systems, eight staff technologists, phones, and computer printers at six workstations. What suggestions would you make to the supervisor in an effort to relieve the technologist's symptoms?

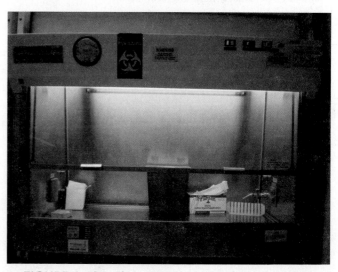

■ **FIGURE 1-10** Class II Biological Safety Cabinet

★ **TABLE 1-7** Three Classes of Biosafety Cabinets and Associated Descriptors

Type	Description
Class I	Face velocity, 75 feet per min
	Open front, exhaust only through HEPA* filter
Class II	Face velocity, 100 feet per min
	Recirculation through HEPA filters and exhaust via HEPA filter
Class III	Supply air inlets and exhaust through two HEPA filters

*HEPA = high efficiency particulate air

to manufacturer's recommendations. Proper procedures and documentation of all maintenance should be described in the laboratory's chemical hygiene plan.

Staff Responsibilities

Some safety practices are the employee's responsibility to address. The following issues represent good safety practices and commonly are supported by laboratory management.

- Do not use personal electronic devices in areas where infectious exposure is likely.
- Do not wear PPE or laboratory coats outside of the laboratory.
- Use splash barriers when capping/uncapping tubes, pipetting or dispensing, vortexing and mixing, and making dilutions.
- Do not eat or drink in the laboratory.
- Do not apply cosmetics in the work area.
- Secure hair back and off the shoulders.
- Do not wear jewelry that can become caught in equipment or come into contact with biological fluids or chemical testing materials.
- Do have the hepatitis B vaccination.
- Do not store personal belongings such as purses, coats, coffee mugs, and other personal items in the technical areas.

Safety Manual

A laboratory safety manual should be written, reviewed, and made available to all laboratory staff. The safety manual should present defined policies, procedures, and job responsibilities for each member of the laboratory staff. The manual may also serve as a training document to teach employees appropriate safe working practices. A list of specific items to include in the laboratory safety manual is shown in Box 1-8.[28]

The laboratory staff can design a checklist of tasks for staff action. Schedules should be developed for each safety topic that requires action, for example, fire drills, new employee orientation, annual required safety sessions on right to know, and bloodborne pathogens. The frequency of this type of review should be in accordance with state and federal regulations.

BOX 1-8   Recommended Topics for Inclusion in a Clinical Laboratory Safety Manual

Institutional Emergency Codes
Emergency Phone Numbers
Biosafety Level 2 Credentials
Standard Operating Procedures (SOP)
Personal Protective Equipment (PPE)
Chemical Handling and Inventory
Safety Data Sheets (SDSs)
Bloodborne Pathogens
Fire Safety
Electrical Safety
Compressed Gases
Signs and Labels
Medical Considerations
Emergency Procedures and Cleanup
Waste Disposal
Record Keeping and Training

Training

Training laboratory staff in safety-related activities should be considered an ongoing event. Safety training needs to be part of a new employee orientation and laboratory staff continuing education and conducted in accordance with local, state, and federal regulations. Safety courseware should include material on safety at work, biosafety, bloodborne pathogens, and right to know. Training of laboratory staff should be conducted on a regular schedule.

Assessment of knowledge and skills should be included in the laboratory safety program. This can be accomplished by developing a competency assessment tool and judgment skills tests. For example, a competency assessment tool would include a scoring system (e.g., 1 = rarely performs through 4 = always performs) and a set of tasks that may include the following:

- Donning gloves
- Donning a lab coat
- Using eyewear when appropriate
- Washing hands
- Cleaning the work area with appropriate materials

A passing score is established by laboratory management, and a staff member who fails would be required to complete some form of remediation.

A skills test may include a combination of questions including both rote memory questions and questions that require assimilation and analysis of facts to provide a safe decision. The skills test could also involve the demonstration of proper techniques to operate a fire extinguisher or eyewash station. The skills test could be graded and a passing grade established. Employees who score below a passing grade would need remediation.

Institutional Alerts

As an example of institutional alerts, the state of New York has established a communication system named "NY-Alert," which is part of the New York State All-Hazard Alert and notification web-based portal. NY-Alert is designed to alert all participants via cell phones, telephones, email, and media outlets of a significant incident occurring within the institution's area of responsibility.[29] For example, if someone within the boundaries of the institution witnesses an occurrence such as an assault, the witness could contact the security staff who in turn can contact the NY-Alert staff to issue a communication to all participants via all of the above devices and outlets that an unsafe event is in progress. Throughout the event NY-Alert will update participants with information regarding response actions being taken by local and state agencies and protective actions that participants should take.

Emergency Codes

Institutional emergency codes represent a means for healthcare facilities to alert their employees that an adverse event is occurring somewhere in or near the facility. The codes were developed using several different designations (e.g., colors, numbers, and names) and these codes are commonly initiated over a facilities paging system. In 1999, a shooting incident occurred in West Anaheim Medical Center, CA, and a wrong emergency code was activated. This brought to light the fact that there was not a standardized emergency code set for the state of California.

During the years following this tragedy in which three people were killed, several initiatives were developed that were designed to rectify this situation, and the Hospital Association of Southern California (HASC) published a model for standardized emergency codes that has been adopted (with modification) by many healthcare facilities across the United States.[30] Examples of possible colors used for each emergency are shown in Figure 1-11 ■.

Emergency Management

An emergency or crisis situation from many possible causes can affect a laboratory at any time. Emergencies range from internal and community-based patient care emergencies, chemical spills, fires, and bomb threats to explosions, natural disasters, and civil disturbances such as riots or labor unrest. Every institution (i.e., hospital, reference laboratory) should create an *Emergency Management Plan* (EMP) in accordance with state and federal mandates. Adoption of the National Incident Management System (NIMS) is typically recommended. The plan should include protocols that discuss how the institution prepares for emergencies; mitigates their potential effects; responds, demobilizes, and recovers from actual events; and then evaluates its effectiveness.

Management of a disaster is effectively mitigated using the Incident Command System. **Incident command system** (ICS) is a standardized on-scene incident management concept designed specifically to allow responders to adopt an integrated organizational structure equal to the complexity and demands of any single incident or multiple incidents without being hindered by jurisdictional boundaries. ICS uses a common organization structure that consists of Command, Logistics, Finance/Administration, Planning, and Operations. Once an incident begins, the Incident Commander, who is positioned at the top of the organization, will delegate duties and responsibilities to the other positions listed above as needed. As an incident evolves, the positions of the ICS organization that are activated will expand and contract based upon need. An individual appointed to an ICS position reports to only one designated person who most likely is not his or her day-to-day supervisor. All departments involved in ICS are expected to manage to common objectives. Once the incident has ended, the participants gather to debrief and discuss what worked well and what did not.

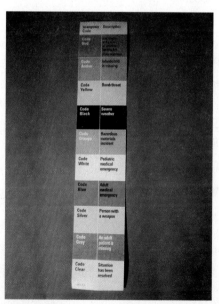

■ **FIGURE 1-11** Emergency Code Color Scheme and Descriptions

---

MINI-CASE 1-4

The emergency department was very busy in a 250-bed hospital when a distraught individual pushed his way into the waiting area and continued into one of the smaller examination rooms. In the room, a patient was being examined for a knife wound when all of a sudden the intruder began yelling and verbally threatening the patient. Denise, the nurse attending to the patient, noticed a handgun protruding from the intruder's pants pocket. Denise asked the intruder to leave and yelled for a code purple, which signaled the need for immediate security (unarmed). The patient pulled out the pistol and threatened to shoot anyone who tried to stop him. He fled the hospital firing one shot at the security guard. Fortunately, he missed the guard and no one was hurt.

1. What code should have been called and why?

Key Points to Remember

- The employer is obligated to provide a safe working laboratory.
- The employee is responsible for adhering to all safety policy and procedures.
- Developing a comprehensive exposure control plan will serve to reduce injuries in the laboratory.
- Proper utilization of chemicals in the laboratory can reduce injuries.
- Knowledge of the behavior of electricity will reduce the possibility of shocks or electrocution.
- Good waste management practices can reduce cost and pollution of the environment.

Review Questions

Level I

1. What is the "A" in the acronym for fire-related emergencies RACE? (Objective 8)

    A. Accident

    B. Activate alarm

    C. Analyze

    D. Answer the phone

2. Liquid nitrogen is an example of which of the following? (Objective 4)

    A. Teratogen

    B. Mutagen

    C. Halogen

    D. Cryogen

3. A class A fire involves which of the following? (Objective 7)

    A. Combustible metals such as sodium

    B. Flammable liquids for example ethanol

    C. Ordinary combustible material including paper and wood

    D. Electrical equipment

4. The letters SDS are defined as which of the following? (Objective 4)

    A. Safety devices schedule

    B. Safety data sheet

    C. Safety design sheet

    D. Systems data sheets

5. Universal precaution is a practice developed to provide guidance in handling which of the following types of materials? (Objective 1)

    A. Toxic chemical

    B. Liquid nitrogen

    C. Human blood

    D. Ionizing radiation

6. Splash shields, self-sheathing needles, and impervious needle boxes are examples of which of the following? (Objective 2)

    A. Engineered controls

    B. Storage containers

    C. Items in a chemical hygiene plan

    D. Items in a waste management plan

7. Proper safety practices including not applying cosmetics in the work area, not using electronic devices in areas where infectious exposure is likely and not wearing your laboratory coat outside of the laboratory are the responsibility of? (Objective 12)

    A. Employer

    B. Employee

    C. Department of human resources

    D. Payroll department

8. A ground fault interrupter (GFI) should be used in which of the following situations? (Objective 5)

    A. Where there is a source of nonionizing radiation

    B. Where there is a source of toxic chemicals

    C. Where there is a source of liquid nitrogen

    D. Where there is a source of water (e.g., sink faucets)

9. The person who directs an emergency response to a catastrophic incident where the incident command systems has been activated is called the (Objective 12)

    A. Commander in chief

    B. Incident Director

    C. Incident Commander

    D. Incident Assistant

10. PASS is an acronym for which of the following?

    A. Responding to a fire

    B. Responding to a mass casualty incident

    C. Proper use of a fire extinguisher

    D. Proper use of an eyewash station

11. An ABC-type fire extinguisher can be used to extinguish which type of materials?

    A. Paper, flammable combustible liquids, and energized electrical equipment

    B. Paper only

    C. Combustible metals such as magnesium

    D. A metal block containing sodium

12. Which of the following hand washing practices is recommended by the Centers for Disease Control (CDC)?

    A. Vigorous rubbing together of all lathered surfaces for at least 15 minutes.

    B. Vigorous rubbing together of all lathered surfaces for at least 15 seconds.

    C. Mild, gentle rubbing together of all lathered surfaces for at least 30 seconds.

    D. Mild, gentle rubbing together of all lathered surfaces using very hot water for at least 20 minutes.

13. A biosafety level 2 (BSL2) agent is described as

    A. Not known to cause diseases in healthy adults consistently.

    B. Associated with human disease.

    C. Indigenous or exotic agents with potential for aerosol transmission.

    D. Dangerous/exotic agents that pose high risk of life-threatening disease.

14. Which of the following is a good practice for storing chemicals?

    A. Store at least three times the amount of chemicals as you would normally use.

    B. Store chemicals alphabetically.

    C. Store chemicals by categories (i.e., acids, bases, oxidizers).

    D. Store chemicals in a hood.

15. The Resource Conservation and Recovery Act (RCRA) identified laboratories as

    A. Large waste generators.

    B. Small waste generators.

    C. Major sources of pollutants for lakes and rivers.

    D. Significant sources of radioactive waste.

16. Compressed gas cylinders should be stored in which of the following manner? (Objective 9)

    A. Upright and chained to the wall or bench

    B. Upright and taped to the wall

    C. Laid flat on the floor

    D. Laid flat on the floor using large bricks to keep them from rolling on the floor.

17. Which of the following statements describes nonionizing radiation? (Objective 5)

    A. Electromagnetic radiation that possess an enormous amount of energy that enables it to remove electrons from atoms and molecules.

    B. Electromagnetic radiation comprised of high-energy gamma radiation capable of causing electrons to be ejected from an atom.

    C. Electromagnetic radiation that does not possess sufficient energy per quantum to ionize atoms or molecules by removing an electron from an atom.

    D. Beta-emitting radionuclides capable of causing the ejection of outer shell electrons from an atom.

Level II

1. The NFPA 704-M identification system is associated with which of the following? (Objectives 4, 5)

    A. Warning labels for mechanical devices

    B. Warning labels for biohazardous materials

    C. Warning labels for chemical hazards

    D. Warning labels for laboratory safety hoods

2. Which of the following statements best describes the proper method of storing chemicals in the laboratory? (Objective 4,3)

    A. According to their chemical properties and classifications

    B. Alphabetically, for easy accessibility

    C. Inside a chemical fume hood

    D. Inside a walk-in type refrigerator

3. Which of the following are examples of sources of nonionizing radiation? (Objective 6)

    A. Microwaves, tungsten-halogen lamps, xenon lamps

    B. X-ray imaging devices

    C. Beta radiation emitting isotopes such as tritium

    D. Gamma radiation emitting isotopes (e.g., ^{125}Iodine)

4. A plan designed to help prevent accidental exposure of laboratory personnel to bloodborne pathogens is called a (an)? (Objective 2)

    A. Chemical Exposure Plan

    B. Carcinogen Exposure Plan

    C. Exposure Control Plan

    D. Universal Precaution Plan

5. Cumulative trauma disorders (CTDs) are described as which of the following? (Objective 10)

    A. Disorders due to blunt trauma injuries to the head caused by an automobile accident.

    B. Disorders associated with the overloading of particular muscle groups from repeated use.

    C. Post-traumatic distress disorders associated with soldiers returning from battle.

    D. Trauma due to emotional stress and anxiety.

6. Which of the following would be the correct interpretation of a NFPA 704-M designation number 3 in the blue diamond? (Objectives 4, 5)

   A. May detonate

   B. Corrosive

   C. Extreme dangers

   D. Radioactive

7. What is the proper storage procedure for compressed gas cylinders? (Objective 8)

   A. Lay the gas cylinders on the floor with the valves against the wall.

   B. Place the gas cylinders in the corner of the room between two benches for stability.

   C. Tie the gas cylinders to the bench with rope or wire.

   D. Store gas cylinders in an upright position and secured to either the wall or the bench, preferably with a chain.

8. A laboratory safety training program should include which of the following? (Objective 11)

   A. Material on safety at work, an assessment of knowledge and skill

   B. Material on health benefits, pension plans, and retirement benefits

   C. No coursework, a 50-question exam, and penalties for employees who fail the exam

   D. Procedure for dismissing an employee who fails to follow safety protocols.

9. Which of the following Codes of Federal Regulations (CFR) would be appropriate to review if there was a concern about hazardous chemicals in the laboratory (Objective 1)

   A. 29CFR 1910.77

   B. 29CFR 1910.1450

   C. 29CFR 1910.1030

   D. 29CFR 1910.155

10. OSHA standards are found in which of the following documents? (Objective 1)

    A. Codes of State Regulations (CSRs)

    B. Codes of Federal Regulations (CFRs)

    C. Safety Data Sheets (SDSs)

    D. National Fire Protection Agency (NFPA)

Endnotes

1. Occupational Exposure to Hazardous Chemicals in Laboratories. Occupational Safety and Health Administration (OSHA) Final Rule. Federal Register, 29CRF part 1910 subpart Z standard 1910.1450.

2. Occupational Exposure to Bloodborne Pathogens. Occupational Safety and Health Administration (OSHA). Federal Register, 56:235: 64004–64182, 1991.

3. National Institute for Occupational Safety and Health (NIOSH). *Guidelines for prevention of transmission of human immunodeficiency virus and hepatitis B virus and health-care and public safety workers.* Centers for Disease Control (NIOSH) publication No. 89-107. Atlanta, GA: Centers for Disease Control, July 1989.

4. CLSI. Clinical Laboratory Safety; Approved Guideline-2nd ed. CLSI document GP17-A2 [ISBN 1-56238-530-5]. CLSI, 940 West Valley Road, Suite 1400, Wayne, PA 19087-1898 USA, 2004.

5. United States Department of Health and Human Services: Recommendations for Prevention of HIV Transmission in Health Care Setting. MMWR 36 no. SU02; 001, 1987.

6. Center for Disease Control and Prevention. Guideline for Hand Hygiene in HealthCare Settings: Recommendations of the Healthcare Infection Control Practices Advisory Committee and the HICPAC/SHEA/APIC/IDSA Hand Hygiene Task Force. MMWR 2002; 51 (No. RR-16): 32–35.

7. The Needlestick Safety and Prevention ACT, Nov. 6, 2000; H.R. 5178.

8. Occupational Exposure to Bloodborne Pathogens; Needlesticks and Other Sharps Injuries; Occupational Safety and Health Administration (OSHA) Final Rule. Document 29 CFR Part 1910 subpart Z standard 1910.1030. 2001; 66: 5318–25.

9. National Institute for Occupational Safety and Health (NIOSH). Alert: Preventing Needlestick Injuries in Health Care Setting. Centers for Disease Control (NIOSH) publication No. 2000-108. Atlanta, GA: Centers for Disease Control and Prevention, 1999.

10. Respiratory Protection. Occupational Safety and Health Administration (OSHA). Document 29CRF part 1910 subpart I standard 1910.134. *Federal Register.*

11. Chosewood LC, Wilson DE. Editors. *Biosafety in Microbiological and Biomedical Laboratories*, 5th ed. U.S. Department of Health and Human Services. CDC. HHS publication No. (CDC) 21-1112. Revised 2009. www.cdc.gov/biosafety/publications/bmbl5/(accessed October 25, 2013)

12. Occupational Exposure to Hazardous Chemicals in Laboratories. Occupational Safety and Health Administration (OSHA) Final Rule. Federal Register, 29CRF part 1910 subpart Z standard 1910.1450.

13. http://www.osha.gov/dsg/hazcom/msdsformat.html (accessed October 25, 2013)

14. NFPA 704: Standard for the Identification of the Fire Hazards of Materials for Emergency Response. National Fire Protection Agency, 2001 Edition, Quincy Mass.

15. Bretherick L, Urben P, Pitt M. *Bretherick's handbook of reactive chemical hazards*, 6th ed. Oxford: Butterworth Heinemann, 1999.

16. Bretherick L, Urben P, Pitt M. *Bretherick's handbook of reactive chemical hazards*, 6th ed. Oxford: Butterworth Heinemann, 1999.

17. Resource Conservation and Recovery Act (RCRA, Pub. L. 94-580). Dept. of Energy (DOE) Washington, DC, 1976.

18. Codes of Federal Regulations. Title 40, Protection of the Environment, Volume 27 & 28, pages 260–299. Revised 2013. (e-CFR at www.ecfr.gov)

19. Nonionizing Radiation. Occupational Safety and Health Administration (OSHA) Document 29 CFR part 1910 subpart G standard 1910.97. *Federal Register*, 2005; 6: 450-58.

20. Automatic Sprinkler Systems. Occupational Safety and Health Administration (OSHA). Document 29 CFR part 1910 subpart L standard 1910.159. *Federal Register* 2005; 5: 501–2.

21. National Fire Protection Association (NFPA) 13: *Standards for Installation of Sprinkler Systems*. Quincy, MA: NFPA, 2001.

22. Compressed Gas Association. *Handbook of Compressed Gases*, 4th ed. New York: Springer Science + Business Media, LLC., 1999.

23. National Institute for Occupational safety and health (NIOSH). *Elements of Ergonomics Programs. A Primer Based on Workplace Evaluation of Musculoskeletal Disorders*. Centers for Disease Control (NIOSH) publication No. 97-117. Atlanta, GA: Centers for Disease Control and Prevention, July 1997.

24. National Institute for Occupational safety and health (NIOSH). *Musculoskeletal Disorders and Workplace Factors: A Critical Review of Epidemiologic Evidence for Work-related Musculoskeletal Disorders of the Neck, Upper Extremities, and Low Back*. Centers for Disease Control (NIOSH) publication No. 97-141. Atlanta, GA: Centers for Disease Control and Prevention, July 1997.

25. Monitoring Noise Levels. Occupational Safety and Health Administration (OSHA). Document 29 CFR part 1910 subpart G standard 1910.95 App I. *Federal Register*, 2005; 5: 211–33.

26. *Primary Containment for Biohazards: Selection, Installation, and Use of Biological Safety Cabinets*, 2nd ed. Centers for Disease Control publication No. 89-107. Atlanta, GA: Centers for Disease Control and Prevention, 2000.

27. Chosewood LC, Wilson DE. Editors. *Biosafety in Microbiological and Biomedical Laboratories*, 5th ed. U.S. Department of Health and Human Services. CDC. HHS publication No. (CDC) 21-1112. Revised 2009. www.cdc.gov/biosafety/publications/bmbl5/(accessed October 25, 2013)

28. Gile TJ. *Lab Safety Training Made Simple*. Marblehead, MA: HCPro, Inc. (www.hcmarketplace.com) accessed March 6, 2013.

29. www.nyalert.gov (accessed March 6, 2013)

30. Truesdell A. Meeting Hospital Needs for Standardized Emergency Codes—the HASC Response. *Journal of Healthcare Protection Management*, 2005; 21(1):77–89.

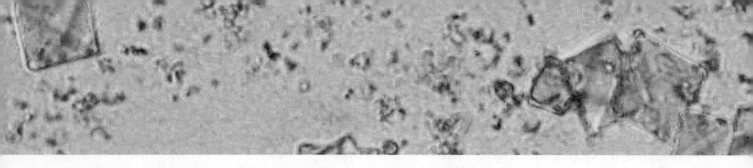

2 Quality Issues in a Clinical Urinalysis Laboratory

Objectives

LEVEL 1

Following successful completion of this chapter, the learner will be able to:

1. Compare and contrast descriptive statistics and inferential statistics.
2. Identify measures of central tendency and dispersion.
3. Define accuracy, precision, calibration, and quality control.
4. List several examples of variables associated with pre-analytical, analytical, and post-analytical stages of testing.
5. Explain the characteristics of a Levey-Jennings chart and include x- and y-axis labels.
6. Define each Westgard rule violation.
7. List nine analytes measured using urine chemistry strips.
8. Identify the measuring principles used to determine urine chemistry on a strip, specific gravity, color, clarity, and formed elements.

LEVEL II

Following successful completion of this chapter, the learner will be able to:

1. Calculate and interpret the results of selected laboratory statistics.
2. Select the appropriate statistic(s) for a given set of measurements.
3. Provide examples of essential elements included in a procedure manual.
4. Describe the variables for pre-analytical, analytical, and post-analytical stages of laboratory testing and indicate the consequences for failure to follow laboratory protocols.
5. Interpret a Levey-Jennings quality control plot.
6. Indicate course of action when a urine chemistry measurement fails a Westgard rule.
7. Discuss the measurement principles for each component of an automated urinalysis system.
8. Select the appropriate calibration and quality control material for manual urine tests.

Key Terms

Accuracy	Inferential statistics	Mode	Range
Calibration	Linearity	Population	Sample
Coefficient of variation	Mean	Precision	Standard deviation
Descriptive statistics	Median	Quality control	

A CASE IN POINT

A laboratory technologist performs a urinalysis and microscopic analysis on a patient urine specimen using the automated urinalysis system. The results for the urine chemistry using a urine chemistry strip were either zero or negative for all tests and deemed unacceptable.

Questions to Consider

1. What steps should be taken to attempt to resolve this problem?
2. Is the instrument calibrated?
3. Is the quality control acceptable?
4. Have there been any electrical power interruptions?

LABORATORY STATISTICS

Statistics (e.g., arithmetic mean, standard deviation, and variance) should be viewed as tools that are available for the laboratory staff to use to assist in making important decisions about data collected during a study. Knowing which tool or statistic to use is important. Selecting the wrong "stat" will most likely result in a wrong assumption being made or an inappropriate action taken. This chapter will present a discussion of the tasks required to produce reliable laboratory data and will describe procedures for these tasks. The text will also discuss guidelines for selecting the proper statistic or "tool" to help make decisions and will discuss appropriate interpretation of data.

Computation of most statistics is performed using any of several computer software packages or calculators. Therefore, derivation and memorization of formulas is not necessary. Most textbooks on clinical chemistry include formulas; thus, only a few will be included in this textbook. What is most important is the selection of appropriate statistics and accurate interpretation of the statistical calculations.

Data Formats

In urinalysis laboratories, data is presented in both numeric and nonnumeric format. For example, the result of a urine specific gravity measurement is reported as 1.013, whereas the result of a qualitative human chorionic gonadotropin (hCG) assay is reported as positive or negative. Some results may be semiquantitative in nature; for example, urine reducing substances are reported as 2+. The value 2+ correlates to an actual urine glucose concentration in milligram/deciliter (mg/dL). This type of data is referred to as ordinal (rank order).

Types of Statistics

Descriptive statistics are used to disclose some characteristic of a sample data set and include the mean, median, mode, range, variability, and distribution of a data set. They represent the commonly used statistical computations in the urinalysis laboratory.

Inferential statistics are used to make estimates of population parameters and to make decisions concerning those parameters.

For example, is the mean of one set of data significantly different from another? If there is a difference between the means of the two samples, what are the probabilities associated with this difference? Examples of inferential statistics include the following:

- *F*-test
- *t*-test
- *Z*-test
- chi square

Two additional important terms are population and sample. A **population** refers to the universe of values or attributes, such as all of the fasting serum cholesterol levels of all apparently healthy males in the United States.

Sample refers to a portion or subset of a population, such as the serum cholesterol levels of all males in the laboratory. Often the distinction between population and sample is not made very clear (e.g., a sampling could be argued to be a population).

Parameters and *statistics* are terms associated with population and samplings, respectively. A parameter describes a quantitative feature of a population. Statistics describes a quantitative feature of a sample.

Measures of Central Tendency

The **mean** is the average for the variable and is commonly used to describe data. For example, what is the mean value of urine sodium for all samples in a study? Summing all data and dividing the sum by the number of data represented by *n* or *N* determines arithmetic means. The **median** in a sample set is the middle value or the 50th percentile value when the data are rank ordered by magnitude. Close observation of the data will show that half the data points are above and half are below the median. The **mode** is the data point that occurs most frequently. Measures of central tendency are illustrated in Table 2-1 ★. Calculations of central tendency allow the derivation of graphical plots that can clearly show modal distributions and skewness or measure of the symmetry of a distribution.

★ **TABLE 2-1** Results of Selected Descriptive Statistics for 10 Replicate Measurements of Glucose in Urine

Replicate Number	Results (mg/dL)
1	20.9
2	20.8
3	20.7
4	20.2
5	20.5
6	20.6
7	20.9
8	20.3
9	20.6
10	20.6
Sum	206.1
Arithmetic mean	20.61
Median	20.60
Mode	20.60
Range	20.2-20.9 or 0.7
Standard deviation	0.233
Variance	0.054
Coefficient of variation (CV)	1.13%

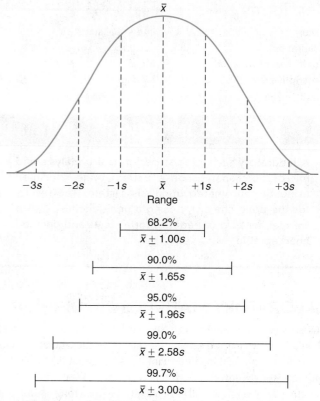

■ **FIGURE 2-1** A Normal Bell-Shaped Curve Showing ± 1, 2, 3s and the Relative Percentages Associated with Each Area Under the Curve

From Sunheimer RL, Graves L. *Clinical Laboratory Chemistry*, 1st ed. (Upper Saddle River, NJ: Pearson Education), 2011.

Measures of Dispersion

Range

Range is a measure of spread or variation in a set of data. The range of data is the difference between the largest and the smallest numbers of the data set or the smallest to the largest number. For example, the data in Table 2-1 show a range of 20.2-20.9 or 0.7.

Standard Deviation

Standard deviation (s, SD) is a commonly used estimator of dispersion because it is predictably related to a common type of data distribution, the Gaussian, or normal distribution. **Standard deviation** is a measure of the dispersion of a group of values around a mean. It is derived from the curve of normal distribution and bears a meaningful relation to the area under the normal distribution curve so that, for example, the area under the center of the curve represented by the mean ± 1.96 is ~95% of the whole area. A plot of a normal curve distribution is shown in Figure 2-1 ■.

Coefficient of Variation

Coefficient of variation (CV) is another way of expressing standard deviation. The term is *relative standard deviation*. It is defined as 100 times the standard deviation divided by the mean. CV is expressed as a percentage. It relates the standard deviation to the level at which the measurements are made. For example, from the data in Table 2-1, the mean and s of the measurements are 20.61 and 0.233, respectively. The CV for the data set is 1.13% (0.233/20.61 × 100).

Many laboratories find CV to be a useful statistic. Because the numbers are in percentage format, it is often easier to relate to percentage CV than to standard deviation. Remember that the lower the CV, the better the performance of the assay.

Variance

When the values of a set of observations lie close to their mean, the dispersion is less than when they are scattered over a wide range. If the laboratory needs to know the measure of dispersion of data relative to the scatter of the values about the mean, a statistic is available to provide this information. The statistic is called *variance* (s^2). Variance is calculated by squaring the standard deviation or by subtracting the mean from each of the values, squaring the resulting differences, and then adding up the squared differences. This value is divided by the sample size minus one ($N - 1$) to obtain the sample variance. The variance of the set of data shown in Table 2-1 is 0.054.

Outliers

An outlier in a sample set is a measurement that belongs to a population other than the one to which most of the measurements belong. Outliers can distort the computed values of statistics and cause incorrect inferences to be made about the population parameters of interest. There are tests to determine whether a value is an outlier. The gap test[1] and Prescott Test for Outliers[2] are two examples used for clinical laboratory statistics.

☑ CHECKPOINT 2-1

As a laboratory technologist, you are asked to determine the descriptive statistics for the data presented in the following table. The data represents replicate measurements of sodium in a random urine sample. Twenty measurements are completed on one sample. Determine the statistics listed for the data shown in the table:

- Mean
- Standard deviation
- Variance
- Percentage coefficient of variation
- Median
- Mode
- Range (mean $\pm$ 2s)

Data Number	Sodium Value (meq/L)	Data Number	Sodium Value (meq/L)
1	180	11	179
2	181	12	178
3	179	13	180
4	180	14	180
5	180	15	181
6	178	16	179
7	182	17	179
8	181	18	181
9	181	19	180
10	180	20	180

Linear Regression and Correlation

Regression

Regression analysis is useful in assessing specific aspects of the relationship between variables, and the ultimate objective is to predict or estimate the value of one variable based on a given value of the second variable. The most commonly used form of regression statistics is linear regression by least squares.

Linear Regression by Least Squares

Regression analysis is commonly used in the comparison of two methods or two instruments and to evaluate the **linearity** of an instrument or method. Regression calculations provide a simple and general descriptive statement relating one set of observations to another.

Linear regression by the method of least squares positions a straight line among the points on the graph in such a way that the sum of the squares of the vertical distances from each point to the fitted line is the smallest value possible. In Figure 2-2 ■, two sets of data, representing variables X and Y, are plotted on a graph. The data sets represented by the closed circle forms a scatterplot. The X-variable is referred to as the *independent variable* because the investigator frequently controls it. The Y-variable is called the *dependent variable*, and the experimenter measures it to determine the effect of the

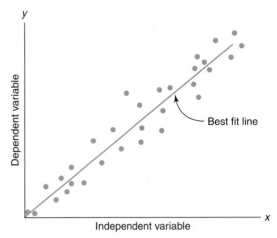

FIGURE 2-2 Plots of Independent Variable and Dependent Variable Using Linear Regression by Least Squares

From Sunheimer RL, Graves L. *Clinical Laboratory Chemistry*, 1st ed. (Upper Saddle River, NJ: Pearson Education), 2011.

independent variable; thus, the terminology refers to the regression of Y on X. The following are the assumptions underlying the simple linear regression model.[3]

A least squares or "best-fit" straight line is included in Figure 2-2. The graph shows that there is an association between the two variables. In such cases, it is often desirable to use a mathematical description of such an X-Y relationship. The simplest such expression is the general equation for a straight line:

$$Y = a + bX \qquad (2\text{-}1)$$

This linear model or simple linear regression formula contains two parameters: the intercept (a) and slope (b). The data presented in Table 2-2 ★ show that a nearly linear relationship between glucose oxidase (X) and glucose hexokinase (Y) exists and is expressed in the following equation for a straight line:
Y (Hexokinase) $= -0.007 + 0.918x$ (Oxidase)
where

$$a \text{ (intercept)} = -0.007$$
$$b \text{ (slope)} \quad = 0.918$$

This equation reveals that the slope (b) is positive; the best-fit line crosses the Y-axis just below the origin at -0.007, and the fitted line shown in Figure 2-3 ■ extends from the lower left-hand corner of the graph to the upper right-hand corner. In addition, for each unit increase in X, $\hat{y}$ (calculated value for Y on the line at each X value) increases by an amount equal to $[0.918(X) + (-0.007)]$. For example, if a given value of $X = 3.0$, then $\hat{y} = [0.918(3.0) + (-0.007)] = 2.75$.

The result for correlation coefficient (r) is 0.996. Refer to the next section for a discussion of (r) statistic.

Correlation Coefficient

The Pearson product-moment correlation coefficient is calculated by setting up a ratio of the sums over all the observed (X, Y) points. Its value does not depend on which variable we identify as X and

★ **TABLE 2-2** Least Squares Regression Analysis of Glucose Measurements in Urine Samples from Adult Females by Two Different Enzyme Methods. The Current Method is Glucose Oxidase and Candidate Replacement Assay is Hexokinase

Sample Number	Glucose Oxidase (x-axis) (mg/dL)	Glucose Hexokinase (y-axis) (mg/dL)
1	0.9	0.9
2	1.1	1.0
3	8.0	8.5
4	4.3	4.2
5	5.4	5.3
6	1.9	1.2
7	15	16
8	52	48
9	8.0	7.8
10	4.0	3.4
11	44	42
12	35	30
13	10	8
14	28	26
15	25	22
16	24	20
17	17	18
18	11	9.0
19	19	17
20	50	46
Sum	363.60	334.30
Average	18.18	16.715
Bias (average of y – average of x)	−1.46	
Intercept	−0.007	
Slope	0.918	

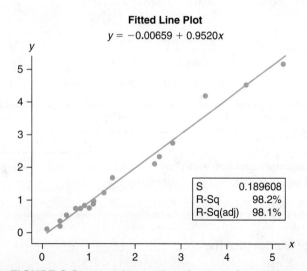

Fitted Line Plot

$$y = -0.00659 + 0.9520x$$

S	0.189608
R-Sq	98.2%
R-Sq(adj)	98.1%

■ **FIGURE 2-3** Fitted Line Plots for Data from Table 2-2

From Sunheimer RL, Graves L. *Clinical Laboratory Chemistry*, 1st ed. (Upper Saddle River, NJ: Pearson Education), 2011.

which we identify as Y. The magnitude of r describes the strength of the association between two variables, and the sign of r indicates the direction of this association: $r = +1$ when the two variables increase together and $r = -1$ when one decreases as the other increases.

☑ **CHECKPOINT 2-2**

As a technologist in a urinalysis laboratory, you are required to correlate a new colorimetric assay for phosphate in urine. The current assay is being phased out by the manufacturer. Calculate the following from the data presented in the table below.
- Linear regression by least squares, including slope and intercept
- Correlation coefficient

Sample Number	iP (mg/dL) Current Method (x-axis)	iP (mg/dL) New Method (y-axis)
1	145	146
2	140	140
3	139	140
4	138	139
5	150	151
6	155	157
7	130	132
8	134	136
9	131	133
10	142	142
11	144	147
12	152	153
13	151	150
14	137	139
15	144	145
16	132	133
17	128	130
18	160	163
19	158	162
20	146	146

Clinical laboratories frequently change methodologies, add new laboratory tests, and replace or add new instruments. The implementation of any of these changes requires proper evaluation and validation. The Centers for Medicare and Medicaid Services (CMS) through the Clinical Laboratory Improvement Amendments of 1988 (CLIA 1988) requires that certain tasks be completed to ensure the quality of laboratory tests resulting from these changes. The quality of laboratory testing is monitored via quality-control procedures and performance on proficiency tests.

Accuracy

The International Federation of Clinical Chemistry (IFCC) defines **accuracy** as the closeness of the agreement between the measured value of an analyte to its "true" value.[4]

Precision

The **precision** of a method is its ability to produce the same value for replicate measurements of the same sample. Precision is also described as the random variation in a population of data. Estimates of precision are determined for within-run and between-run analysis using mean, standard deviation, and coefficient of variation.

Within-run repeatability is described as the closeness of agreement between results of successive measurements carried out under the same conditions. Between-run reproducibility is the closeness of agreement between results of measurements performed under changed conditions of measurement (e.g., time, operator, and calibrator).[5]

Analytical Range

The range of concentration in the sample over which the method is applicable without "modification" is termed *analytical range*.[6] Analytical range is determined by a linearity experiment.[7] The analytical range should be wide enough to include 95 to 99% of the expected samples without predilution. CLIA 1988 states that once the analytical range of a method has been validated, it is termed the *reportable range* of the method.[8]

Reference Interval

Determining the reference interval of an analyte is an issue that requires close attention. CLSI has published a document that provides guidelines on how to define and determine reference intervals in the clinical laboratory.[9]

Method Comparisons of Qualitative Tests

Several assays performed routinely in the clinical laboratory provide qualitative results (e.g., pregnancy tests, where the results of the test are reported as positive or negative, and urine dipstick chemistries that may be reported as 1+, 2+, etc.). Evaluation of qualitative assays cannot be carried out in the same manner as quantitative assays; therefore, a different approach and statistics must be used. An example of a statistical test that is useful for comparing two qualitative assays with nominal-type data is the McNemar test.[10] The results of a study assessing concordance of data between qualitative assays are entered into a 2 × 2 contingency table similar to that of Table 2-3 ★. This test compares paired proportions and focuses on the pairs' discordant data. An example of an application of a McNemar test is shown in Mini-case 2-1.

MINI-CASE 2-1

Janet was asked to evaluate a new qualitative assay kit for urine hCG. She developed a study, and the data presented below shows 100 patient specimens assayed by both hCG kits. The results are entered into a 2 × 2 contingency table, and four results are discordant. A determination of significance is assessed using hypothesis testing and a chi square table of probability. The null hypothesis and alternate hypothesis must be stated:

	Test Kit 2 Positive	Test Kit 2 Negative	Total
Test Kit 1 Positive	28	3	31
Test Kit 1 Negative	1	68	69
Total	29	71	100

H_0 = There is no significant difference in response of both assay kits to patient specimens.

H_A = There is a significant difference in the response of both assay kits to patient specimens.

The level of significance or α for this evaluation is 0.05. Number of degrees of freedom = (2 rows − 1) × (2 rows − 1) = 1

Questions to Consider

1. What is the McNemar statistic for this set of data?
2. Should Janet accept or reject the null hypothesis?

★ **TABLE 2-3** McNemar Statistic for Comparing Results of Test Kit One Versus Test Kit Two

	Test Kit 2 Positive	Test Kit 2 Negative	Total
Test Kit 1 Positive	Number of positive results for test kits 1 and 2	Number of positive results for test kit 1 and negative results for test kit 2	Total tests results for row
Test Kit 1 Negative	Number of negative results for test kit 1 and positive results for test kit 2	Number of negative results for test kits 1 and 2	Total test results for row
Total	Total of number of results in column	Total of number of results in column	Total test results for row

From Sunheimer RL, Graves L. *Clinical Laboratory Chemistry*, 1st ed. Upper Saddle River, NJ: Pearson Education, 2011.

PROCEDURE MANUAL

A laboratory procedure manual must be present in the urinalysis laboratory. The manual provides useful information for laboratory staff and is typically requested for review by visiting accrediting agencies' personnel. The procedure manual should comply with CLSI guidelines and contain the essential elements listed in Box 2-1.[11] Support documents such as package inserts can accompany the procedure in the manual. Laboratories may use electronic copies, provided they are made available to laboratory staff.

The laboratory procedure manual should be reviewed on an annual basis by the supervisor and Pathologist. The reviewing process must be documented along with any changes made during the year.

LABORATORY TESTING STAGES

Testing biological fluid in samples obtained from individuals with or without disease passes through three stages: (1) pre-analytical, (2) analytical, and (3) post-analytical. Different types of mistakes and errors can be made anywhere in the stages of testing with several examples listed in Box 2-2. Many of these mistakes and errors are made while using various pieces of equipment and instruments shown in Box 2-3. There are many different types of "tools" (i.e., statistics), procedures, and practices available to the laboratory worker to assist in reducing errors in laboratory testing.

BOX 2-1 Summary of Essential Elements to be Included in a Laboratory Procedure Manual

Title

Purpose or principle

Procedure instructions including;

    Preparation of reagents, solutions, calibrators

    Calibration procedures

    Quality-control procedures

    Corrective action to be taken when a calibration or quality control is unacceptable

    Interpretation of examination results

    Reporting patient results

Reportable range of patient test results

Reference values, therapeutic or toxic ranges, or other interpretive criteria

Limitations of the procedure, including interfering substances

Preventive maintenance and function checks

Biosafety and chemical safety

Performance criteria for accuracy, precision, reportable range of patient results, linearity, analytical sensitivity, and specificity

References

BOX 2-2 Examples of Mistakes and Errors Made During the Various Stages of Laboratory Testing

Mislabeling of specimens

Drawing the wrong patient

Misinterpreting quality control rules

Mistakes made while running a procedure

Mistakes made while calibrating an assay

Dilution mistakes (e.g., forgetting to multiply results by dilution factor and incorrectly preparing a dilution)

Transcription mistakes

Performing a test on a clotted specimen

Improper sample preparation

Performing the wrong test on a patient specimen

Reporting results that exceeded the method linearity

Calculation mistakes

Performing tests on hemolyzed, lipemic, and icteric specimens

Incorrect decisions made based on incomplete understanding of assay procedure

---

Pre-Analytical

The pre-analytical stage of testing typically begins with a request by a healthcare provider to perform a laboratory tests(s) on a patient. Several additional variables in pre-analytical stage of laboratory testing are presented in Box 2-4 and discussed in more detail below. Test turnaround time (TAT), which addresses the issue of a quantity of time required to present the clinician with test results, encompasses several

---

BOX 2-3 Instruments and Equipment Frequently Found in Urinalysis Laboratories

Automated urinalysis systems

Cytospin

Centrifuge

Slide stainer

Stat spin

Refractometer

Pipettes

Class I or II Biological safety cabinet

Incubator

Refrigerator

Osmometer

Hemocytometer

Thermometers

Microscope

Safety equipment and devices

BOX 2-4 Variables in the Pre-Analytical Stage of Laboratory Testing

Test requests
Patient identification information
Patient preparation
Specimen collection
Specimen transport
Specimen separation, aliquot, and distribution

BOX 2-5 Proper Patient Identification and Labeling Procedures

- Use at least two person-specific identifiers.
- Label all blood in the presence of the patient.
- Verification must be done prior to the start of any invasive procedure.
- Verification process must be active and not passive.
- Label tubes in ink.
- Label after blood is collected in tubes.
- Information needed:
  Patient's name
  Hospital number or birthdate
  Time of collection
  Date
  Phlebotomist's initials
  For blood bank specimens full signature

Outpatient:
- Ask patient to state and spell full name, birthdate or an identification number.

Inpatient:
- Check ID bracelet for identification number.
- Verbally ask the patient's name.
- All inpatients are required to wear an ID bracelet.
- ID bracelet should state patient's name, birthdate, hospital number, physician, and room number.

pre-analytical factors including ordering tests, collecting, and transporting the specimens. The clinical laboratory must strive to reduce TAT, which would then avoid duplication of test orders and ensure an acceptable specimen.

Test Requests

The whole testing process commences with the ordering of a laboratory test by an appropriate licensed healthcare provider. The test request can be initiated via computers and/or handwritten test requisitions. Facilities using paper requisitions can have issues with illegible handwriting and transcription errors. Electronic test ordering can minimize this problem. Another issue that arises is verbal miscommunication of information from the person ordering the test(s) with the person submitting the test request. This occurs more often with complex tests, such as molecular biomarker tests, and test analytes with several variations, such as hepatitis testing. Computerization of all laboratory test requests would decrease the number of mistakes and errors made by healthcare staff. Many computer systems are programmed with limit checks, digits check, test-correlation check, and verification checks.

Patient Identification Information

The most important step in specimen collection is patient identification. Several recommendations are shown in Box 2-5. Most errors involving patient identification occur with the use of handwritten labels and request forms. Bar code identification serves to reduce these types of errors. There are several commercial computer adaptations of positive patient identification products that provide a variety of services, including:

- Software for positive identification of medications, specimen collection, and blood transfusion
- Mother/baby matching
- Software for handheld devices and PCs, including laptops on mobile carts

These positive patient identification products can interface with both hospital and laboratory information systems. In addition, there are electronic health record (EHR) and electronic medical record (EMR) systems available to reduce the frequency of patient/specimen identification errors.

Patient Preparation

There are several factors that can affect laboratory tests: smoking, use of caffeine, exercise, ethanol, drugs, recent food ingestion, stress, posture during specimen collection, diurnal sleep variation, circadian rhythm, and other variables. When a lab test requires special preparation, the patient must be informed and properly instructed. The laboratory is required to provide this information to the healthcare worker responsible for the patient. Failure of the patient to adhere to these instructions can bias the laboratory test results and negatively impact the clinician's interpretation of the data.

Specimen Collection

Essential elements for proper specimen collection include procedures for proper collection, timing, site of collection, containers, specimen type, and volume. Important issues relevant to these elements are shown in Box 2-6.

Specific instructions for unique body fluids should be written clearly and accurately because some fluid removal techniques are more difficult and hazardous than others. For example, CSF aspiration (Chapter 10) requires the clinician to insert a syringe needle into a pressurized column without causing an infection. The CSF must be transferred into appropriate collection containers in a proper sequence. Removal of serous fluids (Chapter 11) often yields a large volume that must be transported to the laboratory in a finite amount of time. Requirements for synovial fluid (Chapter 12) analysis depend on the size of the joint and effusion. Removal of amniotic fluid (Chapter 13) has a certain amount of risk to the fetus and must be completed with

BOX 2-6   Essentials for Valid Specimen Collections

Specific directions for proper procedures for specimen collection

Timing

    24 hours

    Random

    Fasting

Site of collection

    IV line

    Line draw

    Patient with mastectomy

    In-dwelling catheter

Containers

    Blood drawing tubes

    Syringes

    Urine vessels

    Stool collection

    CSF withdraw

    Synovial fluid

    Pericardial, peritoneum

    Additives to collection containers (anticoagulants, acid, clot activators, gel separation)

Specimen type

Specimen volume

---

strict adherence to protocol. Specimen collection for feces (Chapter 15) can be a challenge for the patients. It is important that the patient be properly instructed on how to collect the sample. A deviation from specimen collection protocol may invalidate the laboratory tests and require a second sample from the patient. This can result in an increased risk and certain amount of discomfort for each patient.

Many laboratory tests on body fluids require unique timing intervals, for example, 24-hour collections or 12- to 18-hour fasts before sampling. These timing requirements must be followed and not shortened unless authorized by the clinician.

The site of collection and subsequent preparation is important. There are many issues associated with various sites, and strict adherence to protocols is important. The laboratory needs to communicate with medical staff to determine the appropriate techniques and safety precautions necessary to remove body fluids.

There are many types of containers and collection vessels used to capture body fluids. Some containers require additives to enhance the stability of the body fluid. Failure to use a proper container will invalidate the laboratory tests.

Specimen types and volume are also significant factors relevant to the collection of body fluids. Many of these fluids contain cells and contaminants that must be processed using proper procedures. An insufficient volume may result in the laboratory rejecting the specimen and requesting a new sample.

Specimen Transport

Transporting specimens from the patient to the laboratory is often overlooked as a potential source of error for laboratory tests. Patient specimens are exposed to variable lighting conditions, temperature changes, and length of time differences that can affect sample integrity. The goal of the laboratory should be to limit the exposure of the sample to environmental conditions and complete the processing of the sample as quickly as possible. Failure to do so may cause falsely elevated or depressed analyte concentrations or cell counts.

Another process that may lead to variations in test results is sending samples out to another laboratory. This entire procedure is manual in nature with many opportunities available to make a mistake. Most reference laboratories are quite strict in their specimen requirements and will not accept a sample if their protocols are not followed exactly as written. Mistakes can be made in transcribing information, improperly packaging samples, submitting insufficient sample volume, or placing samples in the wrong containers. The laboratory staff must be knowledgeable and vigilant in processing these "send-outs."

Specimen Separation, Aliquot, and Distribution

Once a body fluid specimen reaches the laboratory, it is the responsibility of the laboratory staff to properly process and distribute the original samples and all aliquots. There are several variables that the laboratory can control to reduce error, including centrifugation, containers, and personnel. Proper maintenance and function checks must be completed on all centrifuges (see below), and containers must be free of contaminants. If glassware is used during sample processing, it must be properly cleaned and tested for contaminants such as calcium. Laboratories that use commercial products and disposables typically will not have a problem with contaminants.

Many body fluid procedures involve physical separation of components and typically use a centrifuge or adaptations such as a cytospin centrifuge. These separation techniques must be completed in a timely manner or risk false testing results. Specimen aliquot preparations can produce errors that can adversely affect laboratory results. For example, (1) two different fluids can be mixed together in one container, (2) aliquot containers can be mislabeled, (3) aliquots may contain cellular debris that can interfere with testing, and (4) subjecting the aliquot to a radically different environment could adversely affect the analyte.

Analytical

The analytical stage of testing includes the variables presented in Box 2-7. There are several options available to reduce errors and enhance quality laboratory testing during this stage of testing. The information provided in Table 2-4 ★ identifies specific tasks that can be initiated for instruments and equipment typically found in urinalysis and body fluid laboratories.

Test Procedures and Methods

The analytical stage of testing depends upon a well-written and accurate documentation of test procedures. All of the necessary steps required to complete a procedure should be in correct sequence, specific, succinct, and thorough. Discussion of test methodologies should include the principal factor that may influence the proper

BOX 2-7   Variables in the Analytical Stage of Laboratory Testing

Test procedures

Test methods

Reagents

Instrumentation

    Analyzers

    Automation

    Preventive maintenance

    Function checks

Equipment

    Preventive maintenance

    Function checks

Quality control

Proficiency testing

Staff competency

Facilities/resources

performance of the assay, instructions for preparation of reagent and calibrator, specimen preparation, and any test limitation that may directly affect the method.

Reagents

Reagents are a key component of all test methods, and the laboratory staff must be completely familiar with each one, including water sources. Instructions for proper preparation of a reagent must be followed exactly as the manufacturer has described. This includes techniques for mixing, time requirements, and storage temperature. If ancillary laboratory equipment (beaker, flask, glass pipets) is required, it must be scrupulously cleaned and volumetrically accurate. Never used expired reagents or calibrators. Failure to follow the above recommendations will typically result in incorrect result of the laboratory tests.

Instrumentation

Analytical instrumentation such as spectrophotometer or an automated system requires continuous care and attention. Preventive maintenance should be performed prior to use, followed by any appropriate function checks (e.g., wavelength accuracy, absorbance check, and electrode drift).

Equipment

Laboratory equipment also requires routine maintenance, and, for some pieces, function checks as highlighted in Box 2-7. Laboratory equipment tends to have a longer functional life when it is properly maintained. Failure to follow preventive maintenance will result in shorter lifespan, more frequent breakdowns, and increased laboratory costs.

Quality Control and Proficiency Testing

Quality control and proficiency testing is discussed in more detail later in the chapter. It provides timely and compelling information relevant to the performance of the laboratory tests. Each laboratory should determine its rules or criteria for accepting or rejecting patient data based on quality control standards. Quality control failure should be assessed immediately, and any corrective action must be documented. Proficiency testing, while utilized by accreditation agencies for assessment of laboratory performance on a regular frequency, can

★ **TABLE 2-4** Maintenance and Calibration Requirements for Laboratory Instruments and Equipment Typically Located in Urinalysis Laboratories

Instruments/Equipment	Maintenance/Calibration
Centrifuge	Cleaning inside of centrifuge, buckets, carriers, and rotor. Calibrate the typical speed (RPM) using a tachometer
Refrigerator	Clean inside and outside of refrigerator. Temperature should be monitored using a temperature-sensing device calibrated with a NIST or other type of reference thermometer
Thermometers	Calibrated with a NIST or other type of reference thermometer
Microscope	Clean lenses and objectives. Check alignment of light source, illumination (Kohler illumination), and resolving power
Refractometer	Cleaning eyepiece and surface of the prism. Calibrate device using pure water and solutions with known particulate concentration
Pipetting devices	Clean the opening at the end of the barrel where the tips are placed. Calibrate pipets for accuracy and precision.
Osmometer	Clean exterior, probe, and thermistor. Replace ethylene glycol bath. Calibrate analyzer using solutions of known osmolality
Safety cabinet	Decontaminate with an appropriate disinfectant. Calibrate air flow
Hemocytometer	Clean surface
Incubator	Clean interior and exterior. Monitor temperature using a temperature sensing device calibrate with a NIST or other type of reference thermometer
Automated urinalysis systems	May require extensive maintenance and staff should refer to the analyzer manual. Reflectometer and refractometer (if used) require calibration

also provide the laboratory with valuable information regarding test performance. Recurring proficiency test failures may result in an order of discontinuation for that particular test.

Staff Competency

Initial assessment and monitoring staff competency is a task that each laboratory is required to complete. The assessment should include the following:

- Direct observation of patient testing
- Monitoring the recording and reporting of results
- Reviewing intermediate test results or QC records
- Direct observation of maintenance/function checks
- Blind testing or proficiency testing
- Assessment of problem-solving skills
- Observation for compliance with safety protocols

Laboratory supervisory staff should provide the technical staff with proper training that serves to teach staff the proper procedures and establish uniformity in techniques. This will reduce the number of mistakes or errors made in the laboratory. Creating a list of objectives that outline the critical tasks and knowledge is useful in training laboratory staff. Another useful tool for enhancing staff competency is in-service and continuing education programs.

Facilities and Resources

Adequate facilities and resources are essential to ensure quality test results. Laboratory staff should have access to current reference material and atlases. A sufficient amount of time should be allotted so that the staff can participate in conferences, webinars, grand rounds, and journal clubs. Laboratory instruments and equipment should be updated, plentiful, and available for use by all staff.

Laboratory facilities should maintain adequate room space, safety equipment, and bench surface area. Additional space for break rooms, conference rooms, computers stations, and personal hygiene facilities typically improve morale among laboratory staff.

Post-Analytical

The post-analytical stage of laboratory testing involves the processes that impact reporting of results, test interpretation, archival procedures, and other tasks shown in Box 2-8. Computer and other technologies have facilitated this stage of laboratory testing. Also, the number of errors has been significantly reduced due in part to bidirectional interfacing of instrument computers and laboratory information systems.

BOX 2-8 Variables in Post-Analytical Stage of Laboratory Testing

Reports generated

Results reported

Clinical responses to results and interpretation

Records and specimen retention

Test Reporting

Presentation of patient information begins once the analytes(s) are measured and "released," or transmitted by the analyzer computer. This information must be "matched" to the correct patient for electronic transmission or hand written documents. The reporting format should be standardized and include reference intervals. Procedures should be established to provide active review of all results reported and timely correction for any errors created. Printers should be cleaned and maintained to prevent poor alphanumeric recognition.

Clinical Response to Results and Interpretation

Test interpretation should appear on the report to the clinician. This information is to be consistent with the FDA-approved information accompanying the test system. Assay sensitivity and specificity should also be included in the procedure manual for correct interpretation of results.

Reports Generated

All ancillary reports generated for internal and external use must be correct and clearly documented. Active review by laboratory staff should be ongoing and documented.

Records and Specimen Retention

Once reports are generated, they must be archived for an extended period of time, depending on guidelines developed by accrediting agencies. Specimens, including blood tubes, slides, and tissues, are required to be saved. A system should be developed within each laboratory to store documents and samples with a focus on cost and space limitations.

QUALITY ASSURANCE AND QUALITY CONTROL

Quality control has its roots in the early automotive industry. Shewhart developed a type of control chart for use in industry.[12] Since that time quality controls have evolved to a level in the laboratory that has served to minimize error, especially in the analytical stage of testing. For a review of the origin of present-day quality-control procedures, refer to the references cited.[13, 14, 15]

Quality Assurance

Total quality management (TQM) is a concept that began in industry and provides a philosophy for organizational development and a process for improving the quality of workmanship[16] Clinical laboratories have incorporated many of the aspects of TQM, especially quality assurance and quality control.[17] TQM programs accomplish the following:

- Monitoring and evaluating the ongoing and overall quality of the total testing process and the effectiveness of its policies and procedures.
- Identifying and correcting problems and ensuring the accurate, reliable, and prompt reporting of test results.
- Ensuring the adequacy and competency of the staff.

Quality assurance (QA) in a healthcare facility encompasses global issues and is the responsibility of everyone involved in the care of patients. There are many essentials for a quality assurance program, including the following:

- Commitment
- Adequate facilities
- Adequate resources
- Competent staff
- Reliable procedures, methods, and instrumentation

The clinical laboratory is an important component of the overall QA within a facility due in part to the volume of testing and the clinical importance of the laboratory data being generated. If an error occurs in any one step during the acquisition, processing, analysis, or reporting of a laboratory test result, it will invalidate the quality of the analysis and the laboratory will not realize its QA goals.

Quality Control

Quality control (QC) refers to the procedures for monitoring and evaluating the quality of the analytical testing process of each method to ensure the accuracy and reliability of patient test results and reports. The purpose of assaying control material is to verify the stability and accuracy of calibration and testing systems. This is an extremely important function supported by several organizations and regulatory agencies.

The International Organization for Standardization (ISO) 9000 series identified ten quality-ensuring items that are common to all quality-control systems:[18]

- Instituting an effective quality system
- Ensuring valid and timely measurements
- Using calibrated measuring and testing equipment
- Using appropriate statistical techniques
- Developing a product identification and traceability system
- Maintaining adequate record-keeping systems
- Ensuring an adequate product handling, storage packaging, and delivery system
- Maintaining an adequate inspection and testing system
- Ensuring adequate personnel training and experience

CLIA 1988 embraces most of these items in its regulations under *subpart K* and *subpart P*, therefore it is incumbent on clinical laboratories to do the same.[19]

Quality-Control Materials.

The best practice when selecting the appropriate material for quality control is to use a matrix that is similar to the test specimens. For example, if the analyte to be measured in a patient specimen requires whole blood, then the quality-control material should be whole blood. Unfortunately, matrixes such as whole blood are difficult to stabilize; therefore, a suitable alternate must be found.

There are several factors to consider when selecting quality-control materials:

- The materials must be stable.
- The materials must be available in aliquots or vials.
- The materials can be analyzed periodically over a long span of time.
- There is little vial-to-vial variation.
- The concentration of analyte should be in the normal and abnormal ranges.

Commercially prepared control materials are manufactured in three different forms: (1) lyophilized or freeze-dried pooled material, (2) liquid pooled material, and (3) frozen pooled material. Lyophilized materials are processed so that the water content is minimal, thus requiring reconstitution and special mixing procedures. This process often results in error because of incorrect pipetting and/or failure to follow mixing procedures exactly as written. A means to alleviate these problems is to acquire control material that is already liquefied and may be stored frozen or refrigerated.

Target Values

Commercial QC material may be assayed or unassayed. Assayed QC material has concentrations or *target values* that are determined by the manufacturer. Unassayed QC material has no predetermined target values, and its ranges must be determined by the laboratory. The target values for the QC material include the mean and standard deviations of the analyte for the particular control material. Each target value must represent a concentration in the normal range and abnormal range for bi-level QC material and an additional abnormal level for tri-level QC material. The decision whether to assay two levels or three levels of QC material depends on the analyte to be measured, the method of measurement, and the clinical significance of the analyte to disease. For example, blood-gas analytes require three levels of controls; general chemistries (e.g., glucose and urea nitrogen) require at least two levels; and immunoassays usually require three levels.

Quality-Control Limits

Levey-Jennings Control Charts

Levey-Jennings (L-J) charts show the difference between the observed values and the expected mean. The charts are created by calculating the mean concentration and up to $\pm 3s$ for a pool of quality-control material. The data are plotted on the Y-axis. The X-axis is divided into days, usually in 30-day intervals. As quality-control data are generated during the month, the values are plotted on the L-J chart. L-J charts are very useful for observing patterns of data (for instance, *trends* and *shifts*). A trend is a pattern of data in which all of the QC values continue to increase or decrease over a period time. QC trends may occur, for example, when reagents begin to deteriorate, a polychromatic light source continually diminishes in luminescent intensity, or when a monochromatic filter becomes delaminated. If a trend is allowed to continue, the QC results will eventually exceed $\pm 2s$. A shift in QC values is described as consecutive data that remain on one side of the mean for at least six days. The presence of a shift in QC results may be due to a change in incubation temperature, contamination of reagents, changes in calibrator values, or changes in pipette volumes. A typical L-J QC chart for blood glucose measurement using bi-level (normal and abnormal) QC material is shown in Figure 2-4 ■.

Level I Control [Normal]

Glucose

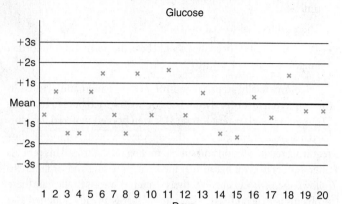

Level II Control [Abnormal]

Glucose

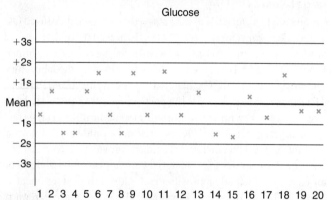

■ **FIGURE 2-4** Levey-Jennings Quality-Control Charts for Normal and Abnormal Concentrations of Glucose in Blood

From Sunheimer RL, Graves L. *Clinical Laboratory Chemistry*, 1st ed. (Upper Saddle River, NJ: Pearson Education), 2011.

★ **TABLE 2-5** Westgard Quality Control Rule Designations and Interpretation

Control Rule Designations	Interpretation
1_{2s}	One control observation exceeding the mean $\pm 2s$. This rule may be used as a **warning** rule that initiates testing of the control data by the other control rules.
1_{3s}	One control observation exceeding the mean $\pm 3s$. The recommendation is to reject patient results; this rule is sensitive to random error.
2_{2s}	Two consecutive control observations exceeding the same mean plus 2s or mean minus 2s limit. The recommendation is to reject patient results; this rule is sensitive to systematic error.
R_{4s}	One observation exceeding the mean plus 2s and another exceeding the mean minus 2s. The recommendation is to reject patient results; this rule is sensitive to random error.
4_{1s}	Four consecutive observations exceeding the mean plus 1s or the mean minus 1s. The recommendation is to reject patient results; this rule is sensitive to systematic error.
$10\overline{X}$	Ten consecutive control observations falling on one side of the mean (above or below, with no other requirement on size of the deviations). The recommendation is to reject patient results; this rule is sensitive to systematic error.

Note: standard deviation (*s*).

From Sunheimer RL, Graves L. *Clinical Laboratory Chemistry*, 1st ed. Upper Saddle River, NJ: Pearson Education, 2011.

Westgard Multirule Procedures

A multirule procedure developed by Westgard and colleagues uses an assortment of control rules for interpreting quality-control data.[20] The procedure requires a chart in which lines for control limits are drawn at the mean; this chart can be adapted to existing L-J charts by adding one or two sets of control limits. This system provides a more structured use than that proposed by Levey-Jennings and shows either random or systematic errors. A summary of the rules is shown in Table 2-5 ★ and is diagrammed in Figure 2-5 ■.

Table 2-6 ★ summarizes the evaluation of QC data in the examples provided in Figure 2-6 ■. The table provides the day, the decision to accept or reject, the control rule violated, and the type of error that may have caused the questionable control value.

Sources of Random and Systematic Errors

Once the possibility of an error has been detected, the next step is to determine the cause of the error. Sources of error vary depending on whether they are random or systematic. Examples of sources of error are shown in Box 2-9.

BOX 2-9 Sources of Random and Systematic Error

Random Error

Power supply

Double pipetting of control samples

Air bubbles in samples or reagents

Incorrect reconstitution of control material

Operator technique

Improper specimen handling

Systematic Error

Improper alignment of sample or reagent pipettes

Drift or shift in incubator chamber temperature

Deterioration of reagent while in use, storage, or shipment

Failing light source

Deterioration of control material

Recent calibration

Change in test operator

Incorrect handling of control product

Change of reagent or calibrator lot numbers

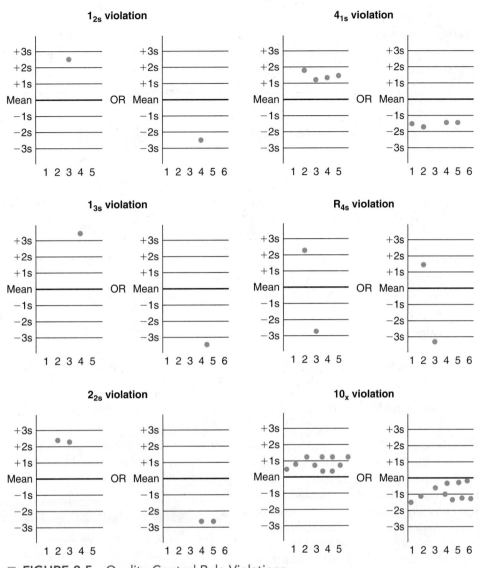

FIGURE 2-5 Quality-Control Rule Violations

From Sunheimer RL, Graves L. *Clinical Laboratory Chemistry*, 1st ed. (Upper Saddle River, NJ: Pearson Education), 2011.

★ **TABLE 2-6** Application of Westgard Multirule System of Quality Control for Data Shown in Figure 2-6

Day	Level I	Level II	1$_{2s}$	1$_{3s}$	2$_{2s}$	R$_{4s}$	4$_{1s}$	10 $\bar{x}$	RE	SE	Accept	Reject	Warning
2	X			X					X			X	
5	X	X			X					X		X	
8	X		X							X			X
9	X				X					X		X	
12	X	X				X				X		X	
16	X						X			X		X	
23	X							X		X		X	

From Sunheimer RL, Graves L. *Clinical Laboratory Chemistry*, 1st ed. Upper Saddle River, NJ: Pearson Education, 2011.

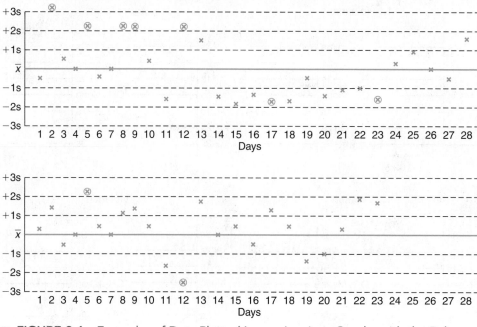

■ **FIGURE 2-6** Examples of Data Plotted Levey-Jennings Graphs with the Rule
Interpretations Presented in Table 2-6

From Sunheimer RL, Graves L. *Clinical Laboratory Chemistry*, 1st ed. (New Jersey: Pearson Education), 2011.

Detecting Quality-Control Problems

Computers

Computer software applications for quality control are available for both PCs and laboratory information systems (LISs). QC results can be entered into these computers either manually by the operator or automatically through data transmission ports. Target values and control limits are established for each analyte and QC level. Levey-Jennings plots and QC rules such as Westgard are also available. QC data can be reviewed by the operator to determine acceptability of the result. If Westgard rules are available, the computer will determine whether any test results in a rule violation and alert the operator. The advantages of using computers for QC include (1) real-time review, (2) early detection of QC problems, and (3) documentation of the QC process.

Steps to Remedy Westgard Rule Violations

If QC results violate any Westgard rules, the laboratory must have a procedure that will resolve these violations. This procedure includes the following: (1) steps to take toward problem resolution, (2) proper documentation of the problem and solution(s), and (3) indications of whom to notify of the rule infractions (e.g., a supervisor or QC officer). The following example identifies steps that may be taken if a problem occurs while assaying quality-control materials.

- If a control value is outside the acceptable range, then reassay a fresh aliquot of the same control material.

- If the control value is still outside the acceptable range, then reconstitute a new vial of control material and reassay.

- If the control value is still outside the acceptable range, then look for obvious problems such as clots in the specimen, low reagent levels, and instrument-related mechanical faults. This may be a good time to replace the reagents.

- If the control value is still outside the acceptable range, then consider recalibrating the assay.

- If the control value is still outside the acceptable range, then the technologist may be directed to consult the QC officer and/or supervisor for further direction.

☑ CHECKPOINT 2-3

The means and standard deviations for urine creatinine levels in quality control pools I and II are shown in the following table:

Creatinine	Level I	Level II
Mean	0.8	6.0
Standard deviation	0.1	0.3

The technologists in the urinalysis laboratory recorded the following quality-control values for a 10-day period:

	Level I	Level II
Day 1	0.9	6.1
Day 2	1.15	6.2
Day 3	0.8	5.9
Day 4	0.7	6.7
Day 5	0.7	6.8
Day 6	0.8	5.5
Day 7	0.9	6.0
Day 8	1.3	6.5
Day 9	0.8	6.2
Day 10	0.9	6.1

Using the data presented do the following:

1. Determine all of the Westgard rule violations.
2. Identify the type of errors associated with each rule violation.
3. Determine a course of action for each rule violation.

Calibration

The purpose of **calibration** as defined by CLIA 1988 is to "substantiate the continued accuracy of the test system throughout the laboratory reportable range of the test results for the test system."[21] Materials used to perform a calibration are called *calibrators*. Calibration material or calibrators are described as "a material—either solutions or a device of known, or assigned quantitative or qualitative characteristics (e.g., concentration, activity, intensity, reactivity)—used to calibrate, graduate, or adjust a measurement procedure or to compare the response obtained with the response of a test specimen and/or sample."[21] Controls and calibrators are different. Calibrators are prepared differently from controls; therefore, controls must not be used as calibrators. Calibrators should not be used as controls unless there are no suitable control materials for a particular test. CLIA 1988 will allow the use of calibrators as controls if that situation occurs. Commercially prepared calibrators have assigned values for each analyte that are determined by a definitive or reference method. The calibrator value assigned for the material is programmed into the analyzer's computer for use as a comparator in measuring an unknown sample.

The values for quality-control material are determined by the laboratory using its respective analyzers to determine the mean and standard deviation. The analyzers used for routine chemistry and urinalysis do not represent the definitive measuring devices that yield highly accurate values for analyses in solutions.

Proficiency Testing in Urinalysis

CLIA 1988 recommends that proficiency testing (PT) be conducted in clinical laboratories. Proficiency tests, also referred to as *surveys*, are an example of external quality control wherein an agency or organization provides biological samples whose concentrations are unknown to the testing clinical laboratory. The clinical laboratory submits its data for the unknown sample to the PT testing service. The results are returned to the laboratory with an evaluation of the laboratory's performance. A commonly used criterion for evaluation of PT results for a given clinical laboratory has been comparing PT test results with the results of peer groups and considering all values that exceed 2*s* to be "unacceptable." PT samples are sent routinely several times a year for analysis, and the overall performances from all the PT samples are used to determine whether a laboratory performance is acceptable or unacceptable. If the laboratory performance is unacceptable, then the laboratory is placed on a probationary status for that category of tests (e.g., electrolytes or blood gases) until the laboratory successfully passes subsequent PT. If the laboratory continues to perform unacceptably, then it will not be allowed to report patient results for that test(s) until the lab is reinstated.

CLIA 1988 regulations specify that PT specimens should be treated the same as patient specimens. Therefore, "special handling" of PT specimens is discouraged. Except for the special instructions for preparing PT specimens, they must be included with the laboratory's daily assay regimens.

MINI-CASE 2-2

Jessica has completed her measurements of both levels of quality control for serum general chemistries. Her analysis of the data reveals a 2_{2s} Westgard rule violation for glucose. This is a first-time occurrence and five patients' samples have been analyzed while assaying the quality control material.

Questions to Consider

1. What is Jessica's course of action for the quality control rule violation?
2. What should Jessica do about the patient samples that were assayed?

AUTOMATED URINALYSIS STYSTEMS

Automated urine systems consist of chemistry and microscopy modules. These systems are designed to provide a complete urinalysis including assessment of color and clarity, measurement of specific gravity, chemistry constituents, and a microscopic analysis of the patient's specimen.

Once instrument maintenance is completed, the chemistry and microscopic modules must be calibrated. The specific method used to calibrate and verify with quality controls differs with each automated system. There may also be variations in procedures and protocol from one state to another, but the purpose and principles remain the same. The following discussion represents a generic approach for calibration and quality-control procedures of all tests performed by similar automated urine systems.

Urine chemistry strips or sticks are used to determine the amount of glucose, protein, bilirubin, urobilinogen, pH, blood, ketones, nitrite, and leukocytes in a specimen. The measuring principle is reflectance spectroscopy. A reflectometer is used to detect and measure reflected light off the surface of a test strip or stick. The light reflected is diffused (i.e., radiates off a non-shiny surface in many directions). Only a fraction of the light reflected is detected by a photodetector and used for measurement. The reflected light passes through a monochromator, either a filter or diffraction grating, to isolate the specific wavelength in the visible region of the electromagnetic spectrum.

An instrument calibration is performed using one or two unique calibration sticks. These calibration sticks create a known percentage of reflectance at several different wavelengths normally used to measure analytes in urine specimens. The percentage of reflectance is determined by loading the calibration strips and performing the "reflectometry calibration." If the results of the calibration measurements fall within the manufacturer's stated tolerance, then the reflectometer is calibrated satisfactorily. If measurements fall outside tolerance, the appropriate troubleshooting steps must be initiated.

Urine specific gravity is estimated by measuring the refraction angles of light passing through a prism. Calibration of the refractometer is accomplished using two specific gravity calibrators containing varying amounts of salt and color substance representing a low and high specific gravity. Tolerance limits are established by the manufacturer; upon completion of the specific gravity calibration, the operator determines whether the measured values are outside the calibration ranges.

Once calibration of the required components of the automated urine chemistry module is complete, proper quality-control procedures must be initiated. Assaying quality-control materials serves to validate the calibration and ensure the likelihood that measurements of urine constituents in patient's specimens will be correct.

The urinalysis laboratory must assay at least two levels of quality-control material representing normal and abnormal ranges. Commercially available materials that have been assayed with established quality control ranges are widely used in all types of clinical laboratories. The quality-control material must include all of the urine constituents that are reported by the laboratory. These typically include color, clarity, specific gravity, pH, protein, glucose, ketones, bilirubin, blood nitrites, urobilinogen, and leukocytes. Analyte results may be reported numerically (e.g., urine pH of 7.0), as text (e.g., negative), and alphanumerically (e.g., 1+) and with appropriate units.

Both color and clarity are also measured by some automated urine systems. The color is determined by comparison to four specific wavelengths of electromagnetic radiation, and clarity is measured by passing a beam of light through the sample and measuring the scattered light. Quality-control testing is performed for both of these urine parameters. Two solutions of different color and clarity (turbidity) representing normal and abnormal characteristics are assayed and compared to the results provided by the manufacturer. In addition, many instrument design formats have a built-in mechanism to compensate for the natural color of urine and its effect on the specific color reactions produced within the absorbent pads on the urine strip.

> ## ☑ CHECKPOINT 2-4
>
> Discuss one reason why quality-control material cannot be used to calibrate a method.

Formed Elements

The urine microscopy module identifies formed elements in a specimen using their size, shape, contrast, and texture to autoclassify them into several categories including erythrocytes, white blood cells, white blood cell clumps, hyaline casts, unclassified casts, squamous epithelial cells, bacterial, yeast, crystals, mucus, and sperm. The identification function involves the use of a flow cytometer system that allows for aspiration of urine samples, which is subsequently sandwiched between enveloping layers of a suspending fluid. This fluid, or "lamina," is positioned exactly within the depth of focus and field of view of the objective lens of a microscope.

Calibration of the microscopy module is performed periodically by assaying prepared samples containing known amounts of formed elements, for example, erythrocytes or other particles per microliter.

The measured number of erythrocytes must fall within the range of values provided by the manufacturer.

Two quality-control samples each containing a specified number of particles (e.g., erythrocytes) representing positive and negative samples are assayed, and the results must lie within the assigned ranges to be acceptable.

Body Fluids

Some urinalysis systems are capable of assaying other body fluids (e.g., cerebrospinal fluid (CSF) and serous fluid). Two levels of controls are required and must include a low and a high level. The control matrix usually contains a mixture of formed elements such as stabilized human erythrocytes and simulated white blood cells in the form of erythrocytes from animal or bird sources.

Automated Urine Chemistries

Quantitative analysis of urine chemistries routinely includes sodium, potassium chloride, calcium, magnesium, phosphate, glucose, creatinine, urea nitrogen, amylase, microalbumin, and proteins. The result of these measurements provides the clinician with significant information necessary to provide optimum care to the patient. Therefore, it is incumbent upon the clinical urinalysis laboratory to ensure that all instruments and methods are providing quality data. Calibration and quality-control procedures must be followed in a consistent and timely fashion.

A majority of the urine analytes mentioned above are assayed on an automated chemistry analyzer. These automated systems provide faster turnaround time, improved precision, and fewer analytical errors. There may be exceptions; for instance, several manufacturers provide non-automated benchtop analyzers, which provide equally reliable results. No matter what instrument platform is used, the whole process begins with calibrating the chemistries.

Calibration of urine chemistry requires at least two levels of calibrants. This material usually consists of a serum-based matrix and is appropriate for blood samples (e.g., serum and plasma sodium). The calibrants are assayed using the calibration mode, which is preprogrammed into the analyzer computer. Upon completion of the calibration, all data is reviewed for acceptability and presence of error. Examples of errors include:

- Measuring values that exceed calibrant target values.
- A small difference between two calibrators with different concentration.
- A significant difference in the standard deviation limits, which is due to an error in the order of the calibrations.

Quality control of urine chemistries requires at least two levels of concentration, normal and abnormal. Control material should contain the analytes to be tested in a urine matrix. If the analyte is to be measured in patient CSF, then the quality-control matrix should be CSF.

MANUAL URINE TESTS

Manual urine testing often presents unique challenges in securing acceptable sources of calibrators, quality-control samples, and PT samples. The menu of tests available in clinical laboratories is

★ **TABLE 2-7** Manual Urine Tests, Calibration, and Quality Control

Test	Calibration	Quality Control (number of levels)	Quality Control (interpretation)	Comments
Qualitative hCG, serum/urine	N/A	Bi-level	Positive and Negative	
Urine/stool reducing substances	N/A	Bi-level	Positive and Negative	
Urine/fluid pH	2-3 aqueous-based standards	Bi-level	Numeric values	
Osmolality (serum, urine)	2-3 aqueous-based standards	Bi-level	Positive and Negative	Calibrator values are low abnormal, high abnormal, and a commercially prepared 290 osmol/kg
Acetone (urine/serum)	N/A	Bi-level	Numeric value	Prepared solution of acetoacetate at a known concentration
Urine bilirubin (Ictotest)	N/A	Bi-level	Positive and Negative	
Urine hemoglobin (Hemastix)	N/A	Bi-level	Positive and Negative	
Specific gravity (refractometer)	One level	Bi-level	Numeric value	Calibrate to 0.0 SG with water and measure distilled water and a 7.5% saline solution for quality control
Urine multistix (manual)	N/A	Bi-level	Positive and Negative	Visual interpretation of color

highly variable and includes examples of waived, moderate, and highly complex tests. Every lab providing manual tests must be familiar with appropriate regulations regarding the number of levels of calibrators and quality-control samples and frequency of testing such materials. A list of body fluid tests are presented in Table 2-7 ★ with recommendation for calibrators, QC levels, and interpretative comments.

☑ CHECKPOINT 2-5

Which part of a urinalysis is determined by (A) reflectance spectroscopy? (B) refractometry? (C) cell identification?

MINI-CASE 2-3

Greg just completed the calibration of his automated urine analyzer. The results of his calibration fell outside the tolerance limits.

Questions to Consider

1. What did Greg do wrong?
2. Can Greg continue on and assay his quality control samples?
3. What should Greg do immediately after failing his calibration?

Key Points to Remember

- Laboratory statistics are the "tools" used in assessing laboratory data created by measuring analyte concentration in biological fluids.
- Selecting and evaluating test methods are dependent upon examination of analytical performance parameters.
- Selection of appropriate statistics and correct interpretation are of paramount importance to good decision making in a clinical laboratory.
- Quality control focuses on periodic monitoring of method performance by measuring analyte concentrations in solutions with known amounts of analytes.

- A complete understanding of Westgard and Stewart quality-control procedures is important in monitoring the performance of laboratory tests.
- Quality assurance is those activities performed by all employees in the institution that serve to provide the best patient care.
- Automated urinalysis systems provide faster turnaround time, improve precision, and reduce error rates for urine chemistries, specific gravity, and microscopic analysis.

Review Questions

Level I

1. The method of least squares is used for (Objective 1)

   A. Linear regression.

   B. Correlation.

   C. Standard deviation.

   D. Precision.

2. Which of the following statements best defines the term *accuracy*? (Objective 3)

   A. A test's ability to produce the same value for replicate measures of the same sample

   B. A test's ability to correlate to another method

   C. The closeness of the agreement between the measured value of an analyte and its true value

   D. Laboratory results that do not agree

3. Which of the following is an example of an inferential statistic? (Objective 1)

   A. Mean

   B. Standard deviation

   C. Student's *t*-test

   D. Correlation coefficient

4. Which of the following statements defines a 2_{2s} quality-control rule violation? (Objective 6)

   A. Two consecutive control values exceed $\pm 2s$

   B. Two non-consecutive control values exceed $\pm 1s$

   C. Four consecutive control values exceed $\pm 2s$

   D. Two control values exceed $\pm 4s$

5. Which of the following instrument principles is used to measure urine chemistries using strips or sticks? (Objective 8)

   A. Absorption spectroscopy

   B. Fluorescence spectroscopy

   C. Reflectometry

   D. Atomic absorption spectroscopy

6. Clarity of a urine specimen is determined by (Objective 8)

   A. potentiometry.

   B. refractometry.

   C. passing a beam of light through the sample and measuring the fluorescent light.

   D. passing a beam of light through the sample and measuring the scatter of light.

7. Which of the following is used in a urine microscopy module to identify formed elements in a urine specimen? (Objective 8)

   A. Specific gravity

   B. Size, shape, contrast, and texture

   C. Molecular weight and particle size

   D. A reflectometer to measure light scatter off the surface

8. The light reflected off the surface of a urine test strip for glucose is described as (Objective 8)

   A. specular.

   B. biphasic.

   C. diffuse.

   D. fluorescent.

9. Which of the following defines mode? (Objective 2)

   A. The average for the variable

   B. The data point that occurs most frequently

   C. The middle value or the 50th percentile

   D. The lowest value in a set of data

10. The "y" axis of a Levey-Jennings quality control chart represents which of the following parameters? (Objective 5)

    A. Mean and coefficient of variation

    B. Mean and standard deviation

    C. Mean and variance

    D. Days of the month

11. Which of the following is an example of an analytic test variable? (Objective 4)

    A. Specimen transport from the emergency department to the laboratory

    B. Test requests from a clinician

    C. Reporting results to the clinician

    D. Reagents used for the analysis

12. Which of the following analytes is tested for in urine using a test strip? (Objective 7)

    A. Glucose

    B. Urea nitrogen

    C. Sodium

    D. Amylase

Level II

1. The following data represents 10 replicate measurements of a random urine potassium level. What are the mean, standard deviation (s), and percentage coefficient of variation (%CV) for the data shown in the table? (Objective 1)

Sample Number	Urine Potassium (mmol/L)
1	50
2	50
3	48
4	51
5	49
6	52
7	50
8	53
9	49
10	48

   A. mean = 48 mmol/L, s = 3.5 mmol/L, %CV = 72.9

   B. mean = 50 mmol/L, s = 3.27 mmol/L, %CV = 1.63

   C. mean = 50 mmol/L, s = 1.63 mmol/L, %CV = 3.27

   D. mean = 52 mmol/L, s = 0.175 mmol/L, %CV = 5.0

2. Linear regression by least squares is useful for identifying which of the following? (Objective 2)

   A. Systematic and proportional error

   B. Quality-control failures

   C. Variation among three or more methods

   D. Cutoff values that maximize both sensitivity and specificity

3. Which of the following actions represents the best course of action for a 1_{3s} quality-control failure? (Objective 5)

   A. Release all patient results but rerun the control material that failed.

   B. Release all patient results and do not rerun control material that failed.

   C. Do not release patient results and rerun the control material that failed.

   D. Do not release patient results, recalibrate the assay, and then rerun all levels of control material.

4. The linearity of a method is characterized by which of the following? (Objective 1)

   A. Slope and bias

   B. Slope and intercept

   C. Intercept and p-value

   D. A large correlation coefficient

5. Quality control samples used for measurement of formed elements in urine samples contain (Objective 8)

   A. a mixture of salts (e.g., sodium chloride and potassium chloride).

   B. a mixture of skin epithelial cells.

   C. a mixture that contains renal epithelial cells.

   D. a mixture that includes erythrocytes.

6. Which of the following statistics is used to evaluate two different tests for determining urine human chorionic gonadotropin? (Objective 2)

   A. Linear regression by the method of least squares

   B. McNemar test

   C. Correlation coefficient (r^2)

   D. Standard deviation

7. Phil has a 10 $\bar{x}$ Westgard rule violation with his normal glucose quality-control sample. Which of the following may cause this rule violation? (Objective 5)

   A. Air bubbles in the tubing

   B. Pipetting mistake

   C. Change in reagent lot

   D. Intermittent power supply problem

8. Which of the following urine tests is determined by measuring the refraction angles of light passing through a prism? (Objective 7)

   A. Glucose

   B. Sodium

   C. Lipase

   D. Specific gravity

9. Which of the following actions should reduce the number of mistakes involving patient identification? (Objective 4)

   A. Purchase a computerized positive patient identification product.

   B. Write the patient's last name on his or her arm.

   C. Have the patient write his or her name on a test request form.

   D. Have the patient recite the body fluid test(s) that are ordered by the clinician.

10. Which of the following statements is correct regarding the urinalysis procedure manual? (Objective 3)

   A. The manual does not have to ever be reviewed once it is written.

   B. The manual must be written in at least three different languages.

   C. The manual should be reviewed on an annual basis by the supervisor and pathologist.

   D. The manual can be reviewed by any clerical staff.

Endnotes

1. Hollander M, Wolfe DA. *Nonparametric statistical methods*, 2nd ed. New York: Wiley-Interscience, 1999.

2. Prescott P. An approximate test for outliers in linear model. *Technometrics* (1975) 17:129–132.

3. Zar JH. *Biostatistical analysis*, 4th ed. Upper Saddle River, NJ: Prentice Hall, 1999:332–333.

4. Buttner J, Broth R, Boutwell JH et al. (IFCC Committee on standards). Provisional recommendations on quality control in clinical chemistry: general principles and terminology. *ClinChem* (1976) 22:532–539.

5. Linnett K, Boyd JC. Selection and analytical evaluation of methods with statistical techniques. *In*: Burtis CA, Ashwood ER, Bruns DE (eds.). *Tietz textbook of clinical chemistry and molecular diagnostics*, 4th ed. Philadelphia: W. B. Saunders, 2006:357–358.

6. Buttner J, Borth R, Boutwell JH, et al. International Federation of Clinical Chemistry. Committee on Standards. Expert Panel on Nomenclature and Principles of Quality Control in Clinical Chemistry. Approved recommendation (1978) on quality control in clinical chemistry. Part 1. General principles and terminology. *ClinChemActa* (1979) 98 (1-2):129F–143F.

7. National Committee for Clinical Laboratory Standards. *Evaluation of the linearity of quantitative analytical methods: Approved guidelines*. NCCLS Document EP6-P. Wayne, PA: National Committee for Clinical Laboratory Standards, 2003.

8. Health Care Financing Administration (42CFR part 493, et al) the Public Health Service, U.S. Department of Health and Human Services: Clinical Laboratory Improvements Amendments of 1988. Final rule. *Federal Register*, (1992)57:7002–7288.

9. National Committee for Clinical Laboratory Standards. *How to define and determine reference intervals in the clinical laboratory: Approved guidelines*, 2nd ed. Document C28-A2. Wayne, PA: National Committee for Clinical Laboratory Standards, 1996.

10. Dawson B, Trapp RG. *Basics and clinical biostatistics*, 4th ed. New York: McGraw-Hill, 2004:119–121.

11. Procedure manual (CLSI). Laboratory documents; *Development and control*, 5th ed. CLSI Document GP-02-A5. Wayne, PA; Clinical and laboratory standard institute, 2006.

12. Shewhart WA. *Economic control of quality of the manufactured product*. New York: Van Nostrand, 1931.

13. Levey S, Jennings ER. The use of control charts in the clinical laboratory. *AmJClinPath* (1950) 20:1059–1066.

14. Henry R, Segalove M. The running of standards in clinical chemistry and the use of control charts. *JClinPath* (1952) 5:305–311.

15. Westgard JO, Groth T, Aronsson T, et al. Performance characteristics of rules for internal quality control: Probabilities for false rejection and error detection. *ClinChem* (1977) 23(10):1857–1867.

16. Berwick DM, Godfrey AB, Roessner J. *Curing health care: New strategies for quality improvement*. San Francisco: Jossey-Bass, 1990.

17. Westgard JO, Burnett, RW, Bowers GN. Quality management science in clinical chemistry: A dynamic framework for continuous improvement of quality. *ClinChem* (1990)36:1712–1716.

18. Breitenberg M. Questions and answers on quality, the ISO 9000 standard series, quality systems registration and related issues, U.S. Department of Commerce, National Institute of Standards and Technology Publication NISTIR 4721, Gaithersburg, MD, 1991, USDC.

19. Health Care Financing Administration (42CFR part 493, et al) the Public Health Service, U.S. Department of Health and Human Services: Clinical Laboratory Improvements Amendments of 1988. Final rule. *Federal Register*, (1992)57:7002–7288.

20. Westgard JO, Barry PL, Hunt MR et al. A multi-rule Shewhart chart for quality controlling clinical chemistry. *ClinChem* (1981) 27:494–501.

21. National Committee for Clinical Laboratory Standards. *Nomenclature and definitions for use in the NRSCL and other NCCLS documents: Proposed standard*. 3rd ed. NCCLS document NRSCL 8-P3. Wayne, PA: National Committee for Clinical Laboratory Standards 1996.

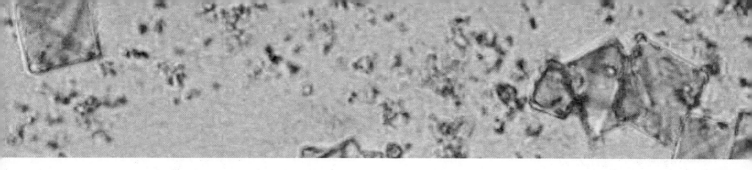

Renal Anatomy and Physiology

Objectives

LEVEL I

Following successful completion of this chapter, the learner will be able to:

1. List and briefly describe the main constituents of the urinary system, including the major components of the nephron.
2. Outline the flow of the urinary filtrate through the nephron.
3. Review the renal blood flow through the nephron.
4. Discuss glomerular filtration and the factors that influence filtration.
5. Summarize the function and regulation of the renin-angiotensin-aldosterone system.
6. Explain tubular reabsorption.
7. Define and compare and contrast active transport and passive transport and the substances reabsorbed by the two cellular transport mechanisms.
8. Define maximal reabsorptive capacity.
9. Describe and discuss the countercurrent mechanism.
10. Explain the role of antidiuretic hormone in controlling the body's level of hydration.
11. Define and describe renal threshold.
12. Describe tubular secretion.

LEVEL II

Following successful completion of this chapter, the learner will be able to:

1. Discuss renal clearance.
2. List three reasons why creatinine is a good indicator of GFR. Discuss the advantages and disadvantages of inulin clearance.
3. Discuss eGFR and review two equations for calculating the eGFR from creatinine.
4. Describe ρ-aminohippurate and its role in measuring tubular secretory capacity.

Key Terms

Active transport
Afferent arteriole
Aldosterone
Angiotensin
Angiotensin-converting
  enzyme (ACE)
Antidiuretic hormone (ADH)
Ascending loop of Henle
Bladder
Bowman's capsule
Cellular transport mechanism
Collecting duct
Cortex

Countercurrent mechanism
Creatinine clearance
Cystatin C
Descending loop of Henle
Distal convoluted tubule
Efferent arteriole
eGFR
Fenestrated endothelium
Glomerular filtration
Glomerulus
Juxtaglomerular apparatus
  (JGA)
Inulin clearance

Macula densa
Maximal reabsorptive
  capacity (T_m)
Medulla
Nephron
p-aminohippurate (PAH)
Passive transport
Peritubular capillaries
Proximal convoluted tubule
  (PCT)
Renal artery
Renal calyces
Renal clearance

Renal threshold
Renal vein
Renin
Renin-angiotensin-aldosterone
  system
Tubular reabsorption
Tubular secretion
Ultrafiltrate
Ureter
Urethra
Visceral epithelial podocytes

A CASE IN POINT

Paul had a history of renal problems. His physician ordered a blood urea nitrogen (BUN) and a 24-hour creatinine clearance test. The following results were reported:

Serum creatinine:	6.5 mg/dL	(0.9–1.2)
Urine creatinine:	120 mg/dL	
24-h urine volume:	1850 ml/24 h	
BUN:	100 mg/dL	(6–20)

Questions to Consider

1. Calculate Paul's creatinine clearance assuming a normal body surface area (1.73 m^2).

2. What does the creatinine clearance measure? What part of the nephron is affected?

3. Does Paul have a decreased, normal, or elevated creatinine clearance?

4. What calculated value is used to predict decreased creatinine clearance?

5. If Paul's body surface area was lower than 1.73 m^2, would his corrected CrCl be lower or higher than the calculated?

The kidney has three major roles. One, it filters toxins (e.g., urea and creatinine) from the blood; two, it maintains homeostasis or balance in the body's chemistry including pH and many salts (e.g., sodium, potassium, chloride, bicarbonate); and three, it produces and modifies hormones, including erythropoietin, vitamin D, angiotensin, and antidiuretic hormone (ADH)/vasopressin.

Understanding the urinary system and the anatomy and physiology of the kidney is vital for comprehending many urinalysis concepts, including grasping and fully understanding the physical components of the urinalysis, the chemical examination of the urine, the microscopic examination of the urine, as well as renal diseases. The kidney's nephrons play a vital role in the formation of urine and the various renal functions described in the previous paragraph. Therefore, the anatomy and physiology of the kidney and its major functions, including glomerular filtration, tubular reabsorption, and tubular secretion, will be reviewed before proceeding to the major components of the routine urinalysis in the subsequent chapters.

RENAL ANATOMY

The urinary system consists of two kidneys, two **ureters**, a **bladder**, and **urethra** as illustrated in Figure 3-1 ■. The kidneys are located on the posterior abdominal wall and are approximately 12 cm long, 6 cm wide, and 2.5 cm in depth; each weighs approximately 140 g. The kidneys are divided into two distinct areas: the outer layer or **cortex** and the inner layer or **medulla**. Each kidney contains approximately 1 million to 1.5 million **nephrons**, the functional unit of the kidney (see Figures 3-2 ■ and 3-3 ■).

Renal blood flow is essential to renal function. Blood is supplied to the kidney by the **renal artery** from the abdominal aorta and enters the nephron through the **afferent arteriole**. It flows through the glomerulus into the **efferent arteriole**. The **glomerulus** consists of a coil of approximately 40 capillary loops referred to as the *capillary tuft* located within the **Bowman's capsule**, the initial section of the nephron. The blood is filtered in the glomerulus, and the filtrate flows through the **proximal convoluted tubule (PCT)**,

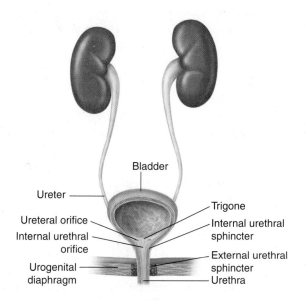

FIGURE 3-1   Urinary System

From Colbert, Ankey, and Lee, *Anatomy and Physiology for Health Professions* (Upper Saddle River, NJ: Prentice Hall, 2007), p. 417.

BOX 3-1   Urinary Filtrate Flow

1. Bowman's capsule
2. Proximal convoluted tubule
3. Descending loop of Henle
4. Ascending loop of Henle
5. Distal convoluted tubule
6. Collecting duct
7. Renal calyces
8. Ureter
9. Bladder
10. Urethra

the *descending loop of Henle*, the **ascending loop of Henle**, the *distal convoluted tubule* (DCT), the *collecting duct* (CD), and *renal calyces*, leading to the *ureter, bladder*, and *urethra* in that order. The **collecting duct** from each nephron combines with other collecting ducts to form the **renal calyces**, where urine collects before passing into the ureters, bladder, and urethra.[1] Box 3-1 outlines the flow of the urinary filtrate.

Renal blood flows from the renal artery to the afferent arteriole to the efferent arteriole, with the smaller diameter of the efferent arteriole resulting in a hydrostatic pressure differential that is important for glomerular filtration, which will be discussed later in this chapter. From the efferent arteriole, the blood enters the *peritubular capillaries* and flows slowly through the cortex and medulla, where the capillaries divide into the vasa recta. The **peritubular capillaries** surround the proximal and **distal convoluted tubules** and are responsible for the immediate reabsorption of essential substances from the fluid in the PCT. The vasa recta lead to the **renal vein** where blood is returned to the body. Renal blood flow is outlined in Box 3-2 and illustrated in Figure 3-4 ■.

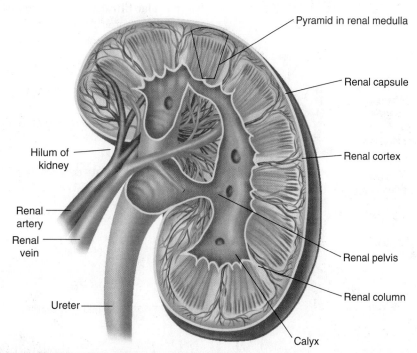

FIGURE 3-2   Kidney

From Colbert, Ankey, and Lee, *Anatomy and Physiology for Health Professions* (Upper Saddle River, NJ: Prentice Hall, 2007), p. 404.

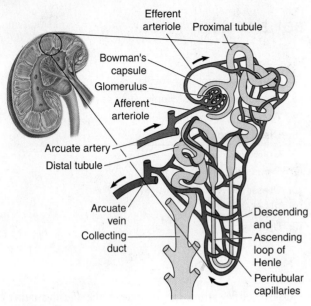

■ **FIGURE 3-3** Nephron

Dorling Kindersley, Ltd.

BOX 3-2   Renal Blood Flow

1. Renal artery
2. Afferent arteriole
3. Glomerulus
4. Efferent arteriole
5. Peritubular capillaries
6. Vasa recta
7. Renal vein

☑ CHECKPOINT 3-1

1. How many nephrons are found in the average kidney?
   - (a) 13.000
   - (b) 130,000
   - (c) 1.3 million
   - (d) 13 million

2. In the nephron plasma filtrate flows from (list in order using numbers 1–6)
   - _____ (a) proximal convoluted tubule
   - _____ (b) distal convoluted tubule
   - _____ (c) descending Loop of Henle
   - _____ (d) ascending Loop of Henle
   - _____ (e) glomerulus
   - _____ (f) collecting duct

3. Blood enters the kidney through the ——————— and leaves through the ———————.
   - (a) renal artery, renal vein
   - (b) renal vein, renal artery
   - (c) hepatic vein, hepatic artery
   - (d) hepatic artery, hepatic vein

RENAL PHYSIOLOGY

The three major renal functions are glomerular filtration, tubular reabsorption, and tubular secretion.

Glomerular Filtration

Glomerular filtration occurs in the glomerulus, which is the first part of the nephron. Approximately 20% of the plasma that enters the glomerulus is filtered and flows into the urinary space inside the Bowman's capsule. The remaining 80% leaves the glomerulus through

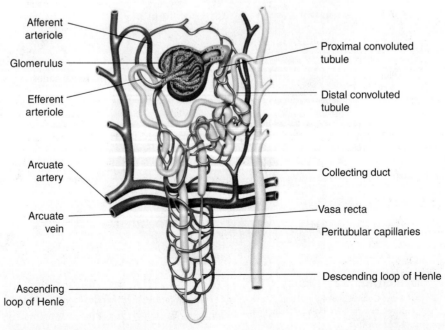

■ **FIGURE 3-4** Renal Blood Flow

the efferent arteriole.[2] Several factors influence the actual filtration process:

1. The cellular structure of the capillary walls and Bowman's capsule.

2. The hydrostatic (pressure exerted by a liquid, e.g., blood pressure) and oncotic pressures (pressure caused by the presence of larger particles—larger proteins in the blood and not in the ultrafiltrate). **Ultrafiltrate** is obtained when a colloidal substance in which the dispersed particles, but not liquid, is held back. The ultrafiltrate is very similar to plasma except that it is free of proteins, with the exception of low molecular weight proteins that make it through the glomerulus. Hydrostatic pressure is caused by the smaller diameter of the efferent arterioles and the smaller size of the glomerular capillaries.

3. The feedback mechanisms of the renin-angiotensin-aldosterone system.

The glomerular membrane consists of three layers. The first layer in the capillary wall membrane are *mesangium* (mesangial cells), made of **fenestrated endothelium**, which differs from those in other capillaries by containing pores. The endothelial cells line the capillaries and provide a smooth surface, allowing blood to flow easily. The pores allow the smaller-molecular-weight proteins to penetrate to the next layer. The second layer is the glomerular basement membrane (GBM) of basal lamina, which has three layers that separate the endothelium from the epithelium. The GBM, composed of collagen and other matrix proteins, is believed to be the major barrier to the passage of proteins in the urinary space. The semipermeable glomerular membrane allows low-molecular-weight molecules of less than 66,000 daltons to pass through into the filtrate. Albumin and other low-molecular-weight proteins, glucose, amino acids, urea, and creatinine are freely filtered and proceed to the proximal convoluted tubules. The basement membrane is also negatively charged, so large, negatively charged molecules (e.g., proteins) are repelled. The third layer is the visceral epithelium comprised of **visceral epithelial podocytes**. These cells contain podo (foot) processes that restrict large molecules, such as larger proteins, from passing through the glomerular membrane (see Figure 3-5 ■).[3]

By increasing or decreasing the size of the afferent arteriole, which is an autoregulatory mechanism within the juxtaglomerular apparatus of the kidney, the kidney maintains the glomerular blood pressure relatively constant regardless of fluctuations in systemic blood pressure. Dilation of the afferent arterioles when the blood

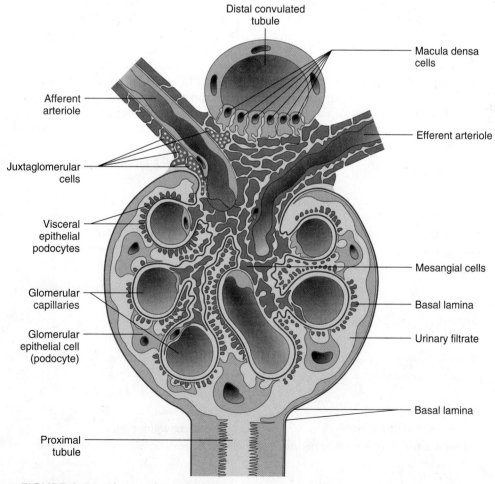

■ **FIGURE 3-5** Glomerular Membrane

pressure drops prevents a marked decrease in blood flowing through the kidneys, thus preventing a rise in blood levels of toxic waste products. Constriction of the afferent arteriole when the blood pressure rises prevents an increase in blood flow.

Additional influence on the blood flow through the kidney is provided by the **renin-angiotensin-aldosterone system**. This system is activated in response to changes in the blood flow to the kidney sensed by the **macula densa** in the **juxtaglomerular apparatus (JGA)**. The JGA is composed of the juxtaglomerular cells of the afferent arteriole and the macula densa of the distal convoluted tubule. The macula densa of the afferent arteriole contains large amounts of secretory granules containing **renin**, which controls the regulation of blood flow to and within the glomerulus. **Aldosterone** is secreted by the adrenal cortex and increases the reabsorption of sodium from the glomerular filtrate. An increase in aldosterone leads to an increase in reabsorption of sodium from the filtrate, which results in a decrease in urine sodium, an increase in plasma sodium levels, and an increase in blood pressure. Conversely, a decrease in aldosterone results in a decrease in reabsorption of sodium from the filtrate, an increase in urine sodium, a decrease in plasma sodium, and a decrease in blood pressure.

Renin is an enzyme produced in the kidney by the cells of the JGA when (1) blood pressure declines (renal artery hypotension), (2) a decrease in blood volume is sensed, or (3) sodium in the distal tubules of the kidney decreases. Renin converts **angiotensin** to angiotensin I, which is converted to angiotensin II by an enzyme, **angiotensin-converting enzyme (ACE)** when passing through the lungs. Angiotensin II triggers the release of aldosterone (see Equation 3-1).

The functions of angiotensin II are listed in Box 3-3. The renin-angiotensin system results in passive water retention, which increases the extracellular fluid volume and intravascular pressure. An increase in blood pressure causes a decrease in renin, resulting in a decrease in angiotensin and aldosterone and a subsequent decrease in blood pressure.[4] When the blood pressure is too low, the opposite occurs (Decrease BP → Increase renin → Increase angiotensin → Increase aldosterone → Increase blood pressure).

MINI-CASE 3-1

Leon experiences an abrupt increase in blood pressure.

1. Discuss the reactions that occur in the kidney to decrease blood pressure in the nephrons.
2. Describe how the responses decrease the blood pressure.
3. How do the kidneys respond when the blood pressure decreases to normal levels?

Tubular Reabsorption

Every minute 120 mL of ultrafiltrate is filtered through approximately 2 million nephrons. Obviously, the body cannot lose 120 mL of water containing essential substances every minute; therefore, in the PCT 80% of the fluid and electrolytes filtered by the glomerulus are reabsorbed through **cellular transport mechanisms**. Cellular transport mechanisms are divided in two major categories: active transport and passive transport.

In **active transport** the substance to be reabsorbed must be combined with a carrier protein contained in the membranes of the renal tubular cells. The substance is reabsorbed against a concentration gradient and requires energy. The electrochemical energy created by this interaction transfers the substance across the cell membranes and back into the blood stream, the peritubular capillaries.

Box 3-4 lists the major sites of active transport and the substances reabsorbed. PCTs reabsorb over 66% of filtered water, Na^+, and Cl^-, in addition to approximately 100% of glucose, amino acids, and proteins.

Passive transport is the movement of molecules across a membrane as a result of differences in their concentration or electrical potential on opposite sides of the membrane. These physical differences are called *gradients* and involve movement from a region of

$$\begin{array}{ccccccc} & \text{Renin} & & \text{ACE} & & & \\ \text{Angiotensin} & \rightarrow & \text{Angiotensin I} & \rightarrow & \text{Angiotensin II} & \rightarrow & \text{Aldosterone} \end{array} \qquad (3\text{-}1)$$

BOX 3-3   Functions of Angiotensin II

1. Dilates afferent arteriole
2. Constricts efferent arteriole
3. Stimulates sodium reabsorption in the proximal convoluted tubule
4. Triggers secretion of aldosterone
5. Triggers release of antidiuretic hormone
6. Stimulates water reabsorption in the collecting duct

BOX 3-4   Active Transport

Proximal convoluted tubule
- Glucose
- Amino acids
- Salts (e.g., Ca^{+2}, Mg^{+2})

Ascending loop of Henle
- Chloride

Distal convoluted tubule
- Sodium (influenced by aldosterone)

BOX 3-5 Passive Reabsorption

Substance	Part(s) of the Nephron
Water	PCT, Descending loop of Henle, Collecting Tubules
Urea	PCT, Ascending loop of Henle
Sodium	Ascending loop of Henle

higher concentration to a region of lower concentration; no energy is required for this process. Passive reabsorption of water takes place in all parts of the nephron except the ascending loop of Henle, whose walls are impermeable to water. Passive reabsorption of sodium accompanies the active transport of chloride in the ascending loop of Henle. Box 3-5 lists the substances reabsorbed by passive transport and the part(s) of the nephron.

In active transport, when the plasma concentration of a substance that is normally completely reabsorbed reaches an abnormally high level, the filtrate concentration exceeds the **maximal reabsorptive capacity** (T_m) of the tubules, and the substance begins appearing in the urine. T_m is the highest rate in mg/dL at which tubules can transfer a substance either from the tubules to the interstitial fluid or vice versa. The plasma concentration at which active transport stops is called the **renal threshold**, which allows for complete reabsorption of the substance when its plasma concentration is within normal limits. For example, normal fasting plasma glucose is less than 100 mg/dL, and the renal threshold is 160–180 mg/dL, which is a leeway of 60–80 mg/dL. At plasma levels above the renal threshold, glucosuria occurs, in other words, glucose is spilt into the urine. Knowledge of renal threshold and plasma concentration can be used to distinguish between excess solute filtration (e.g., high plasma glucose) and renal tubular damage. When renal tubular damage occurs, glucose may be found in the urine with normal plasma glucose levels.

☑ CHECKPOINT 3-2

1. Decreased levels of aldosterone result in
   (a) decreased serum sodium levels.
   (b) decreased potassium levels.
   (c) increased serum sodium levels.
   (d) decreased potassium levels.
2. Which of the following is a characteristic of renin, an enzyme secreted by specialized cells of the juxtaglomerular apparatus?
   (a) Renin stimulates the diffusion of urea into the renal interstitium.
   (b) Renin inhibits the reabsorption of sodium and water in the nephron.
   (c) Renin regulates the osmotic reabsorption of water by the collecting tubules.
   (d) Renin converts angiotensin to angiotensin I and causes the secretion of aldosterone.

3. The renal threshold level for glucose is 160 to 180 mg/dL. This corresponds to the
   (a) rate of glucose reabsorption by the renal tubules.
   (b) concentration of glucose in the tubular lumen fluid.
   (c) plasma concentration above which tubular reabsorption of glucose occurs.
   (d) plasma concentration above which glucose is excreted in the urine.
4. Water reabsorption occurs throughout the nephron except in the
   (a) cortical collecting tubules.
   (b) proximal convoluted tubules.
   (c) ascending loop of Henle.
   (d) descending loop of Henle.

Renal Concentration

Active transport of over two-thirds of filtered sodium out of the PCTs is accompanied by the passive transport of an equal amount of water; therefore, the fluid leaving the PCT still maintains the same concentration as the ultrafiltrate. Renal concentration begins in the descending and ascending loops of Henle where the filtrate is exposed to the high osmotic gradient (salt concentration) of the renal medulla. Water is removed by osmosis in the **descending loop of Henle**, which is the concentrating portion. Sodium and chloride are reabsorbed into the interstitium in the ascending loop of Henle. Excessive water reabsorption as filtrate passes through the highly concentrated medulla is prevented by the water-impermeable walls of the ascending loop.

This selective reabsorption process is called the countercurrent mechanism and serves to maintain the osmotic gradient of the medulla. The **countercurrent mechanism (CM)** is the passive exchange by the diffusion of reabsorbed solutes and water from the nephron's medullary interstitium into the blood of its vascular blood supply. In the medulla the filtrate is diluted by the water from the descending loop of Henle and reconcentrated by sodium and potassium from the filtrate in the ascending loop. In summary, in the countercurrent mechanism the concentration increases in the direction of the flow in the descending loop of Henle, then decreases as flow continues through the parallel ascending loop of Henle.

Reabsorption of sodium continues in the distal convoluted tubule but is now under the control of aldosterone, which regulates reabsorption in response to the body's need for sodium. The final concentration of the filtrate by reabsorption of water begins in the late distal convoluted tubule and continues in the collecting duct. Reabsorption is dependent on two factors: the osmotic gradient in the medulla and the hormone vasopressin or antidiuretic hormone. **Antidiuretic hormone (ADH)** renders the walls of the distal convoluted tubules and collecting ducts permeable or impermeable to water. An increase in ADH causes an increase in reabsorbed water and a decrease in urine volume. The spaces between cells dilate and allow more water to be reabsorbed. ADH has an inverse relationship with urine volume: High levels of ADH are associated with a low urine volume and low levels of ADH with a high urine volume.

ADH is controlled by the body's state of hydration. Dehydration will result in increased secretion of ADH, decreased urine volume, and increased plasma volume due to increased reabsorption of water.

Tubular Secretion

Tubular secretion is defined as the passage of substances from the blood in the peritubular capillaries to the tubular filtrate. It is the opposite of **tubular reabsorption**. Tubular secretion serves two major functions: One, it eliminates waste products not filtered by the glomerulus; two, the acid-base balance in the body is regulated through secretion of hydrogen ions. Many foreign substances (e.g., medications) cannot be filtered by the glomerulus because they are bound to plasma proteins. However, when these protein-bound substances enter the peritubular capillaries, they develop a strong affinity for the tubular cells and dissociate from their carrier proteins. This dissociation results in their ability to be transported into the filtrate by the tubular cells.

The buffering capacity of blood is dependent on the bicarbonate ions that are readily filtered by the glomerulus and must be quickly returned to the blood to maintain proper pH. The secretion of hydrogen ions by the renal tubular cells prevents the filtered bicarbonate from being excreted in the urine and causes a return of bicarbonate ions to the plasma. This process provides for almost 100% reabsorption of filtered bicarbonate and occurs primarily in the proximal convoluted tubules.

All three processes (glomerular filtration, tubular reabsorption, and tubular secretion) occur simultaneously at rates determined by the acid-base balance. One percent of the original plasma ultrafiltrate presented to the renal tubules is eliminated as urine. Glomerular filtration, tubular reabsorption, and tubular secretion have to work together to achieve optimal renal function.

RENAL FUNCTION TESTS

Various renal function tests can be performed to determine the status of the many metabolic functions and chemical interactions that occur in various parts of the nephron. The following are summaries of the most common tests. More in-depth information can be found in chemistry textbooks listed under recommended reading at the end of the chapter.

Glomerular Filtration Tests

Renal clearance is defined as the rate at which the kidneys remove a substance from the plasma or blood or a quantitative expression of the rate at which a substance is excreted by the kidneys in relation to the concentration of the same substance in the plasma, usually expressed as mL cleared per minute. The best markers are freely filtered by the glomeruli, produced at a constant rate, not reabsorbed or secreted by tubules in any appreciable amount, present in stable concentrations in the plasma, and have an inexpensive and rapid assay for detection.[5]

Creatinine Clearance

Creatinine clearance (CrCl) is the most popular and practical method for estimating the glomerular filtration rate (GFR). Creatinine is present in stable concentrations in the plasma and has an inexpensive and rapid assay for detection. It is easily measured and extensive data is available for all age groups. Creatinine is a very good indicator of glomerular filtration rate for three reasons: One, it is freely filtered by the glomeruli; two, it is not reabsorbed by the tubules to any significant extent; and three, creatinine is released into the plasma at a constant rate, resulting in constant plasma levels over 24 hours. A linear decrease in creatinine clearance over time as renal function fails has been documented for different diseases (e.g., chronic glomerulonephritis).

Creatinine levels are measured on serum and urine specimens. A 24-hour urine is usually collected. The CrCl is calculated using the serum and urine creatinine levels and the urine volume as shown in Equation 3-2.

The volume of urine in mL/min is calculated by dividing the 24h volume in mL/day by 1440 min/day. Plasma concentration is inversely proportional to the clearance: the higher the plasma concentration, the lower the clearance.

For example, a laboratory reports the following results for Sharon:

Total 24h volume:	1550 mL/24h
Serum creatinine:	2.0 mg/dL
Urine creatinine:	150 mg/dL

Assuming a normal BSA (Body Surface Area), her clearance would be:

$$\text{Clearance (X)} = \frac{U \times V}{P} = \frac{150 \text{ mg/dL} \times \dfrac{1550 \text{ mL/24h}}{1440 \text{ ml/24h}}}{2.0 \text{ mg/dL}}$$

$$= 81 \text{ mL/min}$$

Creatinine clearance has to be corrected to an adult body surface area (BSA) of 1.73 m^2, which is especially important for small adults, pediatric patients, and obese patients. This can be done in two ways: using the Dubois formula or a nomogram. The Dubois formula is shown in Equation 3-3. The nomogram is much easier. See Appendix E.

The correction or normalization factor for BSA is added to the CrCl equation as shown in Equation 3-4.

$$\text{Clearance (X)} = \frac{U \times V}{P} \tag{3-2}$$

U = urine concentration in mg/dL

P = plasma or serum concentration in mg/dL

V = urine flow in mL/minute (1440 min/24h) → $\dfrac{24\text{h volume in mL/day}}{1440 \text{ min/day}}$

$$SA \text{ (Surface area in m}^2) = W \text{ (kg)}^{0.425} \times H \text{ (cm)}^{0.725} \times 0.007184 \qquad (3\text{-}3)$$

$$\text{Clearance (X)} = \frac{U \times V}{P} \times \frac{1.73 \text{ m}^2}{\text{BSA m}^2} \text{ (normalization formula} = \text{CrCl (mL/minute/1.73 m}^2)) \qquad (3\text{-}4)$$

The reference range for males is 97–137 mL/minute; for females 88–128 mL/min. An increased CrCl is not clinically significant and probably due to an error in specimen collection. Decreased CrCl indicates decreased GFR as a result of acute or chronic damage to the glomeruli. Mild impairment is indicated by a CrCl of 50–79 mL/min, moderate 10–49 mL/min, and severe < 10 mL/min.

The corrected CrCl for a larger or obese individual will be lower because the normalization factor will be less than one. For a pediatric patient or small adult, the corrected CrCl will be increased.

Inulin Clearance

Inulin, a naturally occurring polysaccharide of fructose found in artichokes, is the gold standard for measuring glomerular filtration rate. Inulin, an exogenous substance, is injected and measured in serum and urine in the appropriate time frame. Major disadvantages are that unlike creatinine there is no easily performed methodology for inulin; it is an invasive procedure requiring injection of inulin from outside the body, and it is time-consuming and expensive.[6] **Inulin clearance** is not currently used for glomerular filtration testing.

eGFR

Many studies have recommended the use of an estimating or prediction equation (**eGFR**) to estimate glomerular filtration rate (GFR) from the serum creatinine level in patients with chronic renal disease and those at risk for chronic kidney disease CKD (e.g., diabetes, hypertension, cardiovascular disease, and family history of kidney disease). The primary reasons are that GFR and creatinine clearance are not as accurate as using creatinine alone, and creatinine is more often measured than urinary albumin. Also the Modification of Diet in Renal Disease (MDRD) Study equation has been thoroughly validated and is superior to other methods of approximating GFR. It does not require weight or height variables because it is normalized to 1.73 m² body surface area, which is the accepted BSA.

In patients over 18 years of age the MDRD equation is the best means currently available to use creatinine values as a measure of renal function. The equation has been validated in the Caucasian and African American populations with impaired renal function (eGFR < 60 ml/min/1.73 m²) between the ages of 18 and 70 years

of age. It requires four variables: serum or plasma creatinine, age in years, gender, and race (African American or not).[7]

Two versions of the equation exist depending on whether the serum creatinine has been calibrated to be traceable to an isotope dilution mass spectrometry (IDMS) method (see Equations 3-5 and 3-6). These MDRD equations are recommended by the National Kidney Disease Education program.[8]

Most laboratories have elected to routinely report both the eGRF and the creatinine.

eGFR Pediatric Creatinine Clearance

For children under 18 years of age, the Schwartz formula, Equation 3-7, may be used. Only the height and serum creatinine are required.

Age Group	
Low birth weight infants, age < 1 year	0.33
Term infants < 1 year	0.45
Children, ages 2–12 years	0.55
Girls, ages 13–21 years	0.55
Boys, ages 13–21 years	0.70

• Adapted from MedCalc[9]

Cystatin C

Cystatin C, a single chain, nonglycosylated, low-molecular-weight protein synthesized by all nucleated cells, is a cysteine protein inhibitor. Its most important characteristics, small size and high isoelectric point (pI = 9.2), enable it to be freely filtered by the glomeruli and catabolized in the proximal convoluted tubules. Cystatin C is produced at a constant rate by all nucleated cells, and serum concentrations are not affected by muscle mass, diet, race, age or gender.[10] No Cystatin C is secreted by the tubules, therefore, serum concentration is directly related to the GFR.

Tubular Secretion Test

Tubular secretion must be measured by using a substance that is secreted into the tubules and not filtered by the glomerulus. Secretion involves the passage of substances from the blood in the peritubular capillaries to the tubular filtrate.

Original MDRD Study Equation

When S_{cr} is in mg/dL (conventional units) $\qquad$ (3-5)

$$\text{eGRF (mL/min/1.73 m}^2) = 186 \times (S_{cr})^{-1.154} \times (\text{Age})^{-0.203} \times (0.742 \text{ if female}) \times (1.210 \text{ if African American})$$

IDMS-Traceable MDRD Study Equation	
When S_{cr} is in mg/dL (conventional units)	(3-6)
eGRF (mL/min/1.73 m²) = $175 \times (S_{cr})^{-1.154} \times (Age)^{-0.203} \times (0.742$ if female$) \times (1.210$ if African American$)$	

Schwartz GFE: $\delta \times$ height (cm)*	
P_{cr}	(3-7)
Proportionality Constants (δ)	

ρ-aminohippurate

ρ-aminohippurate (PAH) is approximately 90% cleared by the renal tubules in a single passage through the kidneys and measures tubular secretory capacity. It is also useful in determining total renal blood flow (total renal plasma flow) if the tubular function is known to be normal. One-quarter of the cardiac output flows through the renal arteries.

PAH is exogenous and has to be injected; it is removed from the blood primarily by the peritubular capillaries. It is a nontoxic substance that is loosely bound to plasma proteins; therefore, it can be completely removed as blood flows through the peritubular capillaries. All of the PAH in the plasma is secreted by the proximal convoluted tubules.

Key Points to Remember

- The urinary system consists of two kidneys, two ureters, a bladder, and urethra.
- The nephron, the functional unit of the kidney, is comprised of the Bowman's capsule, proximal convoluted tubule, descending loop of Henle, ascending loop of Henle, distal convoluted tubule, collecting duct, and renal calyces.
- Blood enters the kidney through the renal artery through the afferent arteriole, filtered by the glomerulus, to the efferent arteriole, peritubular capillaries, and vasa recta and leaves the kidney through the renal vein.
- Glomerular filtration is regulated by three major factors: the cellular structure of the capillary walls and Bowman's capsule; the hydrostatic and oncotic pressures; and the feedback mechanism of the renin-angiotensin-aldosterone system.
- The renin-angiotensin-aldosterone system responds to changes in blood pressure. Renin, produced in response to a decrease in blood pressure or volume, converts angiotensin I to angiotensin II, which stimulates the secretion of aldosterone.
- Tubular reabsorption occurs through active transport, when the substance is combined with a carrier protein and requires energy, and passive transport, the movement of molecules across a membrane as a result of differences in their concentration or electrical potential on opposite sides of the membrane.
- Maximal reabsorptive capacity is the plasma concentration of a substance that exceeds the highest rate in mg/dL at which tubules can transfer a substance either from the tubules to the interstitial fluid or vice versa.

- The countercurrent mechanism is the passive exchange by the diffusion of reabsorbed solutes and water from the nephron's medullary interstitium into the blood of its vascular blood supply.
- Antidiuretic hormone renders the walls of the distal convoluted tubules and collecting ducts permeable or impermeable to water; an increase in ADH causes an increase in reabsorbed water and a decrease in urine volume.
- Renal threshold is the plasma concentration at which active transport stops; at plasma levels above the renal threshold the substance is excreted in the urine.
- Renal clearance is the rate at which the kidneys remove a substance from the plasma or blood or a quantitative expression of the rate at which a substance is excreted by the kidneys in relation to the concentration of the same substance in plasma, usually expressed as mL cleared per minute.
- Creatinine clearance is the most popular and practical method for estimating the glomerular filtration. Creatinine is freely filtered by the glomeruli, not reabsorbed by the tubules to any significant extent, and released in the plasma at a constant rate over 24 hours.
- eGFR estimates or predicts the glomerular filtration rate from the serum creatinine level in patients with chronic renal disease and those at risk for chronic kidney disease.
- P-aminohippurate measures the tubular secretory capacity and is approximately 90% cleared by the renal tubules in a single passage through the kidneys.

Review Questions

Level I

1. Each kidney is composed of more than a million urinary units. Each of these is called a: (Objective 1)

   A. glomerulus.

   B. nephron.

   C. photon.

   D. medulla.

2. The order of blood flow through the nephron is: (Objective 3)

   A. afferent arteriole, glomerulus, peritubular capillaries, vasa recta, efferent arteriole.

   B. efferent arteriole, peritubular capillaries, vasa recta, afferent arteriole.

   C. peritubular capillaries, vasa recta, afferent arteriole, efferent arteriole.

   D. afferent arteriole, glomerulus, efferent arteriole, peritubular capillaries, vasa recta.

3. Which of the following components are NOT present in the glomerular filtrate? (Objective 4)

   A. Urea

   B. Large-molecular-weight proteins

   C. Glucose

   D. Water

4. The glomerular membrane consists of three layers in this order: (Objective 4)

   A. Podocytes, fenestrated endothelium, basal membrane

   B. Basal lamina, juxtaglomerular apparatus, podocytes

   C. Fenestrated endothelium, basal membrane, podocytes

   D. Juxtaglomerular apparatus, podocytes, fenestrated endothelium

5. The juxtaglomerular apparatus is comprised of: (Objective 5)

   A. the juxtaglomerular cells of the efferent arteriole and the macula densa of the distal tubule.

   B. the juxtaglomerular cells of the afferent arteriole and the macula densa of the distal tubule.

   C. the macula densa of the afferent arteriole and the juxtaglomerular cells of the distal tubule.

   D. the macula densa of the efferent arteriole and the juxtaglomerular cells of the distal tubule.

6. Substances removed from the blood by tubular secretion include primarily: (Objective 12)

   A. protein, hydrogen, and ammonia.

   B. protein, hydrogen, and potassium.

   C. protein-bound substances (e.g., penicillin), hydrogen, and potassium.

   D. amino acid, glucose, and ammonia.

7. Renin is secreted in response to stimulation by: (Objective 5)

   A. macula densa cells.

   B. angiotensin I and II.

   C. visceral epithelial podocytes.

   D. fenestrated epithelium.

8. The primary chemical affected by the renin-angiotensin-aldosterone system is: (Objective 5)

   A. glucose.

   B. potassium.

   C. chloride.

   D. sodium.

9. Increased production of aldosterone causes: (Objective 5)

   A. decreased urine sodium levels.

   B. decreased glomerular blood pressure.

   C. increased urine sodium levels.

   D. increased urine volume.

10. Glucose is reabsorbed mainly in the: (Objective 6)

    A. proximal convoluted tubule.

    B. descending loop of Henle.

    C. ascending loop of Henle.

    D. distal convoluted tubule.

11. All of the following are reabsorbed from the glomerular filtrate by active transport *except*: (Objective 7)

    A. glucose.

    B. water.

    C. sodium.

    D. amino acids.

12. For active transport to occur, a chemical: (Objective 7)

    A. must combine with a carrier protein to create electrochemical energy.

    B. must be filtered through the proximal convolute tubule.

    C. must be in higher concentration in the filtrate than in the blood.

    D. must be in higher concentration in the blood than in the filtrate.

13. Increased production of antidiuretic hormone causes: (Objective 10)

    A. decreased plasma sodium levels.

    B. decreased urine volume.

    C. increased plasma sodium levels.

    D. increased urine volume.

14. The only area of the nephron that is impermeable to water is the: (Objective 10)

    A. proximal convoluted tubule.

    B. descending loop of Henle.

    C. ascending loop of Henle.

    D. distal convoluted tubule.

15. The normal renal threshold for glucose in adults is approximately: (Objective 11)

    A. 70 mg/dL.

    B. 140 mg/dL.

    C. 160 mg/dL.

    D. 200 mg/dL.

16. When a person's plasma volume is increased: (Objective 10)

    A. ADH secretion is increased.

    B. ADH secretion is decreased.

    C. urine volume is decreased.

    D. aldosterone production is increased.

Level II

17. The creatinine clearance is used to estimate the: (Objective 2)

    A. glomerular secretion of creatinine.

    B. glomerular filtration rate.

    C. tubular reabsorption of creatinine.

    D. renal glomerular mass.

18. Which substance is used to measure tubular secretory capacity? (Objective 5)

    A. Inulin

    B. Creatinine

    C. ρ-aminohippurate

    D. Cystatin C

19. Which of the following clearance substance (s) is exogenous? (Objective 3)

    A. Creatinine

    B. Cystatin C

    C. Inulin

    D. None of the above

20. The eGFR is calculated using all of the following criteria except (Objective 4)

    A. serum creatinine level.

    B. age.

    C. female.

    D. 24h urine volume.

    E. African American.

21. Dolores's serum glucose is 321 mg/dL. What is the renal threshold for glucose? What occurs when the serum glucose is above the maximal reabsorptive capacity?

22. John completed a marathon in 80°F temperature. What affect would this have on his fluid levels? Which hormone regulates water balance and how does it function?

Endnotes

1. Sunheimer R, Graves L. *Clinical Laboratory Chemistry*. Upper Saddle River, NJ: Pearson, 2011: pp. 247–248.

2. National Institute of Diabetes and Digestive and Kidney Diseases. Glomerular Disease Primmer: The Normal Kidney. (www2.niddk.nih.gov/NIDDKLABS/GlomerularDisease_Primer/NormalKidney.htm) Accessed March 2, 2011.

3. Ibid.

4. Klabunde, RE. *Renin-Angiotensin-Aldosterone System*. (www.cvphysiology.com/Blood%20Pressure/BP015.htm) Accessed March 2, 2011.

5. Sunheimer R, Graves L. *Clinical Laboratory Chemistry*. Upper Saddle River, NJ: Pearson, 2011: pp. 247–248.

6. Ogedegbe, HO. Renal function tests: A clinical laboratory perspective. *LabMedicine* (2007) 38(5):295–303.

7. National Kidney Disease Education Program. Estimating GFR. (www.nkdep.nih.gov/labprofessionals/estimated_gfr.htm) Accessed March 14, 2011.

8. Lippi G, et al. Comparison of 2 methods for the calculation of estimated glomerular filtration rate. *LabMedicine* (2008) 39(1):35–37.

9. MedCalc. MedCalc: Pediatric Glomerular Filtration Rate. (www.medcalc.com/pedigfr.html) Accessed February 15, 2013.

10. Tan GD, et al. Clinical usefulness of Cystatin C for the estimation of glomerular filtration rate in Type 1 diabetes. *Diabetes Care* (2002) 25(11):2004–2009.

Suggested Readings

Burtis, C, et al., *Fundamentals of Clinical Chemistry*. St. Louis, MO: Saunders Elsevier, 2008.

Sunheimer R, Graves L. *Clinical Laboratory Chemistry*. Upper Saddle River, NJ: Pearson, 2011.

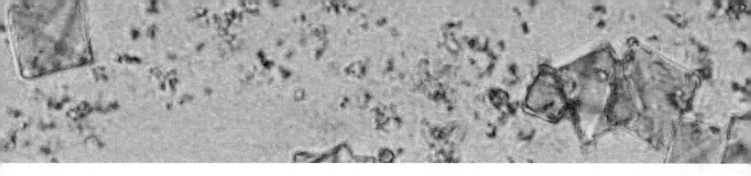

4 Pre-Analytical Urinalysis

Objectives

LEVEL I

Following successful completion of this chapter, the learner will be able to:

1. Describe the containers used for different types of urine specimens.
2. Discuss the various types of urine specimens, the collection process, and the purpose of each specimen.
3. Instruct a patient on the correct procedure for obtaining a clean-catch urine specimen and 24-hour or timed specimens.
4. Describe the changes that occur in an improperly preserved urine specimen.
5. Discuss the most common urine preservatives including their use, advantages, and disadvantages.
6. State the normal range for 24-hour urine volume.
7. List four factors influencing urine volume.
8. Define *oliguria* and list common conditions associated with a decreased urine volume.
9. Define and list common causes and conditions associated with *anuria*, *nocturia*, and *polyuria*.

LEVEL II

1. Explain the prerenal, renal, and postrenal causes of oliguria.
2. Examine the various causes of anuria, nocturia, and polyuria.

Key Terms

Anuria
Catheterized urine
Clean-catch urine

First morning specimen
Nocturia
Oliguria

Polyuria
Random urine
Suprapubic aspiration

Three-glass collection
24-hour specimen
Timed specimen

A CASE IN POINT

A specimen from the emergency room was delivered to the laboratory for a routine urinalysis. It was collected at 2:00 p.m. and it was delivered at 7:00 p.m., and at room temperature when it was received in the laboratory.

Questions to Consider

1. Is the specimen acceptable for a routine urinalysis?
2. What is the **maximum** time allowable before testing?
3. If over the maximum time, how can the urine specimen be preserved?

4. If it is not preserved properly, how will the following tests be affected? (increased, decreased, or no effect)
    a. Clarity/Appearance ——————
    b. Glucose ——————
    c. Urobilinogen ——————
    d. Nitrite ——————

HISTORY

The analysis of urine began 6000 years ago and was called uroscopy until the 17th century when it was renamed urinalysis. Although Hippocrates is often credited with being the first uroscopist, there is evidence that uroscopy predates Hippocrates. Babylonian and Egyptian physicians practiced uroscopy.[1]

Evidence from the late Middle Ages and the Renaissance indicates that many physicians carried uroscopy beyond the "bounds of reason." Physicians were known to prognosticate over the patient by merely examining the urine and without ever seeing the patient. Joannes Actuaris (1275–1328), a physician from Constantinople, and others warned against diagnosis on urine alone.[2] Urine was poured on the ground to see if it would attract ants, which was an indication that the urine was sweet—the first test for the unknown disease: diabetes mellitus.

The predominant theory of the cause of disease, which was accepted into the 1600s, was that four humors—blood, phlegm, yellow bile, and black bile—originated from different parts of the body. Disease was caused by an imbalance of these four humors, and it was the physician's responsibility to keep them in equilibrium.[3]

The misuse of uroscopy caused a backlash that was led by Thomas Brian in his book, *The Pisse Prophet*, published in 1637. Those who used solely urine for diagnosis were called pisse prophets, water-caters, and pissemongers and became objects of ridicule.[4]

In 1694 Frederik Dekkers of Leiden, Netherlands, observed that urine that contained protein would form a precipitate when boiled with acetic acid, the turning point when urinalysis became more scientific and more valuable. Thomas Willis (1621–1675), an English physician and proponent of chemistry, noticed the characteristic sweet taste of diabetic urine, which differentiated diabetes mellitus from diabetes insipidus.[5]

Urinalysis has changed dramatically in over 400 years. Today urinalysis is a widely accepted screening test and an integral part of an annual physical. Two major reasons can be given for its popularity: One, urine specimens are easily available, effortlessly collected, and noninvasive; second, urinalysis tests provide information inexpensively and about many different organs.

Urine specimens should be collected and handled according to strict standards that will be discussed in this chapter. As with all laboratory tests, the results can be no better than the specimen provided.

SPECIMEN COLLECTION

Urine specimens should be submitted in clean, dry, leakproof containers with screw-top containers being the best alternative, because they are less likely to leak. They are disposable and come in a variety of sizes. Disposable containers are preferred because of the chance of contamination from inadequate washing if reusable.

Pediatric containers are plastic *urine collection bags* with adhesive to firmly attach to the infants or small children's genitalia. They are soft and pliable and the easiest way to obtain a urine specimen without contamination from a diaper. Fibers from the diaper can obscure clinically significant sediment structures, e.g., red and white blood cells, or the cells remain in the diaper. Figure 4-1 illustrates a pediatric collection bag.

Routine specimen urine containers are of the 50 mL size. They have a wide mouth that makes it easier for female patients to collect the specimen and a wide, flat bottom to prevent tipping over. Specimen containers should be at least 50 mL for adequate sample size; 12 mL is the minimum sample size. The cup should be a clear plastic

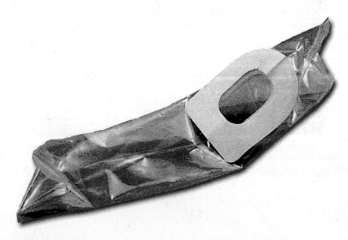

■ **FIGURE 4-1** Pediatric urine collection bag

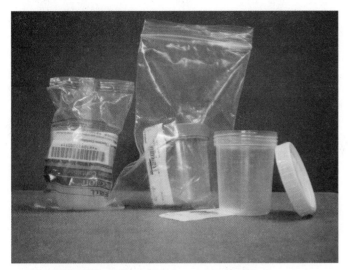

■ FIGURE 4-2   Routine Urine Container

to allow for color and clarity determinations discussed in Chapter 5. An example of a routine urine container is pictured in Figure 4-2 ■.

Containers for *24-hour specimens* are large brown or amber plastic bottles graduated to 3000 mL or 3-liter size. Figure 4-3 ■ illustrates a 24-hour urine container.

All urine specimens should be properly labeled with labels attached to the side of the container, not the lid, to avoid mix-ups if the lid is separated from the container. The label should include the patient's name, identification number, date and time of collection, and physician's name. Additional information would be the location of the patient: outpatient, hospital room number, or physician's office.

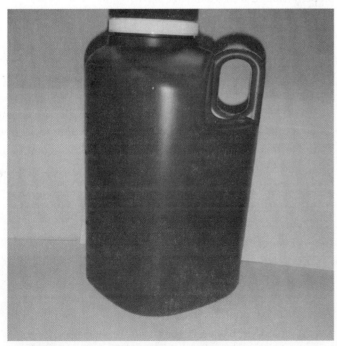

■ FIGURE 4-3   24-Hour Urine Container

TYPES OF SPECIMENS

Urine specimens are collected or obtained various ways, depending on the purpose of the specimen. The containers used are described in the previous section. Samples to be cultured should be collected in sterile containers. Most urine for routine urinalysis are clean-catch midstream specimens.

Clean-catch urines are the specimens of choice when uncontaminated urine is required. They are easy to obtain, and the specimen can be used for culture as well as for routine urinalysis. Before collection, the external genitalia are thoroughly cleansed from front to back with a mild, antiseptic solution. A cleansing towelette is provided for this purpose. Women should spread the labia apart during the entire collection process. Men should hold the foreskin back with one hand and with the other hand take the cleansing towelette and cleanse the meatus (opening from which they urinate) well using a circular stroke from the center outward. During collection the initial urine stream is allowed to go into the toilet while the midstream portion is collected in the urine container. The final urine is also discarded. If a culture is not required, a midstream sample without cleansing is adequate for a routine urinalysis.

Random urine specimens are the most convenient for the patient. They are collected at any time—no specified time, but the time collected should be noted on the container. For example, random specimens are used to screen for obvious abnormal conditions during a routine annual physical. If anything abnormal is detected, a repeat specimen and /or additional testing is ordered to confirm or rule out the initial result.

Three-glass collection is similar to the clean-catch and is used to determine prostatic infection in males. In the three-glass process all portions of the urine—beginning, middle, and end—are collected in three separate containers. The prostate is massaged prior to collection of the third portion. In urinary tract infections the number of white cells and bacteria will be increased in the second and third containers, but in prostatic infections the white blood cells and bacteria will be higher in the third container than in the second.

Catheterized urines are sometimes required to obtain a suitable specimen. A catheter is inserted into the bladder to obtain a specimen that is not contaminated by vaginal fluids or menstruation. However, catheterization always has the risk of introducing bacteria into the urethra or bladder thereby causing an infection; therefore, it should not be used if at all possible.

Suprapubic aspiration of the bladder is sometimes used to obtain a single, uncontaminated sample of urine from the bladder. Using ultrasonography, a needle is inserted directly into the bladder. Suprapubic aspiration is indicated when the patient has urinary retention (e.g., prostate hypertrophy or cancer), urethral stricture, or urethral trauma and cannot be catheterized. Suprapubic aspiration is the method of choice to obtain an uncontaminated specimen in neonates or children under 2 years of age if the previous methods are not successful. Studies suggest that it was superior to catheterization or transurethral collection of bladder urine for bacteriologic study.[6]

First morning specimens are the specimen of choice when concentrated urine is recommended. It ensures that chemicals and formed elements that may not be found in dilute, random specimens are detected, for example, human chorionic gonadotropin to detect early pregnancy. The patient is instructed to collect a sample of the first morning specimen and deliver it to the laboratory within 2 hours.

24-hour specimens or **timed specimens** are required to measure the exact concentration of a urine chemical and not the presence measured semiquantitatively (trace, small, moderate, or large) or by absence. The most commonly performed tests on timed specimens are creatinine, blood urea nitrogen (BUN), glucose, sodium, potassium, or analytes like catecholamines and hydroxysteroids that are affected by diurnal variations (variation in excretion based on the time of day). Timed specimens must be carefully timed and begin and end with an empty bladder. See Box 4-1 for directions for collecting a 24-hour urine. Timing and completeness of collection (collecting ALL urine) are the major obstacles associated with timed specimens. A summary of the types of specimens and their purpose is provided in Table 4-1 ★.

Upon arrival in the laboratory the urine is thoroughly mixed and the volume accurately measured and recorded. Depending on what test or tests are to be performed, an aliquot is saved for testing; the

BOX 4-1   24-Hour or Timed Specimen Collection

- The patient must be given very detailed written instructions and the collection procedure should be explained.
- The proper collection container and preservative (if needed) are provided.
- Day 1 at 8 a.m. patient empties bladder into the toilet and ALL urine from then on is collected for the next 24 hours.
- Cap the container and keep it in the refrigerator or cool place during the entire collection period.
- Day 2 at 8 a.m. the patient voids and collects the final 24-hour urine in the container.
- Deliver the urine to the laboratory.

★ TABLE 4-1 Type of Specimen and Purpose

Type of Specimen	Purpose
Clean-catch	Uncontaminated urine specimen for routine screening and possible culture
Random	Routine screening; convenient, no specified time
Three-glass collection	Prostatic infection in males
Catheterized	Culture; used to obtain urine in cases of difficult collection
Suprapubic aspiration	Bladder urine for culture or cytology; used only when all other methods are unsuccessful
First morning	Concentrated urine for screening, e.g., pregnancy test, and ruling out orthostatic proteinuria
24-hour or timed	Quantitative chemical tests

MINI-CASE 4-1

Heidi's physician ordered a creatinine clearance test, which requires a 24-hour urine collection. She voided her bladder in the toilet at 8 a.m. the first morning and collected all of the urine that day. At 1 a.m. the next morning she went to the bathroom and neglected to save that urine.

1. What is the most common problem with 24-hour urine collection?
2. Would the creatinine clearance be affected by the omission of one sample?
3. How can the laboratory scientist help to prevent these errors?

aliquot must be adequate for repeat testing and also to perform additional tests, if required.

SPECIMEN HANDLING

Urine specimens should be handled as biohazardous substances. Required personal protective equipment consists of a laboratory coat and gloves. All standard precautions described in Chapter 1 should be observed. Specimens should be delivered to the laboratory and tested within 2 hours. If not, the specimen must be refrigerated or an appropriate chemical preservative should be added. Specimens left at room temperature for over 2 hours will decompose. For example, urea-splitting bacteria will convert urea to ammonia, which will cause an increase in pH—the urine will become more alkaline. An alkaline pH will lead to deterioration of red and white blood cells and casts. Changes in the urinalysis tests that can occur if the specimen is not properly handled are listed in Table 4-2 ★.

MINI-CASE 4-2

Twyla, a 20-year-old nursing, student was seen by her physician complaining of lethargy, nausea, and vomiting. Physical examination reveals jaundice, including yellow sclera and hepatomegaly.

The technician reported:

Bilirubin:	2 +
Urobilinogen:	4 mg/dL

A clinical laboratory science student repeated the urinalysis 2 hours later and reported:

Bilirubin:	1+
Urobilinognen:	1 mg/dL

1. How do you explain the difference between the tech results and the student's results? What happens to bilirubin upon standing?
2. What is urobilinogen converted to when a specimen is improperly stored or handled?

★ TABLE 4-2 Changes in Urinalysis Tests in Improperly Preserved Specimens

Analyte	Change	Reason
Color	Darkens/Modified	Metabolites are oxidized or reduced
Clarity/Appearance	Decreases	Precipitation of amorphous crystals; Bacterial growth
pH	Increases/more alkaline	Loss of CO_2; urea metabolized to ammonia by bacteria
Glucose	Decreases	Bacterial utilization/glycolysis
Ketones	Decreases	Volatilization and bacterial metabolism
Bilirubin	Decreases	Photo oxidation to biliverdin by exposure to light
Urobilinogen	Decreases	Oxidation to urobilin
Nitrite	Increases	Increase in nitrate-reducing bacteria
Red blood cells	Decreases	Lyse in dilute, alkaline urine
White blood cells	Decreases	Shrink in hypertonic urine; lyse in hypotonic urine
Red and white blood cell casts	Decreases	Disintegrate in dilute, alkaline urine
Bacteria	Increases	Growth, multiplication
Odor	Increases	Breakdown of urea to ammonia, growth of bacteria

MINI-CASE 4-3

Sarah's physician ordered a serum glucose and a routine urinalysis to rule out diabetes mellitus because the symptoms she described were consistent with diabetes. The serum glucose was 220 mg/dL (Reference range 60–99 mg/dL), but the urine glucose was negative.

1. What is one explanation for the negative urine glucose?

2. How can the technologist determine if it is in fact the cause?

BOX 4-2   Common Urine Preservatives

- Refrigeration (most common)
- Thymol
- Toluene
- Formalin/Formaldehyde
- Boric acid
- Sodium fluoride
- Preservative tablets

PRESERVATIVES

If a specimen is to be kept for over 2 hours, it must be preserved. The most common method is refrigeration at 2°C to 8°C. This decreases bacterial growth and metabolism and minimizes the changes described in Table 4-2. Refrigeration, however, may result in the precipitation of amorphous crystals, phosphates, and urates, which will make it difficult to examine the urine microscopically. The specimen must be brought to room temperature before testing with chemical reagent strips described in Chapter 6. If the specimen is to be transported to a reference laboratory and refrigeration is not possible, chemical preservatives, e.g. preservative tablets, may be utilized. Box 4-2 lists the most common preservatives. The Clinical and Laboratory Standards Institute (CLSI) Approved Guidelines on Urinalysis Collection and Transportation, and Preservation of Urine Specimens states that in general chemical preservatives should be avoided for urinalysis.[7]

Thymol preserves glucose and other chemical tests on the reagent strip well, but it interferes with the acid precipitation test for protein, e.g., sulfosalicylic acid. It also preserves formed elements in the sediment. One small crystal is adequate, but thymol is rarely used as a preservative.

Toluene does not interfere with chemical tests in the routine urinalysis. The usual concentration is 2 mL/100 mL of urine. It preserves ketones, proteins, and reducing substances, but does not eliminate the bacteria already present in the specimen. One disadvantage of toluene is that it floats to the surface of the specimen, which makes it difficult to separate it from the urine.

Formalin/Formaldehyde is an excellent preservative for urine sediments using 1 drop/30 mL of urine. It will, however, act as a reducing substance and interfere with chemical reagent strip tests for glucose, blood, leukocyte esterase, and Clinitest (copper reduction). It will also precipitate protein if present in larger quantities.

Boric acid preserves protein and formed elements and does not interfere with the chemical tests except pH. It may precipitate crystals at higher concentrations. Boric acid is the preservative used in tubes to preserve urine for culture and sensitivity. It is bacteriostatic (inhibits growth), but not bactericidal (capable of killing bacteria).

Chloroform will inhibit bacterial growth, however, it is no longer recommended for routine specimens because it alters the characteristics of the cellular sediment.

Sodium fluoride prevents glycolysis and is a good preservative for drug testing. When the specimen is to be tested with the chemical reagent strip, sodium benzoate may be substituted for fluoride.

Preservative tablets are commercially available and act by releasing formaldehyde, 1 tablet/30 mL of urine. As with liquid formaldehyde, lower concentration will not affect tests for reducing substances, but at higher levels it will cause false positives.

☑ CHECKPOINT 4-1

1. The urine specimen that is most often used for routine urinalysis and culture is
   (a) catheterized,
   (b) suprapubic aspiration.
   (c) clean-catch.
   (d) first morning.

2. Unpreserved specimens should be tested within a maximum of
   (a) 30 minutes.
   (b) 1 hours.
   (c) 2 hours.
   (d) 4 hours.
   (e) 24 hours

3. State whether the following urinalysis tests will increase, decrease, or not change if not properly handled.
   (a) pH _____
   (b) Glucose _____
   (c) Bilirubin _____
   (d) Ketones _____
   (e) Nitrite _____

4. The most common method of preservation is _____.

URINE VOLUME

Urine volume depends on the amount of water that the kidneys excrete, which is determined primarily by the body's state of hydration. One of the most common factors that influences urine volume is fluid intake. A person who is dehydrated will have a low urine volume, whereas a person whose fluid intake is greater than normal will have a higher urine volume. Other factors include fluid loss from non-renal sources, for example, sweating, variations in antidiuretic hormone (ADH), and the excretion of increased amounts of dissolved solids, e.g., glucose and salts. Factors influencing urine volume are summarized in Box 4-3.

BOX 4-3   Factors Influencing Urine Volume

1. Fluid intake
2. Fluid loss from non-renal sources
3. Variations in the secretion of antidiuretic hormone
4. The excretion of increased amounts of dissolved solids

Normal 24-hour urine volume is 1200–1500 mL/day, but it can range from 800–2000 mL/day.[8] The wide range is influenced by the factors in Box 4-3.

Oliguria is a decrease in urine volume to < 400 mL/day. Oliguria is most commonly caused by dehydration due to excessive water loss because of vomiting, diarrhea, perspiration, or severe burns. However, oliguria is often the earliest sign of acute renal failure. Oliguria can also occur as the result of certain medications, renal disease, renal failure, multiple organ failure (MOF), sepsis, and urinary obstruction/urinary retention.[9] Causes of oliguria can be classified in three categories: prerenal, renal, and postrenal. Box 4-4 lists some of the causes under each category.

BOX 4-4   Prerenal, Renal, and Postrenal Causes of Oliguria[10]

Prerenal
- Absolute decrease in blood volume due to hemorrhaging, vomiting, diarrhea
- Relative decrease in blood volume due to sepsis, hepatic failure, nephrotic syndrome
- Myocardial infarction, congestive heart failure

Renal
- Acute glomerulonephritis due to connective tissue disorders (systemic lupus erythematosus), toxemia of pregnancy, poststreptococcal glomerulonephritis, rapidly progressive glomerulonephritis
- Interstitial nephritis related to drugs, infection, or cancer
- Acute tubular necrosis

Postrenal
- Upper urinary tract obstruction, e.g., ureteral obstruction of the kidney(s)
- Lower urinary tract obstruction, e.g., bladder

MINI-CASE 4-4

Bill, a 50-year-old man, called for an appointment with his physician because he had noticed a significant decrease in his urine volume.

1. What is the term for decreased urine volume?
2. List some causes of decreased urine formation.
3. What are some questions the physician is likely to ask to narrow the possibilities?
4. What type of specimen would give the physician a better idea of the severity of Bill's problem?

Anuria is the complete cessation of urine flow to less than 50 mL per day as a result of damage to the kidneys or a decrease in the flow of blood to the kidneys.[11] Oliguria is more common than anuria, but it can progress to complete cessation of urine production.

Nocturia is the increase in urine excretion at night. Normally, plasma levels of antidiuretic hormone (ADH) are higher at night than during the day; therefore, most solutes, e.g., sodium, potassium, and chloride, are excreted during the day. At night the urine is more concentrated with a decreased volume and low solute concentration.[12] Normally, the urine excretion during the day is two to three times the volume at night.

Nocturia increases with age because the size of the bladder decreases and urine production increases with increasing age. Nocturia can be explained by something as simple as drinking large amounts of fluid in the evening or consuming caffeinated drinks. Urinary tract conditions such as bacterial or viral infections of the urinary tract, bladder, or kidney can also result in nocturia.[13] Other conditions associated with nocturia are summarized in Box 4-5.

Polyuria is an increase in daily urine volume over 2000 mL/day. Polyuria, like nocturia, can be artificially induced by consuming large amounts of fluids especially those containing caffeine, alcohol or certain medications, such as diuretics.[14]

Conditions associated with polyuria include diabetes insipidus, diabetes mellitus, and some types of renal failure. Diabetes insipidus (DI) is a condition resulting in polyuria caused by inadequate levels of antidiuretic hormone (ADH) secreted by the hypothalamus (central DI) or failure of the kidneys to respond to ADH (renal DI).[15]

Diabetes mellitus is a result of a defect in the pancreatic production of insulin or in the function of insulin. Insulin is the primary hormone that decreases the level of glucose in the blood. A decrease in insulin results in hyperglycemia (high blood glucose). When the renal threshold of glucose is exceeded, the kidneys respond to the high levels by excreting excess glucose in the urine. Renal threshold is described in more detail in Chapter 3. See Box 4-6 for a list of conditions resulting in polyuria.

BOX 4-6   Causes of Polyuria

- Diabetes mellitus
- Diabetes insipidus—renal
- Diabetes insipidus—central/hypothalamic
- High fluid intake
- Medications, e.g. diuretics
- Renal failure

☑ CHECKPOINT 4-2

1. The following may be causes of oliguria *except*
   (a) congestive heart failure.
   (b) acute glomerulonephritis.
   (c) diabetes mellitus.
   (d) lower urinary tract obstruction.

2. The complete cessation of urine flow or a decrease to less than 50 mL per day is called
   (a) anuria.
   (b) oliguria.
   (c) nocturia.
   (d) polyuria.

3. Nocturia may be caused by
   (a) hepatic failure.
   (b) benign prostatic hypertrophy.
   (c) diarrhea.
   (d) upper urinary tract obstruction.

4. Polyuria is defined as
   (a) an increase in daily urine volume to over 1,000 mL/day.
   (b) an increase in daily urine volume to over 2,000 mL/day.
   (c) a decrease in urine volume to under 400 mL/day.
   (d) a decrease in urine volume to under 50 mL/day.

BOX 4-5   Common Causes of Nocturia

- Advanced age
- Consuming caffeinated or alcoholic drinks at night
- Drinking excess fluids late in the day
- Medication side effects
- Pregnancy
- Menopause
- Benign prostatic hyperplasia (BPH)
- Cystitis
- Congestive heart failure (CHF)
- Type 2 Diabetes mellitus
- Urinary tract infections
- Chronic renal disease
- *Malignant tumor of the bladder
- *Malignant tumor of the prostate

*Serious or life-threatening causes

Key Points to Remember

- Urine specimens should be submitted in clean, dry, leak-proof containers with screw tops usually plastic 50 mL size with a wide mouth.
- Types of urine specimens include random, clean-catch, three-glass, catheterized, suprapubic aspiration, first morning, and 24-hour or timed specimens.
- Clean-catch is the most common and is suitable for both urinalysis and culture.
- Specimens should be delivered to the laboratory and tested within 2 hours.
- At room temperature changes will occur due to urea-splitting bacteria, which will convert urea to ammonia, causing an increase in pH, alkalization. Other examples of changes are a decrease in glucose because of bacterial utilization and a decrease in bilirubin due to oxidation to biliverdin by exposure to light.
- If a specimen is kept for over 2 hours, it must be preserved. The most common method is refrigeration at 2°–8°C. Other preservatives are thymol, toluene, formalin, boric acid, chloroform, sodium fluoride, and preservative tablets. Each has specific uses, and each has specific advantages and disadvantages.

- Urine volume is influenced by a number of factors: fluid intake, fluid loss from nonrenal sources, variations in antidiuretic hormone, and the excretion of increased amounts of dissolved solids.
- The normal 24-hour volume is 1200–1500 mL /day, but it can range from 800–2000 mL/day.
- Oliguria is a decrease in urine volume to <400 mL/day, usually caused by dehydration due to excessive water loss, e.g. vomiting, diarrhea, and perspiration.
- Anuria is the complete cessation of urine flow or a decrease to less than 50 mL/day as a result of renal damage.
- Nocturia is the increase in urine excretion at night. Common causes of nocturia include consuming caffeinated or alcoholic drinks at night, benign prostatic hyperplasia, congestive heart failure, urinary tract infection, and chronic renal disease.
- Polyuria is an increase in daily urine volume over 2000 mL/day. Causes of polyuria are diabetes mellitus, diabetes insipidus, medications, high fluid intake, and renal failure.

Review Questions

Level I

1. Which type of urine specimen is used when a concentrated specimen is required? (Objective 2)

   A. Random

   B. Clean-catch

   C. First morning

   D. Catheterized

2. The most common or specimen of choice for an uncontaminated urine is (Objective 2)

   A. clean-catch.

   B. catheterized.

   C. suprapubic aspiration.

   D. first morning.

3. Which type of urine collection is used to diagnose prostatic infection? (Objective 2)

   A. Clean-catch

   B. Random

   C. Three-glass

   D. First morning

4. A timed or 24-hour urine specimen should include all of the urine the person produced during the timed period. The patient's instructions should include: (Objective 3)

   A. Day 1 @ 8 am: Urinate and discard the specimen, for the next 24 hours, collect all urine and put it in the 24-hour urine container.

   B. Day 2 @ 8 am: Urinate and put the urine in the 24-hour urine container.

   C. a and b.

   D. Collect all urine for the next 24 hours, except any that is voided during the night.

5. After receiving a 24-hour urine for quantitative total protein, the technician must first: (Objective 3)

   A. add the appropriate preservative.

   B. screen the urine for albumin using a reagent strip.

   C. measure the total volume.

   D. subculture for bacteria.

6. The urine specimen label should be attached to (Objective 2)

   A. the lid.

   B. the side of the container.

   C. the bottom.

   D. any of the above.

7. Which of the following tests would not be affected by allowing a urine specimen to remain at room temperature for 3 hours before analysis? (Objective 4)

   A. Occult blood

   B. Glucose

   C. pH

   D. Protein

8. Urine samples should be examined within 1 hour (2 hours maximum) of voiding because: (Objective 4)

   A. ketones will increase due to bacterial metabolism.

   B. bacterial contamination will cause alkalinization of the urine.

   C. urobilinogen will increase after prolonged exposure to light.

   D. RBCs, WBCs, and casts agglutinate on standing for several hours at room temperature.

9. Which of the following may be increased if a sample is not tested within 2 hours? (Objective 4)

   A. Glucose

   B. Ketones

   C. Nitrite

   D. Urobilinogen

10. A urine specimen is delivered to the laboratory 10 hours after it is obtained. It is acceptable if the specimen has been stored: (Objective 5)

    A. at room temperature.

    B. at 2°–8°C (refrigerated).

    C. frozen.

    D. with a preservative additive.

11. The ideal preservative should do all of the following except: (Objective 5)

    A. be bactericidal.

    B. enhance urease activity.

    C. preserve formed elements in sediment.

    D. not interfere with chemical tests.

12. What is the most frequently used method to preserve urine? (Objective 5)

    A. Formalin

    B. Refrigeration

    C. Phenol

    D. Saccamano fixative

13. Which of the following preservative preserves protein and formed elements and is bacteriostatic? (Objective 5)

    A. Sodium fluoride

    B. Boric acid

    C. Chloroform

    D. Toluene

14. The normal range for daily urine excretion is (Objective 6)

    A. 600–1200 ml/day.

    B. 1200–1500 ml/day.

    C. 1200–2000 ml/day.

    D. 800–2000 ml/day.

15. Urine production of less than 400 mL/day is: (Objective 8)

    A. called anuria.

    B. defined as oliguria.

    C. associated with diabetes insipidus.

    D. normal.

16. Cessation of urine flow is defined as: (Objective 9)

    A. diuresis.

    B. anuria.

    C. azotemia.

    D. dysuria.

17. Polyuria is commonly associated with: (Objective 9)

    A. acute pyelonephritis.

    B. tubular damage.

    C. diabetes mellitus.

    D. hepatitis.

Level II

1. A prerenal cause of oliguria would be (Objective 1)

   A. poststreptococcal glomerulonephritis.

   B. lower urinary tract infection.

   C. absolute decrease in blood volume.

   D. acute tubular necrosis.

2. Nocturia may be caused by (Objective 2)

   A. acute glomerulonephritis.

   B. drinking tea or coffee before going to bed.

   C. obstruction of the bladder.

   D. hepatic failure.

3. Which of the following would describe the urine volume of a patient who is taking diuretics? (Objective 2)

    A. Polyuria

    B. Anuria

    C. Oliguria

    D. Normal

4. Jane has noticed an increase in urine production. Her physician ordered a urinalysis and chemistry profile. Abnormal results include:

    Serum glucose: 180 (Reference Range: 70–99 mg/dL)

    Urinalysis Glucose: 2+ (Objective 2)

    A. What is the term for increased urine production?

    B. What is her probable diagnosis?

Endnotes

1. Armstrong, JA. *Urinalysis in Western Culture: A Brief History.* (www.kidney-international.org) Accessed August 2, 2011.
2. White, WI. A new look at the role of urinalysis in the history of diagnostic medicine. *Clin. Chem.* (1991) 37(1):119–125.
3. Armstrong, JA. *Urinalysis in Western Culture: A Brief History.* (www.kidney-international.org) Accessed August 2, 2011.
4. Ibid.
5. Berger, D. A brief history of medical diagnosis and the birth of the clinical laboratory. *MLO.* (1999). (www.mlo-online.com) Accessed August 2, 2011.
6. Rosh, AJ. *Suprapubic Aspiration.* (www.emedicine.medscape.com/article/82964-overview) Accessed July 26, 2011.
7. Baer, DM. Tips from the clinical experts. *Medical Laboratory Observer* (2002) 34:10:38–39.
8. Dugdale, DC. *Urine 24-Hour Volume.* (www.nlm.nih.gov/medlineplus/ency/article/003425.htm) Accessed July 1, 2011.
9. *Oliguria.* (www.oliguria.net) Accessed July 1, 2011.
10. Klahr, S, Miller, S. Acute oliguria. *NEJM* (1998) 338:671–675.
11. *Oliguria.* (www.oliguria.net) Accessed July 1, 2011.
12. Vertuno, LL, Kozeny, GA. *Chapter 183, Nocturia.* (www.ncbi.nlm.nih.gov/books/NBK293/?report=printable) Accessed July 1, 2011.
13. BetterMedicine. *Nocturia.* (www.bettermedicine.com/article/nocturia/causes) Accessed July 1, 2011.
14. Dugdale, DC. *Urination—excessive volume.* (www.nlm.nih.gov/medlineplus/ency/article/003146) Accessed July 1, 2011.
15. Ibid.

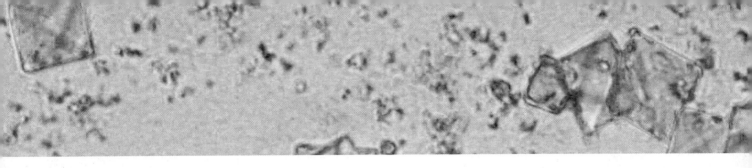

5 Urinalysis: Physical Components

Objectives

LEVEL I

Following successful completion of the chapter, the learner will be able to:

1. List the optimal conditions required to view the physical characteristics of urine.
2. Discuss the cause of normal urine color and the standardized terminology used to report urine color.
3. List and describe the most common causes of abnormal urine color and list variables that may affect urine color.
4. Classify the common causes of urine color as pathologic or nonpathologic.
5. Describe urine clarity/turbidity and the standardized terminology for reporting urine clarity.
6. Discuss the various pathologic and nonpathologic causes of turbid urine.
7. Define and discuss the importance of specific gravity and list the reference range for various specimens.
8. Explain the principle of refractometry and the advantages of using a refractometer.
9. Describe the principle of the reagent strip specific gravity reaction.
10. Calculate the corrected specific gravity given the concentration of protein and glucose and the temperature (for urinometer specific gravities).
11. Define *isosthenuric, hypersthenuric,* and *hyposthenuric.*

LEVEL II

1. Correlate isosthenuric, hypersthenuric, and hyposthenuric with various conditions.
2. Describe the quality control procedures for specific gravity.

Key Terms

Bilirubin	Harmonic oscillation densitometry	Refractive index	Turbidity
Clarity	Hypersthenuric	Refractometer	Urinometer
Isosthenuric	Hyposthenuric	Specific gravity	Urochrome

A CASE IN POINT

Mary had an appointment for her annual physical. The doctor ordered a urinalysis on a random urine sample, and the following results were reported on the physical examination of the urine.

Color: Amber

Clarity: Hazy

Specific Gravity: 1.025

Questions to Consider

1. What are the most common causes of the patient's amber colored urine?

2. Are any of them pathologic?

3. List some of the causes of hazy urine.

4. Would the specific gravity be described as hypersthenuric or hyposthenuric? List three explanations for the specific gravity.

The first part of a routine urinalysis is examination of the physical components. Color is the initial characteristic, followed by turbidity or clarity, and specific gravity. Physical characteristics can provide preliminary information concerning some disorders. For example, specific gravity aids in the evaluation of renal tubular function. Results of the physical examination can also be used to confirm or to explain findings in the chemical and microscopic components of the urinalysis which will be covered in Chapters 6 and 8.

Certain criteria need to be met to view the physical characteristics of urine:

- First, the specimen has to be well mixed. Upon standing, some of the formed elements, e.g., red blood cells and white blood cells, settle to the bottom and would be missed if the specimen isn't well mixed.

- Second, the specimen must be viewed through a clear container as described in the previous chapter on specimen collection.

- Third, specimen must be viewed against a white background to avoid interference from other colors in the background.

- Fourth, there must be adequate room lighting.

COLOR

Urine color can range from colorless to black. Noticeable change in urine color is often the reason a patient seeks medical advice. Variation in urine color may be due to many causes:

1. Normal metabolic functions

2. Physical activity

3. Ingested material or diet

4. Pathological conditions/disease

Normal metabolic functions and physical activity produce waste products that are excreted in the urine and may affect urine color. Remember: Care should be taken to examine the specimen under a good light, looking down through the container against a white background.

Normal Urine Color

Terminology used to describe the color of normal urine may differ slightly among laboratories. It is important that each laboratory has standardized terminology or common descriptions used to report urine color. An example is presented in Box 5-1 with terms in order of decreasing hydration or increased concentration.

The color of urine is caused by a pigment called **urochrome**. Urochrome, the chief pigment in urine, is the product of endogenous metabolism, and under normal conditions it is produced at a constant rate. The actual amount of urochrome produced is dependent on the body's metabolic state, with increased amounts produced in hyperthyroid conditions and fasting states. Urochrome also increases in urine that stands at room temperature. Because it is excreted at a constant rate, dilute urine (diluted in more water) will be pale yellow, and concentrated urine will be dark yellow with the same amount of urochrome diluted in less water. Severe dehydration can result in amber urine. See Figure 5-1 ■ for examples of normal urine color.

Abnormal Urine Color

Many abnormal urine colors are nonpathologic and are caused by ingestion of highly pigmented foods, vitamins, or medications. On the other hand, the urine of patients with significant disease can have a normal color. Color is an important physical characteristic, but

BOX 5-1 Standardized Terminology for Normal Urine Color

1. Pale yellow

2. Straw

3. Light yellow

4. Dark yellow

5. Amber

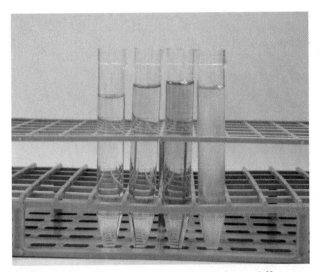

FIGURE 5-1 The first three tubes show different shades of yellow: straw, light yellow, dark yellow. The fourth tube illustrates cloudy urine.

often there is no significant correlation between color and disease. Table 5-1 ★ provides a list of abnormal colors with examples of different causes and descriptions/laboratory results.

Pink/Red/Brown

Some abnormal colors are seen more frequently and have a greater clinical significance than others. One of the most common causes of abnormal urine color is red blood cells (RBCs) (Figure 5-2 ■). The color depends on three factors:

1. The number of RBCs
2. The pH of the urine
3. The length of contact or how long RBCs have been in the urine.

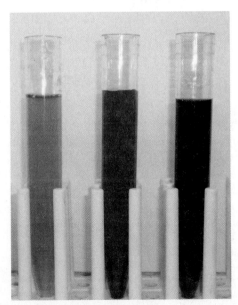

FIGURE 5-2 Blood in the urine

Tube 1 (from the left) is pinkish-small amount of red blood cells/blood. Tube 2 is red showing increased RBCs. Tube 3 is brown/black indicating glomerular bleeding.

Pink urine probably means a small amount of RBCs. Red indicates more RBCs that have been in the urine a relatively short time. Fresh brown/black urine may be indicative of glomerular bleeding—RBCs in the urine for a longer period of time. Red cells remaining in acidic urine for several hours will produce brown/black urine due to the oxidation of hemoglobin in the red blood cells to methemoglobin.

Red/Brown

Hemoglobin and myoglobin are examples of other substances besides RBCs that can result in red or brown urine. Hemoglobin is produced by the hemolysis of RBCs in vivo (in the body) and can be differentiated from intact RBCs by the clarity of the urine and the microscopic examination. Urine with intact RBCs will be red and cloudy; if only hemoglobin is present, it will be red and clear. Urine with hemolyzed RBCs will have no intact RBCs in the sediment.

Myoglobin results from damage to skeletal muscle. It is usually a more reddish-brown color than hemoglobin, and it is rapidly cleared from plasma. Chemical tests can be used to distinguish myoglobin from hemoglobin and will be discussed in Chapter 6.

Nonpathogenic causes of red urine include ingestion of highly pigmented foods with red pigment, menstrual contamination, and certain medications. Beets, blackberries, and rhubarb are known to cause a red color in alkaline urine in genetically susceptible people. Examples of medications that can result in red urine include antipsychotics (chlorpromazine and thioridazine) and the anesthetic propofol (Diprivan).[1]

MINI-CASE 5-1

Jane noticed her urine had a red tinge. She was not menstruating; therefore, that cause of contamination can be ruled out.

1. What are three possible causes of red urine?
2. List four factors that affect urine color.

Dark Yellow/Amber

Dark yellow may not always signify concentrated urine. Dark yellow can also be caused by the presence of an abnormal pigment, **bilirubin**, which may be a sign of liver disease. For example, bilirubin in the urine may indicate that the urine contains the hepatitis virus and is a potentially biohazardous specimen. Remember, however, that ALL specimens should be treated as biohazardous. Another indication that the specimen contains bilirubin is the presence of yellow foam when the specimen is shaken. Bilirubin alters the surface tension of the urine, which results in the production of yellow foam when agitated (Figure 5-3 ■).

Orange

Orange urine can be caused by medications or food or food supplements containing vitamin C, carrots, and carrot juice. Carotene, the orange pigment in carrots, winter squash, and other vegetables (in large amounts), can discolor the palms of the hands and the soles of the feet as well as the urine.

★ **TABLE 5-1** Causes for Urine Color

Color	Cause	Description/Laboratory Results
Pink	Red Blood cells (RBCs)*	Reagent strip for blood: small; few RBCs microscopically
Red	RBCs*	Cloudy urine; reagent strip for blood: moderate to many; moderate to many RBCs microscopically
	Porphyrias*	Reagent strip for blood: negative; Caused by genetic disorders
	Hemoglobin*	Clear urine; reagent strip: positive; No RBCs or few RBCs microscopically
	Beets	Alkaline urine in genetically susceptible people
	Menstrual contamination	
	Phenytoin	Anticonvulsant medication
	Compazine (phenothiazines)	Medication used to treat severe nausea and vomiting.
	Chlorpromazine and thioridazine	Antipsychotics
	Diprivan (propofol)	Anesthetic
	Laxatives (ExLax)	Phenolphthalein—indicator dye
Brown	RBCs*	Hemoglobin oxidized to methemoglobin; reagent strip: positive
	Chloroquine	Antimalarial medication
	Metronidazzole	Antibiotic
	Nitrofurantoin	Antibiotic
Black	Methemoglobin*	
	Melanin*	Urine darkens on standing; may indicate the presence of a melanoma
	Aldomet (methyldopa)	Antihypertensive medication
	Levodopa	Parkinson's medication
	Homogentisic acid*	Alkaptonuria: a metabolic disorder—HGA seen in alkaline urine upon standing
Amber		Dehydration
Amber/Orange	Bilirubin*	Reagent strip test: positive and yellow foam when shaken
	Carrots/Vitamin A	Carotene-orange pigment in carrots
	Acriflavine	Antiseptic yellow fluorescent dye, negative reagent strip for bilirubin
	Nitrofurantoin	Antibiotic prescribed for urinary tract infections
	Rifadin (rifampin)	Antibiotic
	Coumadin (warfarin)	Anticoagulant (blood thinner)
	Pyridium (phenazopyridine)	Medications for urinary tract discomfort
	Serenium (ethoxazene)	
Yellow-Green	Biliverdin*	Bilirubin oxidized to biliverdin, reagent strip negative for bilirubin
Green	Pseudomonas infection*	Bacterial urinary tract infection
Blue-Green	Clorets	Breath mints that contain chlorophyll
	Methylene blue	Medications (Trac Tabs, Urised, Uroblue) used to treat bladder inflammation or irritation
	Asparagus	
	Amitriptyline	Antidepressant medication
	Propofol	Anesthetic
	Tagamet (Cimetidine)	Medication used to treat ulcers and gastroesophageal reflux disease (GERD)
	Phenergan	Antinausea medication
	Familial hypercalcemia	"Blue diaper syndrome"
	Multivitamins	

*Pathologic conditions

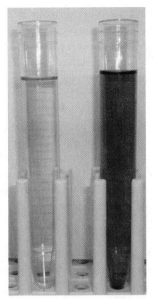

■ **FIGURE 5-3**   Bilirubin causes the urine to become dark yellow.

Certain medications can turn urine orange, including rifampin (Rifadin), an antibiotic; Coumadin (warfarin), a blood thinner (anticoagulant); Pyridium (phenazopyridine); Serenium (ethoxazene) given for pain in urinary tract infections; and certain chemotherapy medications.[2]

Blue/Green

A pathogenic cause of a blue/green color is a bacterial infection, for example, a urinary tract infection by *Pseudomonas* species resulting in urinary indican, which is a potassium salt found in sweat and urine that is formed by the conversion of tryptophan to indole by intestinal bacteria.

Familial hypercalcemia, or blue diaper syndrome, a genetic defect inherited as an autosomal dominant trait, is characterized by an inappropriate secretion of parathyroid hormone. Phenol derivatives found in intravenous medications can produce a green color on oxidation. A number of medications can produce a blue urine, including amitriptyline, indomethacin (Indocin), cimetidine (Tagamet), phenergan (anti-nausea), propofol (anesthetic), and multivitamins. Asparagus can also give urine a greenish tinge.[3]

Brown/Black

In RBCs in acid urine for a few hours the hemoglobin will be oxidized to methemoglobin resulting in a brown/black urine. Melanin and melanogen are found in patients with malignant melanoma. Melanogen will oxidize to melanin, causing the urine to darken upon standing from the air-exposed surface downward. In alkaptonuria, a hereditary disease, the urine will darken over time due to the presence of homogentisic acid. Aldomet (methyldopa), an antihypertensive medication, and Levodopa, used in the treatment of Parkinson's disease, also will impart a black color to the urine.

MINI-CASE 5-2

Linda submitted a urine sample for her routine physical. The technologist reported an amber color.

1. Although all urines are treated as potentially biohazardous which analyte on reagent strip could explain the amber color?

2. If that analyte is negative, what could the specific gravity tell her about the color?

3. What other urine solutes could result in an amber color?

☑ CHECKPOINT 5-1

1. Which of the following criteria should one use to evaluate urine color and clarity consistently?
   1. Mix all specimens well.
   2. View through a clear container.
   3. Evaluate the specimen with adequate lighting.
   4. View the specimen against a dark background with good lighting.
      (a) 1, 2, and 3 are correct.
      (b) 1 and 3 are correct.
      (c) 4 is correct.
      (d) All are correct.

2. A dark yellow urine usually indicates
   (a) a dilute urine.
   (b) a concentrated urine.
   (c) can't tell from the information provided.

3. Which of the following will result in amber or orange-colored urine?
   (a) RBCs
   (b) Bilirubin
   (c) Clorets
   (d) Beets

4. A pale yellow urine will have decreased concentration of which urine pigment?
   (a) Urochrome
   (b) Bilirubin
   (c) Hemoglobin
   (d) Azogantrisin
   (e) Vitamin A

URINE CLARITY/APPEARANCE

Clarity and turbidity are used to describe whether a urine sample is clear or is one of the various degrees of cloudiness. The **clarity** of urine can range from clear to milky (see Box 5-2). Clarity is often described based on whether you can read text (a printed page) through the specimen. This is done by holding a sheet with printed material behind

BOX 5-2   Urine Clarity/Appearance

1. *Clear:* No visible particulates
2. *Hazy:* Few particulates, print easily readable
3. *Cloudy:* Many particulates; print blurred
4. *Turbid:* Print can't be seen
5. *Milky:* May precipitate or clot

the tube and determining how well you can read the print through the urine.

Freshly voided urine is typically clear in a normal patient; however, upon standing the urine can become cloudy because of the precipitation of normal salts that form crystals.

Hazy urine is only slightly cloudy with few particulates; therefore, print is easily readable. It may be caused by precipitation of normal crystals in refrigerated urine (Figure 5-4 ■).

Cloudy urine (Figure 5-4). Normal acid urine can also appear cloudy because of precipitated amorphous urates, calcium oxalate, or uric acid crystals which will be discussed in Chapter 8. Cloudiness may resemble brick dust due to the accumulation of pink pigment, *uroerythrin* or "brick dust," which attaches to the surface of crystals. Uroerythrin is a normal constituent of urine and is most often seen in refrigerated urines.

Milky urine refers to a white, opaque urine that can be caused by phosphaturia, a condition in which excess amorphous phosphate crystals form in the urine. It can also be a result of chyluria, the presence of triglycerides and cholesterol in the urine.

Turbidity refers to the opacity of urine due to the suspension of flaky or granular particles in a normally clear urine and should be reported in a standardized format with everyone in the lab using the same terminology to describe various degrees of turbidity. See Box 5-2 for an example of a reporting format. As with color, turbidity should be determined using a well-mixed specimen in a clear container, against a white background, and with adequate lighting.

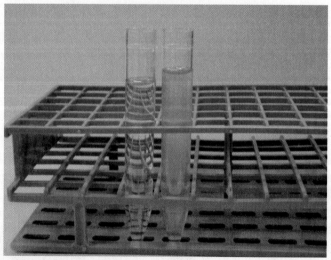

■ **FIGURE 5-4**   The urine in the left tube is clear. Cloudy urine in the right tube.

Many substances can cause turbidity in the urine; some are pathologic, but many are nonpathologic. See Box 5-3 for lists of the most common pathologic and nonpathologic causes of turbidity. White blood cells (WBCs), red blood cells (RBCs), squamous epithelial cells, and bacteria are the most common causes of a cloudy urine. Specimens that are allowed to stand or are refrigerated are more likely to develop turbidity that is nonpathologic.

As with color, turbidity is often nonpathologic. Clear urine can be abnormal, and cloudy urine can be normal. For example, clear urine cannot exclude the presence of a urinary tract infection.[4] However, clarity often provides a key to chemical and microscopic examination and should correspond to the amount of material detected by the reagent strip chemical tests and what is seen under the microscope.

☑ CHECKPOINT 5-2

1. Clarity of a urine sample should be determined
   (a) after the addition of sulfosalicylic acid.
   (b) following thorough mixing of the urine.
   (c) against a colored background.
   (d) after centrifugation.
2. Which of the following is a nonpathologic cause of turbidity in urine?
   (a) WBCs
   (b) RBCs
   (c) Squamous epithelial cells
   (d) Bacteria

BOX 5-3   Causes of Urine Turbidity

Pathologic Causes

1. WBCs
2. RBCs
3. Bacteria
4. Nonsquamous epithelial cells
5. Lipids
6. Lymph fluid
7. Abnormal crystals
8. Yeast

Nonpathologic Causes

1. Squamous epithelial cells
2. Semen
3. Mucus
4. Normal crystals (amorphous urates, phosphates, and carbonates)
5. Fecal material
6. Extraneous contamination (talcum powder, x-ray contrast media)

SPECIFIC GRAVITY

Specific gravity is a measure of the kidney's ability to selectively reabsorb essential chemicals and water from the glomerular filtrate, which is one of the body's most important functions. Therefore, specific gravity is valuable in diagnosing or monitoring a number of conditions. A few conditions where the specific gravity may be clinically significant include

1. Determination of unacceptable specimens due to low concentration.
2. Monitoring hydration or dehydration of a patient.
3. Loss of concentrating ability of the renal tubules.
4. Diabetes insipidus.

Specific gravity (SG) is defined as the density of a substance compared with the density of a similar volume of distilled water at a similar temperature. Since urine is actually water with dissolved chemicals (96% water, 4% solutes), the SG of a urine is a measurement of the density of dissolved chemicals in the urine and is influenced by the size and number of particles.

The specific gravity of distilled water is 1.000, and the greater the solute concentration and the larger the particles, the higher the specific gravity. Equation 5.1 describes specific gravity.

Specific gravity can be measured four ways: urinometer, refractometer, reagent strip, and harmonic oscillation densitometry. Urinometers and harmonic oscillation densitometry will be discussed mainly for historical purposes; in today's laboratories specific gravity is measured by reagent strips and refractometers.

Urinometer

The **urinometer** consists of a weighted float that has a scale calibrated in terms of specific gravity from 1.000 to 1.040. The weighted float displaces a volume of liquid (urine) equal to its weight and is designed to sink to a level of 1.000 in distilled water. In urine the additional mass provided by the dissolved substances in the urine causes the urine to displace a volume of urine smaller than that of distilled water; therefore, it doesn't sink as deep as with distilled water. The level to which the urinometer sinks is representative of the specimen's mass or specific gravity. A urinometer is illustrated in Figure 5-5 ■.

The urinometer is added with a spinning motion so it doesn't come in contact with the chamber, and the scale is read at the bottom of the meniscus. The calibration temperature is printed on the instrument and is usually about 20°C. If the specimen has been refrigerated or is cold, 0.001 must be subtracted for every 3°C that the specimen is below the calibration temperature. For example, if the temperature of the specimen is 17°C and the specific gravity is 1.010, the corrected specific gravity is 1.009. Conversely, 0.001 must be added for every 3°C that the specimen is above the calibration temperature. Specific gravity must also be corrected if large amounts of glucose and/or protein are present. Both are high molecular weight molecules that have no relationship to renal concentrating ability, but will increase the specific gravity; therefore, their contribution to the specific gravity must be

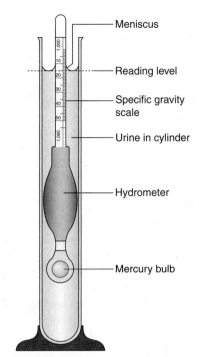

■ **FIGURE 5-5** Urinometers.

subtracted to give a more accurate report of the kidney's concentration ability. This will be discussed later in this section.

The urinometer has three major disadvantages. One, the container must be wide enough to allow the urinometer to float without touching the sides; therefore, a larger volume of urine must be used, 10–15 mL. This can be problematic, especially for pediatric patients. Second, there is a biohazard concern since urine must be poured into the container. Third, it may be necessary to correct the urinometer SG for changes in temperature. Urinometers are very rarely used, are inaccurate, and are no longer recommended by the Clinical Laboratory and Standards Institute (CLSI).

Refractometer

Refractometers measure the concentration of dissolved particles by measuring the refractive index. The **refractive index** is the comparison of the velocity of light in air with the velocity of light in a solution, in this case urine. Velocity is dependent on the concentration of dissolved particles present in the solution and determines the angle at which the light passes through a solution. Clinical refractometers make use of these principles of light by measuring the velocity and angle at which light passes through a solution, enters a prism, and mathematically converts this angle (refractive index) to specific gravity. Refractometer readings are affected by four major variables:

1. Wavelength of light used
2. Size and number of particles
3. Concentration of solution
4. Temperature of solution

$$\text{Specific Gravity} = \frac{\text{Density of urine}}{\text{Density of an equal volume of water}} \qquad (5\text{-}1)$$

A refractometer and scale are illustrated in Figure 5-6 ■.

To measure specific gravity, a drop of urine is placed on the prism. The drop should spread or cover the entire surface of the prism. The refractometer is pointed toward a good light source, and the specific gravity is read from the specific gravity scale. The specific gravity is the value where the boundary line between the light and shaded areas crosses the scale.

The advantages of refractometry are listed in Box 5-4. Specific gravity still has to be corrected for glucose and protein, although the readings are not as affected by particle density as urinometer measurements.

Correction of Specific Gravity

Specific gravities of urines with abnormal levels of glucose and protein have to be corrected. A gram of protein/dL of urine will raise the urine specific gravity by 0.003, and a gram of glucose/dL will raise the specific gravity by 0.004. For each gram/dL of protein present, 0.003 must be subtracted, and for each gram/dL of glucose, 0.004 subtracted from the specific gravity. For example, a specimen with 2 grams of protein/dL and 1 gram of glucose/dL has a specific gravity of 1.030 the corrected specific gravity is $1.030 - [2(0.003) + 1(0.004)]$ for a corrected specific gravity of 1.020.

Quality Control

Calibration of the refractometer is performed using distilled water, which should read 1.000. A zero set screw on most refractometers can be used to adjust the reading if it is slightly higher or lower. Calibration can be further checked by using 4% NaCl, which should read 1.022 ± 0.001, or 9% sucrose with a specific gravity of 1.034 ± 0.001. Two controls must also be run daily and recorded.

Values above 1.035 indicate unusual solutes, e.g., glucose IV or radiopaque compounds used in x-rays. These should be investigated before they are reported out and/or a new specimen requested.

Reagent Strip

The reagent strip specific gravity reaction does not measure total solutes, but only the ionic solutes, (SG_{ionic}), which are the clinically significant components. The nonionic solutes, e.g., glucose, urea, x-ray dyes, plasma expanders, are not measured. Equation 5.2 demonstrates that only two components comprise specific gravity, ionic and nonionic solutes.

Reagent strip specific gravity is measured using a polyelectrolyte, a pH indicator, and an alkaline buffer. Ionic solutes cause hydrogen ions to be released by the polyelectrolyte, e.g., polymethylvinyl ether/maleic anhydride in Multistix, decreasing the pH of the test pad, in other words, making it more acidic. As the pH becomes more acidic the pH indicator, bromthymol blue changes color from blue to green to yellow (acid). Specific gravity is reported out in increments of 0.005, e.g., 1.005, 1.010, and the range is between 1.005 and 1.030.

Reagent strip specific gravities do not need to be corrected for high glucose levels since it is not measured; however, high levels of protein will cause a slight increase in SG since protein may be ionized. Highly buffered alkaline urines may cause falsely low readings; some manufacturers suggest adding 0.005 to urines with a pH higher than 7.0.[5] The reagent strip specific gravity is not reliable for specific gravities over 1.025; these should be confirmed with a refractometer.

$$\text{Specific gravity}_{Total} = \text{Specific gravity}_{ionic} + \text{Specific gravity}_{nonionic} \qquad (5\text{-}2)$$

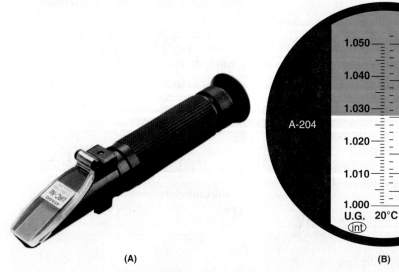

(A)   (B)

■ **FIGURE 5-6**   Refractometer.

Harmonic Oscillation Densitometry

Harmonic oscillation densitometry (HOD) is an older method used in an older version of the Iris 250 and 500 automated systems and not commonly used in today's laboratories. HOD uses sound waves to measure urine concentration. Urine enters a glass tube with an electromagnetic coil at one end. Sonic oscillation is generated when an electric current is applied to the coil. The frequency of the sound waves changes as they are passed through the urine based on the density of the urine. The oscillation detected is proportional to the density of the urine. A microprocessor corrects the specific gravity based on the urine temperature and is accurate to 1.080. HOD measures all dissolved solutes for a total specific gravity of all ionic and nonionic components.[6]

Clinical Correlations of Specific Gravity

The majority of specimens have a specific gravity of 1.015–1.025. Normal random specimens can range from 1.003–1.035 and physiologically the specific gravity can range from 1.002–1.040. Patients with consistently high or low specific gravities should be investigated to determine the cause. For example, abnormally high specific gravities are found in patients who have had kidney x-rays (intravenous pyelogram) when the dye is excreted in their urine.

The specific gravity of plasma filtrate entering the glomerulus is **isosthenuric**, 1.010, neither concentrated nor diluted (*sthenos* means strength). One specific gravity of 1.010 is not a cause for concern, but consistent readings of 1.010 can indicate severe renal disease when the kidneys can no longer concentrate or dilute the urine no matter how dehydrated or overhydrated the patient. The specific gravity of the urine is the same as the plasma.

Urines with a specific gravity below 1.010 are **hyposthenuric**. The lowest specific gravity possible is 1.002, which usually indicates overhydration. **Hypersthenuric** urine has a specific gravity over 1.010.

A specific gravity at the low end of the reference range can be explained by excess fluid intake. This may be an attempt to alter the urine prior to a drug test to make the drug or drug metabolite undetectable. Other causes are renal failure (when there is a loss of ability to reabsorb water), pyelonephritis, and diabetes insipidus (decrease in vasopressin or antidiuretic hormone). Increased blood flow to the kidneys results in a higher urine filtrate and the dissolved solutes excreted in a higher volume of urine. A summary of the causes of decreased specific gravity are in Box 5-5.[7]

A specific gravity at the high end of the reference range may be a result of dehydration, diarrhea, excessive sweating, and vomiting. Conditions resulting in decreased blood flow to the kidneys and decreased glomerular filtrate result in the total dissolved solutes being excreted in lower urine volume. Box 5-6 lists the most common causes of increased specific gravity.[8]

BOX 5-6 Causes of Increased Specific Gravity

Dehydration (water restriction)

Diarrhea

Heart failure

Shock

Excessive sweating

Vomiting

Glucosuria

Syndrome of inappropriate antidiuretic hormone secretion (SIADH)

Addison's disease

MINI-CASE 5-3

Tom's routine urinalysis report indicated a reagent strip specific gravity of 1.030.

1. Would this urine be classified as hyposthenuric, isosthenuric, or hypersthenuric?

2. List four common causes of this SG.

3. What two solutes can be eliminated as contributing to the SG? Why?

4. How should the clinical laboratory scientist confirm the SG?

☑ CHECKPOINT 5-3

1. A specific gravity of 1.015 is called
   (a) hyposthenuric.
   (b) hypersthenuric.
   (c) isosthenuric.

2. Using a refractometer, a urine has a specific gravity of 1.015 and a protein concentration of 1 gm/dL. What is the corrected SG?

3. List three variables that affect the specific gravity using the refractometer.

BOX 5-5 Causes of Decreased Specific Gravity

Renal failure

Severe renal infection (pyelonephritis)

Renal tubular necrosis

Excessive fluid intake

Diabetes insipidus

Aldosteronism

ODOR

Odor is seldom clinically significant and is usually not reported as part of a routine urinalysis unless it is a notable urine property, i.e., clinically significant. Freshly voided urine has a faint odor of aromatic compounds, and as it stands, the odor of ammonia becomes predominant due to the breakdown of urea. In a dehydrated person, the odor has a stronger ammonia smell because the waste products are diluted in less urine.

Unusual odors are found in a number of conditions. In urinary tract bacterial infections, the urine may have a strong, unpleasant, foul, putrid odor. A sweet or fruity odor may be noticed in diabetic ketoacidosis. Onions and garlic can impart a particular odor. Asparagus can cause odor, but only certain genetically disposed people can smell it. Other strong-smelling foods or supplements can contribute to urine odor. Serious metabolic defects, e.g., maple syrup urine disease, which will be covered in Chapter 14 on metabolic diseases, can also impart characteristic odors and definitely should be noted.[9] Table 5-2 ★ summarizes a few of the more common odors and their causes.

★ **TABLE 5-2** Unusual Odors Associated with Urine

Odor	Cause
Strong ammonia	Dehydration
Foul, putrid	Urinary tract infection
Sweet, fruity	Ketones (acetone) associated with diabetic ketoacidosis, nausea and vomiting, anorexia, starvation
Maple syrup	Maple syrup urine disease
Mousy	Phenylketonuria
Asparagus	Smelled only by genetically susceptible people
Rancid	Tyrosinemia

Key Points to Remember

- The physical characteristics of urine are color, clarity or turbidity, and specific gravity. A well-mixed specimen should be viewed through a clear container, against a white background, and with adequate room lighting.

- Color can range from colorless to black. Variations in color are due to normal metabolic functions, physical activity, ingested material or diet, and pathological conditions.

- Urochrome, the chief pigment in urine, is yellow and is the product of endogenous metabolism. It is produced at a constant rate; therefore, dilute urine will be pale yellow, whereas in a dehydrated patient the urine will be a darker yellow.

- One of the most common causes of abnormal urine color is blood, which can range from pink to brown/black. Many abnormal urine colors are nonpathological. Various medications, ingestion of highly pigmented foods, and menstrual contamination are nonpathologic causes of urine color.

- Turbidity refers to the clarity of the urine. Terminology should be standardized with the same words used to describe various degrees of turbidity from clear with no visible particulates to milky when the particulates may precipitate or clot.

- Pathologic causes of urine turbidity include WBCs, RBCs, bacteria, and yeast. Examples of nonpathologic causes are squamous epithelial cells, mucus, normal crystals, and extraneous contamination. As with color, turbidity is often nonpathologic; clear urine can be abnormal and cloudy urine can be normal.

- Specific gravity is the density of a substance compared with the density of a similar volume of distilled water at a similar temperature. It is a measurement of the density of dissolved chemicals in the urine and is influenced by the size and number of particles.

- Specific gravity can be measured four ways: urinometer, refractometer, reagent strip, and harmonic oscillation densitometry.

- The refractometer measures the refractive index, which compares the velocity of light in air with the velocity of light in a solution (urine). Refractometer readings are affected by the wavelength of light used, size and number of particles, concentration of the solution, and temperature of the solution.

- Specific gravities of urines with abnormal levels of glucose and protein should be corrected. For each gram/dL of protein present, 0.003 must be subtracted, and for each gram/dL of glucose 0.004 must be subtracted from the specific gravity.

- Reagent strip specific gravity is measured using a polyelectrolyte, a pH indicator, and an alkaline buffer. Ionic solutes cause hydrogen ions to be released by the polyelectrolyte, e.g., polymethylvinyl ether/maleic anhydride in Multistix, decreasing the pH of the test pad, in other words making it more acidic. The color of bromthymol blue, the pH indicator, changes from blue to green to yellow depending on the acidity and therefore the specific gravity of the urine.

- The specific gravity of plasma filtrate entering the glomerulus is isosthenuric, 1.010, neither concentrated nor diluted. Urines with a specific gravity below 1.010 are hyposthenuric. The lowest specific gravity possible is 1.002, which usually indicates overhydration. Hypersthenuric urine has a specific gravity over 1.010. The majority of specimens have a specific gravity of 1.015–1.025. Normal random specimens can range from 1.003–1.035, and physiologically the specific gravity can range from 1.002–1.040.

- A specific gravity at the low end of the reference range can be explained by excess fluid intake. Other causes are certain renal diseases, renal failure, pyelonephritis, diabetes mellitus, and diabetes insipidus. A specific gravity at the high end of the reference range may be caused by dehydration, diarrhea, excessive sweating, vomiting, water restriction, glucosuria, congestive heart failure, liver disease, and nephrosis.

- Odor is seldom clinically significant and not part of the routine urinalysis, but it can indicate serious metabolic disorders.

Review Questions

Level I

1. The clarity of a urine sample should be determined (Objective 1)

   A. using glass tubes only, never plastic.

   B. following thorough mixing of the specimen.

   C. after addition of sulfosalicylic acid.

   D. after the specimen cools to room temperature.

2. The yellow color of urine is primarily due to (Objective 2)

   A. urochrome.

   B. methemoglobin.

   C. bilirubin.

   D. homogentisic acid.

3. A dark yellow urine producing yellow foam *may* contain (Objective 2)

   A. hemoglobin.

   B. protein.

   C. red blood cells.

   D. bilirubin.

4. A dark yellow urine probably indicates (Objective 2)

   A. high fluid intake.

   B. glucose is present.

   C. protein is present.

   D. concentrated urine.

5. After eating beets purchased at the local farmer's market, two of the four members of a family notice that their urine is red. The family should (Objective 3)

   A. be concerned about contamination of the beets.

   B. not be concerned because only the male family members have red urine.

   C. be concerned because red urine always indicates bleeding.

   D. not be concerned because producing red urine after ingesting beets is a nonpathologic genetic trait.

6. Which urine color is correlated correctly with the pigment-producing substance? (Objective 4)

   A. Smoky red urine with homogentisic acid

   B. Dark amber urine with myoglobin

   C. Deep yellow urine and yellow foam with bilirubin

   D. Red-brown urine with biliverdin

7. A brown or black pigment in the urine can be caused by (Objective 3)

   A. gantrisin.

   B. phenolsulonphthalein.

   C. rifampin.

   D. melanin.

8. Which of the following is a nonpathologic cause of urine turbidity? (Objective 6)

   A. RBCs

   B. WBCs

   D. Mucus

   C. Bacteria

9. The normal range of specific gravity of urine is (Objective 7)

   A. 1.000–1.040.

   B. 1.003–1.035.

   C. 1.025–1.050.

   D. 1.010–1.015.

10. The specific gravity of urine is directly proportional to its (Objective 7)

    A. turbidity.

    B. dissolved solids.

    C. salt content.

    D. glucose content.

11. The refractometer operates on a principle of (Objective 8)

    A. light bending.

    B. color gradient.

    C. column chromatography.

    D. molecular motion.

12. Refractive index compares (Objective 8)

    A. light velocity in solutions with light velocity in solids.

    B. light velocity in air with light velocity in solutions.

    C. light scattering by air with light scattering by solutions.

    D. light scattering by particles in solution.

13. The reading of distilled water on the refractometer should be (Objective 8)

    A. 1.000.

    B. 1.001.

    C. 1.010.

    D. 1.100.

14. Reagent strip specific gravity measures (Objective 9)

    A. ionic solutes.

    B. nonionic solutes.

    C. total solutes.

    D. none of the above.

15. What is the principle of the colorimetric reagent strip determination of SG in the urine? (Objective 9)

    A. Ionic strength alters the pH of a polyelectrolyte resulting in the release of hydrogen ions.

    B. Sodium and other cations are chelated by a ligand that changes color.

    C. Anions displace a pH indicator from a mordant, making it water soluble.

    D. Ionized solutes catalyze oxidation of an azo dye.

16. What would the corrected specific gravity of urine with a refractometer SG of 1.022 that had 1 gm of protein/dL and 1 gm of glucose/dL? (Objective 10)

    A. 1.005

    B. 1.010

    C. 1.015

    D. 1.020

Level II

1. Isosthenuria is defined as a specific gravity that is usually (Objective 1)

    A. fixed around 1.005.

    B. fixed around 1.010.

    C. fixed around 1.015.

    D. variable between 1.010 and 1.020.

2. The specific gravity of plasma and urine leaving the glomerulus is (Objective 1)

    A. 1.005.

    B. 1.010.

    C. 1.015.

    D. 1.020.

3. Calibration of refractometers is done by measuring the specific gravity of distilled water and 4% _____. (Objective 2)

    A. sodium chloride

    B. protein

    C. urea

    D. glucose

4. Which of the following conditions would result in hypersthenuria? (Objective 1)

    A. Diabetes insipidus

    B. Pyelonephritis

    C. Dehydration

    D. Renal failure

5. A student performed Margaret's routine urinalysis in lab. Her report indicated the specific gravity with a refractometer was 1.020 and the reagent strip specific gravity was 1.015. What are two solutes that would cause the discrepancy and why?

Endnotes

1. Mayo Clinic staff. *Urine Color*. (www.mayoclinic.com/health/urine-color/DS01026/METHOD) Accessed April 11, 2011.

2. Terris, M.K. *The Significance of Abnormal Urine Color*. (http://urology.stanford.edu/about/articles/abnormal_urine.html) Accessed June 10, 2014.

3. Ibid.

4. Bulloch, B, Tauscher, JC, Operant, W, Connors, MJ, Mahabee-Gittens, and Dowd, MD. Can urine clarity exclude the diagnosis of urinary tract infection? *Pediatrics* (2000) 106 (5).

5. Roche. *Chemstrip 6, 7, 9, 10 with SG*. [Package insert].1999.

6. Terry, M. Body gluids: Manual and automated urinalysis. *Advance* (2005) 17(20):23–27.

7. U.S. National Library of Medicine NIH National Institutes of Health. Dugdale, DC. *Urine Specific Gravity*. (www.nlm.nih.gov/medlineplus/ency/article/003587.htm) Accessed June 23, 2011.

8. Ibid.

9. Bora, C. *Urine Odor Causes*. (www.buzzle.com/articles/urine-odor-causes.html) Accessed May 27, 2011.

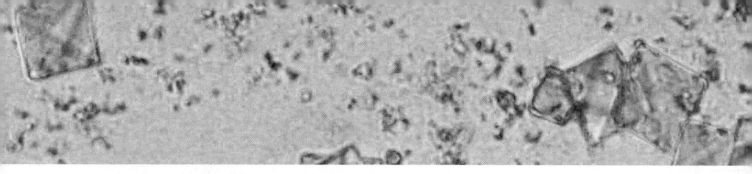

6

Urinalysis: Chemical Examination:
The Reagent Strip

Objectives

LEVEL I

1. Discuss the proper handling and storage of reagent strips and list three possible causes of their deterioration.
2. Describe the proper technique for reagent strip testing.
3. State the quality control procedures for reagent strips and tablet tests.
4. Explain the principle of pH testing by reagent strips.
5. List five factors that affect the pH of urine.
6. Discuss two reasons for measuring pH, including their clinical significance.
7. Differentiate between prerenal, renal, and postrenal proteinuria and list three examples in each category.
8. Explain "protein error of indicators" and the confirmatory sulfosalicylic acid precipitation tests for protein.
9. List four causes of benign proteinuria.
10. Discuss renal threshold as it applies to glucose testing and diabetes mellitus.
11. Explain the glucose oxidase/peroxidase reagent strip reaction for glucose including causes of false positive and false negative reactions.
12. Describe the copper reduction method (Clinitest) for testing reducing substances and discuss the "pass through" phenomenon.
13. List four causes of prerenal and renal glucosuria.
14. List three ketone bodies and discuss their formation.
15. Identify four causes of ketonuria.
16. Discuss the principles of the reagent strip test for ketones, Legal's reaction, and the Acetest tablet confirmatory procedure.
17. Correlate glucose and ketone results with specific conditions.
18. Outline the steps in bilirubin metabolism from heme to urobilin and list three causes of prehepatic, hepatic, and posthepatic jaundice.
19. Discuss the principles of the bilirubin reagent strip reaction and the Ictotest reaction.

Chapter Outline

Objectives (continued)

20. Discuss the clinical significance of urobilinogen.
21. Describe the principle of the urobilinogen reagent strip reaction and list causes of false positive and false negative reactions.
22. Define and list four conditions associated with hematuria and hemoglobinuria.
23. Discuss the principle of the reagent strip reaction for blood and discuss causes of false positive and false negative reactions.
24. Define and list four conditions associated with leukocyturia and pyuria.
25. Discuss the principle of the leukocyte esterase reagent strip test and two conditions resulting in false positives and two resulting in false negatives.
26. Explain the principle of the nitrite reagent strip reaction and list five causes of a false negative nitrite.

LEVEL II

1. Discuss the clinical significance of Bence-Jones protein and orthostatic proteinuria.
2. Explain discrepant results of protein reagent strip reactions and sulfosalicylic acid precipitation.
3. Explain discrepant results between glucose oxidase/peroxidase and the Clinitest/copper reduction methodologies.
4. Correlate between various tests in the routine urinalysis, e.g., glucose and ketones.
5. Correlate urine bilirubin and urine urobilinogen results and prehepatic, hepatic, and posthepatic jaundice.
6. Correlate leukocyte esterase results with the microscopic interpretation.

Key Terms

Acetoacetic acid
Acetest
Acetone
Alkaline tide
β-hydroxybutyric acid
Bence-Jones protein
Benign proteinuria
Bilirubin
Bilirubinuria
Clinitest
Conjugated bilirubin
Diazo reaction
Direct bilirubin
Ehrlich's reaction

False positive
False negative
Glucose
Greiss reaction
Haptoglobin
Hematuria
Hemoglobinuria
Hepatic jaundice
Ictotest
"Inborn error of metabolism"
Indirect bilirubin
Jaundice
Ketonemia
Ketones

Ketonuria
Ketosis
Legal's test
Leukocyte esterase
Leukocyturia
Myoglobin
Myoglobinuria
Nitrite
Orthostatic proteinuria
"Pass-through" phenomenon
pH
Posthepatic jaundice
Postrenal proteinuria
Precipitation test

Prehepatic jaundice
Prerenal glucouria
Prerenal proteinuria
Protein error of indicators
Proteinuria
Pyuria
Reagent strip
Renal glucosuria
Renal proteinuria
Rhabdomyolysis
Specific gravity
Unconjugated bilirubin
Urobilin
Urobilinogen

A CASE IN POINT

Heidi, a 15-year-old girl, was brought into the emergency room in a comatose state. Her parents reported that she had had the flu and had been nauseated and vomiting for the past 24 hours. The ER physician noted a fruity odor to her breath, and her skin and mucous membranes were dry.

Urinalysis

Macroscopic:

Color:	Straw
Appearance:	Clear
Specific Gravity:	1.013
pH:	6.0
Glucose:	4+ {Clinitest: (5 drop): >2000 mg/dL} → pass-through phenomenon {Clinitest (2 drop): 3000 mg/dL }

Bilirubin:	Neg
Ketones:	2+ (Acetest: 2+)
Blood:	Neg
Protein:	Neg
Urobilinogen:	Normal
Nitrite:	Neg
Leukocyte Esterase:	Neg

Microscopic:

WBCs:	0-1/HPF
RBCs:	0-2/HPF
Epithelial Cells:	Rare Squamous/HPF
Casts:	Neg
Bacteria:	Neg

Blood Chemistry

Glucose: 410   RI: (70–99 mg/dL)

Questions to Consider

1. Circle or highlight the abnormal or discrepant result(s).

2. What metabolic disorder is most commonly associated with glucosuria and ketonuria?

3. What is the cause of the "the fruity odor" on Heidi's breath?

4. Explain the difference in the strength of reaction between the reagent strip glucose and the Clinitest reaction.

5. What is the pass-through phenomenon reported in the Clinitest reaction?

6. What would have happened if the tech had not observed/monitored the Clinitest reaction during the reaction period? What would have been reported?

7. Discuss the specificity of the reagent strip glucose and Clinitest reaction.

8. Which two ketones are measured by the reagent strip reaction? Which ketone is NOT measured?

9. Is Heidi exhibiting any signs of renal damage? Why or why not?

10. What test could the physician order to monitor this teenager for any signs of nephropathy? Why is this important?

In Chapter 5, the first part of the routine urinalysis, the physical components were reviewed: color, appearance, and specific gravity. The chemical examination of the urine is the second part of a routine urinalysis. Chemical tests are performed using a reagent strip with pads for each analyte tested. The results of the analytes tested provide information about many different organs and tissues. Bilirubin and urobilinogen can detect liver diseases, e.g., hepatitis and cirrhosis. Abnormal levels of protein in the urine may help diagnose renal disease.

Although this part of the urinalysis may at first seem simple and straightforward, care should be taken in specimen collection and handling and testing techniques to provide the most accurate results. The chemical reactions are also subject to false positive and false negative reactions; therefore, interpretation should be made with as much information as possible.

THE REAGENT STRIP

Urinalysis testing has changed radically since the days of "pisse prophets" described in Chapter 4. Modern urinalysis is performed using a reagent strip to test for 10 clinically significant analytes: pH, protein, glucose, ketones, blood, bilirubin, urobilinogen, nitrite, specific gravity, and leukocytes. Before the 1950s all tests were done individually in test tubes! Two of the major brands of reagent strips are Chemstrip* (Roche Diagnostics, Indianapolis, IN) and Bayer* Multistix (Siemens Medical Solutions Diagnostics, Tarrytown, NY). These are available in a variety of types including single, double, 9 test, and 10 test. Variations in chemical reactions, specificity, sensitivity, and interfering substances exist between the two brands that will be discussed as each analyte is covered. See Figure 6-1 ■ for an illustration of a reagent strip container.

Reagent strips are plastic strips with chemical-impregnated absorbent pads for each test. When the pad comes in contact with a urine sample that contains the substance, a color is produced depending on the concentration of the analyte. The color is compared to a color chart on the container supplied by the manufacturer. Several colors are provided for each analyte corresponding to semiquantitative values of trace, 1+, 2+, 3+, or 4+ or small, moderate, or large, which is reported. Under the color block is also an estimate of the amount of the substance present, e.g., milligrams per deciliter. Semiquantitative values are between qualitative and quantitative. Qualitative tests are reported as simply positive or negative, and quantitative are reported numerically with a specific quantity. Semiquantitative assays are reported as an *approximate* amount of the analyte—more sensitive than positive or negative but less than a quantitative result. Figure 6-2 ■ is a picture of a reagent strip.

Handling and Storage of Reagent Strips

Reagent strips should be stored in a cool, dry area, and they should be kept at room temperature, below 30°C and not frozen. Protect strips from light, moisture, heat, and volatile chemicals. Reagent strip containers are opaque to protect the strips from light and contain a desiccant to absorb moisture. Containers should be opened to remove the number of strips required and then closed immediately using the original stopper, which contains the desiccant. Strips are stable until the expiration date on the container.[1] When the container is opened, it should be dated and initialed by the technologist; opened containers should be discarded after six months.

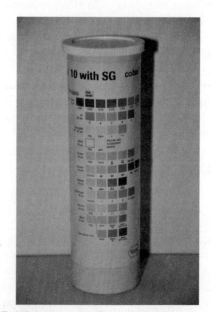

■ **FIGURE 6-1** Reagent Strip Container

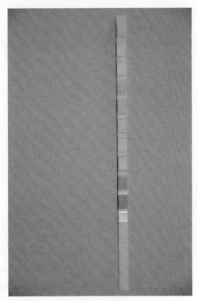

■ **FIGURE 6-2**   Reagent Strip

Reagent Strip Technique

The reagent strip should be dipped briefly (1 second) in the urine, making certain all of the pads are completely moistened. If the strip is left in the urine too long, there may be leaching of reagents from the pad into the urine. When removing the strip from the urine, draw it along the edge of the container to remove excess urine. Turn the strip on its side and tap on a piece of gauze to remove any remaining urine and also to prevent the mixing of chemicals from adjacent pads, which may cause color distortion. After the appropriate time, hold the strip close to the color blocks but not touching, make sure the strip is properly aligned with the correct position on the container, read and record the results. Every test can be read at 60 seconds except for leukocytes, which can be read between 60-120 seconds. If the leukocyte pad indicates a trace result at 60 seconds, it should be read again at 120 seconds.[2] Trace is used to indicate a very small quantity of the analyte. Always follow the manufacturer's directions.

As with determining the physical characteristics of urine in Chapter 5, a good light source is essential for accurate interpretation of color reactions. The color chart from the manufacturer of the reagent strip must be used; color charts are not interchangeable. Also specimens that have been refrigerated for preservation must be allowed to return to room temperature before testing because the enzymatic reactions on the reagent strip are temperature dependent. See Box 6-1 for a summary of the reagent strip procedure.

Quality Control

Reagent strips must be checked with positive and negative controls, or two levels for each analyte, a minimum of once every 24 hours. The lot number and control results must be recorded. Follow hospital protocol; some hospital laboratories require reagent strip control every shift. Positive and negative controls should be within the critical detection levels for each parameter or test. All negative tests should be negative and all positive tests should be within ± one color block. Controls are also run when a new container of reagent strips is opened or when there is a questionable result.

BOX 6-1   Reagent Strip Procedure

- Dip the reagent strip into a well-mixed, uncentrifuged, room-temperature urine.
- Draw the edge of the strip along the rim of the specimen container to remove excess urine.
- Turning the strip on its side, blot the excess urine on a piece of gauze to remove any remaining urine and to prevent mixing of chemicals from adjacent test pads.
- Following the manufacturer's directions read the strip by holding it close to the color blocks but DO NOT TOUCH THE CHART/CONTAINER.
- Read and record the results.

Acceptable QC results do not rule out the possibility of erroneous results. Technical negligence and interfering substances can cause errors. Manufacturers include information about interfering substances and the limitations of the chemical reactions on the package inserts, and technologists should be aware of these and include them in their laboratory's procedure manual. Interfering substances and other information affecting the chemical reactions will be discussed with each analyte covered in this chapter.

Positive reactions or questionable results on reagent strip tests are also verified by tablet tests or liquid reagents. For example, a highly pigmented urine may mask the reagent strip reactions; therefore, confirmatory tests are needed to verify the reaction as positive or negative. Confirmatory tests will be discussed in this chapter, and they also require positive and negative controls. It is important to know the limitations of the chemical reactions of the reagent strips and when to perform confirmatory tests as per the laboratory's protocol. It is essential to make correlations between patient history, the individual test, and the confirmatory test to try to explain discrepant results (e.g., the screening test is positive or negative and the confirmatory indicates the opposite).

SPECIFIC GRAVITY

Measurement of specific gravity (SG) by the reagent strip methodology as well as with a refractometer and urinometer are discussed in Chapter 5, Urinalysis: Physical Components.

pH

The kidneys, in collaboration with the lungs, are the major regulators of the acid-base balance in the body. **pH** is a measure of the hydrogen ion concentration of a solution in this case urine. A solution that is neither acid nor alkaline has a pH of 7; increasing acidity is indicated by a number less than 7, and alkalinity by a number greater than 7. When the body produces too much acid, the kidneys selectively excrete the excess hydrogen ions as hydrogen phosphate, ammonium ions (NH_4^+), and weak organic acids (e.g., pyruvic, lactic, and citric acids) and reabsorb bicarbonate from the filtrate in the convoluted tubules. The kidneys conserve hydrogen ions when the body's pH increases or becomes more alkaline. Alkaline urine, usually containing bicarbonate-carbonic acid buffer, is excreted when there is an increase of base or alkali in the body.

BOX 6-2 Factors Affecting pH of the Urine

- Acid-base content of the blood
- Patient's renal function
- Presence of a urinary tract infection (UTI)
- Diet
- Age of specimen

BOX 6-3 Conditions Associated with Acid Urine

- High-protein diet
- Dehydration
- Emphysema/Respiratory acidosis
- Diarrhea
- Medications
- Cranberry juice
- Diabetes mellitus
- Starvation

The range of the body's blood pH is 7.35–7.45, and the pH of a first morning specimen is 5.0–6.0, slightly on the acidic side. Following meals there is an **alkaline tide**, a temporary decrease in the acidity of urine from an increase of base in the blood following the secretion of HCl into gastric juices. The pH range of normal specimens is 4.6–8.0. Urine pH has no set range of normal values and is dependent on many variables including the acid-base content of the blood and the patient's renal function. See Box 6-2 for a list of the most common variables which affect the pH of the urine.

Diet affects pH with a high-protein or high-meat diet associated with acid urine and vegetarian or low-carbohydrate diet a more alkaline pH because of the formation of bicarbonate by many fruits and vegetables. One exception is cranberry juice, which will keep the urine acidic and is a well-known treatment for mild urinary tract infections (UTIs). A diet high in meat, beans, corn, fish, and grains will result in acid urine. Wine, liver, eggs, and milk increase the alkalinity of the urine.[3]

Clinical Significance

The pH of the urine is important in diagnosing various conditions, e.g., acid-base disorders, and in maintaining the proper pH in certain conditions that require either an acid or alkaline pH. Acid-base imbalances can be caused by respiratory or metabolic diseases or conditions. If the patient is in acidosis and the urine pH is acid (less than 7), the kidneys are functioning normally and excreting excess acid. If the blood and urine pH do not agree, then the problem may be with renal function and the kidneys, e.g., the kidneys are not able to secrete or excrete acid or base in the presence of excess hydrogen or bicarbonate.

Medications can be used to induce either an acid or alkaline urine. Control of pH is important in managing several diseases, e.g., renal calculi and UTIs. An acid urine prevents the formation of alkaline kidney stones and the development of urinary tract infections. Bacteria do not multiply as fast in an acid medium; therefore, in patients susceptible to urinary tract infections, an acidic urine will prevent or minimize UTIs. Ascorbic acid can be used to facilitate the production of acid urine. An alkaline pH will prevent precipitation and enhance the excretion of various drugs, e.g., sulfa drugs and streptomycin.[4] Sodium bicarbonate and potassium citrate are used to alkalinize urine. See Box 6-3 for conditions associated with an acid urine and Box 6-4 for conditions associated with alkaline urine.

Reagent Strip Reactions

Reagent strips usually measure pH in 1 unit increments between 5 and 9. Both Chemstrip and Multistix use a double indicator system to span the range from acid to alkaline. Methyl red covers the acid range from 4 to 6, changing from red-orange to yellow. Bromthymol blue, the alkaline indicator, changes from green to blue and covers the pH from 6 to 9. No known substances interfere with these pH indicators.

A pH below 4.5 or above 8.0 may be due to a problem with specimen handling—investigate for possible problems with the specimen. The pH of freshly voided urine doesn't reach pH 9.0 in either normal or abnormal urine. A new sample should be obtained and the urinalysis repeated.

Erroneous results can be due to improper storage, e.g., increased bacteria causing an increased pH. Contaminated containers can increase or decrease pH depending on the contaminant, although this is not a problem when using disposable specimen containers. Improper technique—allowing the reagent strip to remain in the urine too long and not removing excess urine—will lead to contamination of the pH test mat by the acid buffer of the adjacent protein test mat.

PROTEIN

Protein in the urine can be an important indicator of renal disease. **Proteinuria**, an increase in the loss of protein in the urine, is often associated with early renal disease. Normal urine has very little protein (<10 mg/dL or 100–150 mg/24h). Protein found in urine is mostly low-molecular weight (LMW) protein that has been selectively filtered out by the glomerulus. Protein is categorized in two groups—albumin and globulin. Albumin is small enough to go through the pores of the glomerular membrane and makes up most of the urinary protein. Other proteins found in urine are small amounts of serum and tubular microglobulins, Tamm-Horsfall mucoprotein produced by tubular secretion and important in cast formation, and prostatic, seminal, and vaginal proteins, which are contaminants.

BOX 6-4 Conditions Associated with Alkaline Urine

- Chronic renal failure
- Respiratory diseases associated with hyperventilation
- Urinary tract infection
- Urinary tract obstruction
- Treatment for salicylate overdose
- Pyloric obstruction

Clinical Significance

Proteinuria doesn't always indicate renal disease, and further testing is required to verify whether it is a pathological cause. Clinical proteinuria is defined as ≥ 30 mg/dL. Causes of proteinuria can be categorized as prerenal, renal, or postrenal.

Prerenal proteinuria, also referred to as overflow proteinuria, is proteinuria that occurs before the kidney and is not due to renal disease. Increased levels of LMW proteins in the serum, e.g., acute phase reactants found in inflammation or irritation, can cause prerenal proteinuria. Bence-Jones protein (associated with multiple myeloma, which will be discussed in the next section) and myoglobin are other proteins that are related to prerenal proteinuria.

Renal proteinuria may be associated with glomerular membrane damage by toxic substances and renal infections, e.g., pyelonephritis. It may also be caused by disorders affecting tubular reabsorption of filtered protein such as Fanconi syndrome. Patients with diabetes mellitus may excrete small but measurable amounts of albumin due to diabetic nephropathy.

Postrenal proteinuria is a result of proteins produced by the urinary or genital tract due to inflammation, malignancy, or injury. See Box 6-5 for a summary of prerenal, renal, and postrenal causes of proteinuria.[5]

Benign proteinuria can be associated with dehydration, emotional stress, inflammatory process, fever, intense activity, and orthostatic proteinuria. Benign proteinuria is not associated with increased morbidity or mortality. For the most part, after the cause has subsided, the protein will return to negative. See Box 6-6 for a list of causes of benign proteinuria.

BOX 6-5   Causes of Proteinuria

Prerenal
- Increased LMW proteins, acute phase reactants
- Multiple myeloma/Bence-Jones protein
- Albumin
- Myoglobinuria
- Congestive heart failure

Renal
- Glomerular
  - Primary glomerulonephritis
  - Secondary glomerulonephropathy
    - Diabetes mellitus
    - Amyloidosis
    - Pre-eclampsia (complication of pregnancy)
    - Heavy metals
    - Drugs, e.g., NSAIDs, penicillamine
    - Infections, e.g., HIV, syphilis, hepatitis
- Tubular
  - Tubulointerstitial disease
    - Fanconi syndrome
    - Uric acid nephropathy
    - Heavy metals

BOX 6-6   Causes of Benign Proteinuria

- Dehydration
- Emotional stress
- Fever
- Intense activity
- Inflammatory process
- Orthostatic proteinuria

Orthostatic or postural proteinuria is diagnosed in young adults following periods spent in a vertical position (standing up) and disappears when a horizontal position is resumed. Orthostatic proteinuria accounts for the majority of cases of proteinuria present in childhood or adolescence, 60 and 75% respectively. It is uncommon in patients over the age of 30. Two samples are needed for diagnosis. The first morning urine will be negative for protein (supine), but after a few hours, the urine will be positive for protein (upright). The pathogenesis is not well understood. Several explanations are (1) increased pressure on the renal vein while standing up, (2) subtle glomerular abnormality, and (3) a normal variant.[6] The 24-h protein is usually less than 1 g/24 h. Orthostatic proteinuria is typically a benign condition but should be monitored periodically.

Bence-Jones Protein

Bence-Jones (B-J) protein is associated with multiple myeloma, a proliferative disorder of immunoglobulin-producing plasma cells. The serum contains a marked increase of immunoglobulin light chains, either kappa or lambda, called Bence-Jones protein, which are LMW proteins filtered and excreted in the urine. A simple screening test uses the unique solubility characteristics of B-J protein. B-J protein coagulates at a temperature between 40 and 60°C and redissolves when the temperature reaches 100°C. All other proteins remain coagulated once they have coagulated. B-J protein is not positive in all people with multiple myeloma, 30–40% of multiple myeloma patients are negative for B-J protein.

Protein Testing

Screening Tests

Abnormal amounts of protein in the urine results in the production of foam when the urine is shaken. The production of white foam is caused by the alteration of the surface tension of the urine by protein. Reagent strip protein and the confirmatory acid precipitation tests are the common tests for proteinuria.

Reagent Strip Reactions

Reagent strips utilize the **"protein error of indicators"** to produce a visible colorimetric reaction. This is based on the property of some pH indicators to change color in the presence of protein. At a constant pH they are one color when protein is absent and another color when protein is present. Tetrabromphenol blue (Multistix) and 3′, 3″, 5′, 5″ tetrachlorophenol-3,4,5,6-tetrabromsulfonphthalein (Chemstrip) are two of the indicators used depending on the manufacturer. The indicator releases hydrogen ions, which are accepted by the protein in the urine, and an acid buffer is added to keep the pH constant at 3.0. At this pH level both indicators are yellow in the absence of protein and change from green to blue as protein levels increase.

Readings are negative, trace, 1+, 2+, 3+, or 4+. The sensitivity for trace reactions is 15–30 mg/dL for Multistix and 6 mg/dL for Chemstrip; both are higher than normally present in the urine or high normal. Reagent strips detect mostly albumin and may not detect tubular proteins and Bence-Jones proteins, which are globulins. If those proteins are suspected, confirmatory tests with heat or acid precipitation discussed later in this section must be performed.

Interfering Substances

The major source of interfering substances with reagent strips is highly buffered alkaline urine. The high pH overrides the buffering system and the positive reaction is due to a rise in pH, and the color change is unrelated to protein concentration. This is a **false positive**, a positive reaction when the analyte tested for is not present, but an interfering substance or condition leads to a positive reaction. Other false positives are allowing the pad to stay in contact with the urine too long, which may leach out the buffer meaning that the color change is due to the increase in pH and not protein; contamination of the container with ammonium compounds or detergents (alkaline cleaning agents); and urine with a high specific gravity.

False negative reactions are a result of the reaction being more sensitive to albumin than globulin. The false negative reaction means that the analyte is actually present and the reaction should be positive. The reagent strip reaction is more sensitive to albumin than globulin; therefore, when globulin, myoglobin, hemoglobin, or Bence-Jones protein are present, they may not be detected. Highly acidic or dilute urine may yield a false negative result. Highly colored substances (e.g., pyridium, beets) may mask the color and can result in either false positive or false negative reactions.

Precipitation Test (Confirmatory Test)

A cold **precipitation test** using sulfosalicylic acid (SSA), 3 to 7% weight/volume (w/v), is used as a confirmatory test in some labs, usually with special criteria such as the presence of an alkaline pH, to rule out false positives. The clear supernatant following centrifugation is used, because turbid urine can be difficult to interpret and can lead to false positives. Different methodologies are performed but the most common is to mix equal amounts of urine and SSA and let stand for 10 minutes. It is graded negative, trace, 1+, 2+, 3+, or 4+ according to standardized criteria. The sensitivity of SSA precipitation, the lowest amount it can detect, is 5–10 mg/dL.

False positive reactions are caused by substances that will be precipitated by acid. Radiographic (x-ray) dyes and medications including penicillin, cephalosporins, tolbutamide, sulfasoxazole, and ρ-aminosalicylic acid are associated with false positives.

Discrepant Results

Discrepant results are when the results of one test for an analyte do not agree with the results of another, e.g., one test is positive and another is negative. For example, the reagent strip has a positive reaction for protein, and the sulfosalicylic acid precipitation is negative. Table 6-1 ★ provides possible explanations for discrepant results.

★ **TABLE 6-1** Discrepant Results for Reagent Strip and SSA Urine Protein Tests

Reagent Strip (RS)	Sulfosalicylic acid (SSA)	Possible Explanation
1+	2+	• Protein present, RS more sensitive to albumin than globulin • SSA more sensitive than RS
Negative	1+	• Globulin present • Bence-Jones protein • False Positive SSA: radiographic dyes, drugs (tolbutamide, antibiotics) • False Negative RS → Highly colored substances mask color
1+	Negative	• Highly buffered alkaline urine • False positive RS: Detergent contamination • Improper technique RS: Buffer eluted from protein mat

MINI-CASE 6-1

John had a routine urinalysis performed as part of his annual physical. The following significant results were reported.

pH: 8.0
Protein: 2+ (RS) Precipitation Test: neg

Questions to Consider

1. What is the discrepant result?
2. What are two possible explanations?

☑ CHECKPOINT 6-1

1. Chemstrip reagent strips use which of the following **two** indicators to measure pH (circle two)?
   (a) Phenolphthalein
   (b) Methylene blue
   (c) Bromthymol blue
   (d) Methyl red

2. A vegetarian diet will most likely yield a urine sample with which pH?
   (a) Acid
   (b) Neutral
   (c) Alkaline
   (d) Variable

3. A false positive reagent strip for protein may be caused by
   (a) radiographic dyes.
   (b) highly buffered alkaline urine.
   (c) ascorbic acid.
   (d) salicylates.

4. A false positive sulfosalicylic acid precipitation test can be caused by
   (a) ascorbic acid.
   (b) contamination of the container with detergent.
   (c) radiographic dyes.
   (d) aspirin.

GLUCOSE

Glucose testing is one of the most frequently ordered chemical analyses performed on urine. It is used to detect and monitor diabetes mellitus. Due to the nonspecific symptoms associated with the onset of diabetes, it is estimated that half of the world's cases are undiagnosed; therefore, serum glucose is ordered in routine physical exams and mass health screening programs.

Clinical Significance

As discussed in Chapter 3 almost all of the glucose filtered by the glomerulus is reabsorbed by the proximal convoluted tubules through active transport. This is in response to the body's need to maintain an adequate concentration of glucose. The normal serum glucose is 70–99 mg/dL.

In diabetes mellitus there is a deficiency or relative deficiency in the production of insulin, which leads to hyperglycemia. If the serum glucose is high, as in diabetes, tubular reabsorption of glucose cannot handle the glucose levels, and glucose appears in the urine. The serum level at which tubular reabsorption is unable to handle the glucose load is called the "renal threshold" (160–180 mg/dL).

The causes of glucosuria can be categorized into prerenal and renal glucosuria. Unlike proteinuria there is no postrenal glucosuria. The most common cause of **prerenal glucosuria** is diabetes mellitus. Other hormonal disorders, e.g., hyperthyroidism and Cushing syndrome, increase in the secretion of hormones (thyroxine, cortisol, epinephrine), which can lead to glucosuria. Liver disease, pancreatic disease (pancreatitis, pancreatic cancer), and central nervous system damage (CVA or stroke) are also associated with prerenal glucosuria.[7] Certain drugs, including diuretics and steroids, may have glucosuria as a possible side effect. Heavy exercise, physical stress, acute emotional stress, and anxiety are physiological causes of glucosuria. Gestational diabetes may occur during the last trimester of pregnancy and requires careful monitoring. Hormones secreted by the placenta block the action of insulin, and there may be temporary lowering of the renal threshold. Another cause of prerenal glucosuria is diet—the ingestion of large amounts of sugar or food containing glucose.

Renal glucosuria is caused by conditions that affect tubular reabsorption. Fanconi syndrome is a result of major defects in renal tubular reabsorption, especially glucose. Inborn errors of metabolism, e.g., cystinosis and hereditary tyrosinemia, are also associated with glucosuria.[8] See Box 6-7 for a summary of the conditions associated with prerenal and renal glucosuria.

BOX 6-7 Causes of Prerenal and Renal Glucosuria

Prerenal
- Diabetes mellitus
- Hyperthyroidism (thyrotoxicosis)
- Acromegaly
- Cushing syndrome
- Pancreatic disease (pancreatitis, pancreatic cancer)
- Central nervous system (CNS) damage, cerebrovascular accident (CVA) (stroke)
- Acute emotional stress, anxiety
- Heavy exercise, physical stress
- Drugs, e.g., diuretics, steroids
- Gestational diabetes
- Liver disease
- Ingestion of large amounts of sugar or food containing sugars

Renal
- Fanconi syndrome
- Wilson disease
- Cystinosis
- Hereditary tyrosinemia

Glucose Testing

Two methods commonly utilized for testing for urine glucose are reagent strip (glucose oxidase reaction) and Clinitest (copper reduction). Reagent strips are used as the screening test and Clinitest is the confirmatory test.

Reagent Strip: Glucose Oxidase Reaction

The glucose test pad is impregnated with a mixture of glucose oxidase, peroxidase, chromogen, and buffer. A two-step reaction illustrated by Equations 6.1 and 6.2 occurs.

$$\text{Glucose} + O_2 \xrightarrow[\text{oxidase}]{\text{Glucose}} \text{gluconic acid} + H_2O_2 \qquad \textbf{(6-1)}$$

$$H_2O_2 + \text{chromogen} \xrightarrow{\text{peroxidase}} \text{oxidized \textbf{colored} compound} + H_2O \qquad \textbf{(6-2)}$$

The oxidation of the chromogen indicates the presence of glucose. Different chromogens can be used, e.g., tetramethylbenzidine (Chemstrip) and potassium iodide complex (Multistix). Reagent strips provide semiquantitative measurements: negative, trace, 1+, 2+, 3+, and 4+ associated with approximate glucose levels from 100 mg/dL to 2 grams/dL—levels depend on the manufacturer and the particular reaction, chromogen, involved. Normal urine glucose levels are <20 mg/dL. Therefore, it is important that the sensitivity of the reagent strip is higher than 20 mg/dL, because the reagent strip reaction should be negative at normal levels.

Interfering Substances

False Positive

Glucose oxidase is specific for glucose and will not react with other constituents in the urine, including other sugars that may be present. A container contaminated with chlorine bleach, peroxides, or other strong oxidizing detergents will result in a false positive reaction. This was a problem when disposable containers were not readily available, and urine specimens were submitted in a variety of containers. The sensitivity of the glucose oxidase/peroxidase reaction is increased with low specific gravity or dilute urine, which means the reagent strip will react with lower glucose levels in dilute urine.

False Negative

The greatest source of false negative error is *improperly stored urine.* If urine is allowed to remain unpreserved at room temperature for extended periods of time, the glucose is lowered by the rapid glycolysis of glucose by bacteria. Substances that will interfere with the enzymatic reaction or are reducing agents that prevent the oxidation of the chromogen, including ascorbic acid (Vitamin C), tetracycline, aspirin, Levodopa (drug used in treating Parkinson's disease), will result in falsely low or negative results. A specific gravity >1.020 combined with a high pH may reduce the sensitivity of the test at low concentrations. Cold, refrigerated urine specimens inhibit enzyme activity; therefore, specimens should be allowed to come to room temperature before testing. High levels of ketones can also affect the glucose oxidase reaction at low glucose concentrations because of decreased sensitivity. However, since ketones are often accompanied by glucosuria, this is not a problem.

Clinitest

Although not as sensitive as glucose oxidase, **Clinitest** is one of the earliest tests performed on urine. It relies on the ability of glucose and other substances to reduce copper sulfate (CuII) cupric to cuprous oxide (CuI) in the presence of heat and alkali. The reagents are in tablet form and contain copper sulfate, sodium hydroxide, citric acid, and sodium bicarbonate. Equation 6.3 is the reaction.

Upon addition of water, heat is produced by the hydrolysis of NaOH ($NaOH + H_2O \rightarrow$ heat) and its reaction with citrate acid. Carbon dioxide is released from citric acid and sodium bicarbonate to prevent interference from room air.

The procedure is outlined in Box 6-8.

The five-drop method is sensitive to 200 mg/dL. Clinitest tablets are very hygroscopic and should be stored in a tightly closed container, or individually wrapped. As discussed in Chapter 2 positive and negative controls should be performed and documented.

The **"pass-through" phenomenon** occurs when large amounts of glucose or other reducing substances are present in the urine, and the reaction goes throughout the entire color range very quickly and back to dark greenish-brown. During the pass-through phenomenon the cuprous oxide is reoxidized to cupric oxide. If the reaction is not monitored throughout the reaction period, this can be missed and a negative

---

BOX 6-8   Clinitest Procedure

1. Add 5 drops of urine and 10 drops of water in a tube.
2. Add a Clinitest tablet.
3. Place in rack and watch while boiling. DO NOT SHAKE OR TOUCH. IT IS HOT!
4. Watch for the "pass through" phenomenon.
5. Compare color to the color chart.

---

or lower glucose may be reported. If the pass-through phenomenon occurs, the test may be repeated with two drops of urine and 10 drops of water, which is sensitive to 350 mg/dL. A second color chart is used to interpret the results of the two-drop method.

Interfering Substances

False Positive

False positive reactions are caused by nonglucose-reducing substances. Other carbohydrates will reduce copper and yield a positive Clinitest reaction. Galactose may present in the urine of a newborn with a deficiency of galactose-1-phosphate uridyl transferase, an **"inborn error of metabolism,"** also called galactosemia. This occurs when an infant does not inherit the gene to produce a particular enzyme. The infants cannot metabolize galactose, which can lead to growth that is slower than normal, failure to thrive, or even death. Cataracts, hepatic dysfunction, and extreme mental retardation are other complications of galactosemia.[9] Lactose in milk is metabolized to galactose and glucose; galactose is not metabolized, therefore galactose builds up and the infant is not able to use one of its important sources of energy. All infants should be screened because dietary restrictions can control the condition and greatly reduce the complications. Most hospitals have routine Clinitest testing on urines of all infants less than 3 years of age. Galactose is a reducing sugar and will result in a positive Clinitest and a negative glucose oxidase.

Other reducing sugars that will yield a positive Clinitest are lactose (found in nursing mothers), fructose, and, although not commonly found, pentose and maltose. Sucrose is a nonreducing sugar and will not react with either glucose oxidase or Clinitest. Other substances found in urine that can lead to false positives are ascorbic acid (vitamins, fruits, and some medications), and drugs, e.g., salicylates, penicillin, cephalosporins, which will reduce copper. Box 6-9 lists reducing substances that will result in a positive Clinitest.

Discrepant Results

Clinitest will detect 250 mg/dL sugar. It is less sensitive than glucose oxidase; therefore, if a small amount of glucose is present, the reagent strip may be positive and Clinitest negative. See Table 6-2 ★ for other possible explanations for discrepant results.

$$CuSO_4 \quad + \quad \text{reducing substance} \quad \xrightarrow[\text{alkali}]{\text{heat}} \quad Cu_2O \quad + \quad \text{oxidized substance} \qquad (6\text{-}3)$$

(cupric ions)   (e.g., glucose)   cuprous oxide

BOX 6-9 Reducing Substances Other than Glucose Resulting in a Positive Clinitest

- Sugars
  - Fructose
  - Pentose
  - Galactose
  - Lactose
  - Maltose
- Ascorbic acid (fruits and medications)
- Drugs and Their Metabolites
  - Salicylates
  - Penicillin
  - Cephalosporins

★ TABLE 6-2 Discrepant Results Glucose Oxidase and Clinitest Reactions

Reagent strip (RS) Glucose Oxidase	Clinitest	Interpretation
Positive	Positive	• Glucose present
1+	Negative	• Small amount of glucose (glucose oxidase is more sensitive than Clinitest)
Negative	2+	• Nonglucose-reducing substance, e.g., galactose • Reagent strips defective/outdated • Interfering substances cause false negative RS reaction (Vitamin C, increased specific gravity (SG), cold urine)
4+	Negative	• False positive RS: oxidizing agent contaminant (bleach, peroxide, detergent) • Clinitest tablets outdated/defective

KETONES

Ketones are the intermediate products of fat metabolism formed during the catabolism or breakdown of fatty acids. The three ketones are **acetone**, **acetoacetic acid (diacetic acid)**, and **β-hydroxbutyric acid**. Normally, measurable amounts of ketones do not appear in the urine because all of them are completely metabolized to CO_2 and H_2O. However, when the use of carbohydrates as the body's source of energy is compromised, e.g., in diabetes mellitus, the body turns to stores of fat for energy. The body's metabolism cannot break down fat as quickly or efficiently as carbohydrates, leading to faulty or incomplete fat catabolism and an increase in ketones.

Small amounts of ketones are normally present in the blood (2–4 mg/dL), and they are always present in the following proportions: 20% acetoacetic acid, 2% acetone, and 78% β-hydroxybutyric acid. An increase in ketones in the blood is called **ketonemia**. **Ketonuria** is an increase in urinary ketones and an early indicator of diabetes mellitus. **Ketosis** is a condition with increased ketones in the blood and urine.

MINI-CASE 6-2

A newborn baby girl was bought into the pediatrician's office with failure to thrive, vomiting, and diarrhea.

Urinalysis

Macroscopic:

Color:	Yellow
Appearance:	Clear
Specific Gravity:	1.013
pH:	7.0
Glucose:	Neg (Clinitest: 2+)
Bilirubin:	Neg
Ketones:	Neg
Blood:	Neg
Protein:	Neg
Urobilinogen:	Normal
Nitrite:	Neg
Leukocyte Esterase:	Neg

Microscopic:

WBCs:	0-2/HPF
RBCs:	0-1/HPF
Epithelial cells:	Few squamous/HPF
Casts:	Neg
Bacteria:	Neg

Blood Chemistry

Glucose: 91 mg/dL   RI: 20–110 mg/dL (full term newborn)

Questions to Consider

1. Circle or highlight the abnormal or discrepant result(s).
2. What are three possible explanations for the discrepant result?
3. What is the probable diagnosis in this case?
4. How would you rule out the other two explanations in question 2?
5. List four possible complications of babies born with this disorder.
6. What is the treatment for this condition?

Clinical Significance

Testing for urinary ketones is most valuable in the management and monitoring of diabetes mellitus. Diabetics are unable to metabolize glucose for energy because of a deficiency or lack of insulin, so their bodies use fats, which they can only catabolize to ketones. Typical urine in uncontrolled diabetes mellitus (diabetic ketoacidosis) is pale due to high volume, has a high specific gravity (due to glucosuria), has a low pH (acidic), and is positive for ketones.

Increased accumulation of ketones in blood leads to the following: (1) electrolyte imbalance due to decreased pH (caused by the ketones) and (2) dehydration due to polyuria in order to excrete the excess glucose and ketones. The decrease in pH, if not corrected, can lead to acidosis (diabetic ketoacidosis) and eventual diabetic coma.

Positive ketones unrelated to diabetes can be caused by increased loss of carbohydrates from vomiting and diarrhea and digestive disturbances. Other conditions that can result in ketonuria are inadequate intake of carbohydrates associated with starvation and weight loss, anorexia, starvation, eating disorders, and malabsorption. Strenuous exercise and high-protein or low-carbohydrate diets may also be associated with positive ketones.[10]

Ketone Testing

Reagent Strip

The reagent strip test for ketones is based on **Legal's test**, the reaction of acetoacetic acid with nitroprusside/ nitroferricyanide. In an alkaline medium, acetoacetic acid reacts with sodium nitroprusside to form a purple color. Glycine is added to allow acetone to react. The test does not measure β-hydroxybutyric acid, but since the ketones are always in the same proportion, the presence of β-hydroxybutyric acid can be assumed. Equation 6.4 illustrates the sodium nitroprusside reaction.

Results are reported as negative, small, medium, and large or negative, 1+, 2+, 3+.

Acetest Tablets

Acetest is a confirmatory test for ketones in tablet form. The tablet contains sodium nitroprusside, glycine, disodium phosphate, and lactose (for better color differentiation). The tablet is placed on white paper, and 1 drop of urine is pipetted on the tablet and allowed to run off the side. A purple color surrounding the tablet is positive for ketones. Acetest tablets can also be used to test serum, plasma, or whole blood for the presence of ketones. Quality control must be performed with controls both positive and negative for ketones. An advantage of Acetest tablets is they can be used on serial dilutions in cases of severe ketosis to obtain a more accurate semiquantitative value.

Interfering Substances

False Positive

False positives can be caused by phthalein dyes, e.g., bromsulphthalein used in liver function tests or any medication that may lead to a highly pigmented urine. High concentrations of medications with sulfhydryl groups, e.g., levodopa (Parkinson's disease), methyldopa, and captopril (antihypertensives) will result in a false positive reaction.[11]

False Negative

The most common cause of false negative reactions is improperly stored specimens resulting in volatization of acetone and the breakdown of acetoacetic acid by bacteria.

★ TABLE 6-3 Correlation between Glucose and Ketones

Glucose	Ketones	Explanation
+	+	Diabetes mellitus
+	0	Diabetes mellitus with high glucose but negative ketones
0	+	Starvation, anorexia (eating disorders) dieting, GI disturbance

Correlation of Glucose and Ketones

Glucose and ketones can be related in diabetes mellitus, since they are found in diabetic ketoacidosis and are present in uncontrolled diabetics. However, conditions are found when one is present and the other is negative. Table 6-3 ★ summarizes these conditions.

MINI-CASE 6-3

Cassandra, a 13-year-old girl, was scheduled for a routine physical because her mother was worried about her recent weight loss. A physical was performed and a detailed medical history was obtained. Neither were "remarkable." The routine urinalysis provided the following significant results:

Glucose: neg

Ketones: 2+

Questions to Consider

1. List five possible explanations for the positive ketones.
2. Which ketones are measured? Which one does not react?
3. What conditions would have a negative glucose and a positive ketone?
4. What is the most likely explanation in this case?

☑ CHECKPOINT 6-2

1. The reagent strip glucose reaction is based on
   (a) glucose oxidase/peroxidase.
   (b) glucose mutase.
   (c) copper reduction.
   (d) protein error of indicators.
2. What is one explanation for a positive reagent strip glucose and a negative Clinitest?

Alkaline

(Acetoacetic acid + Acetone) + Na nitroprusside + (glycine) → Purple color   (6-4)

3. The glucose reagent strip test is more sensitive and specific for glucose than the Clinitest reaction because it detects
   (a) other reducing substances and higher concentrations of glucose.
   (b) no other substances and higher concentrations of glucose.
   (c) other reducing substances and lower concentrations of glucose.
   (d) no other substances and lower concentrations of glucose.

4. Which of the following substances if present in the urine results in a negative Clinitest?
   (a) Fructose
   (b) Lactose
   (c) Galactose
   (d) Sucrose

5. Ketones are formed from the incomplete metabolism of _____.

6. Why are ketones associated with diabetes?

7. Ketones are detected by
   (a) sodium ferricyanide.
   (b) copper reduction.
   (c) sodium nitroprusside.
   (d) ketone oxidase.

BILIRUBIN

Bilirubin provides information regarding metabolic and systemic disorders, especially liver function. **Bilirubin** is a degradation product of hemoglobin with 85% of serum bilirubin derived from the breakdown of old red blood cells (RBCs). The normal lifespan of RBCs is 120 days, after which they are catabolized to iron, protein, and protoporphyrin and replaced by new RBCs. Iron and protein are stored and reused to synthesize new RBCs. Protoporphyrin is converted to bilirubin in the mononuclear phagocytic system (macrophages and circulating monocytes from the liver, spleen, and bone marrow).

The bilirubin formed is **unconjugated** or **indirect bilirubin**, which binds to albumin and is carried to the liver. It is not soluble in water and cannot be excreted in the urine; the indirect bilirubin-albumin complex is too large to make it through the glomerular filtrate. In the liver an enzyme, bilirubin glucuronide, adds two glucuronic acid molecules to the indirect bilirubin and converts it to **conjugated** or **direct bilirubin** which is water soluble. Urine does not normally contain bilirubin, or it is present in undetectable amounts.

Direct bilirubin goes through the bile ducts and is concentrated and stored in the gallbladder. After meals the gallbladder secretes bile into the intestine where it is reduced by the intestinal bacteria to **urobilinogen**. It continues through the intestine and is excreted in feces oxidized as **urobilin**, which is responsible for the brown color of feces. Figure 6-3 ■ summarizes the metabolism of bilirubin.

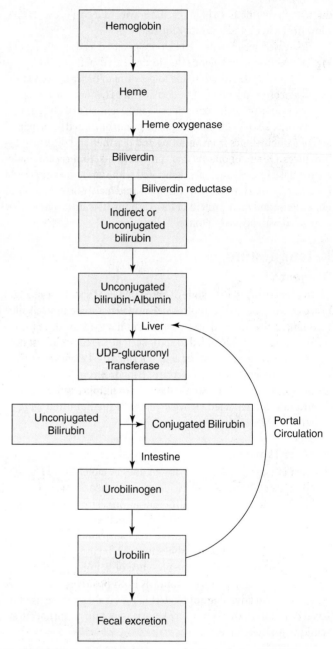

■ FIGURE 6-3   Bilirubin metabolism from Sunheimer and Graves, Clinical Laboratory Chemistry. (2011) Pearson.

Clinical Significance

Bilirubinuria is an early indicator of liver disease that may be present before jaundice. **Jaundice** is an accumulation of bilirubin in the body, leading to yellow pigmentation of the skin, sclera (white of the eyes), and mucous membranes. Jaundice is present when the serum bilirubin is 2–3 mg/dL, two to three times the reference range.

A positive bilirubin can be classified as prehepatic, hepatic, or posthepatic jaundice. **Prehepatic jaundice** is caused by increased RBC destruction or hemolysis, e.g., hemolytic anemia. **Hepatic jaundice** is usually seen in liver damage and is an early warning sign of liver disease. Hepatitis, cirrhosis, and other liver disorders are associated

BOX 6-10 Prehepatic, Hepatic, and Posthepatic Jaundice

Prehepatic
- Hemolytic anemias
- Exposure to chemicals
- Transfusion reaction
- Congestive heart failure
- Disease states, some cancers

Hepatic
- Viral hepatitis
- Cirrhosis
- Alcoholic liver disease
- Hepatocellular carcincoma
- Toxic liver injury

Posthepatic jaundice
- Common bile duct stones, e.g., gallstones
- Cancer of the bile ducts
- Bile duct stricture or stenosis

BOX 6-11 Ictotest Procedure

1. Ten drops of urine are added to the mat, which has special absorbent properties that cause the bilirubin to remain on the surface as urine filters into the mat.
2. Add the tablet to the mat.
3. Add 2 drops of water—1 drop and then 5 seconds later a second drop, making certain that it runs down the side of the tablet.
4. Note the reaction between the tablet and bilirubin on the test mat surrounding the tablet.
5. Read and record results.

Bilirubin will produce a purple color on the test mat within 60 seconds. Colors other than blue or purple are negative. Reaction is graded negative, trace, 1+, and 2+.

Ictotest is four times more sensitive than the reagent strip, will detect 0.05–0.1 mg/dL, and is less affected by interfering substances. Low concentrations of bilirubin may result in a positive Ictotest and a negative reagent strip bilirubin. The test mat minimizes pigment interference because interfering substances are filtered into the mat and will not react.

Interfering Substances

False Positive

Drugs and medications, e.g., pyridium, which produce urine pigments or a colored urine, may cause a false positive reaction. Indican, formed when tryptophan is converted to indole by intestinal bacteria, is another source of false positives. Microscopic examination should be performed on all urines with a positive bilirubin reaction.

False Negative

Improper storage is the most frequent cause of false negative reactions. Bilirubin is rapidly destroyed when exposed to light; bilirubin is oxidized to biliverdin, which will yield a negative reaction with the diazonium salt. High concentrations of ascorbic acid are another cause of false negatives. Nitrite also lowers the sensitivity of the test because it reacts with the diazonium salt; therefore, the diazonium salt cannot react with bilirubin. Medications, e.g., thorazine and selenium, may result in false negative results.

with hepatic jaundice. **Posthepatic jaundice** is caused by bile duct obstruction, e.g., gallstones or cancer.[12] Box 6-10 lists common conditions associated with prehepatic, hepatic, and posthepatic jaundice.

Bilirubin Testing

Screening Test

Urine containing bilirubin usually appears dark yellow or "vivid yellow" and produces a yellow foam when shaken. This may be the first sign of liver disease, because bilirubin alters the surface tension of urine, which leads to the production of yellow foam.

Reagent Strip

The **diazo reaction** is used in reagent strips to detect bilirubin. Bilirubin is coupled with a diazonium salt in an acid medium to form azobilirubin, a colored compound. Bilirubin and 2,4 dichloroaniline diazonium salt or 2,6 dichlorobenzene-diazonium-tetrafluoroborate in an acid medium will produce a pink to violet color. The semiquantitative results are negative, small, moderate, large, or 1+, 2+, 3+.

The sensitivity of the reaction, or the lowest quantity it will detect, is ~0.5 mg/dL. The diazonium reaction is difficult to interpret and easily influenced by other pigments that may be present. Positive results or questionable results should be confirmed with the Ictotest.

Ictotest

Ictotest is a tablet test that yields a more sharply colored diazo reaction. It consists of a mat and tablet. The tablet contains: (1) p-nitrobenzene-diazonium-p-toluencsulfonate, (2) sulfosalicylic acid (acidic environment), (3) sodium carbonate, and (4) boric acid. The mat is an asbestos-cellulose mixture. The procedure for the Ictotest is outlined in Box 6-11.

UROBILINOGEN

Urobilinogen, a bile pigment that is formed from the degradation of hemoglobin, is produced in the intestine from the reduction of bilirubin by the intestinal bacteria. Approximately half of the urobilinogen is reabsorbed from the intestine back into the portal circulation and recirculated to the liver where it is secreted back into the intestine through the bile duct. Urobilinogen remaining in the intestine is oxidized to urobilin, the pigment responsible for the characteristic brown color of feces, and is excreted in the feces. See Figure 6-3 for a diagram of bilirubin metabolism.

Urobilinogen appears in the urine because, as it circulates in the blood going to the liver, it passes through the kidney and is filtered by the glomerulus. Therefore, a small amount of urobilinogen, less than 1 mg/dL is normally present in the urine. Urobilinogen excretion peaks between 2:00 and 4:00 PM, so screening for liver damage should be performed on urine obtained during this period. Diurnal excretion is the term for increased or decreased excretion during a certain period during the day. Urobilinogen is enhanced in the alkaline tide that occurs 2 hours after lunch.

Clinical Significance

Increased urine urobilinogen is seen in liver disease, e.g., hepatitis and cirrhosis, which results in the impairment of liver function and the liver's ability to process urobilinogen recirculated from the intestine. Therefore, the excess urobilinogen remains in the blood after being filtered by the kidneys. Hemolytic disorders, resulting in increased destruction of RBCs, also cause an increase in urobilinogen. Examples of hemolytic disorders are hemolytic anemias and transfusion reactions.

Urobilinogen Testing

Reagent Strips

The reagent strip reaction is a modification of **Ehrlich's reaction**, *p-dimethylaminobenzaldehyde* turns a cherry red color in the presence of urobilinogen. The Multistix is a modified Ehrlich's aldehyde reaction with a color chart going from tan to orange. The Chemstrip reaction is more specific than Multistix and uses an azo-coupling reaction: 4-methoxybenzene-diazonium-tetrafluoroborate in an acid medium resulting in a red azo dye with the color chart from pink to red.

Interfering Substances

False Positive

Both Multistix and Chemstrip color reactions are obscured by highly pigmented urine, e.g., from dyes and beets. Multistix Ehrlich's reaction yields false positive reactions with Ehrlich's reactive substances, e.g., porphobilinogen, indican, sulfonamides, aldomet, and methyldopa.

★ **TABLE 6-4** Prehepatic, Hepatic, and Posthepatic Jaundice

	Urine Bilirubin	Urine Urobilinogen
Prehepatic (hemolytic disease)	Negative	+++
Hepatic (liver damage (hepatitis)	+/−	++
Posthepatic (Bile Duct Obstruction)	+++	Normal

Chemstrip is more specific and won't react with Ehrlich's reactive substances. Phenazopyridine, a medication, can cause a false positive. However, neither reaction can detect the complete absence of urobilinogen, which may be present in biliary obstruction. Note: The first block in the color chart for urobilinogen is labeled *normal* not *negative* (Figure 6-4 ■). The normal urine urobilinogen is 0.05 – 2.5 mg/day. The sensitivity of the test pad is approximately 0.4 mg/dL; therefore, most normal urines give a slight pink color because of the minimal amount of urobilinogen.

False Negative

The most common cause of false negative reaction is improper handling and storage. Urobilinogen is photo-oxidized to urobilin, which does not react. High concentrations of nitrite interfere with the azo-coupling reaction on the Chemstrip. Preservation of the specimen with formalin may also cause a false negative reaction.

Correlation of Bilirubin and Urobilinogen

Bilirubin and urobilinogen results can point toward prehepatic, hepatic, or posthepatic jaundice. See Table 6-4 ★ for a summary of urine bilirubin and urine urobilinogen results in the different types of jaundice.

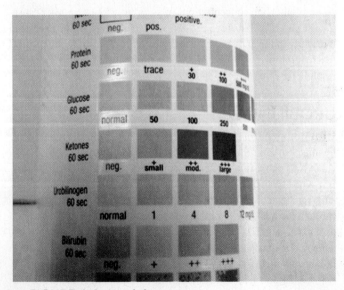

■ **FIGURE 6-4** Urobilinogen

☑ **CHECKPOINT 6-3**

1. Most bilirubin is formed from
   (a) urobilinogen.
   (b) old RBCs.
   (c) myoglobin.
   (d) ascorbic acid.

2. Direct or conjugated bilirubin is produced in the
   (a) kidney.
   (b) bone marrow.
   (c) liver.
   (d) spleen.

3. Bilirubin is increased in _____ disease.
   (a) kidney
   (b) liver
   (c) bone marrow
   (d) pancreatic

4. The bilirubin reagent strip and Ictotest are based on
   (a) Ehrlich's aldehyde reaction.
   (b) the oxidation of bilirubin to biliverdin.
   (c) the reduction of bilirubin to azobilirubin.
   (d) the coupling of bilirubin with a diazonium salt.
5. What is the major cause of false negative results for bilirubin?
6. What gives feces its normal brown color?
   (a) Urobilinogen
   (b) Urobilin
   (c) Bilirubin
   (d) Nitrite

BLOOD

Hematuria is the presence of blood present in the form of intact RBCs in the urine. **Hemoglobinuria** is the presence of hemoglobin from hemolyzed RBCs in the urine. Blood in large quantities can be detected visually due to the pink or red color and an increase in turbidity. Hematuria results in a cloudy red specimen, whereas hemoglobinuria is usually characterized by a clear, red specimen.

Since any amount of blood greater than 5 RBCs/μL is considered significant, visual examination is not adequate for detection. Chemical tests provide the most accurate method for determining the presence of blood (RBCs or hemoglobin), and microscopic examination will differentiate between hematuria and hemoglobinuria. Microscopic examination will also detect intact RBCs, but free hemoglobin produced by hemolytic disorders and lysis of RBCs in the urinary tract will not be identifed.

Clinical Significance

Hematuria is always of major clinical importance. It is most closely associated with disorders of the renal or genitourinary tract resulting from trauma, irritation, or bleeding. Renal diseases such as glomerulonephritis, pyelonephritis, and cystitis and renal calculi (stones), tumors, or trauma to the kidneys are renal causes of hematuria. Exposure to toxic chemicals or drugs, strenuous exercise, and acute febrile episodes are also associated with hematuria. People who smoke tend to have increased levels of RBCs in the urine. Menstrual contamination should be ruled out in premenopausal women.[13]

Hemoglobinuria may occur as hemolysis of RBCs produced in the urinary tract or as a result of intravascular hemolysis. If hemolysis occurs in the urine, a mixture of hematuria and hemoglobinuria will be present. If no RBCs are seen in the microscopic examination, the cause is most likely intravascular hemolysis. Under normal conditions glomerular filtration of hemoglobin is prevented by the formation of large hemoglobin-haptoglobin complexes in circulation that are too large to pass into the glomerular filtrate. **Haptoglobin** is the protein carrier of hemoglobin in the bloodstream; however, when the amount of hemoglobin present exceeds the haptoglobin, free hemoglobin will be present in the glomerular filtrate. Hemoglobinuria may be seen in hemolytic anemias, transfusion reactions, severe burns, infections, and strenuous exercise. See Box 6-12 for a list of conditions associated with hematuria and hemoglobinuria.

Myoglobin

Myoglobin, a muscle hemoglobin, is a well-known interfering substance for blood. Its low molecular weight (<17,000 Dalton) allows it to pass through the glomerular filtrate. Myoglobin should be suspected in conditions associated with muscle destruction, **rhabdomyolysis**. Box 6-13 list conditions associated with **myoglobinuria**, myoglobin in the urine.

Myoglobin is more toxic to renal tubules than hemoglobin and can lead to acute renal failure. The color of the patient's serum may help differentiate between hemoglobin and myoglobin; patients with hemoglobinuria usually have a pink or red serum, patients with myoglobinuria have a normal yellow serum because myoglobin is rapidly cleared from serum, Myoglobin can be measured by specific immunochemical tests.

A simple chemical screen can differentiate myoglobin from hemoglobin. Add 80% ammonium sulfate to urine, centrifuge, and test for blood using the reagent strip discussed below. If it's positive, myoglobin is present; if negative, it's hemoglobin because hemoglobin is precipitated by ammonium sulfate. After centrifugation, myoglobin will be present as a red supernatant; a clear supernatant indicates hemoglobin. Precipitated hemoglobin is centrifuged to the sediment at the bottom of the tube.

BOX 6-12 Conditions Associated with Hematuria and Hemoglobinuria

Hematuria
- Renal disease/dysfunction
  - Glomerulonephritis
  - Pyelonephritis
  - Cystitis
- Systemic lupus nephritis
- Renal calculi
- Tumors/Cancer (kidney, bladder, prostate)
- Trauma, e.g., contact sports
- Exposure to toxic chemicals or drugs, e.g., NSAIDs, cyclophosphamide (Cytoxan)
- Benign prostatic hypertrophy
- Strenuous exercise, e.g., marathon running
- Generalized bleeding disorders
- Anticoagulant therapy
- Acute febrile episodes
- Appendicitis
- Contaminant during menstruation
- Smoking

Hemoglobinuria
- Hemolytic anemias
- Transfusion reactions
- Severe burns
- Infections, e.g., syphilis, malaria
- Strenuous exercise

BOX 6-13 Conditions Associated with Myoglobinuria

- Trauma
- Crushing injury
- Convulsions, seizures, epilepsy
- Muscle-wasting diseases, e.g., muscular dystrophy
- Extensive exertion
- Alcoholic myopathy, alcoholic overdose
- Drug abuse, e.g., heroin addiction
- Cholesterol-lowering medications, e.g., statins

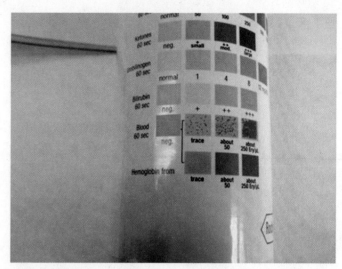

■ FIGURE 6-5 Blood and Hemoglobin

Blood Testing

Reagent Strip Reactions

The chemical tests for blood utilize the peroxidase activity of hemoglobin to catalyze a reaction between hydrogen peroxide and a chromogen, *tetramethylbenzidine*, to produce an oxidized chromogen, which is blue-green. The peroxidase activity of heme releases oxygen from the peroxide contained in the reagent strip, and the released oxygen reacts with the reduced chromogen to yield an oxidized, colored chromogen. The reaction is illustrated in Equation 6.5.

Two color charts correspond to reactions with hematuria and hemoglobinuria (Figure 6-5 ■). With hematuria, intact RBCs are lysed when they come into contact with the pad, and the liberated hemoglobin produces an isolated reaction, resulting in a speckled pattern. The degree of hematuria can be estimated by the intensity of the speckled pattern. In hemoglobinuria the pad is a uniform color with yellow, a negative reaction, to green to blue corresponding to the amount of hemoglobin present.

The reaction is graded negative, small, moderate, or large, or $1+, 2+, 3+$. The peroxidase reaction can detect 5 to 10 RBCs/μL and is slightly more sensitive to free hemoglobin.

Interfering Substances

False Positive

False positive reactions can be caused by menstrual or hemorrhoidal contamination. Vegetable peroxidase in the urine will react like heme and give a positive reaction. Bacterial enzymes or microbial peroxidases, e.g., *Escherichia coli* peroxidase, also react with the chromogen. Contamination with providone-iodine used in surgical procedures will result in a positive reaction due to the strong oxidizing property of iodine.

False Negative

High levels of ascorbic acid (Vitamin C), which is a reducing substance, react with the H_2O_2 so it cannot react with the chromogen, but usually there is no interference at reasonable (normal) levels. High urinary nitrite from a severe UTI may result in a false negative reaction. Urine with a high specific gravity and protein has a reduced sensitivity to the heme peroxidase reaction and may not react at lower levels. A pH less than 5.0 may inhibit hemolysis on the pad, leading to a negative reaction. The presence of Captopril and formalin are known to cause false negatives. False negatives may also be caused by poor technique and using an unmixed urine with the RBCs settled to the bottom of the container, resulting in a negative or falsely low reaction.

MINI-CASE 6-4

Cassandra, a 20-year-old long distance runner went to the Health Center for her physical following the first practice of the season.

Routine Urinalysis

Macroscopic:

Color:	Amber
Appearance:	Clear
Specific Gravity:	1.028
pH:	7.0
Glucose:	Neg
Bilirubin:	Neg
Ketones:	Neg
Blood:	1+
Protein:	Trace (SSA = trace) 5-20 mg/dL
Urobilinogen:	4 mg/dL

$$\text{H}_2\text{O}_2 + \underset{\text{(tetramethylbenzidine)}}{\text{Chromogen}} \xrightarrow[\text{(peroxidase activity)}]{\text{heme}} \text{Oxidized chromogen} + \text{H}_2\text{O} \qquad (6\text{-}5)$$

Nitrite:	Neg
Leukocyte Esterase:	Trace

Microscopic:

WBCs:	10-20/HPF
RBCs:	30-40/HPF
Epithelial cells:	Rare squamous/HPF
Casts:	10-20 Hyaline/LPF
	10-15 Granular/LPF
Bacteria:	Neg
Crystals:	Neg

Questions to Consider

1. What are the abnormal or discrepant results?
2. List five possible explanations for these abnormal results.
3. Should Cassandra be concerned about these results?
4. What is the most likely explanation for the abnormal results?
5. What would the physician do to follow up with this athlete?

LEUKOCYTES

Leukocyturia or **pyuria** is the presence of white blood cells in the urine and often indicates the presence of an infection in the upper or lower urinary tract. **Leukocyte esterase (LE)** is an enzyme found in the primary granules of polymorphonuclear neutrophils (PMNs), which are the most common leukocytes found in response to a bacterial infection. Leukocyte esterase is positive whether the WBCs are lysed or intact.

Clinical Significance

The leukocyte esterase reaction should be interpreted in conjunction with nitrite, which is present in UTIs or bacteriuria. Both are useful in screening urine specimens for culture. Leukocyte esterase is also present in urinary tract infections not caused by gram negative bacteria, e.g., gram positive bacteria, yeast, and viruses.

Sterile pyuria, leukocytes with no bacteria, may also be associated with urethritis, bladder tumors, viral infections, nephrolithiasis, exercise, glomerulonephritis, and use of corticosteroids.[14]

Leukocyte Testing

Reagent Strip

The leukocyte esterase reaction is based on an acid ester and a diazonium salt. An indoxylcarbonic acid ester is cleaved by LE to indoxyl, and the aromatic compound reacts with the diazonium salt to form a purple azo dye, as shown in Equation 6.6.

★ **TABLE 6-5** Leukocyte Esterase and Sediment Interpretation

Reagent Strip	Sediment	Interpretation
+	+	• WBCs in sediment

0	+	• False negative reagent strip
		  • > glucose, > protein, >>SG
		  • Ascorbic acid
		  • Antibiotics
		• Defective/outdated reagent strips
		• NOT WBCs

+	0	• Lysed WBCs • Strong oxidizers, bleach (false positive) • Highly pigmented urines

The sensitivity of LE is 5–15 cells /hpf. It also has the longest reaction time of the reagent strip analytes, 2 minutes.

Interfering Substances

False Positive

Urine containers contaminated with strong oxidizing agents such as bleach and formalin will give a false positive reaction. Another source of false positives is contamination with vaginal discharge that contains leukocytes. Pigmented urine due to food or drug metabolites may mask the color or resemble a positive reaction.

False Negative

Urine with increased glucose, a high specific gravity, and high protein has a decreased sensitivity and will yield a negative or falsely low result. The presence of antibiotics, e.g., cephalexin, tetracycline, and gentamicin, may also cause falsely low or negative results. Ascorbic acid reacts with the diazonium salt, interfering with the leukocyte esterase reaction. Table 6-5 ★ differentiates between reagent strip and microscopic results for WBCs.

☑ **CHECKPOINT 6-4**

1. Following precipitation of a clear, red urine with ammonium sulfate, a clear, colorless supernatant (neg: blood) indicates the presence of
   (a) hemoglobin.
   (b) myoglobin.
   (c) RBCs.
   (d) leukocytes.
2. A speckled pattern on a blood pad points to
   (a) hemoglobin.
   (b) myoglobin.
   (c) RBCs

Leukocyte Esterase

Indoxylcarbonic acid ester $\rightarrow$ indoxyl + diazonium salt $\rightarrow$ purple azo dye (6-6)

3. High levels of ascorbic acid may cause false negative results in all of the following EXCEPT:
   (a) blood.
   (b) glucose.
   (c) protein.
   (d) nitrite.
   (e) leukocytes.

4. Why is it possible to have a positive LE reaction and NOT see any leukocytes in the microscopic sediment?

NITRITE

Nitrite is produced by the reduction of nitrate by the enzyme nitrate reductase by gram negative bacteria. Nitrite is not normally present in urine. The presence of nitrite in the urine can be used to detect bacteria; therefore, it can be used to screen for UTIs.

Clinical Significance

Nitrite can detect UTIs. Cystitis, inflammation or infection of the bladder, is the most common. Bacteria travel up the urinary tract through the urethra to the bladder. UTIs are eight times more prevalent in women than men due to the shorter urethra, providing a shorter distance for the bacteria to travel. Pyelonephritis is inflammation or infection of the kidney, most commonly with gram negative bacteria such as *Escherichia coli*, Klebsiella, or Proteus species.

Nitrite can be used to monitor or evaluate the effectiveness of antibiotic therapy. Nitrite is valuable in monitoring patients at high risk for developing UTIs: patients with recurring infections; patients with diabetes mellitus; and pregnant women.

Nitrite Testing

Reagent Strip

The nitrite test pad is based on the **Greiss reaction**, which involves diazotization of nitrite with an aromatic amine to form a diazonium salt. Any shade of pink is interpreted as a positive reaction (see Equation 6.7).

Interfering Substances

False Positive

Improperly collected or stored specimens containing bacteria will yield a false positive or a stronger positive result. Containers contaminated with strong oxidizing agents will also give a false positive reaction. Azo-containing compounds or dyes, which turn urine red, may mask the color reaction.

False Negative

Not all bacteria produce nitrate reductase, although the bacteria most commonly associated with UTIs do reduce nitrate. Gram negative bacteria are nitrite positive; Gram positive bacteria and yeast are nitrite negative. Bacteria need time to reduce nitrate (at least 4 hours); therefore, first morning specimens, which have been in the bladder a longer period of time, are more likely to be positive. Random specimens may produce a false negative reaction because the bacteria have not had sufficient time to reduce nitrate to nitrite. Nitrate, from vegetables in the diet, has to be present in the urine in sufficient quantities to be reduced to nitrite. In severe infections, bacteria may reduce all of the nitrate to nitrite and all the way to nitrogen, which is not detected and yields a negative result.

Another cause of false negatives is the presence of antibiotics, which inhibit bacterial metabolism. Ascorbic acid may interfere with the diazo reaction, causing a false negative or delayed reaction. See Box 6-14 for a list of conditions associated with false negative nitrite reactions.

BOX 6-14   Causes of False Negative Nitrite

- Bacteria that do not produce nitrate reductase, e.g., Gram positive bacteria, yeast
- Random urine that has not been in the bladder at least 4 hours
- Insufficient nitrate in the urine
- Severe infection with high levels of bacteria reducing nitrate to nitrite to nitrogen
- Antibiotic that inhibits bacterial metabolism
- Ascorbic acid

$$\text{Acid pH}$$
$$\text{Nitrite + para-arsanilic acid (or sulfanilamide)} \rightarrow \text{diazonium compound (pink)} \tag{6-7}$$

Key Points to Remember

- The chemical examination component of the routine urinalysis is comprised of a number of chemical reactions on the test pads of reagent strips.

- The pH of the urine is affected by many factors, e.g., diet, age of specimen, and renal function. It can help to diagnose various conditions associated with acid-base imbalances. Acid urine is associated with a high-protein diet, dehydration, and emphysema (respiratory acidosis); alkaline urine is found in urinary tract infections, chronic renal failure, and respiratory diseases associated with hyperventilation. The pH is measured using a double indicator system: methyl red for the acid range 4 to 6, and bromthymol blue covers the alkaline range 6-9.

- Proteinuria is an important indicator of renal disease. Proteinuria can be prerenal, renal, or postrenal. Prerenal proteinuria, or overflow proteinuria, occurs before the kidney, and is usually associated with low molecular weight proteins. Renal proteinuria may be caused by damage to the glomerular membrane by toxic substances and renal infections, e.g., pyelonephritis. Postrenal proteinuria is as a result of protein produced by the urinary or genital tract due to inflammation, malignancy, or injury.

- The protein reagent strip reaction is based on the protein error of indicators. At a constant pH, tetrabromphenol blue and other pH indicators are one color in the presence of protein and another color when protein is not present.

- Glucose testing, for the screening and monitoring of patients for diabetes mellitus, is one of the most common procedures. Glucosuria can be categorized into prerenal or renal causes. Prerenal glucosuria is related to diabetes mellitus, pancreatic disease, heavy exercise or physical stress, drugs/medications, and hyperthyroidism. Renal glucosuria is associated with conditions affecting tubular reabsorption, e.g., Fanconi's syndrome. The reagent strip test for glucose is based on the glucose oxidase/peroxidase reaction and is specific for glucose. The confirmatory test is Clinitest, a copper reduction method, which reacts with all reducing substances including glucose.

- Ketones, comprised of acetone, acetoacetic acid, and β-hydroxybutyric acid, are formed as a result of incomplete fat metabolism. In diabetes mellitus, glucose cannot be metabolized for energy because of a deficiency or lack of insulin; therefore, fats are metabolized for energy. Examples of other conditions that are characterized by an increased loss or intake of carbohydrates are digestive disturbances, anorexia, starvation, and malabsorption. The reagent strip reaction for ketones is Legal's test based on the reaction of acetoacetic acid with sodium nitroprusside. Glycine is added to the test pad to allow acetone to react; therefore, the only ketone not detected is β-hydroxybutyric acid.

- Bilirubinuria may indicate liver disease, e.g., hepatitis and cirrhosis. Bilirubin is formed from the catabolism of hemoglobin from old RBCs, and conjugated or direct bilirubin can be excreted in the urine. Bilirubinuria can be classified as prehepatic, hepatic, or posthepatic jaundice. Prehepatic jaundice is caused by increased RBC destruction or hemolysis, e.g., hemolytic anemia. Hepatic jaundice is often seen in liver diseases, including hepatitis and cirrhosis. Posthepatic jaundice is caused as a result of bile duct obstruction by gallstones or cancer. The reagent strip reaction for bilirubin is based on the diazo reaction, whereby bilirubin is coupled with a diazonium salt to form azobilirubin, a colored compound. The Ictotest tablet test is the confirmatory test based on a more sharply defined diazo reaction.

- Urobilinogen, also a degradation of hemoglobin, is produced in the intestine by a reduction of bilirubin by the intestinal bacteria. It is important in monitoring liver disease and also hemolytic disorders. The reagent strip reaction is a modification of Ehrlich's reaction: ρ-dimethylaminobenzaldehyde turns a cherry red color in the presence of urobilinogen and other Ehrlich's reactive substances.

- Hematuria, the presence of blood in the urine, and hemoglobinuria, the presence of hemoglobin in the urine, are very important tests to detect renal disease and other conditions. Examples of conditions associated with hematuria are renal disease, renal calculi, trauma, tumors, and exposure to toxic chemicals or drugs. Hemolytic anemias, transfusion reactions, severe burns, and strenuous exercise can result in hemoglobinuria. The reagent strip reaction is based on the peroxidase activity of hemoglobin to catalyze a reaction between hydrogen peroxide and a chromogen, tetramethylbenzidine, to produce an oxidized chromogen, which is blue green.

- Leukocyturia or pyuria, the presence of white blood cells in the urine, indicates the presence of an infection in the upper or lower urinary tract. The primary granules of polymorphonuclear neutrophils (PMNs) contain leukocyte esterase, which cleaves an indoxylcarbonic acid ester to form an aromatic compound that reacts with a diazonium salt to form a purple azo dye.

- Nitrite detects the presence of Gram negative bacteria in the upper or lower urinary tract and is used to detect urinary tract infections. It useful to monitor patients at high risk for developing urinary tract infections: patients with recurring infections, diabetes mellitus, and pregnant women. The reagent pad is based on the Greiss reaction, which involves the diazotization of nitrite with an aromatic amine to form a diazonium salt.

Review Questions

1. To ensure the precision and accuracy of the reagent test strips used for the chemical analysis of urine, it is necessary that (Objective 3)

   A. positive controls be run on a daily basis.

   B. negative controls be run on a daily basis.

   C. positive and negative controls be run on a daily basis.

   D. positive controls be run on a daily basis and negative controls on a weekly basis.

   E. positive controls be run on a daily basis and negative controls be run when opening a new bottle of test strips.

2. The double indicator system employed by commercial reagent strip companies to determine pH uses which two indicator dyes? (Objective 4)

   A. Methyl orange and bromphenol blue

   B. Methyl red and bromthymol blue

   C. Phenol red and thymol blue

   D. Phenolphthalein and litmus

3. A urine with a low pH contains a (Objective 5)

   A. high concentration of chloride ions.

   B. high concentration of hydrogen ions.

   C. low concentration of chloride ions.

   D. low concentration of hydrogen ions.

4. Which statement regarding urine pH is true? (Objective 5)

   A. High protein diets promote an alkaline urine pH.

   B. pH tends to decrease as urine is stored.

   C. Contamination should be suspected if urine pH is less than 4.5.

   D. Bacteriuria is most often associated with a low urine pH.

5. The range of urinary pH for healthy individual varies from (Objective 5)

   A. 4.6 to 8.0.

   B. 2.0 to 5.5.

   C. 6.0 to 9.0.

   D. 7.0 to 10.0.

6. Which of the following is most likely to cause a false-positive reagent strip test for protein? (Objective10)

   A. Urine of high SG

   B. Highly buffered alkaline urine

   C. Bence-Jones proteinuria

   D. Salicylates

7. The protein section of the reagent strip is MOST sensitive to (Objective 8)

   A. albumin.

   B. mucoprotein.

   C. Bence-Jones protein.

   D. globulin.

8. Which of the following is a cause of prerenal proteinuria? (Objective 7)

   A. Prostatitis

   B. Multiple myeloma

   C. Pre-eclampsia

   D. Diabetes mellitus

9. The labstix (reagent strip) determination for protein in urine is based on (Objective 8)

   A. precipitation of protein on a mat.

   B. protein error of indicators.

   C. nitrogen binding with acid.

   D. albumin salting out.

10. The sulfosalicylic acid reaction with urine detects (Objective 8)

    A. protein.

    B. glucose.

    C. ketone.

    D. bilirubin.

11. The two enzymes used in the Chemstrip reagent strip for urine glucose are (Objective 11)

    A. glucose dehydrogenase and glucose oxidase.

    B. glucose oxidase and peroxidase.

    C. glucose dehydrogenase and peroxidase.

    D. none of the above.

12. Clinitest tablets measure (Objective 12)

    A. all reducing substances.

    B. only glucose.

    C. glucose and galactose.

    D. galactose.

13. Which of the following is the primary reagent in the copper reduction tablet (Clinitest)? (Objective 12)

    A. Sodium carbonate

    B. Copper sulfate

    C. Glucose oxidase

    D. A polymerized diazonium salt

14. The normal renal threshold for glucose is (Objective 10)

    A. 75–85 mg/dL.

    B. 100–115 mg/dL.

    C. 130–145 mg/dL.

    D. 160–180 mg / dL.

15. While performing a Clinitest, you observe that the color changes rapidly from blue to orange and then back to blue. You should (Objective 12)

    A. report the test as negative because the final reaction color is blue.

    B. report the test as negative because the brief orange color probably was from detergent in the tube.

    C. repeat the test using fewer drops of urine to check for "pass through phenomenon."

    D. repeat the test using more drops.

16. Ketone bodies are excreted in the urine in ketosis. The disease most commonly responsible for this condition is (Objective 15)

    A. leukemia.

    B. diabetes mellitus.

    C. acute pancreatitis.

    D. multiple myeloma.

    E. gout.

17. The active ingredient in Acetest for the detection of ketones is (Objective 16)

    A. iodine.

    B. p-dimethylaminobenzaldehyde.

    C. potassium permanganate.

    D. sodium nitroprusside.

18. Ketones in the urine are due to (Objective 15)

    A. complete utilization of fatty acids.

    B. faulty fat metabolism.

    C. high-carbohydrate diets.

    D. renal tubular dysfunction.

19. Tests for urine bilirubin may be used to assess (Objective 18)

    A. hormone function.

    B. kidney function.

    C. liver function.

    D. white cell destruction.

20. The conjugation of bilirubin occurs mostly in the (Objective 18)

    A. kidney.

    B. pancreas.

    C. liver.

    D. reticuloendothelial system.

    E. erythrocyte.

21. Bilirubin is the breakdown product of (Objective 18)

    A. taurocholate.

    B. glycocholate.

    C. cholesterol.

    D. hemoglobin.

    E. stercobilin.

22. Which of the following is NOT true about the Ictotest? (Objective 19)

    A. Bilirubin is concentrated on the surface of an absorbent pad.

    B. Interfering pigments can be washed into the pad.

    C. It uses the same principle as the reagent strip.

    D. It is less sensitive than the reagent strip test.

23. Urobilinogen excretion is greatest in (Objective 20)

    A. a first morning specimen.

    B. any random specimen.

    C. a specimen collected during the hours of 2–4 p.m.

    D. there is no diurnal variation.

24. Which of the reagents below is used to detect urobilinogen in urine? (Objective 21)

    A. p-dinitrobenzene

    B. p-aminosalicylate

    C. p-dimethylaminobenzaldehyde

    D. p-dichloroaniline

25. Reagent strip reactions for blood are based on the (Objective 23)

    A. peroxidase activity of hemoglobin.

    B. oxidation of hemoglobin peroxidase.

    C. reaction of hemoglobin with bromthymol blue.

    D. reduction of a chromogen by hemoglobin.

26. A reagent strip test for blood is reported positive. No red blood cells are seen on the microscopic examination. The patient's condition is called (Objective 22)

    A. oliguria.

    B. hemoglobinuria.

    C. hemosiderinuria.

    D. hematuria.

27. Leukocyte reagent strips are used to detect leukocyte (Objective 25)

    A. peroxidase.

    B. esterases.

    C. hydroxylase.

    D. phosphatase.

28. A false-negative leukocyte esterase reaction may be caused by (Objective 25)

    A. the presence of eosinophils and basophils.

    B. increased bacteria.

    C. lysed leukocytes.

    D. failure to wait 2 minutes to read the reaction.

29. Nitrite testing is used to detect (Objective 26)

    A. WBCs.

    B. RBCs.

    C. bilirubin.

    D. bacteria.

30. Detection of the presence of nitrite in the urine is useful (Objective 26)

    A. in the detection of asymptomatic urinary tract infection.

    B. in the detection of infection by Gram positive organisms.

    C. in the prevention of kidney damage by treatment of early infection.

    D. a and c.

Level II

1. A condition characterized by increased excretion of protein in the urine during the day while at night there is normal excretion of protein is known as (Objective 1)

    A. functional proteinuria.

    B. Bence-Jones proteinuria.

    C. orthostatic proteinuria.

    D. isosthenuria.

    E. hyposthenuria.

2. Bence-Jones proteins are found in (Objective 1)

    A. pneumonia.

    B. infectious hepatitis.

    C. multiple myeloma.

    D. galactosemia.

    E. normal individuals.

3. A negative glucose oxidase test and a positive test for reducing sugars (Clinitest) indicates (Objective 3)

    A. true glycosuria.

    B. the presence of a nonglucose-reducing sugar such as galactose.

    C. false negative glucose oxidase reaction.

    D. a trace quantity of glucose.

4. The following urinalysis results are obtained: (Objective 3)

    Glucose by reagent strip: positive

    Ketones by reagent strip: positive

    These results are *most* consistent with

    A. starvation.

    B. polydipsia.

    C. diabetes mellitus.

    D. diabetes insipidus.

5. Linda's routine urinalysis report indicated a 1+ glucose, and her plasma glucose was 99 mg/dL. Explain the clinical significance of the positive urine glucose and a normal plasma glucose.

6. Diana's routine urinalysis reported a 1+ positive bilirubin on the reagent strip and a 2+ Ictotest. Four hours later a clinical laboratory scientist student reported a negative bilirubin.

    A. Discuss one reason for the discrepant result.

    B. Explain why the CLS student reported a negative result.

Endnotes

1. Chemstrip 6,7, 8, 9, 10 with SG Product Insert. Roche Diagnostics, Indianapolis, IN (1999).

2. Ibid.

3. Pandey, K. Acidic Urine. 2011. www.buzzle.com/articles/acidic-urine.html. Accessed September 16, 2011.

4. Urine pH. www.rnceus.com/ua/uaph.html. Accessed September 16, 2011.

5. Carroll, Michael F. *Proteinuria is Adults: A Diagnostic Approach.* American Family Physician. (September 15, 2000). www.aafp.org/afp/20000915/1333.html. Accessed September 22, 2011.

6. Rose, Burton, and Herron, John. *Orthostatic or postural proteinuria.* www.uptodate.com/contents/orthostatic-or-postural-proteinuria. Accessed October 5, 2011.

7. *Causes of Glycosuria.* www.rightdiagnosis.com/symptoms/glycosuria/causes.htm. Accessed October 12, 2011.

8. Willacy, Hayley MD. *Glycosuria.* www.patient.co.uk/printer.asp?doc=40001080. Accessed September 29, 2011.

9. Haldeman-Englert, Chad. *Galactosemia.* www.nim.nih.gov./medlineplus/ency/article/000366.htm. Accessed November 1, 2011.

10. Dugdale, David C. *Ketones-urine.* www.nlm.nih.gov/medlineplus/ency/article/003585.htm. Accessed October 12, 2011/

11. Rull, Gurvinder. *Urine Ketones-Meanings and False Positives.* www.patient.co.uk/printer.asp?doc=40001083. Accessed October 12, 2011.

12. Sunheimer, Robert & Graves, Linda. *Clinical Laboratory Chemistry.* Upper Saddle River: Pearson (2011), 417-419.

13. Mayo Clinic. Blood in Urine (hematuria). www.mayoclinic.com/health/blood-in-urine/DS01013/METHOD. Accessed November 9, 2011.

14. Simerville, Jeff A. *Urinalysis: A Comprehensive Review.* American Family Physician. 2005 March 15.

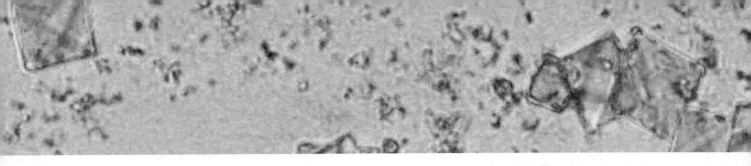

7

The Microscope

Objectives

LEVEL I

1. List the components of the light microscope.
2. List the engraved numbers and markings on the objectives and define each with respect to the magnification of a specimen.
3. State the importance of the condenser in microscope illumination.
4. Calculate overall magnification as the product of objective and ocular magnification values.
5. Explain the reason for adjusting the microscope to attain Köhler illumination. List the steps to adjust the microscope for this method of illumination.
6. Recall important steps in proper microscope maintenance and handling.
7. Explain the basic principles of phase contrast, polarizing, dark field, and fluorescent microscopy.

LEVEL II

1. Discuss the principles of chromatic aberration, spherical aberration, resolution, and resolving power.
2. State the important factors involved in adjusting a phase contrast microscope to obtain the proper phase image.
3. Define birefringence with regard to crystal structure and polarized microscopy.

Chapter Outline

Key Terms

Achromatic
Abbé condenser
Annulus
Birefringence
Brightfield microscopy
Chromatic aberration
Compound microscope

Condenser
Condenser diaphragm
Contrast
Depth of field
Diffraction
Focal length
Focal point

Iris diaphragm
Köhler illumination
Numerical aperture (NA)
Optical tube length
Parfocal
PLAN
Resolution

Resolving power
Reticle
Rheostat
Spherical aberration
Working distance

A CASE IN POINT

A laboratory microscopist consistently had problems focusing the microscope causing breakage to both the coverslip and slide and specimen contamination of the objective. Consequently, the next tech to use the microscope would find a dirty and damaged objective that must be attended to before use of the microscope.

Questions to Consider

1. What is the technique for properly focusing a microscope using the 100× objective?

2. What are some maintenance and clean-up procedures that can be completed to keep the objectives in good condition for the next user?

The microscope in use today is far different from the instruments of the 16th and 17th centuries. One of the earliest working microscopes, which was developed by Anton van Leeuwenhoek in 1673,[1] used a single lens and enabled the user to see living organisms invisible to the naked eye. The modern microscope achieves much higher magnification by using a multiple lens system.

The image in Figure 7-1 ■ of the microscope illustrates the outer structure and components of the basic microscope. A heavy base designed to decrease vibration of the specimen from the surrounding surface supports the optical components. The lens system within the tube resides at either end: the objective lens at the base and the ocular or eyepiece opposite to the base. The specimen or object is placed on a movable mechanical stage beneath the objective lens to allow the user the ability to position it easily for maximum visualization.

The **condenser**, located beneath the stage, focuses the light emitted from within the base of the microscope onto the specimen and influences the quality of the image seen. In **brightfield microscopy** light passes directly onto the objective and produces a brightly lit background. Increasing or decreasing the aperture size of the **iris** and **condenser diaphragms** can modify the amount of light to achieve optimum visualization of the specimen (Figure 7-2 ■). Additional components or alternate light sources may be used depending on the type of microscopy needed, such as polarization using special filters, interference or phase contrast, or dark field or fluorescence to produce different visual effects of the object.

CARE AND USE OF MICROSCOPES

The microscope is an expensive and useful tool in identifying cells and elements found in urine sediments and body fluids examined in the laboratory. It is essential that this tool be treated with utmost care and respect in order to use it to its maximal capacity. Each microscopist should follow the steps outlined in Box 7-1 to achieve the best results. What is seen microscopically is the result of good specimen preparation and intelligent use of the instrument.

Use both hands when transporting the instrument to another space. One hand firmly grasps the microscope arm while the other hand supports the heavy base. The workspace used should not be in close proximity to centrifugal vibration, which may cause harm to

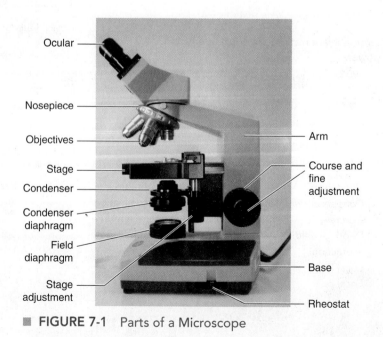

Ocular

Nosepiece

Objectives

Stage

Condenser

Condenser diaphragm

Field diaphragm

Stage adjustment

Arm

Course and fine adjustment

Base

Rheostat

■ **FIGURE 7-1**   Parts of a Microscope

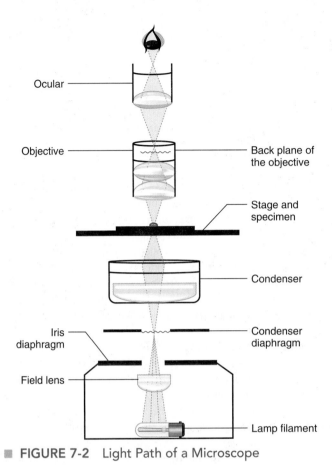

Ocular

Objective

Back plane of
the objective

Stage and
specimen

Condenser

Iris
diaphragm

Condenser
diaphragm

Field lens

Lamp filament

■ **FIGURE 7-2** Light Path of a Microscope

the instrumentation and poor visualization of the specimen. Place a dust cover over the instrument when not in use to keep dust from all surfaces because it abrades the glass surfaces and wears off the anti-reflection coatings.

For the sharpest images and maximal illumination attained, all glass surfaces in the optical path must be clean and highly polished. Objective lenses and eyepieces should be cleaned using proper lens cleaner and lens paper. Other forms of tissues or cloths may contain fibers that will scratch the lens surface and interfere with proper visualization of the specimen.

Controlling illumination in the microscope is the major procedure that must be mastered by the microscopist. Using **Köhler illumination** will provide uniform illumination of the field and maximal resolution of the microscopic detail. This is accomplished by focusing the image of the field diaphragm simultaneously in the same plane of focus as the image of the specimen using the steps provided later in this chapter.

Focusing the objective should be done in a manner that avoids damage to both the specimen slide and the objective. Placing the low objective close to the slide surface while viewing from the side and not through the oculars will avoid catastrophic results. The objective is now in a position closest to the slide and can be focused upward and away from the slide. Once the next highest objective is put into place, it is now easily focused using the fine adjustment for proper visualization.

MAGNIFICATION AND LIGHT

A simple handheld lens will magnify an object about six times. In a **compound microscope** the object is magnified by the first set of lenses, the objective, which is further enlarged by the second lens system, the ocular. The lens system of the light microscope displays detail in very small objects using light to perform the task.

The ability to view an object with no visual aid is limited by how much detail can be concentrated on the retina of the eye. Each ray of light projected onto the retinal surface must fall on a separate receptor in order to be seen as separate and distinct. When the object is brought closer to the eye, the object's image will cover more retinal receptors, more detail will be evident, and the **resolution** will improve. Unfortunately, as the object comes to within 10 inches of the eyes, both the ability to focus and the detail of the object are lost. The use of a magnification lens can increase the focus by spreading the image of a tiny

BOX 7-2   Köhler Illumination

1. Set the light source to approximately two-thirds brightness and focus the specimen using the 10× objective.

2. Open the iris diaphragm in the substage condenser to the largest setting and raise the condenser vertically to the highest point beneath the stage.

3. Close the field diaphragm to approximately one-third of the opening. This limits the size of the lighted field seen through the oculars. The edges of the field (the diaphragm image) encircle the lighted field, which should be centered. If the field is not centered, then the screws holding the condenser can be adjusted to center the image.

4. Lower the condenser until the edges of the field are focused.

5. Open the field diaphragm until the dark edges just disappear from view and the light from the condenser fills the field of vision. Opening the diaphragm too much will over-fill the field with light and cause glare and loss of contrast. **Contrast** is described as the difference in light intensity between the image and adjacent background relative to the overall background intensity. While viewing specimens through a microscope, difference in intensity and/or color create image contrast and will allow definitive features and details of the specimen to become visible. Using the lever (if available) on the condenser diaphragm, adjust the opening to match the objective in use.

6. Adjust the brightness of the light.

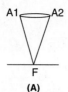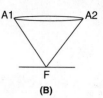

■ FIGURE 7-4   Angle of Aperture
Angle A1FA2 defines the angle of aperture and the cone of light which enters the lens and defines its resolving power.

The illumination system is the most important aspect of ensuring visualization of the specimen through the chosen objective. This system consists of the light source, usually a tungsten-halogen lamp or low voltage light bulb, the lens collector system placed in front of the light, and the substage condenser lens system. The light-gathering ability of the objective lens is proportional to the diameter of the cone of light entering the lens. This cone of light, called the *angle of aperture*, defines the resolving power of the lens. As the cone's angle increases, more light is allowed to enter the lens, and the resolving power increases (Figure 7-4 ■). Each objective lens is engraved with the value of its **numerical aperture (NA)**. This value is calculated using the angle of aperture, the resolving power, and the numerical value of light refraction, or the refractive index (RI). The refractive index is required in the calculation because different media refract, or bend, light rays to a different degree as they travel the path to the retina where the final image is formed.

Light refraction is an important concept when considering lenses and microscope systems. The lenses of the microscope are curved, and light will have a different refraction pattern passing through different areas of the curved surface. If the rays pass through the exact center of a convex or concave glass, there will be no **diffraction** of the light path. However, light passing through the outer edge of a convex glass will be diffracted inward to the center (converging) while light passing in the same area of a concave glass will bend the light rays out (diverging) (Figure 7-5 ■). The **focal point** of the converging rays of the

object over a larger area of the retina by increasing the visual angle (Figure 7-3 ■). The **resolving power** of a magnifying lens allows the observer to see separate and distinct points within the specimen. For example, what would be the resolving power of an image consisting of 100 lines drawn side by side within a one-centimeter space using a lens that allows the viewer to observe 100 separate lines? The answer is 100 lines per centimeter. A lens allowing less individual lines to be distinguished per centimeter would have lower resolving power.

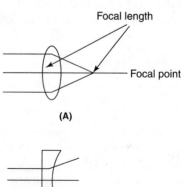

(A)

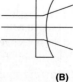

(B)

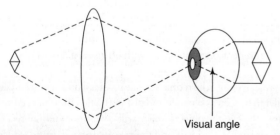

■ FIGURE 7-3   Visual Angle
Using magnification, the image of the tiny object is spread over a large retinal area. The increase in visual angle allows more detail to be seen.

■ FIGURE 7-5   Concave/Convex Lens and Refraction
(A) Convergence of light rays to a center focal point after passing through the center and outer edges of a convex lens. (B) Divergence of light rays after passing through a concave lens.

convex lens is the point at which the rays intersect. The distance from the focal point to the center of the lens describes the **focal length**.

The focal point and focal length are two aspects necessary to understand types of aberrations seen in images. When a lens fails to focus all wavelengths to the same convergence point, a color distortion occurs called **chromatic aberration**. Each wavelength of light has a different angle of refraction and therefore will converge at a slightly different focal point. The blue and red wavelengths are of concern because these will produce a colored halo effect and will distort the image projected through the microscope. **Spherical aberration** is due to the increased refraction of light rays when they strike a lens nearer to the edge rather than the center. This effect produces an imperfect image. The focus may be adjusted to view detail in either the outer edges or the center of the field but not both at once. To correct the distortion, concave and convex lenses are used together within the objective lens system to counteract both chromatic and spherical aberration. Objective lenses that correct chromatic aberration are termed **achromatic**.

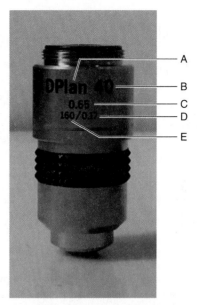

■ **FIGURE 7-6** Objective Lens With Engraving
(A) Plan/plano describes an objective corrected for lens curvature. (B) The lens magnification is 40 with (C) a numerical aperture of 0.65. This lens is appropriate for (E) an optical tube length of 160 mm and will accommodate (D) a coverslip thickness of 0.17 mm.

CHECKPOINT 7-1

1. The value of the resolving power, the angle of aperture, and the refractive index are used to calculate
   (a) the light intensity of the lamp.
   (b) the refraction ability of the lamp.
   (c) the numerical value of the objective.
   (d) the numerical aperture of the objective.

2. The resolving power of a magnification lens allows the observer to
   (a) add more light to the field.
   (b) see separate and distinct points within the specimen.
   (c) view the whole specimen with no detail.
   (d) add more depth of field to the sample.

3. The most important aspect of ensuring visualization of the specimen is
   (a) the objective.
   (b) illumination.
   (c) depth of field.
   (d) size of the object viewed.

4. Objectives are corrected for both
   (a) spherical and optical aberration.
   (b) light and dark.
   (c) spherical and chromatic aberration.
   (d) chromatic and optical aberration.

COMPONENTS

Objectives

A number of objectives are fitted to a rotating nosepiece, each of which is engraved with pertinent information about its specifications and capability (Figure 7-6 ■).

The *magnification factor* of the objective indicates the ratio of the size of the original image to the size of the image projected into the tube. Commonly encountered objectives have magnification powers of 4×, 10×, 20×, 40×, 50×, and 100×. These objectives are threaded at one end so that they can be screwed into the nosepiece, which rotates through the position directly above the stage. The objectives are maneuvered into position above the specimen by turning the knurled ring on the nosepiece. The objectives may be damaged or become misaligned if strained and should not be used as "handles."

The *numerical aperture (NA)* of the objective is by far the most important indication of the quality of the image obtained by any objective. The number inscribed pertains to the light-gathering ability of the objective and relates to its resolving power. Low magnifications of 4× and 10× (low power) do not require fine detail and high resolution, therefore the value of the NA is relatively low. Conversely, higher magnifications will have a higher NA value. Almost all objectives are designed for "dry" use, meaning the material or medium between the front end of the objective lens and the upper surface is air. Remember, the NA is related to the refractive index (RI) of the medium. Air has an RI of 1.0. At the higher magnifications, due to the limitations of manufacturing lenses, the highest available theoretical value for NA is 0.95. Other objectives of high magnification are designed for use as a "wet" lens if fluid lies between the lens and specimen. These immersion objectives will most often use oil as the medium, which has an RI of 1.5. The oil helps to curtail the loss of light rays by refracting them toward the lens aperture. This allows more light to enter (a larger cone of light to the lens) and thus will increase the resolution (Figure 7-7 ■).

Depth of field is another area of specimen magnification that is affected by the NA of the objective. The depth of field of a specimen will range from 0.01 mm with an objective of lower NA to 0.004 mm

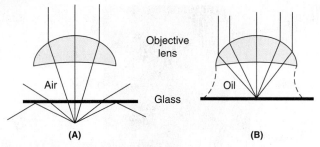

■ **FIGURE 7-7**   Oil Immersion
(A) Air resides in the space between the objective lens and the glass slide resulting loss of light rays and, therefore, lower resolution. (B) Oil immersion allows for more light rays to be captured by the objective resulting in higher resolution. Lens (B) has a higher numerical aperture than lens (A).

with an objective of an NA that is much higher. In each case a different level of the specimen is being viewed. Examining urine sediments involves a liquid specimen, which is dispersed between the glass slide and the coverslip. This requires a lower magnification (10× and 40×) and therefore an objective of lower NA so the elements within the space can be seen. It is important to remember to allow any specimen contained in a fluid to settle to the surface of the slide in order to limit the depth of field where the elements are located. In contrast, when examining any dried and stained preparation that has minimal depth of field, it is in the best interest of the microscopist to use a high magnification (100×), high NA objective, and oil immersion to view the specimen.

The **optical tube length** and the thickness of the coverslip used in slide preparation are indicated on the objective. The length of the tube dictates the distance between the two objective systems and is standardized at 160 mm for most microscopes. This is the measured length described as the distance between the objective read focal plane and the intermediate or primary image at the fixed diaphragm of the eyepiece. This will affect the magnification power of the microscope and thus the correct objective lens must be used.

The thickness of the cover glass to be used in slide preparation is marked on the objective separated by a slash mark from the *optical tube length*. The cover glass is like another lens through which the light passes; it will affect the path of the light that enters the objective. A very thick cover glass will also affect the **working distance** between its surface and the surface of the objective. If the mechanical means to raise and lower the objective is hindered while attempting to focus, the cover glass may be shattered and the objective ruined or damaged. Therefore, the correct cover glass is essential to allow the objective to get close enough to bring the specimen into focus.

Optical correction is the final piece of information engraved on the objectives and refers to correction for spherical or chromatic aberration. The most commonly used terms to indicate color correction are (1) achromat, (2) apochromat, and (3) fluorite. In instances of chromatic correction, the more expensive lenses correct for more colors of the spectrum (red, green, blue) and will provide an image

of true color and no distortion. The PLANO or **PLAN** objective is corrected for curvature of the objective and produces an image that appears flat. These objectives provide a larger field of view without distortion of focus to either the edge or center of the field. In some cases, there may also be a notation for "oil" or "water" to indicate the medium used with an immersion lens. In addition, the objective may indicate "phase" or "ph," which means it contains the annular rings required within the objective for use with phase contrast microscopy. The notation "pol" indicates the use of the objective with polarized light.

MINI-CASE 7-1

A student carefully focuses the low power objective on a specimen. After rotating the next higher power objective into position, the student cannot bring the specimen into focus using the fine adjustment. After careful inspection, the student notices that the objective has been loosened in the nosepiece socket.

Questions to Consider

1. What is the likely reason for the loose objective?

2. How can this be avoided in the future?

Most manufacturers currently produce objectives that are described as **parfocal**. This means that as the objectives are switched from one to another, only a very slight adjustment is needed to restore optimum focus of the image. This is important when using an oil immersion lens. The specimen can be focused using a dry lens of lower magnification. When the oil drop is added to the specimen before moving the oil immersion lens into use, there is very little focal adjustment needed to see the image at high magnification clearly. This keeps the objective safe within its small working distance.

Ocular Lens

The ocular lens system contains the eye lens and the field lens. The latter receives the light rays from the objective to form the image inside the ocular itself. A diaphragm exists within the ocular, which forms the field of vision and is the space where a tool for measurement, or **reticle**, may be placed. This reticle may be a micrometer scale useful for measurement, which is superimposed on the image. Ocular lenses are manufactured in several different magnifications, including, 6×, 10×, or 15×. It is important that the ocular lens be optically compatible with the objective lens used in order to achieve the best quality image projected by the objective lens system.

Once the magnification power of both the objective and ocular lenses are known, the overall magnification of the specimen can be calculated. For a microscope with an optical tube length of 160mm the magnification of the image is calculated using Equation 7.1.

(Objective Magnification) × (Ocular Magnification) = Overall Magnification   (7-1)

Light Source, Condenser, Diaphragm

The light source, condenser, and diaphragm affect the illumination of the specimen, which is the most important aspect of the working microscope.

Methods of illumination have progressed from using reflected sunlight, candles, or an oil lamp to placing a light source within the base of the instrument. The **rheostat** located on the microscope base controls the light intensity. Several different types of light sources are used in microscopy, including halogen, light-emitting diode (LED), or tungsten-halogen, which produce a more intense "white light." Microscopes using tungsten-only lamps require a blue filter usually placed on the outer surface of the field diaphragm in order to compensate for the yellow light produced by the tungsten filament.

A substage condenser is used to focus the transmitted light from the base of the microscope onto the specimen. The construction of this lens system is similar to that of the objective. This system contains two or more lenses to achieve focus of the specimen and may correct for optical aberration. The NA of the condenser should match that of the objective in use to achieve maximum resolution. A very common type of condenser, the **Abbé condenser**, consists of two lenses and has no correction for either spherical or chromatic aberration. This is the least expensive condenser and works fine in student microscopes at the lower magnifications of 10× and 40× (NA ≥0.75). As the NA of the objective increases, the aberrations in the Abbé condenser will not produce a cone of light large enough to fill the objective in use (NA = 0.95), thus producing improper illumination. Some condensers are equipped with a lens that swings out and away from the substage field. When used, this auxiliary lens increases the NA of the condenser to approximately 0.95 and will provide proper illumination for 100× objectives.

The condenser can be properly aligned with the objectives above the stage by use of the setscrews located on the condenser if needed. This allows the light to fill the objective properly. Misalignment of the condenser causes uneven illumination and a refractile quality to the image in brightfield microscopy. The available transmitted light projected to the specimen is also increased or decreased via the field diaphragm located in the base of the microscope and the iris diaphragm within the substage condenser.

Köhler Illumination

Optimum specimen illumination is obtained by properly focusing the light through the technique of Köhler illumination, which is recommended for all laboratory microscopes.

The collector lens in the base of the microscope enlarges and projects the image of the lamp filament onto the aperture diaphragm of the substage condenser. This allows the light source to be focused below the condenser, permitting illumination of the specimen using the condenser. The vertical adjustment of the condenser obtains the correct cone of light corresponding to the aperture of the objective resulting in optimum resolution of the specimen image. Proper alignment of the condenser can be achieved for Köhler illumination by using the method outlined in Box 7-2 each time the microscope is used.

These adjustments have corrected the light path and focused the light to obtain maximum illumination for the best resolution of the specimen. Further adjustments to light level are made by the rheostat and not by altering the vertical position of the substage condenser.

Wet Preparation of Specimens

Köhler illumination is the preferred method for microscopic evaluation of fixed and stained specimens. However, wet preparations of transparent or translucent objects as seen in urine sediment are often hard to visualize using this method. The specimen is prepared by placing a drop of sediment in urine on a glass slide with a coverslip. The sample is viewed under low power (10×). By increasing the light and lowering the condenser, light rays reflect in a more oblique pattern from the objects in the field producing more contrast. In this way transparent objects that have the same refractive index as the surrounding medium are easier to see. The condenser is raised when switching to high power (40×) to introduce more light into the field.

CHECKPOINT 7-2

1. To limit depth of field and find an element in a liquid medium it is important to
   (a) increase the light.
   (b) let the specimen settle to the slide surface.
   (c) use an objective of higher NA.
   (d) decrease the light.

2. The blue filter located on the field diaphragm corrects yellow light produced by
   (a) tungsten lamps.
   (b) halogen lamps.
   (c) lithium lamps.
   (d) iron lamps.

3. To achieve maximum resolution, the NA of the condenser should be
   (a) the same as the NA of the objective.
   (b) higher than the NA of the objective.
   (c) lower than the NA of the objective.
   (d) any NA value; it does not matter.

4. The inexpensive condenser that has no correction for either spherical or chromatic aberration is called
   (a) Abbot.
   (b) Abbé.
   (c) achromat.
   (d) PLANO.

TYPES OF LIGHT MICROSCOPY

The following section describes different types of light microscopy. These techniques may not be available in all laboratories; however, each has special advantages for viewing microscopic specimens (Table 7-1 ★).

★ **TABLE 7-1** Comparison of Light Microscope Methods

	Use	Microscope Objective	Special Equipment Required	Comments
Brightfield	Commonly used method in most laboratories Location, identification, and differentiation of casts and cells are perfected with practice and technique	PLAN/PLANO	None	Wet preparations best viewed by lowering condenser for contrast
Phase Contrast	Contrast produced in wet preparations allow for ease of identification and differentiation of casts, epithelial cells, blood cells	Phase (pol) or (ph)	Annular plate	
Polarizing	Identification of crystals, fats; differentiation from artifact	PLAN/PLANO	Analyzer and polarizer	
Fluorescence	Very tiny objects are viewed easily using fluorescence against a dark background	Fluorescent (fl)	Short wave radiation source; exciter and barrier filters; fluorochrome specimen treatment	Brightfield microscope may be converted for use, but may be less effective; Darkroom necessary for best results

Phase Contrast Microscopy

The cells and objects viewed in urine sediment have the unfortunate characteristic of having only slightly different refractive indices while occupying the same field. In brightfield microscopy, many of these structures may not be easily seen without much focusing or use of stains. A stained specimen will absorb some wavelengths of light, and opaque objects will block light, causing a decrease in the brightness of the object. This allows the eye to detect the change and see the objects in the field. Phase contrast technique uses the differences in refractive indexes of the objects and allows them to be visually brighter in the field. For example, the difference between the refractive indices of cell contents and the liquid environment can be seen more easily with phase contrast microscopy (Figure 7-8 ■) than with bright field microscopy (Figure 7-9 ■). The development of phase contrast microscopy in 1935 earned a Nobel Prize for Frederick Zernicke.

A "phase object" is one that is transparent and colorless. The object will not alter the amplitude of light waves but will diffract and change the phase (wavelength) of some light rays as they pass through it. The two waves are separated by the medium through which they pass: one passes through air and the other passes through some object. The object in the light path will change the amplitude of the wave such that the two waves are "out of sync," meaning that the waves peak and trough at different times.

Zernicke used the difference in the wave amplitudes of the rays that pass through and those waves that are refracted to form an image of transparent objects more easily seen when contained in a similarly transparent medium. This was accomplished through a combination of transmitted and reflected light to enhance the diffraction of a particular set of light waves (Figure 7-10 ■). A ring of light produced by an **annulus** covering the condenser passes through the outer edges of the condenser lens and is focused only on the center of the objective. The phase objective contains a phase plate, which allows diffracted light and non-diffracted light to pass through different zones of the plate. This changes the amplitude of the two light waves in such a way that they interfere with each other. The image is formed by the combination of the two light rays at the plane of the eyepiece and is

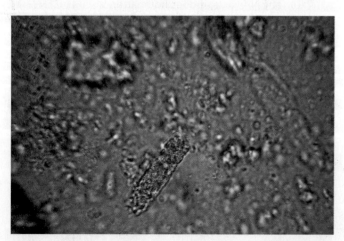

■ **FIGURE 7-8** Hyaline Cast, Phase Contrast, 40X

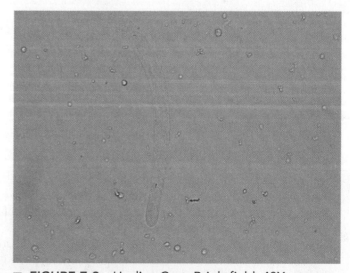

■ **FIGURE 7-9** Hyaline Cast, Brightfield, 40X

tube with the ocular removed. This should be done before each use of the microscope.

Polarizing Microscopy

Polarized light microscopy is another method of manipulating light wave characteristics to distinguish similar microscopic urine elements such as crystals. Glass allows the equal refraction of light waves in all directions, because the molecules are uniform and evenly spaced. The waves will retain the same vibration both entering and leaving the glass or crystal. Some crystals will have a non-uniform spatial orientation of the molecules that cause the light waves to diverge into two rays and exit as such due to the uneven arrangement. This phenomenon is called double refraction or **birefringence** since the two rays vibrate in different planes, either vertically or horizontal, and travel at different velocities.

Birefringence of crystalline specimens can be analyzed with the use of polarizing filters that block light waves in either the horizontal or vertical plane. Two polarizing filters are used in polarization microscopy: one is placed between the light source and the specimen (polarizer), while the second is placed between the specimen and the ocular (analyzer). The polarizer is rotated until the field becomes completely dark. At this point the filters' components are perpendicular to each other because no light is transmitted through the second filter to the observer (Figure 7-11 ■).

If an object is placed in the field having no birefringent properties, the field will remain dark. However, if an object in the field has these properties, it will appear bright on a dark background. This means that the vibration of the waves passing through the first filter strikes the object, and the perpendicular wave vibration is able to pass through the second filter, allowing the observer to view the object (Figure 7-12 ■).

A red compensator (Figure 7-13 ■) placed at a 45° angle to the axis of the polarizer can be added to the system to change the velocity of the transmitted light. This will allow the birefringent crystals to display specific color depending on their orientation in relation to the axis of the compensator.[2] The compensator is rotated on top of the light source until the field background is a red color. The lever on the compensator is manipulated between the arrows as the observer sees the crystals in the field. Crystals seen are compared to the arrows as being in either parallel orientation or perpendicular orientation with relation to the compensator. The color of the crystal is noted when it is oriented in each compensator position and used to identify particular

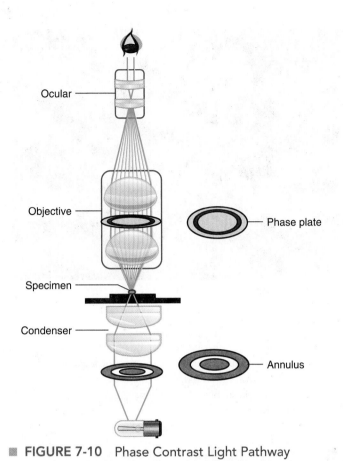

■ **FIGURE 7-10**   Phase Contrast Light Pathway

more easily seen because of the marked difference in wave change in each set of waves. In phase contrast microscopy it is important that the condenser annulus be matched perfectly with the phase plate within the phase objective to see the effect in the specimen. The annulus is an opaque plate containing a ring of transparency that is placed in the condenser. The transparent ring transmits light obliquely to the specimen, which is diffracted to the outer regions of the objective lens. The phase plate within the objective further diffracts the light waves causing visual differences that are detected by the observer. When setting up the microscope for phase contrast microscopy, the condenser can be adjusted using the setscrews to achieve the proper position of the annulus on the phase plate within the objective. This is performed while viewing the back field of the phase objective through the ocular

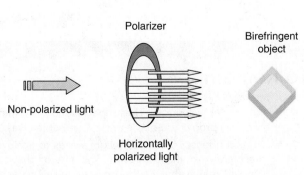
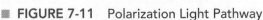
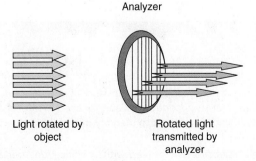

■ **FIGURE 7-11**   Polarization Light Pathway

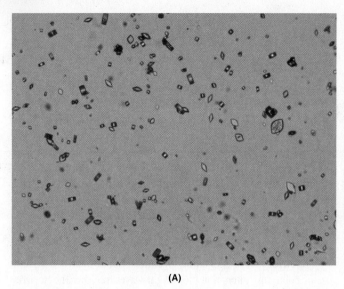

(A)

(B)

■ **FIGURE 7-12**   (A) Uric Acid Crystals. (B) Uric Acid Crystals Polarized

crystal forms. Some crystals contain no colored waves but will normally appear as white against a dark background.

Fluorescence Microscopy

Fluorescence is used to great advantage by using fluorochrome stains to envision microscopic specimens. Fluorochromes are substances capable of emitting radiant energy in the visible range after being illuminated by light of a shorter wavelength in the ultraviolet range. The principles of the reaction involved in the production of this secondary emission concern the excitation of electrons that emit energy as they return to their normal, non-excited state. A major advantage of fluorescence microscopy is the high degree of visibility produced by specimens stained with fluorescent dyes on a very dark background.

The overall composition of the microscope elements used in fluorescent technique is similar to that of regular brightfield microscopy. A mercury or xenon light source, which emits radiation in a narrow range within the ultraviolet spectrum, is located below the substage condenser. Special filters are inserted to select the proper wavelength needed to excite and transmit the visible effect of the fluorochrome used. The exciter filter is placed below the substage condenser, while the barrier filter is placed into the path of the fluorescent image in the ocular to remove the ultraviolet exiting light and allow only the visible wavelengths through to the observer protecting the eye from damaging radiation. The objectives used in brightfield microscopy can also be used for fluorescent images. Generally, objectives that provide a high numerical aperture should be selected so the maximum amount of emitted light from fluorescing specimens can be captured. There are special objectives labeled "fluorite" to identify those specifically designed for fluorescence microscopy.

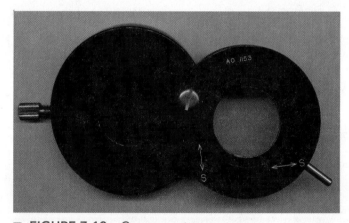

■ **FIGURE 7-13**   Compensator.
The lever is shifted from the right position (perpendicular to the crystal axis) to the left position (parallel to the crystal axis). If the crystal has birefringent properties, it will appear as different colors in each orientation.

Key Points to Remember

- The light microscope is composed of a compound lens system that uses condensed and focused light and objectives of various powers to magnify microscopic objects for identification.

- Each objective is engraved with specifications pertaining to resolving power, correction for lens aberrations, and use in special techniques. These specifications aid the technologist in proper use of the microscope objectives.

- The condenser focuses the light waves to achieve proper resolution of the specimen. The NA of the condenser should match that of the objective used to achieve the best image.

- Köhler illumination is a technique used to align the sub-stage condenser and focus the light for best resolution by the objective. Each microscope should be adjusted before use.
- Microscopes are expensive and valuable tools used in the laboratory for identification of pathologic elements in patient specimens. Proper transport and storage ensures the instrument will be maintained properly. Careful attention should be used when focusing objectives in order not to damage them.
- Special techniques in microscopy have utilized alteration of light wave characteristics to achieve special visualization effects. These techniques include phase contrast, polarizing, dark field, and florescent microscopy.

Review Questions

Level I

1. The most important aspect of the working microscope is (Objective 3)

   A. the light source.

   B. the condenser.

   C. the diaphragm.

   D. all of these are important.

2. The microscope component that focuses the light emitted from the microscope base is (Objective 3)

   A. the diaphragm.

   B. the condenser.

   C. the objective.

   D. the rheostat.

3. The ability of the eye to see separate and distinct points within a specimen is defined as (Objective 2)

   A. the focal point.

   B. refraction.

   C. resolution.

   D. reflection.

4. This number is engraved on each objective and is calculated using the angle of aperture, the resolving power, and the refractive index. (Objective 2)

   A. Numerical aperture (NA)

   B. Microscope coverslip thickness

   C. Optical tube length

   D. Total magnification allowable

5. Optical tube length of a microscope has an effect of the magnification produced by the lenses situated at either end of the tube. The length of the tube is standardized at what length for most microscopes? (Objective 2)

   A. 100 mm

   B. 120 mm

   C. 160 mm

   D. 360 mm

6. An engraved objective correction for curvature of the lens that will provide for a large, flat field without distortion of focus to the field is indicated by the term (Objective 2)

   A. PLANO.

   B. ACHROMAT.

   C. APOCHROMAT.

   D. PHASE.

7. Objectives manufactured to allow interchange between objectives without losing focus are termed (Objective 2)

   A. phase contrast.

   B. parfocal.

   C. interfocal.

   D. phase focus.

8. A microscope using the objective with magnification of 40× and an ocular magnification of 10× will have total magnification of the specimen of (Objective 4)

   A. 4000×.

   B. 400×.

   C. 40×.

   D. 4×.

Level II

1. Which of the following describes the change in resolution as the angle of aperture increases? (Objective 1)

   A. Less light is allowed to enter the lens.

   B. Resolving power decreases.

   C. Resolving power increases.

   D. Nothing will change unless the angle of aperture changes.

2. To view the proper specimen effect with phase contrast microscopy, the annulus ring within the condenser must be aligned with (Objective 2)

   A. the phase plate within the ocular.

   B. the phase plate within the objective.

   C. the light source from the microscope base.

   D. the phase plate within the condenser.

3. Light passing through the outer edge of a convex piece of glass will be diffracted in what directions? (Objective 1)

   A. Inward toward the center

   B. Outward and away from the center

   C. Neither, because all the light will be absorbed by the convex piece of glass

   D. Back toward the source of the light

4. A type of distortion in which there is a failure of a lens to focus all colors to the same convergence point is termed (Objective 1)

   A. resolution.

   B. achromatic.

   C. spherical aberration.

   D. chromatic aberration.

5. The uneven arrangement of molecules within a crystal can cause light rays to diverge into two rays. This phenomenon is called (Objective 3)

   A. bipolar.

   B. bithermal.

   C. biphasic.

   D. birefringence

6. An optical effect due to the increased refraction of light rays as they strike a curved lens at its outer edge is (Objective 2)

   A. spherical aberration.

   B. refractive aberration.

   C. reflective distortion.

   D. chromatic aberration.

Endnotes

1. Freeman JA, Beeler FB. *Laboratory Medicine/Urinalysis and Medical Microscopy.* 2nd ed. Philadelphia: Lea & Febiger, 1983.

2. Harmening, DM. Body fluid examination: Qualitative, quantitative, and morphologic analysis. In: *Clinical Hematology and Fundamentals of Hemostasis.* 5th ed. Philadelphia: FA Davis, 2009: 748.

Additional Reading and Resources

Abramowitz M, et al: Olympus Microscopy Resource Center. Online. Available: http://www.olympusmicro.com (accessed May 28, 2012).

Bradbury P. *An Introduction to Microscopy.* British Columbia, Canada: Steveston Scientific Publications, 1990.

Bradbury S. *An Introduction to the Optical Microscope.* New York: Oxford University Press, 1984.

Brunzel NA. *Fundamentals of Urine and Body Fluid Analysis.* 2nd ed. Philadelphia: Saunders Elsevier, 2004.

Hoppert, M. Light microscopy. In: *Microscopic Techniques in Biotechnology.* Weinheim, Germany: Wiley-VCH Verlag GmbH& Co. KGaA, 2003.

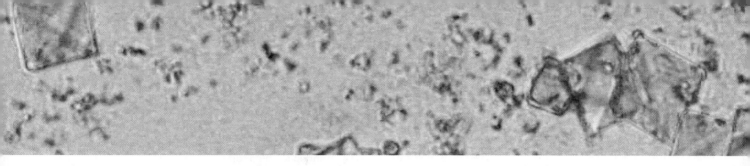

8

Urinalysis: Microscopic Urine Sediment Examination

Objectives

Following successful completion of this chapter, the learner will be able to:

LEVEL I

1. List the changes that occur to cells and formed elements in urine samples during storage and recognize the importance of relating chemical testing to the presence or absence of cells and formed elements in a urine sample.
2. Describe the procedure for preparing urine sediment and wet mount for microscopic examination.
3. State the cells and formed elements reported at both low-power and high-power magnification and recognize the importance of scanning the edges of the microscopic field for larger cells and formed elements during microscopic evaluation.
4. List the sediment stains available and the elements stained by each.
5. Describe the different forms red blood cells may have and the cause of each. Define *hematuria* and list the conditions that cause it.
6. Recognize the differences in morphology between white blood cells and renal tubular epithelial cells and between polymorphonuclear cells and the parasite *Trichomonas vaginalis*.
7. List three types of epithelial cells found in urine sediment. Describe each type of epithelial cell and state the origin in the urinary tract and its clinical significance.
8. Define *pyuria, pyelonephritis, cystitis,* and *urethritis.*
9. Define *urinary cast* and state the location of formation in the renal tubule.
10. List the various forms of renal casts and state the clinical significance of each.
11. List the crystals that may be found in urine sediment at acid, neutral, or alkaline pH.
12. Recognize normal and abnormal crystals that may be found in urine sediment and state the clinical significance of each.

Objectives (continued)

13. Recognize mucus and mucin threads and differentiate them from hyaline casts.
14. Recognize artifacts such as fibers and differentiate them from urinary casts.

LEVEL II

1. Given the relative centrifugal force (g), calculate the revolutions per minute required to prepare urine sediment preparation in a given centrifuge.
2. State the clinical significance of each type of cell found in urine sediment examination including red blood cells, white blood cells, and epithelial cells.
3. State the clinical significance of dysmorphic red blood cells found in urine sediment.
4. Define *pyruria* and *pyelonephritis* and differentiate between them regarding cells and formed elements found in each condition.
5. Relate the presence of oval fat bodies to nephrotic syndrome.
6. State the clinical significance of each type of crystal, parasite, and cast found in urine sediment examination.
7. State the causes for the formation of urinary calculi.

Key Terms

Amorphous crystals	Glomerulonephritis	Oval fat bodies	Tamm-Horsfall glycoprotein
Casts	Granular casts	Polarizing microscopy	Transitional epithelial
Clue cells	Hematuria	Pyelonephritis	Trichomonas vaginalis
Crystalluria	Hemosiderin	Pyuria	Urethritis
Cystitis	Hyaline cast	Renal tubular cells	Uromodulin epithelial
Dysmorphic	Maltese cross formation	Sternheimer-Malbin stain	Urothelial nonsquamous
Glitter cells	Mucus	Suprapubic collection	epithelial

A CASE IN POINT

Maureen, a 37-year-old pregnant female with gestational diabetes, is instructed by her obstetrician to collect a clean-catch urine specimen for urinalysis at her 28-week check-up.

Urinalysis

Color:	Dark Yellow
Appearance:	Cloudy
Specific Gravity:	1.030
pH:	6.0
Glucose:	2+
Bilirubin:	negative
Ketones:	1+
Blood:	1+
Protein:	negative
Urobilinogen:	normal
Nitrite:	negative
Leukocyte Esterase:	2+

Microscopic

WBCs:	5-10/HPF
RBCs:	>100/HPF
Epithelial Cells:	Many squamous/HPF
Casts:	neg
Bacteria:	neg

Blood Chemistry

Fasting Plasma Glucose 210 (70–99 mg/dL)

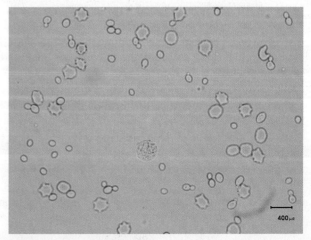

Identify the Cells Present. (200×, Brightfield) (High Power)

Questions to Consider

1. Circle or highlight the abnormal or discrepant result(s) between the dipstick and microscopic analyses.

2. What metabolic disorder is most commonly associated with glucosuria and ketonuria?

3. Study the figure provided. Identify elements present.

4. Explain the result of the Nitrite test on the dipstick considering the answer to question 3.

5. What are the possible causes of the high red blood cell count by the technologist considering the low Blood result on the dipstick?

History has shown that the advent of the microscope was of great importance to the physicians interested in performing urine microscopy to investigate the mechanisms and the manifestations of renal tract disease. Examining urinary sediments is a practice that dates back to the 17th century when Rayer and Vigla introduced it as a routine practice. They made important contributions to the procedures for proper specimen processing and subsequent microscopic examination, and it was their recommendation that the microscopic findings and the urine chemical tests be matched to each other. They described many important urine sediment elements including crystals, squamous and globular cells, as well as mucus, pus, blood, lipids, sperm, and yeasts.[1,2,3]

Collection of a urine specimen is usually noninvasive for the patient and will provide valuable information for the physician regarding the urinary tract and the kidney. In this chapter we will discuss the elements found in the urine sample, the causes of their formation, and methods of detection and enumeration used in the modern laboratory.

PREPARATION OF URINE SEDIMENT FOR EXAMINATION

Many individuals who visit their physicians or patients in a hospital setting are requested to provide a sample of urine for analysis. There are instances in which the physician may need to catheterize the patient for collection or perform a **suprapubic collection** using a needle and syringe. The properly labeled sample is sent in a tightly sealed container to the laboratory for analysis in a timely fashion. Once the specimen arrives in the laboratory, a clinical laboratory scientist will accurately perform the test requested using appropriate techniques and available equipment. The physician uses the laboratory test results to assess the condition of the patient.

The sample should be processed and tested within two hours because cells and casts begin to degrade within this time period. "Casts, erythrocytes and leukocytes are especially susceptible to lysis in urine specimens with a low specific gravity (<1.010) and in urine specimens with an alkaline pH (>7.0).[4] Refrigerating the sample can help preserve these elements if analysis must be delayed; however, **amorphous crystals** are precipitated in the cold temperatures and may obscure detection of pathologic elements that could be important diagnostic information for the physician.

Macroscopic Examination

Urine microscopy begins with appropriate knowledge of the sample *before* centrifugation and sediment examination. The urine is observed for color and clarity and tested for urine chemistries by dipstick. The results of the chemical analysis are confirmed by the presence and enumeration of the microscopic elements seen. A sample with a moderate to high amount of protein measured by dipstick may indicate the presence of **hyaline casts** in the sediment. This is an example of the dipstick results aiding the laboratorian in the observation of an element that may be hard to see if using only a brightfield microscope. Of course, there may be no casts in the urine; however, being clued in by the dipstick (regeant strip) analysis to look a bit closer may make the difference between finding an important pathologic finding and missing it.

There are many variables associated with preparation of urine sediment for analysis. The age and volume of the specimen collected, mixing of the specimen prior to pouring off for centrifugation, and finally the proper resuspension and volume of sediment produced and examined are important factors in producing a good sample for microscopic analysis. The recommended sample size for routine manual microscopy is 12 milliliters (mL) of well-mixed urine.[4] A consistent sample volume ensures reproducibility between technologists in microscopic evaluation. If the sample volume is less than 5 mL, some clinical laboratories may allow microscopic evaluation without concentration of the sediment. When a smaller volume is collected from patients, including pediatrics or neonates, a notation should be made on the physician's report. Accommodations should be made for sample volumes that lie outside laboratory protocols and guidelines for testing and reporting results must be established.

MINI-CASE 8-1

A 6-month-old infant is brought to the Emergency Department (ED) having had high fever and vomiting for the last 48 hours. The physician requests that a urine sample be collected for stat analysis. The nursing staff is able to collect 3 mL of urine using an external pediatric collection bag.

Questions to Consider

1. What is the recommended sample size for routine manual microscopic analysis?

2. What accommodations can be made for a sample size of ≤5mL?

3. How will the physician be made aware of nonstandard results of the testing?

Centrifugation

The sample is centrifuged at $400 \times g$ (400 RCF), which is equivalent to 1500 RPM, in a conical tube for 5 minutes at ambient temperature.[4] Conversion nomograms for converting $\times g$ (RCF) to revolutions per minute (RPM) can be found in most clinical chemistry textbooks or computed using the equation in Box 8-1.

BOX 8-1 Converting RPM to ×g(RCF)

$$RCF(g) = 1.118 \cdot 10^{-5} \cdot r \cdot (RPM)^2$$

RCF — Relative centrifugal "force"

g — The acceleration due to gravity at the Earth's surface

1.118×10^{-5} — an empirical factor

r — Radius in centimeters from the center of the spindle to the bottom of the tube in the rotor bucket

RPM — Number of rotation in revolutions per minute

Sediment Preparation

After centrifugation, sufficient supernatant is removed for resuspension of the sediment in 0.5–1.0 mL of urine. The sediment is gently but briskly mixed with the remaining urine in the bottom of the tube to obtain a homogenous mixture. A wet mount preparation consists of one drop of the resuspended sediment mixture placed on a clean glass slide to which a 22 × 22 mm coverslip is added. It is important to place the coverslip carefully so as not to capture air bubbles causing artifacts in the field.[4] All the possible variables should be accounted for in preparation of urine sediment in order to assure consistency of testing that will produce results that can be reported with confidence and accuracy.

Currently, there are several commercial plastic slide systems available as an alternative to the manually prepared wet mount previously discussed. These commercial systems allow for standardization of microscopic evaluation by ensuring that the same amount of urine and sediment are poured and prepared. This is accomplished by including centrifuge tubes, pipettes, and slides, which contain individual sections manufactured to a specific area and depth (Table 8-1 ★). Using the slide specifications provided in the manufacturer's package inserts, it is possible to calculate the number of elements per mL for the physician's report.

Microscopic Examination

Once the wet mount is prepared or the sediment is loaded into a counting chamber or slide, the urine is allowed to settle for 30–60 seconds. The preparation is viewed with both low power (10× objective) and high power (40× objective). When using a brightfield microscope, decreasing the light and lowering the condenser will provide contrast to view those casts and other elements with low refractive index. This will allow for recognition of translucent structures and identification of hyaline casts, some crystals, and mucin threads (**mucus**). It is essential to scan the outer edges of the preparation in order to find casts, especially if they are rare or few in numbers. Scanning toward the center of the preparation at low power will reveal other large elements such as epithelial cells, **casts**, crystals, and other smaller unidentifiable cells. Amorphous crystals will be evident but will need to be identified along with the smaller cells at a higher power (40×). All of the microscopy work done in the urinalysis laboratory for sediment analysis is done with a dry objective and never with oil immersion.

Several fields are scanned under low power (10×) to identify and quantitate crystals, casts, and epithelial cells. Subsequently, ten high-power (40×) fields are scanned for quantitation of red cells, white cells, and **renal tubular cells**, as well as the presence of bacteria, yeast, trichomonads, and mucus. There are some cells, elements, or organisms that are identified at high-power magnification and reported according to the number seen at low-power magnification.

In each case, 10 fields are counted and the average number of cells per milliliter (mL) can be calculated (Box 8-2) and reported to the physician. The numbers of cells may also be reported as an average number per either low- or high-power field. For example, 50 squamous epithelial cells counted in 10 fields at low power (10×) are averaged and reported as 5 cells per low-power field (LPH). Many clinical laboratories devise a standardized method to report the numbers of elements and use a reference range to describe the possible pathological significance. Some laboratories may report epithelial cells as few, moderate, or many depending on the criteria dictated by their standard operating procedure (SOP). Creating a report for urine sediment results should be standardized in each laboratory so that each person

★ TABLE 8-1 Commercial Plastic Slide Systems for Sediment Evaluation

	COUNT 10™ System Myers-Stevens	UriSystem Fisherbrand	KOVA Hycor
Amount of urine sample	12 mL	12 mL	12 mL
Centrifugation speed (RPM) for 5 minutes	~1500	1800	1500
Amount of sediment prepared	0.80 mL	0.40 mL	1.0 mL
Slide chamber volume	6 μL	14 μL	6.6 μL

BOX 8-2 Standard Variables Used for Calculating Sediment Elements per mL

Clinical and Laboratory Standards Institute (Formerly NCCLS) recommends the following procedure to produce a calculated result for urine sediment taking into account the following variables:

The amount of urine to be centrifuged is measured.

Centrifugation speed is standardized.

The amount of supernatant removed is measured.

A standard cover slip (22 × 22) whose area is 484mm²

A high-power field area of 0.096mm²

A high-power field diameter of 0.35 mm

A measured amount of urine sediment of 0.020 mL placed on the slide

Using 12 mL of urine, it is possible to calculate the number of high-power fields per mL of urine sediment viewed and, therefore, the count of sedimentary elements to report per mL.[4]

performing microscopic examination uses the same terminology, reporting format and reference intervals.[5]

Sediment Stains

Urine sediment analysis may be enhanced by the use of chromatic stains or solutions to identify particular elements (Table 8-2 ★). The supravital **Sternheimer-Malbin Stain** (Box 8-3) can aid in identifying these elements (Figure 8-1 ■), along with leukocytes, epithelial cells, and, especially, casts. In general, one drop of stain is added to 0.5–1.0 ml of prepared urine sediment before placing on a slide for evaluation. Alkaline urine can cause precipitation of Sternheimer-Malbin stain that may obstruct the visualization of formed elements.

Methylene blue or toluidine blue in a 2% solution may be used as a simple, quick supravital stain. These dyes can help delineate the nucleus from cytoplasm in leukocytes, which may make them easier to distinguish from renal cells of similar size. Another technique for identifying leukocytes is the addition of 1–2 drops of 2% acetic acid to a few drops of sediment. The nuclei of white cells and epithelial cells are defined and easily identified, while red blood cells are lysed.

Fats or lipids rarely appear in urine samples unless they are contained within the matrix of casts (fatty casts) or inside renal cells or macrophages (**oval fat bodies**). When neutral fats (triglycerides) are found in the urine of patients with nephrotic syndrome, Oil Red O or Sudan III can be used to stain the elements yellow-orange or red-orange. It is important to recognize that neither cholesterol nor cholesterol esters will be stained by this method. These must be verified by use of **polarizing microscopy**, which will identify both neutral fats and cholesterol.

Eosinophils, not normally found in urine, can be present due to a hypersensitivity reaction to penicillin or its analogs. If the numbers of these white cells are more than 1% of the leukocytes found, it can be a significant finding and should be reported. In order to positively distinguish these bilobed cells from polymorphonuclear cells, a stain such as Hansel secretion stain can be used. Hansel stain is a combination of methylene blue and eosin-Y in methanol and may be purchased or prepared. Eosinophils can also be present in the case of renal transplant rejections.[7]

Prussian blue stain is used to stain iron granules that may be present in patients who have an increased destruction of red blood cells. This occurs in hemolytic anemia and transfusion reactions causing **hemosiderin**, or ferritin aggregates, to be deposited in tubular epithelial cells. As these cells degenerate, the hemosiderin will be incorporated in urinary casts as well.[8]

BOX 8-3 Preparation of Sternheimer-Malbin Stain[6]

Solution I:

Crystal violet	3.0 g
95% (v/v) ethyl alcohol	20.0 mL
Ammonium oxalate	0.8 g
Distilled water	80.0 mL

Solution II:

Safranin O	1.0 mL
95% (v/v) ethyl alcohol	40.0 mL
Distilled water	400.0 mL

Working Solution Preparation: Three parts of Solution I is mixed with 97 parts of Solution II and then filtered. The working solution is filtered every two weeks and then discarded after three months. Storage temperature is 25°C. The stock solutions I and II are good indefinitely.

Prepared working stain may also be purchased from several companies.

★ **TABLE 8-2** Staining Techniques for Identification of Sediment Elements

Stain	Enhancement	Limitations of Method	Specific Diseases or Conditions
Sternheimer-Malbin	Stains leukocytes, epithelial cells, casts, and mucus for better visualization of structures	Precipitation of stain in urines with alkaline pH may obscure important elements	
2% Methylene blue 2% Toluidine blue	Delineates nuclear structure of leukocytes and renal epithelial cells for proper identification		
2% Acetic acid	Defines nuclear structure of leukocytes and epithelial cells		
	Lyses red blood cells; aids in identification of other elements in gross hematuria		

Neutral fat stains
  Oil Red O
  Sudan III
	Stains free neutral fats or those within casts, macrophages, or renal tubular epithelial cells	Cholesterol and cholesterol esters not stained	Possible nephrotic syndrome, increased proteinuria.

Hansel Stain	Stains eosinophils		Renal transplant rejection, hypersensitivity reaction to penicillin
Prussian blue reaction	Stains free hemosiderin granules or those within epithelial cells or casts		Hemolytic anemia

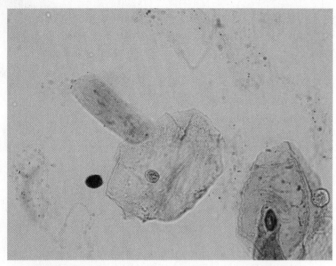

■ **FIGURE 8-1** Sternheimer Malbin Stain. Squamous Epithelial Cells, Hyaline Cast, White Blood Cell, Mucin Threads (200×)

Reporting of Specific Formed Elements in Urine Sediment

The clinician uses the results of urine sediment examination to support diagnoses and monitor the progress of urinary tract diseases. Therefore, it is important to consider which formed elements are normally present in urine. It is normal for healthy individuals to have a few red cells, white cells, and epithelial cells in the urine. These elements originate in the bloodstream and the epithelial lining of the renal tract. Bacteria or sperm can be present due to contamination, and urinary crystals may be present as the result of products of metabolism. Casts are formed within the renal tubules and are composed of Tamm-Horsfall protein and may contain other elements including cells, crystals, bacteria, or hemoglobin. Hyaline and granular casts may be present in increased numbers in physically active individuals. Even healthy individuals who are not physically active produce a few casts and, in both cases, the findings have no clinical significance.

☑ CHECKPOINT 8-1

1. The amount of well-mixed urine recommended by Clinical and Laboratory Standards Institute (CLSI) for routine manual microscopy is
   (a) 2 mL.
   (b) 10 mL.
   (c) 12 mL.
   (d) 20 mL.

2. A urine sample is centrifuged at 400× (g) in a centrifuge having a radius of 15.9 cm. Calculate the rotations in revolutions per minute (RPM) for the centrifuge.
   (a) 5 RPM
   (b) 1500 RPM
   (c) 500 RPM
   (d) 350 RPM

3. The urine sediment is loaded into the counting chamber or prepared as a wet mount. The first important step in microscopic evaluation is
   (a) scanning the urine sediment using oil immersion.
   (b) enumeration of white blood cells and red blood cells using the 40× objective.
   (c) allowing the preparation to settle for 30–60 seconds before proceeding with the counts.
   (d) increasing the light level to view casts at the outer edges of the preparation.

4. The best stain to use for identification of eosinophils is
   (a) Sternheimer-Malbin.
   (b) Prussian blue.
   (c) Hansel stain.
   (d) crystal violet.

5. True or False: It is normal for healthy individuals to have a few red cells, white cells, and/or hyaline casts in the urine.

IDENTIFICATION OF CELLULAR ELEMENTS IN URINE

Red Blood Cells

There are both renal and non-renal causes for the presence of red blood cells (RBC) in urine, which is referred to as **hematuria**. Although red cells are non-motile, they can pass through pores of only 500 nanometers (nm) and can pass out of the blood vessels during inflammation in the same manner as inert, insoluble substances. Normal, healthy individuals may have 0–5 RBC seen per high power field (0–5 per HPF).

Description

Red blood cells are approximately 7.0 micrometers (μm) in size. In unstained sediment from fresh slightly acid urine they appear as pinkish- or tan-colored biconcave discs (Figure 8-2A ■). The state of the urine specimen can have physiologic effects on the shape and color of the red cells (RBCs). A hypotonic specimen having an alkaline pH will cause disintegration of RBCs. The RBCs will swell and burst or may lose their hemoglobin, become faint, and appear as ghost cells (Figure 8-2B). A specimen with a high specific gravity (hypertonic) will cause the RBCs to shrink, crenate, and take on a spikey appearance. This is due to the loss of cellular fluid through osmosis into the surrounding medium.

Dysmorphic RBCs are often oddly shaped and distorted and, when present in increased numbers, can be an indication of glomerular damage in the patient. In glomerular bleeding, the RBCs can take on dysmorphic characteristics due to passage through the glomerular basement membrane. Constant changes in osmotic pressure and pH within the renal tubules cause the RBCs to lose membrane skeleton proteins.[9]

Clinical Significance

Hematuria can originate from the upper or lower urinary tract or can be caused by contamination from other sources during collection by the patient. Conditions that will cause hematuria can be as benign

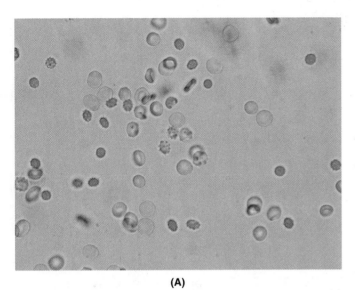
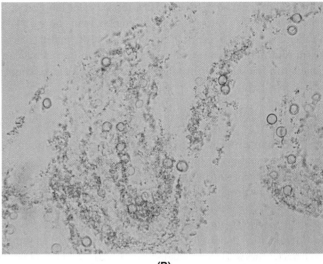

(A)   **(B)**

■ **FIGURE 8-2** **(A)** Red Blood Cells, Normal and Crenated (200×, Brightfield); **(B)** Ghost Red Blood Cells in Hypotonic Urine; Amorphous Phosphate Crystals. (200×, Brightfield)

as normal exercise or pathologic as in glomerular disease, urothelial cancer, renal cancer, prostate cancer, urinary calculus, cystitis, prostatic hypertrophy, renal arteriovenous malformation, and renal cysts.[10] Inflammation and drugs or drug reactions can also cause RBCs in the urine. Contaminating sources can include rectal bleeding or vaginal secretions.

It is possible to see few or no red blood cells in the microscopic and have a very positive test on the dipstick. This may be caused by lysis of the red blood cells in hypotonic or alkaline urine and a strong positive result for hemoglobin. On the other hand, there may be RBCs present, but a negative chemical result. The technologist should investigate either the possibility of an interfering substance in the chemical testing or the presence of an element such as yeast or fat droplets that may be mistaken for RBCs.

White Blood Cells

Urine microscopy of the normal patient will reveal small numbers (0–5 per HPF) of white blood cells (WBCs), the most common of which are polymorphonuclear leukocytes (Figure 8-3 ■). These multi-lobed leukocytes may also be referred to as neutrophils or polys. **Pyuria** is defined as increased numbers of WBCs, most often polymorphonuclear leukocytes, and indicates inflammation or infection involving the kidneys or lower urinary tract. Urine chemistry results in patients with pyuria will be a positive test for leukocyte esterase, which detects the enzyme in the patient's intact or lysed neutrophils.

Other WBCs present in urine sediment are mononuclear cells including lymphocytes and macrophages (histiocytes). These WBCs are easily differentiated from the multi-lobed neutrophils by using staining methods discussed previously. The presence of these cells may indicate chronic inflammation. Increased numbers of small lymphocytes may be found during renal transplant rejection.[11]

MINI-CASE 8-2

Joy, 20-year-old female, stops at the outpatient laboratory clinic to drop off her first-voided urine sample for routine urinalysis on the way to her annual physical exam. The results of the testing showed marked blood (4+) on the dipstick, >100 red blood cells per high-power field (HPF), and an otherwise normal result for all other chemical and microscopic analyses.

Questions to Consider

1. What are the possible contaminating sources causing the increased red cells in the sample?

2. What are some possible solutions to prevent unnecessary cost to the patient and time spent for the laboratory staff in analysis of contaminated samples of this kind?

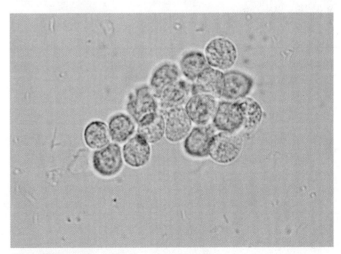

■ **FIGURE 8-3** Large Clump of Polymorphonuclear Cells (WBC) (200×) (High Power)

Eosinophils are rarely observed in urine sediment; however, clinicians may request a special sample preparation technique and stain in patients suspected of experiencing hypersensitivity to drugs such as penicillin. In this case, a cytospin preparation of urine sediment is stained with Hansel's stain, making it easier to recognize and count these bi-lobed white cells.

Description

The most common WBCs seen in urine sediment are neutrophils. They are counted under high power and measure approximately 12–15 μm in diameter. The multi-lobed nucleus and granules in the cytoplasm of neutrophils will react with Sternheimer-Malbin stain (Figure 8-4 ■), which will help distinguish them from red blood cells and epithelial cells (Figure 8-5 ■) under brightfield microscopy.

In fresh urine the smaller size of the neutrophils and their staining characteristics will help distinguish them from renal or transitional epithelial cells, which are large (14–60 μm in diameters) and contain only a single centralized nucleus (Figure 8-6 ■). A urine sample that becomes more alkaline due to prolonged storage at room temperature may show a deterioration of WBCs and will not stain as well. In this case, WBCs may be harder to distinguish from the renal epithelial cells they resemble. Another method useful to enhance the nucleus of both neutrophils and epithelial cells is the addition of one drop of 2% acetic acid to two drops of sediment; this preparation will also lyse red blood cells that are present.

Hypotonic urine will cause the white cells to take up fluid from the surrounding medium and swell. These swollen cells exhibit a "glittering" state due to Brownian motion, which is described as random moving of particles, of the cytoplasmic granules, thus they are referred to as **glitter cells**. These have no pathologic significance.

Clinical Significance

Small numbers of WBC are normally found in the urine of healthy individuals. These cells are motile and will pass through vessel walls

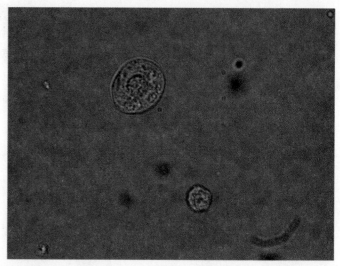

■ **FIGURE 8-5** Polymorphonuclear Cells (WBC) (Lower) Compared to Renal Tubular Epithelial Cell (200×, Brightfield)

in response to inflammation. Pyuria is an indication of infection and/or inflammation in the urinary tract.

Pyelonephritis is a symptomatic infection involving the upper portion of the urinary tract (renal parenchyma), which presents with large numbers of neutrophils and cellular casts (Figure 8-7A ■ and 8-7B). Significant proteinuria often accompanies this disease. In contrast to pyelonephritis, **cystitis** (urinary bladder), prostatitis (prostate gland), and **urethritis** (urethra) are localized inflammations of the lower tract caused by bacterial infection characterized by high numbers of neutrophils, an absence of cellular casts, and a lower or negligible amount of protein.

Causes of increased white blood cells other than bacteria include **glomerulonephritis**, systemic lupus erythematosus (SLE), interstitial nephritis, and tumors, mycoplasmosis, tuberculosis, trichomonads, and chlamydia.[11]

Trichomonas vaginalis can be extremely hard to identify in sediment with WBC and renal epithelial cells because they are similar

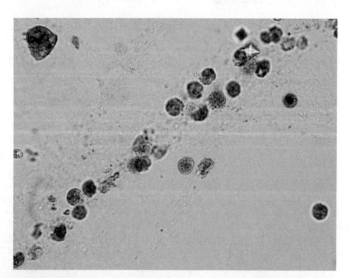

■ **FIGURE 8-4** Polymorphonuclear Cells (WBC), Sternheimer Malbin Stain (200×, Brightfield)

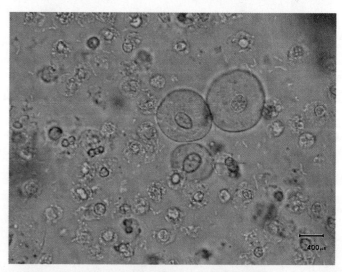

■ **FIGURE 8-6** WBCs with Renal Epithelial Cells(Arrow) (200×, Brightfield)

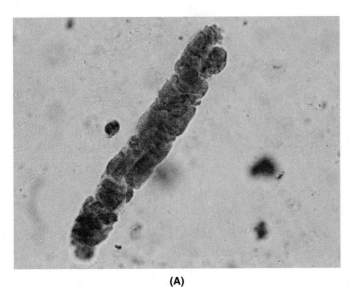

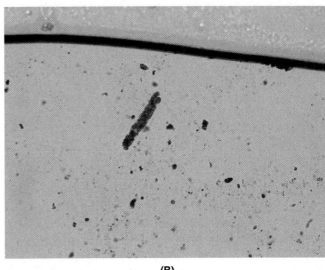

(A)   **(B)**

■ **FIGURE 8-7** **(A)** Cellular Cast Containing Polymorphonuclear Cells (WBC) (200×, Brightfield); **(B)** Cellular Cast. (50×, Brightfield) (Low Power)

in size (Figure 8-8 ■). Their beating flagella and motility in a wet prep of urine sediment is a significant characteristic for proper identification. Trichomonads will stain using Gram stain or giemsa; however, they will not stain using Sternheimer-Malbin.

Epithelial Cells

The urinary tract is lined with different types of epithelial cells, each performing different functions that appear in urine of diseased and non-diseased individuals as the result of normal exfoliation. There are three types of epithelial cells that can be present in urine, including squamous epithelial cells (SQEP), **transitional** or **urothelial non-squamous epithelial** cells (NSE), and renal tubular epithelial cells (RTE). Of these, renal tubular cells are the most clinically significant.[12] The cells are arranged in sheet-like structures covering the basement membrane in the renal tract. Normal sloughing-off of the surface epithelium occurs as the cells are renewed. Increased removal of these cells can be caused by mechanical (catheterization) inflammation, chemical toxins, infection, or disease and can cause an increase in the numbers of these cells seen in urine sediment.

MINI-CASE 8-3

A urine sample sent from an outpatient OB/GYN clinic is refrigerated for one hour before the urinalysis is started. The reagent strip shows 1+ reactivity for both leukocyte esterase (LE) and blood.

Questions to Consider

1. In the figure accompanying this mini-case, what structure is indicated on one of the elements?

2. What must the tech look for in order to differentiate these elements from the white blood cell in the lower left of the image?

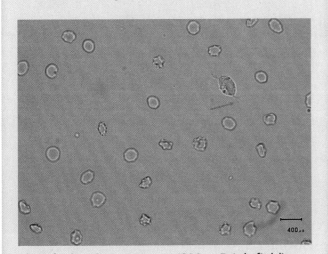

Identify the elements seen (200×, Brightfield)

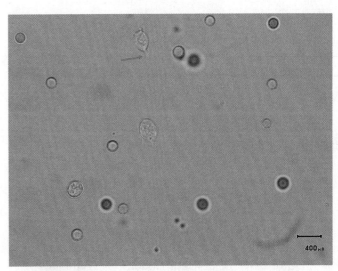

■ **FIGURE 8-8** *Trichomonas Vaginalis* (Arrow). Note the Round WBC in Lower Left. (200×, Brightfield)

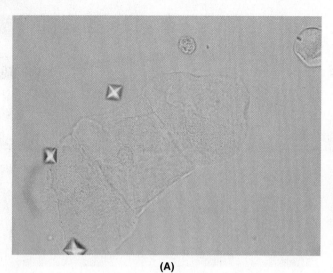

(A)

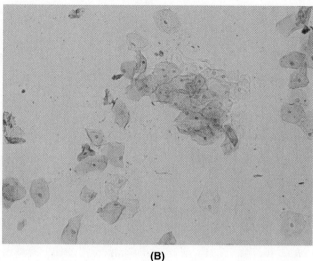

(B)

■ **FIGURE 8-9** **(A)** Squamous Epithelial Cells. (200×, Brightfield); **(B)** Squamous Epithelial Sheet, Sternheimer-Malbin Stain. (50×, Brightfield)

Squamous Epithelial Cells

Squamous epithelial cells (SQEP)are located in the distal third of the male and female urethra. These are the most frequently observed epithelial cells because they are easy to see at low power (10×) due to their large size (40–60 μm). The nucleus is small and centrally located within a flat, granular cytoplasm having edges that are rolled or wrinkled. They have a fried egg appearance with the nucleus as the yolk (Figure 8-9A ■ and 8-9B). Urine specimens from females may contain many SQEP cells due to contamination from the vagina or vulva, which is lined with these cells. **Clue cells** are another form of squamous epithelial that may be seen in urine sediment. The cells are usually a contaminating element from vaginal secretions and are covered with bacteria (*Gardnerella vaginalis*) (Figure 8-10 ■). These cells may or may not be reported depending on laboratory protocol.

Transitional or Urothelial Cells

Transitional epithelial cells (also referred to as nonsquamous epithelial) line the tract from the upper urethra to the renal pelvis. These cells, averaging about 30μm, are smaller than SQEP cells and can have many different shapes, including pear-shaped, oval, or columnar (Figure 8-11 ■). In hypotonic urine, transitional epithelial cells can absorb (imbibe) water, causing them to swell, become more spherical, and have an appearance similar to neutrophils. The acentric, single nucleus (occasionally binucleate) will help distinguish them as transitional epithelial cells in stained or unstained preparations.

It is normal to see a few transitional cells in urine sediment. Occasionally, these cells can appear as sheets or groups caused by invasive catheterization or other scoping procedures (e.g., cystoscopy, ureteroscopy, and ureteropyelscopy). In the absence of mechanical manipulation, the presence of large numbers of transitional epithelial cells can suggest a pathologic process that requires further investigation of the cells using select cytological stains.

■ **FIGURE 8-10** Clue Cells: Squamous Epithelial Covered with Bacteria, Sternheimer-Malbin Stain (200×, Brightfield)

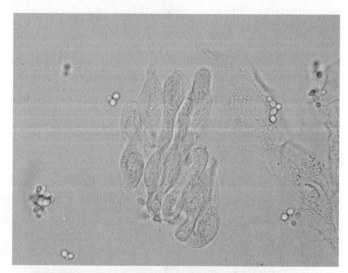

■ **FIGURE 8-11** Transitional Epithelial Cells. Note the Oval and Pear-shaped Appearance (200×, Brightfield)

Renal Tubular Epithelial Cells

Large numbers of renal tubular epithelial (RTE) cells in a urine specimen present a more clinically significant condition than other the presence of other epithelial cells (Figure 8-12A ■ and 8-12B). RTE cells indicate renal tubular damage in cases of acute tubular necrosis or toxic insult to the kidneys due to the presence of drugs or heavy metals such as copper.

RTE cells are present in the proximal and distal convoluted tubules and collecting duct. Distinguishing RTE cells can be quite difficult in wet preparations for urine microscopic examination, and their identification should be confirmed using cytological staining. Usually, RTE cells from the proximal tubule (measuring about 13 μm) are oval or rectangular with a central nucleus and granular cytoplasm, whereas RTE cells from the collecting duct are more polygonal or columnar and smaller in size.[13]

Oval Fat Bodies

Oval fat bodies (Figure 8-13 ■)are renal tubular cells that have taken up fat globules from the tubular lumen and are associated with nephrotic syndrome and markedly increased proteinuria. These cells appear to contain retractile droplets within the cytoplasm. The drops exhibit a **Maltese cross formation** with polarized light and thus can be positively identified as fat. Neutral fats (triglycerides) will stain orange-red on addition of Sudan III or Oil Red O stain.

☑ CHECKPOINT 8-2

1. The oddly shaped or distorted forms that red blood cells can assume due to glomerular bleeding are called
   (a) crenated.
   (b) dynamic.
   (c) dysmorphic.
   (d) polymorphic.

2. Because of their size and shape, red blood cells can often be mistaken for what similarly shaped element seen in urine?
   (a) Spermatozoa
   (b) Yeast
   (c) Bacteria
   (d) *Trichomonas vaginalis*

3. Of the three main types of epithelial cells found in urine, these appear as fried-egg shaped with wrinkled edges.
   (a) Squamous epithelial
   (b) Renal tubular epithelial
   (c) Transitional epithelial

4. This type of epithelial cell can be seen in large numbers in cases of acute tubular necrosis due to heavy metals such as copper.
   (a) Squamous epithelial
   (b) Renal tubular epithelial
   (c) Transitional epithelial

5. Which of the following statements is true concerning transitional epithelial cells?
   (a) Transitional epithelial cells are smaller in size than squamous epithelial cells but are the same shape, having wrinkled edges.
   (b) Transitional epithelial cells have a single central nucleus and will absorb water in hypertonic urine to become large and spherical.
   (c) Transitional epithelial cells can appear as sheets in urines collected by catheterization.
   (d) Presence of large numbers of transitional epithelial cells in urine are common and never pathological.

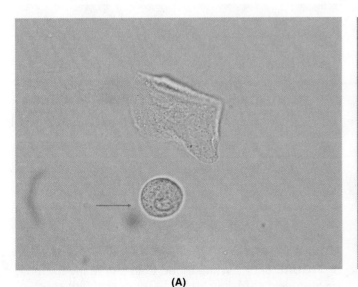

(A)

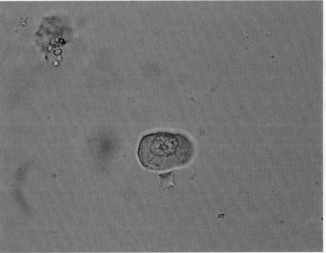

(B)

■ **FIGURE 8-12** **(A)** Renal Tubular Epithelial (Arrow) and Squamous Epithelial Comparison (200×, Brightfield); **(B)** Renal Tubular Epithelia Cell, Calcium Oxalate Crystal (200×, Brightfield)

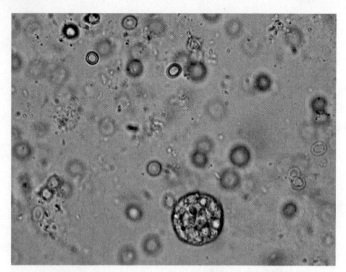

■ **FIGURE 8-13** Oval Fat Body (200×, Brightfield)

Spermatozoa

Spermatozoa may be present in the urine of both men and women. They appear as oval bodies with long, thin tails and are usually not motile (Figure 8-14 ■). In male specimens these appear as the result of nocturnal emissions or ejaculation. In female specimens they are considered a contaminant from vaginal secretions. It is clinically insignificant in cases other than molestation or rape, and reporting the presence of sperm in urine sediment should be handled according to laboratory protocol.

Bacteria

Bacteria are viewed with the high-power objective; however, they are not identified specifically as either rods or cocci. Identification of

bacteria is done by Gram stain and is only reported as few to many per high-power field (HPF). The actual source of bacteria in urine could be contamination during collection; therefore, it is important to check the chemical dipstick results for verification and correlation. For example, urine with normal numbers of WBC and significant bacteria should be considered a suspicious finding. It is possible the sample was improperly collected or stored too long before testing. True urinary tract infection (UTI) will show significant number of both elements in the sediment (Figure 8-15 ■).

Yeast

Candida albicans is the most common yeast found in the urine sediment. Yeast does not take up supravital stain that would help differentiate them from RBCs of similar size and shape. The characteristic budding of yeast will distinguish it from red blood cells.

Although yeast can be a skin contaminant or simply from the air, it can also be present in the sediment due to contamination from vaginal infection found in pregnancy and diabetes mellitus. *Candida* infections are common in immunosuppressed patients (Figure 8-16A ■ and 8-16B).

Parasites

Parasites are often found in urine sediment due to contamination from vaginal or fecal sources. If not motile, *Trichomonas vaginalis* can be difficult to differentiate from WBC or RTE in the microscopic field. These parasites are not stained by supravital stains; however, phase contrast microscopy can enhance the flagella and the movement of the outer membrane. It is imperative that movement of the flagella be visualized to identify and report the presence of the parasite (Box 8-4). Other parasitic infections such as *Entamoeba histolytica*, *Enterobius vermicularis* (pinworm), and *Giardia lamblia* can be found as result of fecal contamination of the sample.

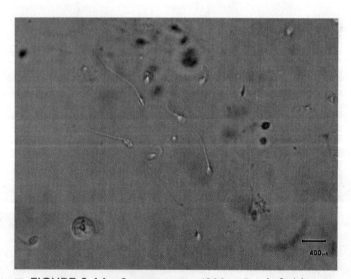

■ **FIGURE 8-14** Spermatozoa (200×, Brightfield)

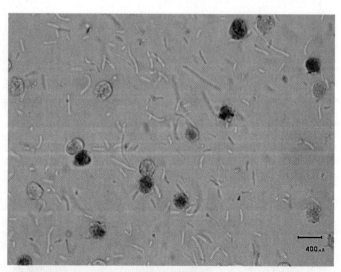

■ **FIGURE 8-15** White Blood Cells and Many Bacteria, Sternheimer-Malbin Stain (200×, Brightfield)

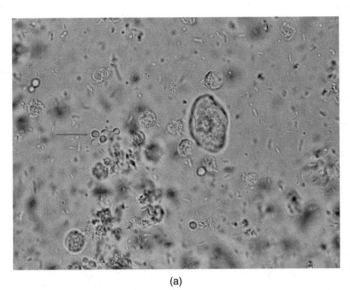

(a)

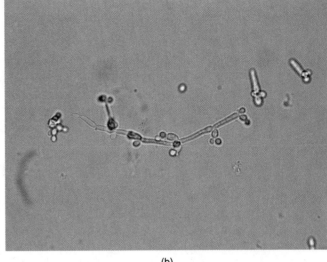

(b)

■ **FIGURE 8-16** **(A)** White Blood Cells, Bacteria, Yeast (Arrow) (200×, Brightfield); **(B)** Yeast, Hyphae (400×, Brightfield)

Schistosoma hematobius ova can be shed directly into urine from the bladder wall.

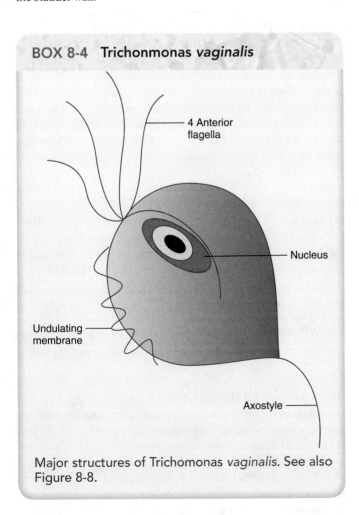

BOX 8-4 Trichonmonas *vaginalis*

4 Anterior flagella

Nucleus

Undulating membrane

Axostyle

Major structures of Trichomonas *vaginalis*. See also Figure 8-8.

IDENTIFICATION OF FORMED ELEMENTS IN URINE

Casts

Urinary casts are named for the molded structure resembling the distal renal tubules or collecting ducts where they are produced. On examination with a high-power objective they appear to have parallel sides and rounded ends, much like a cigar-shaped object (Figure 8-17A ■). **Tamm-Horsfall glycoprotein** (THP) or **uromodulin** is a mucoprotein that is exclusively produced in the cells of both the thick ascending loop and distal convoluted tubule of the nephron. The precipitation of protein is favored by acid pH and higher ionic concentration of urine within the nephron. As the flow of urine becomes static, cast formation occurs in the distal tubule, and various elements may be included within the protein matrix. These elements include RBCs, WBCs, RTEs, bacteria, and crystals.

At very high stasis, the cast may distend the tubule and cause the diameter of the cast to increase, thus causing the cast to grow in diameter (broad cast) within the tubule and cause obstruction. The cast moves very slowly through the tubule as the inclusions within it degrade, progressing from cellular to coarse granular to fine granular and finally to waxy. Waxy casts are an indication of severe end-stage renal disease. The pathologic implications of casts in sediment can be negligible or serious depending on the types and numbers found.

Finding and identifying hyaline casts can be hard for the new microscopist. These casts are more easily identified with a phase contrast microscope or using supravital stain with brightfield technique. Hyaline casts and their cell inclusions will be stained pink with Sternheimer-Malbin stain (refer to Figure 8-1).

Hyaline Casts

Hyaline casts are composed solely of the precipitated mucoprotein uromodulin and have a low refractive index. These types of casts

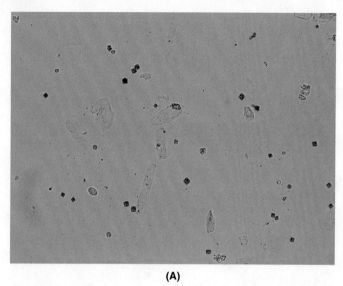

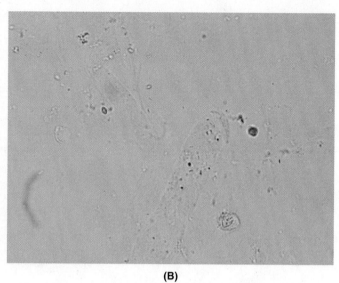

(A)   **(B)**

■ **FIGURE 8-17** **(A)** Hyaline Cast. Note Parallel Sides and Cigar Shape. There are at Least Five Casts in the Field (50×, Brightfield); **(B)** Hyaline Casts. (200×, Brightfield)

are a normal finding in low numbers in the urine of normal healthy individuals. The number of hyaline casts will increase after strenuous exercise, stress, dehydration, or fever (Figure 8-17B).

Cylindroids (Figure 8-18 ■), a form of hyaline cast, may be very long with tapering tails and are clinically insignificant.

Cellular Casts

Cellular casts may be composed of any cells that occur within the tubular system of the nephron: red cells, white cells, epithelial cells or a mixture of these. Cells are incorporated into the matrix and transported through the nephron. These casts are categorized by the cellular inclusions within the protein matrix and are always clinically significant (Figure 8-19A ■ and 8-19B).

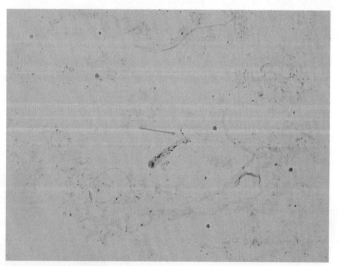

■ **FIGURE 8-18** Cylindroid with Tapering Tail (Arrow) in a Field of Mucin Threads, Sternheimer-Malbin Stain (50×, Brightfield)

Red Blood Cell Casts

Red blood cell casts (RBC casts) are a significant finding that indicate bleeding within the nephron. As red cells enter the tubule due to glomerular damage, they are included in cast formation within the distal tubule. Viewing the red cells inside the casts under a brightfield microscope may be difficult; however, supravital staining or the use of phase contrast microscopy will help. There should be red cells visible in the surrounding microscopic field as well. As the red cells within the matrix degenerate, the cast will take on a yellowish or brown hue from the hemoglobin contained within the cells. The most common diseases associated with the formation of RBC casts include acute glomerulonephritis, systemic lupus erythematosus, and immune complex disorders.

White Blood Cell Casts / Bacterial Casts

White blood cell casts (WBC casts) (Figures 8-20A ■ and 8-20B) are most generally composed of neutrophils and are usually associated with pyelonephritis. An infection of the lower urinary tract would produce many WBC in the urine; however, the formation of WBC casts indicates infection within the kidney itself. Some of these casts also include bacteria if high numbers of microorganisms are present. These may be identified as bacterial casts by Gram stain.

WBC casts are also seen in conjunction with interstitial nephritis or lupus nephritis owing to the chemotaxic effects of complement components.

Renal Tubular Epithelial Casts

Increased exfoliation of renal tubular epithelium caused by viral diseases, chemical toxins, and acute tubular necrosis will enable RTE to become embedded in the cast matrix. Both WBC and RTE casts are a serious pathological finding and every attempt should be made to identify the cells within. As with all microscopic analyses, it is important to correlate the chemical dipstick result with the sediment elements seen. Therefore, a negative result for leukocyte esterase on the dipstick may help identify the cast as RTE and not WBC.

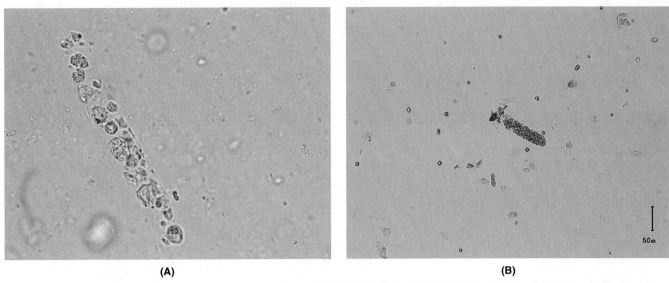

■ **FIGURE 8-19** **(A)** Mixed Cellular Cast (200×, Brightfield); **(B)** Mixed Cellular Cast (50×, Brightfield)

Granular Casts

These casts are of the same composition as hyaline casts; however, there are granular inclusions within the matrix. The granules seen in these casts are graded as fine or coarse and are usually reported under the general term **granular cast**. These inclusions may form from the serum proteins or lysosomes of the surrounding epithelium of the nephron (fine granulation) or the degeneration of red cells, white cells, or epithelial cells (coarse). In either case, the formation of this type of cast can indicate urinary stasis and, therefore, tubular disease. Because granular casts remain static in the nephron tubules, over time the granules can degrade further to produce waxy casts (Figure 8-21A ■ and 8-21B, Figure 8-22 ■).

Waxy Casts / Broad Waxy Casts

The appearance in urine sediment of waxy casts suggests nephron obstruction or renal stasis,[14] and are associated with chronic renal failure. They appear much like hyaline casts; however, these are easier to view with brightfield microscopy due to their high refractive index. In addition, waxy casts have sharp squared edges and cracks or fissures in their sides (Figure 8-23A ■ and 8-23B).

Waxy casts may be broad in diameter due to the static nature of the urine flowing through the nephron. In general, the wide diameter of the cast is due to the distended collecting tubule where they are formed, which indicates urine stasis (Figure 8-24A ■ and Figure 8-24b). Granular or waxy casts may be classified as broad casts.

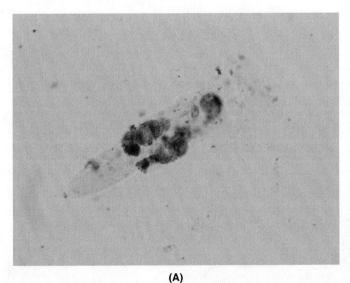

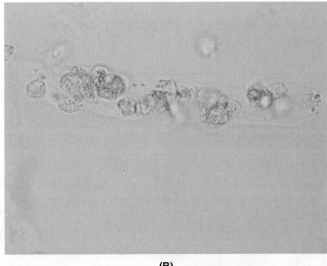

■ **FIGURE 8-20** **(A)** White Blood Cell Cast, Sternheimer-Malbin Stain (200×, Brightfield); **(B)** Mixed Cellular Cast (200×, Brightfield)

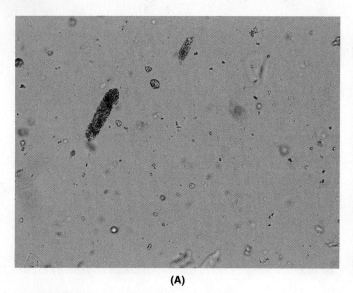

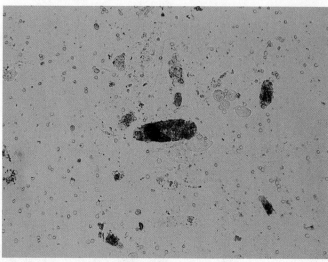

(A)   (B)

■ FIGURE 8-21   (A) Granular Cast (50×, Brightfield); (B) Granular Casts (50×, Brightfield)

Fatty Casts

These are associated with oval fat bodies and globules of fat incorporated into the cast matrix. As with oval fat bodies, confirmation of neutral fats can be done by Sudan III or Oil Red O stain. All types of fats may be viewed as having a Maltese cross formation under a polarizing microscope.

Fatty casts are associated with nephrotic syndrome, diabetic nephropathy, or toxic renal poisoning[15] (Figure 8-25 ■).

Pigmented Casts

Hemoglobin / Myoglobin

Casts containing myoglobin may form as a result of acute muscle damage and appear as dark brown or red from the pigment. Hemoglobin casts may result from the breakdown of red cells within casts or as a result of acute hemolytic episode. In both cases the dipstick results will be positive for hemoglobin.

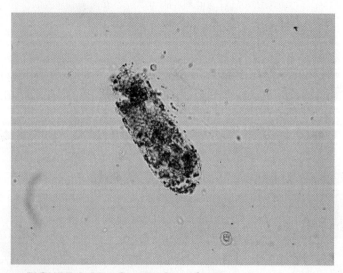

■ FIGURE 8-22   Coarse Granular Cast, Sternheimer-Malbin Stain (200×, Brightfield)

MINI-CASE 8-4

Adeline, a 70-year-old female, has a history of chronic foot ulcerations and diabetes. The patient has a urinalysis performed regularly; however, the patient suffers from oliguria and voids less than 400 mL per day. Refer to the image below.

Questions to Consider

1. Identify the element indicated by the arrow.

2. What causes this type of element to appear in urine?

3. Considering the daily urine volume excreted by the patient and the elements seen in the sediment, what is the likely renal diagnosis?

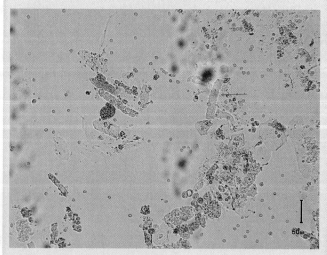

What Type of Cast is Indicated by the Arrow? (50×, Brightfield)

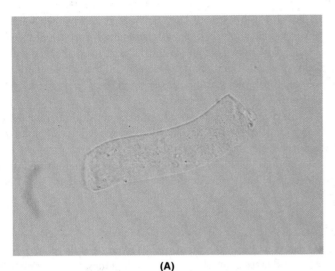 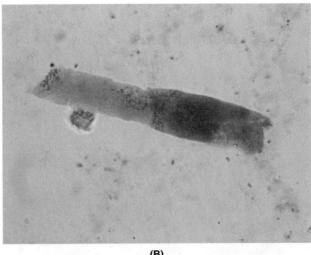

(A)   (B)

■ **FIGURE 8-23** **(A)** Waxy Cast (200×, Brightfield); **(B)** Waxy Cast, Sternheimer-Malbin Stain (200×, Brightfield)

Hemosiderin Casts

Acute hemolytic episode may produce hemosiderin casts, which contain yellow-brown iron granules. Staining the cast with Prussian blue stain will turn the iron granules blue.

Bilirubin and Drug Casts

The color from bilirubin caused by obstructive jaundice will impart a deep yellow-brown color to elements in the urine, including casts. Drugs such as phenazopyridine (Pyridium) cause a bright yellow-orange color in acid urine and will also color casts and cells.[16]

Crystal Casts

On occasion, crystals will be deposited in the tubule or collecting duct, producing crystal casts. These crystals are most often urates, calcium oxalate, and some drugs (sulfonamides). Due to irritation of the epithelial cells, these casts can be accompanied by hematuria. It is possible to confuse crystals adhering to mucin threads for this type of cast, and it is important to look for the cast matrix and outline.

Crystals

Crystalluria is produced by the precipitation of urinary salts due to changes in pH, temperature, and the concentration of urine either *in vivo* or *in vitro*. When crystal formation occurs *in vivo*, the cause is most often due to increased solute concentration, therefore crystals present in freshly voided urine are clinically significant. In the renal tubules, the glomerular ultrafiltrate is concentrated as it moves through the nephron. In cases of dehydration, dietary excess, or medication, the solute concentration may cause supersaturation of some crystal-forming compounds and cause crystal precipitation within the tubule.

Crystals are identified and reported on the basis of the pH of the urine in which they are found, their shape, microscopic appearance, and solubility characteristics (Table 8-3 ★). This differential

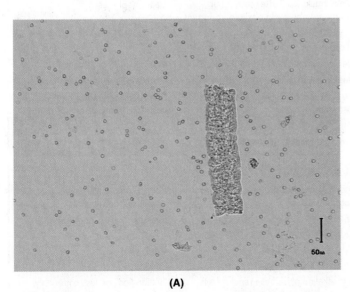 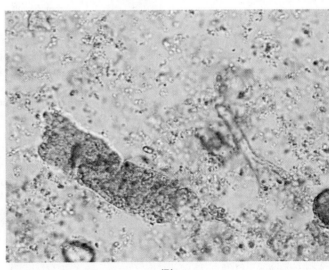

(A)   (B)

■ **FIGURE 8-24** **(A)** Broad Cast, Red Blood Cells (50×, Brightfield); **(B)** Broad Cast Stained with Bilirubin (200×, Brightfield)

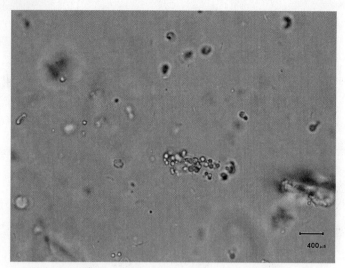

■ **FIGURE 8-25** Fatty Cast (200×, Brightfield)

solubility affords a means of identification for crystals that resemble one another.

Crystal precipitation also readily occurs in stored urine according to changes in pH and temperature. Amorphous forms of some crystals can occur in abundance and obscure clinically significant reportable elements.

Normal Crystals: Acid and/or Neutral Urine

Amorphous Urates

The salts of calcium, magnesium sodium, and potassium will precipitate from a saturated solution in acid pH. Their appearance at the bottom of the tube after centrifugation is pink in color and has been referred to as "brick dust." They can be identified by their solubility in alkali or at 60°C. These clinically insignificant crystals are actually small yellow-brown granules and, in large numbers, they can obscure cells, casts, and other reportable elements in the sediment. Addition of acetic acid will, overtime, convert the granules to uric acid crystals (Figure 8-26A ■ and 8-26B).

Acid urates and monosodium urates have similar characteristics, but the crystals have a different appearance compared to amorphous urates. Acid urates appear as small yellow-brown balls or spheres (Figure 8.27 ■), while the monosodium form appears as slender straight prisms; neither is clinically significant.

Uric Acid

These are the most commonly observed crystals in acid urine. Uric acid takes many shapes: diamonds, cubes, rosettes, or barrels (Figure 8-28A ■–8-28F). The flatter forms may have a layering or lamination that appears on the surface as if they are stacking up on one another. The most common form is the four-sided diamond; however, occasionally these crystals will form with six sides. It is important to differentiate these from cystine crystals, also six-sided, which are clinically significant.

Uric acid crystals are normal and originate from the catabolism of purine nucleotides of both ribonucleic acids (RNA) and deoxyribonucleic acid (DNA). Patients undergoing chemotherapy for leukemia or lymphomas can have a high cell turnover rate, resulting as increased purine breakdown and high uric acid excretion in urine. This is also seen in gout.

Uric acid crystals can exhibit birefringence using polarizing microscopy.

★ **TABLE 8-3** Normal Crystals Found in Urine According to pH

Crystal	Color	Comments	Shape
Acid or Neutral pH			
Amorphous urates	Yellow-brown	Precipitate as pink "brick dust" after settling or centrifugation. Large numbers can obscure important elements. Soluble in alkali or at 60°C.	Balls or spheres
Calcium oxalate-monohydrate	Colorless	Birefringent. Seen in patients post ethanol ingestion.	Oval or dumbbell shapes
Calcium oxalate-dihydrate	Colorless	Birefringent; cause of renal calculi.	Octahedral or "envelope"
Uric acid	Yellow to yellow-brown	Birefringent; crystals exhibit layering or surface lamination. Cause of renal calculi.	Diamonds or spades, barrels, cubes, rosettes; rarely six-sided.
Alkaline pH			
Amorphous phosphate	Colorless	White precipitate after settling or centrifugation. Large numbers can obscure important elements. Soluble acid; insoluble at 60°C.	
Ammonium biurate	Yellow to yellow-brown	Most often found in urine after prolonged storage; however, may form in vivo.	Round sphere. May have spicules ("thorny apples").
Calcium carbonate	Colorless	Forms CO_2 with addition of acetic acid. Large amounts may form pseudocasts under coverslip.	Granular. Rarely, dumbbells.
Calcium biphosphate	Colorless	Form in alkaline to slightly acid pH.	Large Plates
Calcium di-basic phosphate	Colorless		Rosettes
Triple phosphate	Colorless	Form in neutral to alkaline pH. Cause renal calculi.	"Coffin lids" or, less commonly, in leaf-like form

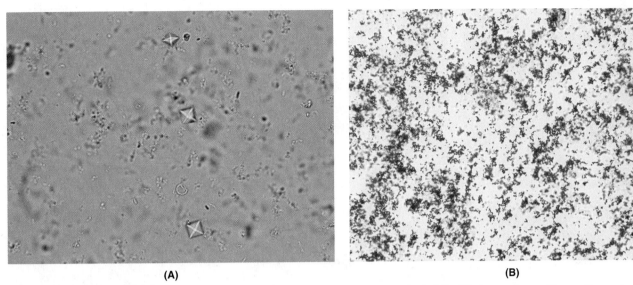

(A)   **(B)**

■ **FIGURE 8-26   (A)** Amorphous Urates, Calcium Oxalate (50×, Brightfield); **(B)** Amorphous Urate Crystals (50×, Brightfield)

Calcium Oxalate

Calcium oxalate crystals are also a common finding at acid or neutral pH. The most common shape is the octahedral form. These appear as envelopes or, more simply, a box containing a three-dimensional "×" (Figure 8-29A ■ and 8-29B). They are colorless and vary greatly in size.

Both calcium and oxalate, derived from ascorbic acid (vitamin C), are found in normal healthy individuals. Foods that contain high levels of vitamin C include many vegetables (asparagus, tomatoes) and citrus fruits. Individuals prone to formation of calcium oxalate crystals are encouraged to eliminate these foods from their diet and increase fluid intake. This will decrease the precipitation of calcium oxalate crystals and the chance that renal calculi will form.

The monohydrate form of calcium oxalate appears either as small dumbbells or as small, ovoid crystals (Figure 8-29C and 8-29D).

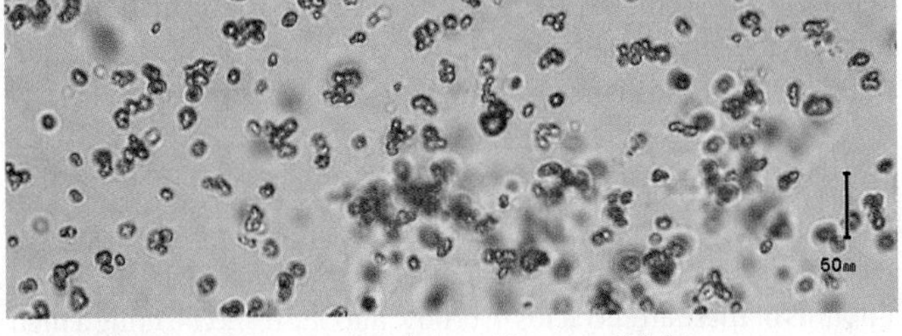

Heavy calcium oxalate crystalluria presenting in the monohydrate form may also provide a striking clinical indicator of ethylene glycol ingestion.[13] It is important for clinical laboratory scientists to recognize this less commonly seen form of the crystal to avoid delay in this diagnosis.

Normal Crystals: Alkaline Urine

Amorphous Phosphate

These clinically insignificant crystals are found in alkaline urine and resemble amorphous urates that are found at acid pH. They differ in the precipitate color, white, as well as their solubility in acid and inability to dissolve at 60°C. They are equally benign and obscure microscopic evaluation when in grossly high amounts.

Calcium Phosphate

These crystals exist in two forms. Calcium biphosphate crystals are large and assume a thin, plate-like shape containing granules. In contrast, dibasic calcium phosphate appears as small prisms that may cluster in groups or rosettes. These can form in a range of pH from alkaline to slightly acidic. Both forms are clinically insignificant.

Triple Phosphate

Described as "coffin lids," the most common form, these crystals can precipitate in neutral to alkaline urine (Figure 8-30 ■). An alternative form of this crystal found in normal individuals is feathery or leaf-like. Little clinical significance is attributed to the presence of these crystals; however, they have been implicated in the formation of renal calculi.

Ammonium Biurate

Rounded forms that may have spicule projections provide the reason for the peculiar shapes of these normal alkaline crystals named "thorny apples." Most often the precipitation of these crystals indicates over-prolonged storage; however, because they can precipitate *in vivo*,

■ **FIGURE 8-27   Amorphous Urates (200×, Brightfield)**

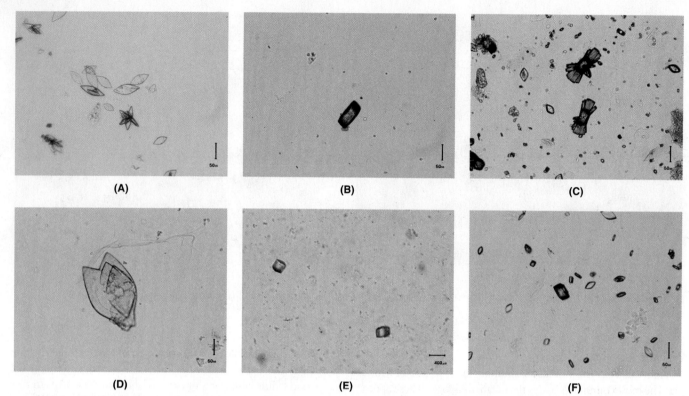

■ FIGURE 8-28 **(A)** Uric acid Crystals (50×, Brightfield); **(B)** Uric Acid Crystal, Barrel Form (50×, Brightfield); **(C)** Uric Acid Crystals, Rosettes and Diamond Forms (50×, Brightfield); **(D)** Uric Acid Crystals. Note the Layering or Lamination of the Structures (50×, Brightfield); **(E)** Uric Acid Crystals, Rhomboid (50×, Brightfield); **(F)** Uric Acid Crystals, Barrel and Diamond Forms (50×, Brightfield)

their presence should be investigated. These crystals dissolve in acetic acid or at 60°C (Figure 8-31 ■).

Calcium Carbonate

These small, colorless granules can form a dumbbell shape when seen in pairs. They resemble amorphous phosphates and are also clinically insignificant. Positive identification for these crystals is the addition of acetic acid and the formation of carbon dioxide gas.

Abnormal Crystals Found in Acidic or Neutral Urine

Cholesterol

Cholesterol crystals are clear, colorless crystals that form large flat plates containing a notch or having a "stair-step" appearance at acid pH (Figure 8-32 ■). A high concentration of cholesterol is found in patients with nephrotic syndrome or those with tumors causing lymphatic rupture into the renal tubules. The microscopist may also see oval fat bodies, fatty casts, and fat globules in the sediment containing cholesterol crystals. Using a polarizing microscope will reveal both Maltese cross formations in the fat globules as well as birefringence of the crystals.

Bilirubin

Rarely seen, these crystals appear in patients with jaundice. Bilirubin can precipitate out of solution upon refrigeration, but the crystals are not formed *in vivo*. They appear as a small tight cluster of fine needles

at acid pH. Of course, these are only seen if the patient's chemical results are positive for bilirubin. Their clinical significance is related to the metabolic disease process causing increased bilirubin in the urine and not the appearance of the crystals.

Cystine

Cystine crystals appear as colorless plates having six sides (hexagonal). Like urine acid crystals, they appear in acid urine and have a laminated "stacked" appearance. Remember, uric acid crystals can also have a six-sided form; however, these are birefringent, which is not true of cystine. Chemical confirmation of cystine in urine is based on the cyanide-nitroprusside reaction forming a purple color when positive.

Uric acid is the end product of purine metabolism. Increased uric acid levels occur in individuals with a diet high in protein or with defects causing an increased purine production. Cystinuria is an inheritable autosomal recessive disorder of amino acid transport.[18] Renal damage occurs in patients with crystal deposition in the tubules and subsequent formation of renal calculi. Therefore, identification and report of these to the clinician is extremely important.

Leucine and Tyrosine

These amino acid crystals are considered together due to their appearance in the urine of patients with rare inherited disorders. Increased amounts of these amino acids overflow into the urine, forming a high blood concentration. Tyrosine crystals appear as sheaves of colorless fine needles. Leucine crystals take the form of "wagon wheels" that look

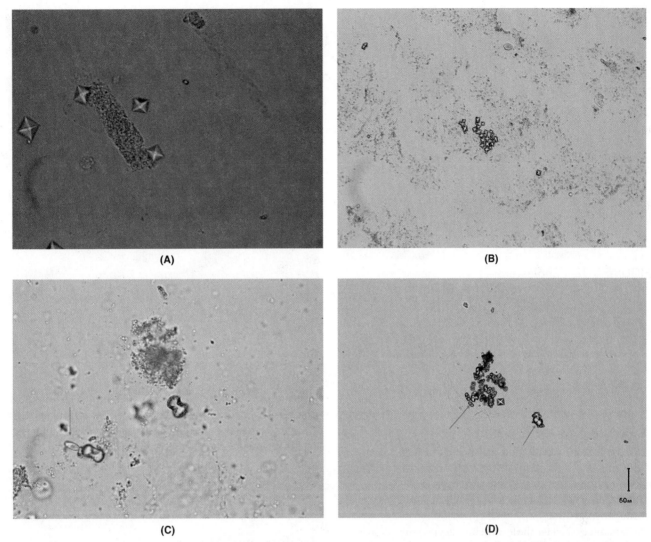

(A)

(B)

(C)

(D)

■ **FIGURE 8-29** **(A)** Calcium Oxalate Dihydrate Crystals, Granular Cast (200×, Brightfield); **(B)** Calcium Oxalate Crystals, Amorphous Urates (50× Brightfield); **(C)** Calcium Oxalate Monohydrate Crystals, Dumbbell and Oval (Arrow) Forms (50×, Brightfield); **(D)** Calcium Oxalate Crystal. Note that the Monohydrate (Arrows) and Dihydrate Forms are Both Present (50×, Brightfield)

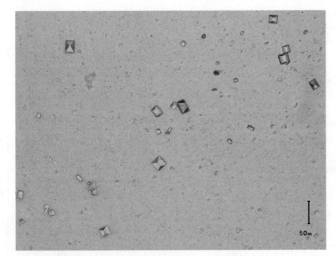

■ **FIGURE 8-30** Triple Phosphate Crystals (50×, Brightfield)

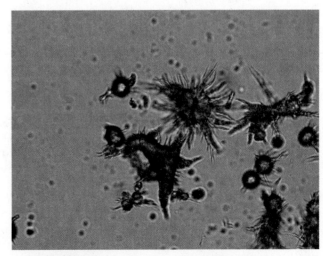

■ **FIGURE 8-31** Ammonium Biurate Crystals (200×, Brightfield)

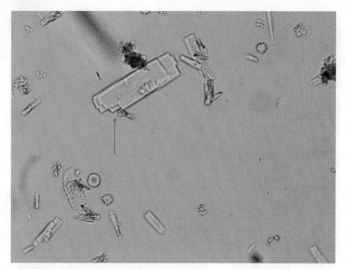

■ **FIGURE 8-32**   Cholesterol Crystal. Characteristic Notch Indicated by Arrow (200×, Brightfield)

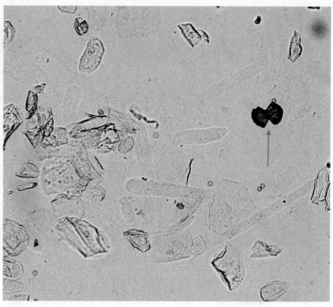

■ **FIGURE 8-33**   Sulfur Crystal (Arrow) with Many Hyaline Casts (50×, Brightfield)

like concentric circles and radial striation (Table 8-4 ★). They sometimes may resemble fat globules. Leucine crystals do not form Maltese crosses with polarization; however, they are birefringent.

Rarely, tyrosine and leucine crystals can be found in patients with severe liver disease.

Sulfonamides and Ampicillin

Excreted by the kidney, medications and their metabolites can exist in high concentrations and precipitate out as crystals. Crystal formation *in vivo* within the kidney can cause renal damage.

Ampicillin crystals appear as long needles and may occur singly or in groups in acid urine.

Sulfonamides can take the form of bundles resemble sheaves of wheat (sulfadiazine) (Figure 8-33 ■) or as brown rosettes or spheres (sulphamethoxazole (Bactrim or Septra)). Their appearance at acid pH differentiates them from ammonium biurates, which form in alkaline urine.

Radiographic Dyes

Media used for radiographic examination include diatrizoate dyes, which may cause crystal formation at acid pH in patients not well hydrated. These crystals appear as flat, notched plates or longer rectangles resembling cholesterol crystals. The crystals can be verified as dye crystals if there is an absence of lipiduria commonly seen with high cholesterol. In addition, the high urine specific gravity seen in patients after injection of radiographic dye is rarely seen in patients with cholesterol crystal formation.

Artifacts and Mucus

Mucin threads can be seen in variable amounts and have no clinical significance. The untrained microscopist may mistake clumps or large threads to be hyaline casts in unstained urine (Figure 8-34A ■).

★ **TABLE 8.4** Abnormal Crystals Found in Urine at Acid or Neutral pH

Crystal	Color	Comments	Shape
Cholesterol	Colorless	Birefringent. May be found in nephrotic syndrome.	Stair-step or notch; flat plates
Bilirubin	Yellow-orange to orange	Crystals form in vitro.	Tight clusters of needles; small spiky spheres.
Cystine	Colorless	Not birefringent. Forms renal calculi.	Hexagonal plates.
Leucine	Colorless	Inherited amino acid disorder. Birefringent. May resemble fat globules; however, crystals do not exhibit Maltese cross formation.	"Wagon wheels."
Tyrosine	Colorless to brown to black depending on concentration.	Inherited amino acid disorder. May rarely be seen in liver disease.	Fine needles, sometimes forming sheaves.
Medications and Dyes			
Sulfonamides	Dark orange	May cause kidney damage if formed in vivo.	Bundles of wheat. Brown rosettes or spheres.
Ampicillin	Colorless		Fine needles
Radiographic dyes	Colorless	Distinguished from cholesterol by absence of lipiduria.	Flat plates, rectangles, notched plates.

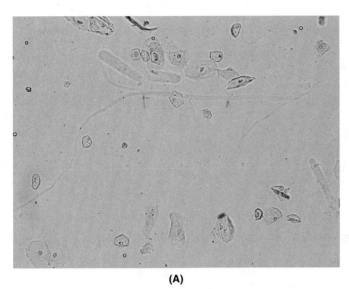

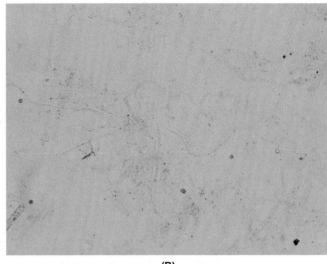

(A)　　　　　　　　　　　　　　　　　　　(B)

■ **FIGURE 8-34** **(A)** Mucin Thread (Arrows) with Hyaline Casts in the Same Field (50×, Brightfield); **(B)** Mucus. Sternheimer-Malbin Stain (50×, Brightfield

Mucus stains very lightly; however, a better method of differentiation from casts is the use of phase contrast or interference contrast microscopy (Figure 8-34B).

Pollen, starch granules, and fibers are common inclusions in the urine sediment examination that pose no clinical significance. Starch granules often are intruded as result of gloved healthcare workers. They can be somewhat difficult to differentiate from fat globules if polarizing microscopy is used. Starch granules will exhibit a Maltese cross pattern; however, under brightfield microscopy these granules appear ragged at the edge and imperfectly round (Figure 8-35 ■).

Fibers can cause some uninitiated microscopists to mistake them for casts. Fibers are usually very large and flat compared to rounded-end casts and can be introduced from diapers, toilet paper, and cotton clothing into the urine sample (Figure 8-36A ■ and 8-36B).

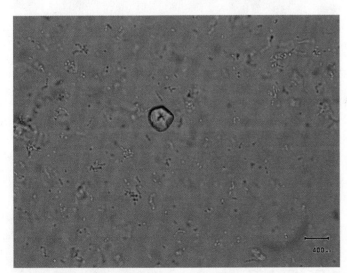

■ **FIGURE 8-35** Starch granule. Note the Small Indentations in the Center of the Granule (200×, Brightfield)

☑ CHECKPOINT 8-3

1. These formed elements are renal tubular cells that have taken up fat globules from the tubular lumen.
   - (a) Oval fat bodies
   - (b) *Trichomonas vaginalis*
   - (c) Polymorphonuclear cells
   - (d) Red blood cells

2. This type of cast is associated with chronic renal failure.
   - (a) Hyaline cast
   - (b) Granular cast
   - (c) Crystal cast
   - (d) Waxy cast

3. Because of the neutral fats incorporated into fatty cast matrix, these casts stain well with
   - (a) Stermheimer Malbin stain.
   - (b) Prussian blue stain.
   - (c) Oil Red O stain.
   - (d) Gram stain.

4. The technologist notes a large amount of pink sediment immediately upon removing the tube from the centrifuge. This "brick dust" appearance is most likely indicative of
   - (a) amorphous phosphates.
   - (b) uric acid crystals.
   - (c) amorphous urates.
   - (d) calcium oxalate crystals.

5. These crystals can appear in patients with jaundice, but appear after precipitation in refrigerated urine. These crystals do not form in vivo.
   - (a) Ammonium biurate
   - (b) Uric acid
   - (c) Calcium oxalate
   - (d) Bilirubin

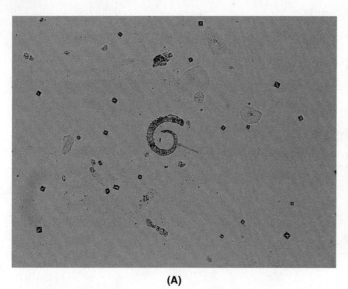

(A)

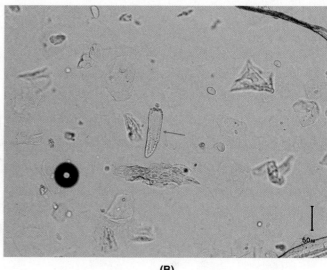

(B)

■ **FIGURE 8-36** **(A)** Artifact (Arrow). Note the Hyaline Cast Directly Under the Fiber (50×, Brightfield); **(B)** Large Air Bubble and Plant Material (Arrow) Artifact Resembling a Cast (50×, Brightfield)

URINARY CALCULI

Crystal formation in both acid and alkaline states can lead to the formation of urinary calculi or stones within the urinary tract. As crystals precipitate from supersaturated urine, they adhere to the urothelium, which provides the location for nucleation and growth of the stone. Stone size can range from grains of sand that can be passed uneventfully to that of a golf ball causing severe pain and urinary obstruction. Approximately 10% of people will develop kidney stones, and nearly half of those individuals will have a recurrence. The type of stone formed is caused by factors influencing the patient to have increased urine excretion of calcium (hypercalcinuria), oxalate (hyperoxaluria), uric acid (hyperuricosuria), or cystine (cystinuria).

Seventy-five percent of stones formed consist of calcium oxalate. In the normal individual most dietary calcium is reabsorbed from the gastrointestinal (GI) tract with a small amount used to bind oxalate for intestinal excretion. Calcium can be bound instead to excess fat and bile salts in those individuals with inflammatory bowel disease. In this case, an excess of unbound oxalate will be reabsorbed into the bloodstream and be excreted in the urine. A diet high in spinach, rhubarb, and nuts can increase oxalate levels and hyperoxaluria. Calciuria can be caused by defects in intestinal reabsorption, increased bone demineralization in hyperparathyroidism, or renal tubular reabsorption of calcium. A combination of both increased calcium and oxalate excretion caused by defects in absorption or dietary changes may cause those individuals at risk to form these stones. In addition, nearly half of all calcium stone-formers also have low urine citrate levels. Normally, crystallization can be impeded by citrate and Tamm-Horsfall protein present in urine. There are some inherited defects that cause the kidney to lose the ability to acidify urine to a pH of 5.5 or less. Calcium oxalate stones are formed in acid urine. Excess calcium may also bind with phosphate, producing calcium phosphate stones.

Uric acid and cystine stones, also formed in acid urine, are less common and are formed by only 10% and 1% of stone-forming patients respectively.[19] Individuals with a low urine pH, low urine volume, and increased uric acid levels are at risk to form uric acid stones.

Struvite stones, produced in alkaline urine, are associated with chronic urinary infections. These stones contain a mixture of magnesium, phosphate, and ammonium and can be seen in the crystalline form as triple phosphate in urine. The stones can take on the shape of the renal pelvis and appear to have horns. These are referred to as staghorn calculi (Figure 8.37 ■). Bacteria such as *Proteus* and

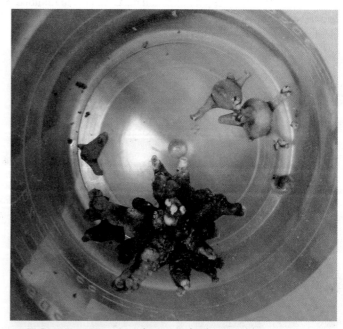

■ **FIGURE 8-37** Staghorn Calculi.
Source: used by permission of E. Wahrendorf.

Pseudomonas hydrolyze urea to produce ammonium and hydroxyl ions, producing alkaline urine, which is needed for the supersaturation of triple phosphate crystallization.

Urinalysis and evaluation of 24-hour urine volume and pH are important factors to consider in patients prone to stone formation. The urine may be tested for mineral excretion as well. Serum levels of calcium, phosphate, uric acid, and parathyroid hormone can be key in helping the physician to diagnose and treat these patients. Urinalysis can be used to detect the presence of red or white blood cells, protein, and crystals.

Stone examination will help define the patient's risk for particular diseases or conditions leading to stone formation. Techniques for analyzing urinary stones include wet chemical analysis, x-ray diffraction, and infrared spectroscopy.

Key Points to Remember

- Urine samples are processed in a timely manner to produce the most reliable results of urine testing. Variables that may affect the stability of urine analytes and solids include length and temperature of storage and exposure to light.

- A well-mixed urine sample is analyzed for urine chemistries and the presence of solid elements by microscopy. The microscopist uses the chemical report as an aid to verification of elements seen in the microscopic evaluation.

- Red blood cells, white blood cells, and urinary casts are counted within a defined space and calculated to give the clinician a precise report of these sometimes pathological elements.

- Examination of the sediment is done using brightfield or phase contrast microscopy at both low power (10×) and high power (40×) magnification.

- Identification of some urine solids such as casts, epithelial cells, white blood cells, and cellular inclusions (fat or iron) can be enhanced through the use of supravital stains.

- It is important to recognize that some elements such as red blood cells, white blood cells, and renal tubular epithelial cells may occur in both benign and disease states.

- Hematuria can originate from the upper or lower urinary tract and be a symptom of conditions ranging from strenuous exercise to glomerular disease or cancer.

- Large numbers of white blood cells, or pyuria, indicate inflammation or infection.

- Squamous, transitional, and renal tubular epithelial cells can be found in urine sediment. Although both squamous and transitional epithelium may be clinically insignificant, renal tubular epithelial cells present in high numbers are a sign of tubular necrosis and severe disease.

- Urinary casts formed from uromodulin or Tamm-Horsfall glycoprotein in the distal renal tubules or collecting ducts are called hyaline casts and may include other elements such as red cells, white cells, or epithelial cells within the matrix, which give indication of renal health. These elemental inclusions may indicate glomerular damage, pyelonephritis, acute tubular necrosis, and severe renal pathologic disease.

- Granular casts are the product of disintegration of matrix elements as the casts pass through the renal tubule. As renal stasis increases, the granules within the cast will fragment and solidify further to create the smooth, opalescent appearance of the waxy cast, indicating severe renal obstruction and impending renal failure.

- Crystalluria is produced by the precipitation of urinary salts due to changes in pH, temperature, and concentration or urine either *in vivo* or *in vitro*.

- Crystals are identified according to shape, color, their ability to polarize light, and the pH of the urine specimen. Abnormal crystals, such as cystine, leucine, and tyrosine, are an indication of rare inherited disorders.

- Urinary calculi can be caused by a dietary excesses, absorption defects, and amino acid disorders as well as by bacterial infection.

- Knowledge of the urine chemistry, specific gravity, and urine pH can help distinguish elements that appear similar to each other, as well as those elements that may be artifacts.

Review Questions

Level I

1. A positive protein result on dipstick procedure for a urine sample can indicate the presence of which of the following? (Objective 1)

    A. Hyaline cast

    B. Uric acid crystals

    C. Vitamin C

    D. Red blood cells

2. A urine sample arrives in the laboratory for routine testing. The sample is placed at room temperature at 7 a.m. and will be tested with the next large batch of samples due to arrive from the outpatient clinic at 11 a.m. How will the sample be affected by the storage time and temperature? (Objective 1)

    A. Cells and casts will degrade in the sample.

    B. There will be no change in the sample since it is stored at room temperature.

    C. The pH of the sample will become more acidic.

    D. The sample will not need to be centrifuged since the elements will settle naturally.

3. The presence of red blood cells in urine is termed (Objective 5)

    A. leukopenia.

    B. hematuria.

    C. icterus.

    D. uricemia.

4. Pyuria is defined as (Objective 8)

    A. increased number of red blood cells in urine.

    B. increased number of white blood cells in urine.

    C. decreased concentrations of protein in urine.

    D. decreased number of hyaline casts in urine.

5. Which of following terms describes a symptomatic infection involving the upper portion of the urinary tract (renal parenchyma)? (Objective 8)

    A. Acute renal failure

    B. Cystitis

    C. Urinary bladder cancer

    D. Pyelonephritis

6. Squamous epithelial cells are located in which part of the urinary tract? (Objective 7)

    A. Urinary bladder

    B. Prostate gland

    C. The distal third of the male and female urethra

    D. Nephrons

7. Which of the following should be completed on every urine specimen prior to chemical and microscopic analysis? (Objective 1)

    A. Observe urine for color and clarity

    B. Smell each urine specimen for the presence of ketone bodies

    C. Centrifuge the urine specimen and observe the precipitate for color

    D. Accurately measure each urine specimen for total urine volume

8. Urine specimens should be processed within two hours to prevent (Objective 1)

    A. obnoxious odor from developing.

    B. significant changes in urine pH values.

    C. cells and cast from degrading.

    D. spontaneous crystal formation, especially calcium oxalate crystals.

9. Microscopic examination of urinary sediment should begin by scanning the preparation with subdued light or phase-contrast illumination at the outer edges to allow the microscopist to identify which of the following? (Objective 3)

    A. Artifacts

    B. Parasites

    C. Oval fat bodies

    D. Casts with low refractive indexes that settle in those areas

10. Hyaline casts are visible using (Objective 3)

    A. electron microscope.

    B. Oil red O stain solution.

    C. brightfield microscopy using a subdued light level.

    D. brightfield microscopy using the highest light level possible.

11. Sternheimer-Malbin, metachromatic dyes, and Sudan III are all examples of (Objective 4)

    A. protein staining compounds.

    B. urinary sediment stains.

    C. white blood counting procedures.

    D. red blood stains.

12. A specimen with a high specific gravity will cause a red blood cell to (Objective 5)

    A. shrink, crenate, and take on spiky appearance.

    B. swell or burst.

    C. form a Maltese cross.

    D. sickle.

13. Which of the following is the most common white blood cell found in urine sediment? (Objective 6)

    A. Monocytes

    B. Lymphocytes

    C. Leukoblasts

    D. Polymorphonuclear leukocytes

14. A patient with an acute tubular necrosis may show a large number of which of the following? (Objective 7)

    A. Transitional epithelial cells (NSE)

    B. Squamous epithelial cells (SQEP)

    C. Renal tubular epithelial cells (RTE)

    D. Spermatozoa

15. "The drops exhibit a Maltese cross pattern with polarized light" describes which of the following formed elements? (Objective 7)

    A. Spermatozoa

    B. Calcium oxalate crystals

    C. Uric acid crystals

    D. Oval fat bodies

16. Hyaline casts are composed of (Objective 10)

    A. the mucoprotein, uromodulin.

    B. fat.

    C. hemoglobin.

    D. red blood cells.

17. A patient whose condition results in hemorrhaging within the nephron will show which of the following in his or her urine? (Objective 10)

    A. White blood cell casts

    B. Red blood cell casts

    C. *Trichomonas vaginalis*

    D. *Candida albicans*

18. Which of the following crystals appear in neutral to alkaline urine and are shaped like "coffin lids"? (Objective 11)

    A. Ammonium biurate

    B. Calcium oxalate

    C. Uric acid

    D. Triple phosphate

19. A patient with gout can have which of the following crystals in his or her urine specimen? (Objective 12)

    A. Cholesterol

    B. Bilirubin

    C. Tyrosine

    D. Uric acid

20. A patient who ingests medications containing sulfonamides may form crystals in his or her urine that resemble which of the following? (Objective 12)

    A. Coffin lids

    B. Large six-sided crystals

    C. Sheaves of wheat or brown rosettes

    D. Large flat plates containing a notch or have a "stair step" appearance at acid pH

Level II

1. A microscopic examination of urine sediment from a patient reveals the presence of dysmorphic red blood cells. Which of the following is a cause of these oddly shaped cells? (Objective 3)

    A. Obstruction of the urethra

    B. Glomerular damage due to physical injury to the kidney

    C. Infection of the urinary bladder

    D. Kidney's response to a patient taking sulfonamide-containing medication

2. Which of the following urinalysis result(s) is consistent with a patient who has a bacterial infection of the kidneys? (Objective 2)

    A. Pyuria and a positive test for leukocyte esterase

    B. Glucosuria and a negative test for leukocyte esterase

    C. Pyremia and a positive test for ketones

    D. Positive identification of *Trichomonas vaginalis*

3. A patient with Wilson's disease, which is characterized by high blood levels of copper, may present with the following results of a urinalysis: (Objective 2)

    A. large number of granular casts.

    B. large number red blood cells and white blood cells.

    C. slight increase in copper oxide crystals.

    D. large number of renal tubular epithelial cells.

4. A microscopic examination of a urine specimen from an adult female using phase contrast microscopy reveals the movement of an organism that has flagella. This organism is an example of which of the following? (Objective 6)

   A. *Candida albicans*

   B. Spermatozoa

   C. *Trichomonas vaginalis*

   D. Mucin threads

5. Which of the following urinalysis results are consistent with nephritic syndrome? (Objective 5)

   A. Negative protein using a dipstick procedure

   B. Cells with Maltese cross pattern using polarized light and a 3+ protein using a dipstick procedure

   C. Clue cells are present

   D. Crystals formed due to the presence of diatrizoate dyes

6. What is the relative centrifugal force (*g*) produced when centrifuging a urine sample at 2500 revolutions per minute. The centrifuge rotor has a radius of 10 centimeters? (Objective 1)

   A. 599

   B. 699

   C. 1699

   D. 1899

Endnotes

1. Fogazzi GB, Garigali G.The clinical art and science of urine microscopy. *Curr opin in nephrol and hypertens.* 2003;12;6:625–632.

2. Fogazzi GB, Cameron JS, Ponticelli C. The History of urinary microscopy to the end of the 19th century. *Am J of Nephrol.* 1994;14(4-6):452–457.

3. Fogazzi GB, Cameron JS.Urinary Microscopy from the seventeenth century to the present day. *Kidney Int.* 1996; 50; 3:1058–1060.

4. Clinical and Laboratory Standards Institute (CLSI). Urinalysis and Collection, Transportation, and Preservation of Urine Specimens. *CLSI Document GP16-A2 (ISBN 1-56238-448-1).* Approved guideline-second edition ed. Vol. 21, No.19940 West Valley Road, Suite 1400, Wayne, Pennsylvania 19087-1898 USA, 2001: Clinical and Laboratory Standards Institute, 2001, p. 12.

5. Clinical and Laboratory Standards Institute (CLSI). Provider-Performed Microscopy Testing; Approved Guideline. *CLSI Document GP16-A2 (ISBN 1-56238-448-1).* Approved guideline-second edition ed. Vol. 23, No.5. 940 West Valley Road, Suite 1400, Wayne, Pennsylvania 19087-1898 USA, 2001: Clinical and Laboratory Standards Institute, 2003, p. 23.

6. Freeman JA, Beeler MF. *Laboratory Medicine/Urinalysis and Medical Microscopy.* 2nd ed. Philadelphia: Lea & Febiger,1983, p. 259.

7. McPherson RA, Ben-Ezra J, Zhao S. Basic examination of urine. *Henry's Clinical Diagnosis and Management by Laboratory Methods.* Eds. McPherson RA, Pincus, MR. 22nd Ed. Philadelphia: Elsevier Saunders, 2011. p. 465.

8. Ibid., p. 468.

9. Nagahama D, Yoshiki K, Watanabe M, et al. A useful new classification of dysmorphic urinary erythrocytes. *Clin and exp nephrol.*2005;9;4:304–309.

10. Higashihara E, Nishiyama T, Horie S, et al. Hematuria: definition and screening test methods. *Int J of Urol.* 2008;15;4:281–284.

11. McPherson RA, Ben-Ezra J, Zhao S. Basic examination of urine. *Henry's Clinical Diagnosis and Management by Laboratory Methods.* Eds. McPherson RA, Pincus, MR. 22nd Ed. Philadelphia: Elsevier Saunders, 2011, p. 465.

12. Ringsrud, KM. Cells in urine sediment. *Lab Medicine,* 2001b; 32;3:153–155.

13. Fogazzi GB, Grignani S, Coluccio P. Urinary microscopy as seen by nephrologists. *Clin chem and lab med.* 1998; 36;12:919–924.

14. Ringsrud KM. Casts in the urine sediment. *Lab Medicine* 2001a;32;4:191–193.

15. Ibid.

16. McPherson RA, Ben-Ezra J, Zhao S. Basic examination of urine. *Henry's Clinical Diagnosis and Management by Laboratory Methods.* Eds. McPherson RA, Pincus, MR. 22nd Ed. Philadelphia: Elsevier Saunders, 2011, p. 469.

17. Terlinsky AS, Grochowski J, Geoly KL, et al. Identification of atypical calcium oxalate crystalluria following ethylene glycol ingestion. *Am J of Clin Pathol.* 1981;76;2:223–226.

18. Mishra V, Wong K. Kidney stones, biochemical evaluation of risk factors. *Clinical Laboratory News, AACC.* 2012;38;12:8–10.

19. Ibid.

Suggested reading:

Brunzel, NA. *Fundamentals of Urine and Body Fluid Analysis.* 3rd ed. Philadelphia: Elsevier 2013, 167–210.

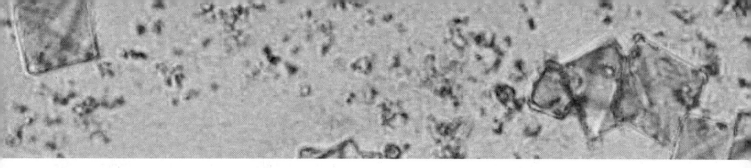

9 Renal Diseases

Objectives

LEVEL I

1. List and give examples of the four categories of renal diseases.
2. Define glomerulonephritis and list examples of primary and secondary causes of glomerulonephritis.
3. Discuss the findings in the routine urinalysis in acute glomerulonephritis.
4. Define crescentic or rapidly progressive glomerulonephritis and describe the common causes of this condition.
5. Define chronic glomerulonephritis and discuss the abnormal laboratory results, and conditions, associated with chronic glomerulonephritis.
6. Describe minimal change disease including the etiology and population incidence.
7. Discuss membranoproliferative glomerulonephritis, including the etiology, and list some of the most common conditions associated with MPGN.
8. Discuss IgA nephropathy, including the clinical course, symptoms, and significant laboratory findings.
9. Describe nephrotic syndrome including primary and secondary causes, symptoms, and laboratory findings.
10. Name the pathognomonic urinalysis finding in acute poststreptococcal glomerulonephritis, chronic glomerulonephritis, nephrotic syndrome, acute pyelonephritis, and chronic pyelonephritis.
11. Define renal tubular disease.
12. Describe acute tubular necrosis and state two examples of ischemic causes and toxic substances that are associated with acute tubular necrosis.
13. Define Fanconi syndrome and give examples of the most common causes in children and adults.
14. Define tubulointerstitial nephritis and list five common conditions and medications associated with this condition.
15. Define acute pyelonephritis and the typical urinalysis findings.

Objectives (continued)

16. Describe chronic pyelonephritis and discuss the findings on a routine urinalysis.

17. Define cystitis, the types of cystitis, and typical urinalysis findings.

18. List prerenal, renal, and postrenal causes of acute renal failure.

19. Describe the four main types of renal calculi and the most common causes associated with each.

LEVEL II

1. Compare and contrast the four categories of renal diseases: glomerular, tubular, interstitial, and vascular.

2. Compare and contrast type 1 to type 4 renal tubular acidosis including conditions and laboratory findings associated with each type.

3. List and describe the five stages of chronic kidney disease.

4. Differentiate the causes and laboratory results associated with prerenal, renal, and postrenal acute renal failure.

Key Terms

Acute glomerulonephritis (AGN)
Acute pyelonephritis
Acute renal failure (ARF)
Acute tubular necrosis (ATN)
Berger's disease
Chronic glomerulonephritis (CGN)
Chronic kidney disease (CKD)
Chronic pyelonephritis
Classical distal renal tubular acidosis

Crescentic (rapidly progressive) glomerulonephritis (RPGN)
Cystitis
Diabetic nephropathy
Fanconi syndrome
Glomerulonephritis
Hyperkalemic renal tubular acidosis
IgA nephropathy
Kimmelstiel-Wilson disease

Membranoproliferative glomerulonephritis (MPGN)
Minimal change disease (MCD)
Nephrolithiasis
Nephrotic syndrome (NS)
Noninfectious glomerulonephritis
Non-streptococcal glomerulonephritis
Pathognomonic
Primary glomerulonephritis

Renal lithiasis
Renal tubular acidosis
Renovascular disease
Secondary glomerulonephritis
Type 1 Distal renal tubular acidosis
Type 2 Proximal renal tubular acidosis
Tubulointerstitial nephritis
Vesicourethral reflux (VUR)

A CASE IN POINT

Mary, a 40-year-old woman, presented with the following symptoms: flank pain (pain in the side of the trunk between the right or left upper abdomen and the back), fever of 102°F, chills and diaphoresis (sweating), dysuria, nocturia, and increased frequency and urgency of urination. A routine urinalysis is performed.

Urinalysis

Macroscopic:

Color:	Yellow
Appearance:	Cloudy
Specific Gravity:	1.019
pH:	6.0
Protein:	1 + (30 mg/dL)(SSA: 1+)
Glucose:	Neg
Ketones:	Neg
Bilirubin:	Neg
Blood:	1+
Urobilinogen:	Normal
Nitrite:	Pos
Leukocyte Esterase:	2+

Microscopic:

WBCs:	40–60/HPF
	2–4 clumps/HPF
RBCs:	0–3/HPF
Epithelial Cells:	Few Squamous/HPF
	Rare Renal Epithelial/HPF
Casts:	3–6 WBC/LPF
	0–2 Granular/LPF
	0–1 Bacterial Casts/LPF
Bacteria:	Moderate/HPF

Questions for Consideration

1. What are the abnormal value(s) or discrepant result(s) in this urinalysis?

2. Are these findings consistent with an upper or lower urinary tract infection (UTI)? Why?

3. Which renal disease/condition is suggested by these urinalysis results? How would you differentiate an acute from a chronic condition?

4. What type of leukocytes are usually associated with pyuria?

5. Which urinalysis finding is pathognomonic (characteristic) of this disease?

6. What are some two common physiological causes for this condition?

7. What follow-up test(s) should be ordered and what would be the most common findings?

8. How is this condition treated?

9. What conditions lead to an increased incidence of this disease—make people more prone to these infections?

10. What is Mary's prognosis?

Renal diseases resulting from damage to the kidneys themselves are primary renal diseases. Secondary renal diseases are disorders and conditions that affect other organs or systems of the body and the kidney secondarily. Renal diseases can occur as a result of many disorders in the body. Glomerular filtration, tubular reabsorption, and tubular secretion are the three most important functions of the kidney that are affected by various renal diseases. This chapter will discuss the most common renal diseases and relate them to the laboratory findings used to diagnose these disorders, concentrating especially on the abnormal results on the routine urinalysis.

CLASSIFICATION OF RENAL DISEASES

Renal diseases can be classified in four categories based on the area of the nephron most affected: glomerular, tubular, interstitial, and renovascular. The most common diseases will be covered by a discussion of the etiology (the cause(s)), symptoms, laboratory findings, and treatment and prognosis.

GLOMERULONEPHRITIS

Acute glomerulonephritis was initially described by Bright in 1927. **Glomerulonephritis** is defined as a sterile (no bacteria), inflammatory process that affects the glomerulus or a group of nephrotic conditions characterized by damage and inflammation of the glomeruli. Changes in the glomeruli include (1) cellular proliferation of the endothelial cells, (2) leukocyte infiltration, (3) glomerular basement membrane thickening, and (4) hyalinization with sclerosis described as loss of structural detail and transformation of a tissue to a glassy appearance.

Glomerulonephritis is caused by the deposits of antigen–antibody complexes on the glomerular membrane. **Primary glomerulonephritis** specifically affects the kidney. **Secondary glomerulonephritis** principally involves other organs and the kidney secondarily.

Acute Glomerulonephritis

Acute glomerulonephritis (AGN) is characterized by a rapid onset of symptoms that indicate damage to the glomerular membrane. AGN is defined as the sudden onset of hematuria, proteinuria, and red blood cell casts. It is most often seen in children and young adults following a group A streptococcal infection, e.g., strep throat or a respiratory infection. Acute poststreptococcal glomerulonephritis usually occurs 1 to 2 weeks following a streptococcal infection of the throat or skin. Glomerulonephritis is antibody-mediated; it is believed that immune complexes (antigen–antibody complexes) form and deposit on the glomerular membrane, causing damage to the integrity of the membrane.[1] AGN is more frequent in children 2–12 years of age, with a peak in 5- to 6-year-olds; however, it has been diagnosed in babies as young as 1 year old and in 90-year-old adults.

Non-streptococcal glomerulonephritis can be caused by other bacteria (e.g., diplococci, other streptococci, staphylococci, and mycobacteria). *Salmonella typhosa, Brucella suis, Treponema pallidum, Corynebacterium bovis*, and actinobaccilli have also been associated with AGN. Viruses including mumps, hepatitis B, cytomegalovirus (CMV), Epstein-Barr virus (EBV), rubella, and rickettsia can be acknowledged as the cause only if a group A beta-hemolytic streptococcal infection cannot be verified. Parasitic or fungal etiologies include *Plasmodium falciparum, Plasmodium malariae, Schistosoma mansoni, Toxoplasma gondii*, filariasis, trichinosis, and trypanosomes. Another etiology that has been identified is chemicals that are nephrotoxic (e.g., hydrocarbon solvents).[2]

Noninfectious glomerulonephritis can be caused by multisystem diseases: vasculitis (e.g., Wegener's granulomatosis), collagen-vascular disease (systemic lupus erythematosus (SLE)), diabetic nephropathy, Henoch-Schonlein purpura, IgA nephropathy, and Goodpasture syndrome. Guillain-Barré syndrome, diphtheria-pertussis-tetanus (DPT) vaccine and serum sickness are also miscellaneous noninfectious causes of AGN[3]. See Box 9-1 for a list of the more common causes of acute glomerulonephritis.

BOX 9-1 Causes of Acute Glomerulonephritis

Poststreptococcal AGN

- **Other Bacteria**
  - Diplococci
  - Other streptococci
  - Staphylococci
  - Mycobacteria
  - *Salmonella typhosa*
  - *Brucella suis*
  - *Treponema pallidum*
  - *Corynebacterium bovis*
  - Actinobacilli
- **Viruses**
  - Mumps
  - Hepatitis B
  - Cytomegalovirus
  - Epstein-Barr virus
  - Rubella
  - Rickettsia
- **Parasitic or Fungal**
  - *Plasmodium malariae*
  - *Schistosoma mansoni*
  - *Toxoplasma gondii*
  - Filariasis
  - Trichinosis
  - Trypanosomes
- Nephrotoxic chemicals

- **Noninfectious**
  - Wegner's granulomatosis
  - Systemic lupus erythematosus (SLE)
  - Diabetic nephropathy
  - Henoch-Schonlein purpura
  - IgA nephropathy
  - Guillain-Barré syndrome
  - Diphtheria-pertussis-tetanus (DPT) vaccine
  - Serum sickness

Symptoms

Symptoms of AGN include sudden onset of fever, malaise, nausea, oliguria, hematuria, and proteinuria. Other clinical findings in AGN are hypertension, edema (e.g., face, eyes, ankles, feet, and legs), azotemia, and renal salt and water retention.

Laboratory Findings

The routine urinalysis is characterized by hematuria, often with dysmorphic RBCs, and a mild increase in protein (<1.0 g/24h). The increased protein may alter the surface tension of the urine resulting in abnormally foamy urine. RBCs (see Figure 9-1 ■ and 9-2 ■) and hemoglobin casts are **pathognomonic** (indicative of or characteristic of a particular disease) of AGN. Hyaline and granular casts and WBCs may also be reported. See Box 9-2 for a summary of laboratory findings.

Elevated renal function tests, Blood Urea Nitrogen (BUN) and creatinine, are a sign of decreased renal function. Creatinine clearance will be decreased, which is indicative of decreased glomerular filtration rate (GFR).

Treatment and Prognosis

Treatment usually involves management of the secondary complications until the inflammation has subsided. Restriction of fluids and/or diuretics are used to treat edema especially of the knees and ankles. Medications, e.g., beta-blockers or angiotensin-converting enzyme (ACE) inhibitors, with diuretics and vasodilators are used to treat severe hypertension, and electrolyte imbalance.[4]

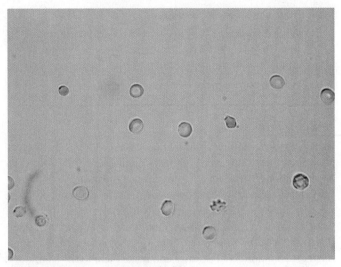

■ **FIGURE 9-2** Red Blood Cells, Normal and Dysmorphic in AGN

Children with poststreptococcal AGN usually recover completely (95%), but the recovery rate is not as high for adults (60%). The prognosis for nonstreptococcal forms is also not as good, with some patients progressing to chronic glomerulonephritis. In elderly patients, especially with debilitating conditions (e.g., malnutrition, alcoholism, diabetes, and other chronic conditions) the incidences of azotemia (60%), congestive heart failure (40%), and significant proteinuria (20%) are high.[5]

MINI-CASE 9-1

Kate, a high school basketball player, has been hospitalized with a severe throat infection, fever, and a question of pneumonia. She had been taking antibiotics. Her physician noted edema and elevated blood pressure.

The following are selected abnormal urinalysis results.

Color:	Red
Protein:	2+ (160mg/dL) (SSA: 2+)
Blood:	2 + (~50 RBCs/µL)
Microscopic	
RBCs:	30–60/HPF (dysmorphic forms present)
Casts:	
	1–3 hyaline/LPF
	0–3 RBC/LPF
	0–1 hemoglobin/LPF
	1–3 granular/LPF

Questions to Consider

1. What is the probable diagnosis?
2. Which urinalysis results is/are pathognomonic (characteristic) of this condition?
3. What is the probable causative agent (organism) in this case?
4. List five other possible causes for this condition.

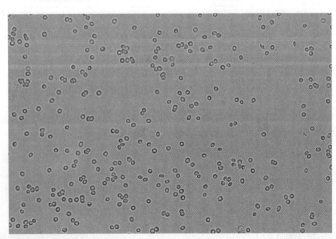

■ **FIGURE 9-1** RBCs Associated with Acute Glomerulonephritis

BOX 9-2 Acute Glomerulonephritis Abnormal Laboratory Findings

- **Blood: moderate to many RBCs***
- **Dysmorphic RBCs**
- Proteinuria: variable, usually mild (<1.0 g/day)
- Leukocytes
- Renal tubular cells
- **RBC casts**
- Hemoglobin casts
- Granular casts
- BUN: elevated
- Creatinine: elevated
- Creatinine clearance: decreased
- Antistreptolysin O titer (ASOT): positive

*Bolded results are the pathognomonic for AGN.

BOX 9-3 Three Categories of Crescentic Glomerulonephritis

- **Anti-GBM Antibody**
  - Goodpasture syndrome
  - Anti-GBM disease
- **Immune Complex**
  - Lupus nephritis
  - Henoch-Scholein purpura
  - Membranoproliferative glomerulonephritis
  - Postinfectious (staphylococci/streptococci)
  - Immunoglobulin A nephropathy
  - Collagen-vascular disease
  - Idiopathic
- **Pauci-immune**
  - Wegner granulomatosis (WG)
  - Renal-limited necrotizing crescentic glomerulonephritis (NCGN)

Crescentic (Rapidly Progressive) Glomerulonephritis

Crescentic or rapidly progressive glomerulonephritis (RPGN) causes permanent damage to the glomeruli due to fibrin deposits that break down the basement membrane inside the Bowman's capsule. Cellular proliferation results in the characteristic crescent-shaped epithelial cells. RPGN is antibody-mediated often by anti-glomerular basement membrane (GBM) antibodies, and the glomeruli are infiltrated with WBCs and fibrin deposits.

Crescentic glomerulonephritis can be classified in three categories: (1) Anti-GBM (~ 3% of cases), (2) Immune complex disease (45%), and (3) Pauci-immune (50%). Immunologic classification is based on the presence or absence of antineutrophil cytoplasmic antibodies (ANCAs). See Box 9-3 for a list of some of the more common conditions under each category.[6]

Symptoms
Common symptoms include edema, hypertension, oliguria, dark- or smoke-colored urine (hematuria), oliguria, and a general malaise.

Laboratory Findings
The urinalysis becomes more abnormal as the disease progresses. Marked hematuria, dysmorphic RBCs, WBCs, increased protein (variable), oliguria, and hyaline, RBC, and granular casts are present. The glomerular filtration rate decreases as the disease progresses and as toxicity subsides, the urinalysis returns closer to normal.

Treatment and Prognosis
Prognosis and appropriate treatment depend on the immuno-pathologic category and disease severity at the time of initial treatment. Immunosuppressive therapy, e.g., cyclophosphamide and azothioprine, should be considered for patients with Anti-GBM and antineutrophil cytoplasmic antibodies (ANCAs). However, IgA nephropathy and acute postinfectious glomerulonephritis may not require extensive immunosuppression.[7]

If renal failure is present at initial visit, there is an increased risk for end-stage disease and death despite immunosuppressive therapy. Death or dialysis occurs in 73% of patients who are treated with conventional therapy and in 88% of patients if they are oliguric upon initial visit.[8]

Chronic Glomerulonephritis

Chronic glomerulonephritis (CGN) is defined as the end stage of persistent glomerular damage associated with irreversible loss of renal tissue and chronic renal failure. Chronic GN can be associated with a variety of conditions that cause continual or permanent damage to the glomerulus. Chronic glomerulonephritis is the third leading cause of end stage renal disease (ESRD) and accounts for 10% of patients on dialysis in the United States.[9] Acute glomerulonephritis, membranoproliferative glomerulonephritis, rapidly progressive glomerulonephritis, idiopathic membranous glomerulonephritis, and IgA nephropathy have all been known to progress to chronic glomerulonephritis.[10] Rapidly progressive glomerulonephritis is the most common condition that progresses to CGN. Chronic GN has also been associated with other disorders such as amyloidosis, multiple myeloma, or immune disorders including AIDS.[11]

Symptoms
CGN causes hypertension and chronic renal failure. The presenting symptom is often edema, followed by fatigue, anemia, metabolic acidosis, and oliguria, which can progress to anuria as renal function is lost and the patient progresses to chronic renal failure.

Laboratory Findings
Routine urinalysis results include hematuria, which is usually milder than with AGN, and heavy proteinuria (>2.5 g/day). Increased WBCs and renal tubular epithelial (RTE), glucosuria, and many types of casts including broad, granular, and waxy casts may also be present. The specific gravity is often isosthenuric at 1.010, indicating a loss of renal concentrating and diluting ability.

BOX 9-4 Chronic Glomerulonephritis Abnormal Laboratory Findings

- Blood: mild to moderate
- Protein: heavy (>2.5 g/day)
- Glucose: positive
- Isosthenuric
- Cellular and granular casts
- Waxy and broad casts
- BUN: increased
- Serum creatinine: increased
- Creatinine clearance: decreased
- Electrolytes

The chemistry results include an increased BUN and creatinine, a decreased creatinine clearance indicating a markedly decreased glomerular filtration rate, and electrolyte imbalance. Box 9-4 lists significant laboratory findings in chronic glomerulonephritis.

Treatment and Prognosis

The treatment for chronic glomerulonephritis focuses on therapy for the underlying disease that precipitated the condition. The physician then addresses the particular symptoms with various medications. Diuretics are used to treat edema and angiotensin-converting enzyme (ACE) inhibitors to lower blood pressure. Anti-inflammatory drugs, e.g., corticosteroids, may be used to decrease the immune response. Usually dietary salt (sodium) and water are restricted. Dialysis may be needed if the condition worsens.[12]

Minimal Change Disease

Minimal change disease (MCD) (also called Nil disease, lipoid nephrosis) can lead to nephrotic syndrome. It is the most common cause of nephrotic syndrome in children (80%) but only 10–15% of nephrotic syndrome cases in adults. In minimal change disease the cellular structure of the glomeruli is not altered to any significant extent (hence the name), but it is postulated that a disorder of T cells (lymphocytes) release a cytokine that injures the glomerular epithelial foot processes of the podocytes. This allows leakage of albumin and results in further damage.[13]

Minimal change disease occurs twice as frequently in boys than in girls with the peak incidence in 2-year-olds; 80% are younger than 6 years of age at the time of diagnosis. In adults the frequency is the same between sexes and the mean age of onset is 40 years.[14] The cause of MCD is unknown, but it can occur or be related to allergic reactions, non-steroidal anti-inflammatory drugs (NSAIDs), tumors, vaccinations, and viral infections.

Symptoms

Patients with minimal change disease may exhibit symptoms of nephrotic syndrome: foamy urine due to increased protein, edema especially around the eyes, feet, and ankles, weight gain from fluid retention, and fatigue. MCD does not reduce the amount of urine produced and rarely progresses to renal failure.[15]

Laboratory Findings

Minimal change disease may show evidence of the following signs of nephrotic syndrome: high cholesterol, marked proteinuria, and hypoalbuminemia.

Treatment and Prognosis

Diuretics may be used to treat the fluid retention, and blood pressure medication, angiotensin-converting enzyme inhibitors, to reduce the blood pressure's pushing protein through the glomerular cell wall. Corticosteroids, e.g., prednisone, can cure minimal change disease in most children. Some patients may need to remain on steroids to keep the disease in remission. Adults do not respond as well to steroids, but they are effective. Adults tend to have more frequent relapses and become dependent on steroids. Cytotoxic therapy, e.g., cyclophosphamide, cyclosporine, or chlorambucil, may be required in patients with three or more relapses.[16]

Membranoproliferative Glomerulonephritis

Membranoproliferative glomerulonephritis (MPGN I) is inflammation of the glomeruli caused by an abnormal immune response. It is an uncommon cause of chronic glomerulonephritis occurring in children and young adults. *MPGN* is characterized by two different alterations in the cells of the glomerulus and peripheral capillaries. Type I has increased cellularity in the mesangial and endothelial cells and expansion of the mesangial matrix as well as, a thickening of the capillary walls by subendothelial immune deposits. The immune complexes in the mesangium trigger complement activation and release of cytokines and chemokines resulting in the increased cellular proliferation.

Immune complex-mediated conditions, autoimmune diseases, chronic infections, and malignant neoplasms (malignant tumors) are associated with MPGN. See Box 9-5 for a list of the more common causes of membranoproliferative glomerulonephritis.[17]

BOX 9-5 Causes of Membranoproliferative Glomerulonephritis

- **Immune Complex Disease**
- Idiopathic
- **Autoimmune Diseases**
  - Systemic lupus erythematosus
  - Rheumatoid arthritis
  - Scleroderma
  - Celiac disease
- **Chronic Infections**
  - Viral: hepatitis B, hepatitis C, cryoglobulinemia
  - Bacterial: endocarditis, multiple visceral abscesses, leprosy
  - Protozoan: malaria, schistosomiasis
- **Malignant Neoplasms**
  - Lymphoma
  - Leukemia
  - Carcinoma

MPGN II or *dense deposit disease* is systemic and characterized by dense deposits in the glomerular basement membrane and splenic sinusoids. It has a high incidence in renal transplant patients. MPGN II is associated with multiple complement abnormalities including a persistent reduction in C3 levels. One hypothesis is that the dense deposits cause complement activation.[18]

Symptoms

Membranoproliferative glomerulonephritis is characterized by hematuria, cloudy urine, dark urine (smoke-, cola-, or tea-colored), oliguria, edema, hypertension, and changes in mental status (decreased alertness or decreased concentration).

Laboratory Findings

The routine urinalysis report will indicate blood, dysmorphic RBCs, and RBC casts. Proteinuria is also present, with 50% of patients exhibiting marked proteinuria. Elevated serum BUN and creatinine levels and a decreased estimated glomerular filtration rate are found in 20–50% of patients. Complement protein levels are decreased in MPGN due to activation of the complement cascade. In type I there is evidence of the activation of the alternative pathway with low C4, C2, C1q, B, and C3 levels. C3 levels are low in 70–80% of patients with MPGN type II.[19]

Treatment and Prognosis

Treatment is based on the symptoms with the primary goals being to reduce symptoms, prevent complications, and slow the progression of the disorder. Limiting salt, fluids, and proteins may help to control blood pressure. Medications may be prescribed to lower blood pressure, diuretics to decrease fluid volume, immunosuppressants (e.g., cyclophosphamide) and steroids to decrease the immune response. Treatment is more effective in children than adults. Dialysis and kidney transplants may be needed to manage kidney failure.[20]

MPGN often slowly gets worse and eventually results in chronic renal failure. The main predictors of an adverse outcome are nephrotic syndrome and hypertension at presentation, a low glomerular filtration rate 1 year following diagnosis, and older age.[21] Fifty percent of patients develop chronic kidney failure within 10 years.

IgA Nephropathy (Berger's Disease)

IgA nephropathy or **Berger's disease** is the most common type of glomerulonephritis. IgA, an antibody that helps the body fight infection, is increased after a mucosal infection of the respiratory, gastrointestinal, or urinary tract by bacteria or viruses. Immune complexes of IgA deposit on the glomerular membrane where they cause inflammation and eventually block the flow of blood through the glomeruli. Glomeruli become damaged through inflammation and loss of blood resulting in scarring. This disorder can appear acute (rapidly) or worsen slowly over many years (chronic glomerulonephritis). IgA nephropathy may run in families or be related to respiratory infections. No consistent trigger for the disease has been discovered.[22] Berger's disease can be asymptomatic for 20 years, then gradually progress to chronic glomerulonephritis and end stage renal disease in 50% of patients.

Symptoms

Recurrent hematuria, especially following infection or strenuous exercise, is characteristic of IgA nephropathy. Patients may exhibit edema or swelling of the hands and feet and other symptoms (e.g., fatigue, hypoalbuminemia, hypercholesterolemia) of chronic kidney disease.

Laboratory Findings

IgA nephropathy is usually discovered when a person with no other symptoms of kidney problems has one or more episodes of bloody urine. Hematuria can be macroscopic (visible to the naked eye) or microscopic. For the majority of patients microhematuria is always detected. Proteinuria may or may not be present and vary from mild to heavy depending on the stage of the disease. Increased serum IgA levels help to narrow the diagnosis.[23]

Treatment and Prognosis

Treatment of IgA nephropathy is focused on slowing the progression of the disease and addressing the complications. Hypertension is treated with two types of medications: angiotensin-converting enzyme (ACE) inhibitors and angiotensin receptor blockers (ARBs). Statins may be recommended for patients with high cholesterols. Steroids, e.g., prednisone, may decrease the inflammation. Mycophenolate mofetil (MMF) is a new immunosuppressive agent being tested for IgA nephropathy.[24]

Diabetic Nephropathy (Kimmelstiel-Wilson Disease)

Since the 1950s kidney disease has been recognized as a complication of diabetes mellitus (DM) with diabetic nephropathy found in as many as 50% of patients with DM of more than 20 years duration. **Diabetic nephropathy**, also called **Kimmelstiel-Wilson disease**, is a clinical syndrome characterized by (1) persistent albuminuria (>300 mg/dL) that is confirmed on at least two occasions 3–6 months apart, (2) progressive decline in the glomerular filtration rate (GFR), and (3) hypertension. Three histological changes in the glomeruli are described. First, cellular proliferation of the mesangium is directly stimulated by hyperglycemia. Second, the glomerular membrane is thickened. Third, glomerular sclerosis is caused by intraglomerular hypertension.[25]

The exact cause of diabetic nephropathy is unknown, but hyperglycemia (leading to hyperfiltration and renal injury), deposition of glycosylated proteins, and activation of cytokines are possible mechanisms. Familial or genetic factors may also play a role. For example, certain ethnic groups, particularly African Americans, Hispanics, and Native Americans are more disposed to renal disease as a complication of diabetes. Diabetic nephropathy is currently the most common cause of end-stage renal disease.

Symptoms

Often there are no symptoms as the kidney damage begins and slowly progresses. Patients with type 2 diabetes mellitus should be tested for microalbumin at the time of diagnosis. Individuals with type 1 should be screened 5 years after diagnosis.

Laboratory Findings

Monitoring glucose levels and renal function is important in preventing or slowing diabetic nephropathy. Screening for microalbumin should be done annually after the initial test. After the diagnosis of microalbuminuria is made, the physician can either continue annual testing to monitor progression or use creatinine clearance to follow the decrease in the glomerular filtration rate.

Treatment and Prognosis

A low fat diet and careful monitoring of glucose levels can decrease or delay the progression of renal disease. The Diabetes Control and Complications Trial (DCCT) has shown definitively that intensive diabetes therapy can reduce the risk of diabetic nephropathy. Hypertension should be controlled (under 130/80) with angiotensin-converting enzyme (ACE) inhibitors and angiotensin II receptor blockers (ARBs).

When caught in the early stages, the progression of kidney damage can be delayed. Once the proteinuria is heavier, the damage to the kidney may require dialysis or transplant.

Nephrotic Syndrome

Nephrotic syndrome (NS) may occur as a complication of glomerulonephritis or as a result of circulatory disorders that affect blood pressure and flow of blood to the kidney, e.g., diabetes mellitus, lupus erythematosus. Changes in the permeability of the glomerular membrane allow high molecular weight proteins and lipids into the glomerular filtrate, resulting in damage to the glomeruli and tubules.

Nephrotic syndrome can be the primary disease specific to the kidneys, or it can be secondary, with renal complications of a systemic general illness. In adults diabetic nephropathy and membranous nephropathy are the most common causes of secondary nephrotic syndrome. Nephrotic-range proteinuria (>3 g/day) in the third trimester of pregnancy is a classical finding in preeclampsia. Frequently the cause of NS is unknown-idiopathic. Box 9-6 lists the common causes of primary and secondary nephrotic syndrome.[26]

BOX 9-6 Primary and Secondary Causes of Nephrotic Syndrome

Primary
- Minimal-change nephropathy
- Focal glomerulosclerosis
- Membranous nephropathy
- Hereditary nephropathies

Secondary
- Diabetes mellitus
- Lupus erythematosus
- Viral infections, e.g., hepatitis B, hepatitis C, HIV
- Preeclampsia
- Drugs of abuse, e.g., heroin

BOX 9-7 Laboratory Findings in Nephrotic Syndrome

- Hematuria
- Urinary fat droplets*
- Oval fat bodies*
- Renal tubular epithelial cells
- Casts: renal tubular, waxy, and fatty casts
- Hypoalbuminemia*
- Hyperlipidemia*

*Pathognomonic

Symptoms

Symptoms include swelling or edema (periorbital, feet, and hands), foamy urine due to proteinuria, and unintentional weight gain. Nephrotic syndrome is characterized by massive proteinuria (>3.5 gm/day). Pitting edema is caused by the decreased excretion of sodium and unintentional weight gain from fluid retention. Hyperlipidemia and hypoproteinemia are the hallmarks of nephrotic syndrome. The body cannot compensate for the substantial loss of protein in the urine.[27]

Laboratory Findings

The routine urinalysis will exhibit marked proteinuria, increased RBCs (may be microscopic), increased urinary fat droplets (lipiduria), oval fat bodies, renal tubular cells, and casts especially renal tubular epithelial, waxy, and fatty casts.

Serum albumin and total protein are decreased, and cholesterol and triglycerides are increased. See Box 9-7 for a summary of laboratory findings.

Prognosis and Treatment

Patients with nephrotic syndrome are more susceptible to infection due to decreased protein levels, especially gamma globulins (antibodies). Blood pressure should be controlled usually with angiotensin-converting enzyme (ACE) inhibitors or angiotensin receptor blockers (ARBs). Corticosteroids or other medications may be used to suppress the immune system. Cholesterol should be lowered by diet or medications (statins) to reduce the risk of heart disease. Diuretics and a low salt diet will address the edema.[28]

The prognosis is variable. Nephrotic syndrome may be acute and short-term or chronic and not respond to treatment. Nephrotic

---

MINI-CASE 9-2

Bonnie, a 40-year-old woman with a past history of kidney infections, was seen by her physician because she had felt lethargic for a few weeks. She also complained of decreased frequency of urination and a bloated feeling. The physician noted periorbital swelling and general edema including a swollen abdomen.

The following significant urinalysis results were reported:

Appearance:	yellow, frothy
Protein:	3 + (SSA: 4+)
Microscopic:	
Casts:	

0–3 hyaline/LPF

0-1 renal tubular epithelial/LPF

0-1 granular. LPF

0-1 waxy/LPF

0-1 fatty/LPF

Occasional oval fat bodies

Questions to Consider

1. What types of disease/condition would be characterized by this urinalysis?

2. What is the primary problem/defect found in this condition?

3. What urinalysis result(s) led to your probable diagnosis?

4. List four diseases/conditions that are associated with this condition.

---

syndrome may disappear once the underlying cause is known and treated. In children minimal change disease, which accounts of 80% of cases, can be successfully treated with prednisone. In adults about half of patients with nephrotic syndrome progress to end-stage renal disease and eventually need dialysis and a renal transplant.

☑ CHECKPOINT 9-1

1. Which of the following disorders occurs following a bacterial infection of the skin or throat?
   (a) Acute glomerulonephritis
   (b) Chronic glomerulonephritis
   (c) Acute pyelonephritis
   (d) Rapidly progressive glomerulonephritis

2. Which of the following statements regarding IgA nephropathy is true?
   (a) It often follows a mucosal infection.
   (b) It is associated with nephrotic syndrome.
   (c) It is characterized by leukocyte infiltration of the glomeruli.
   (d) It occurs secondary to systemic lupus erythematosus.

3. Which of the following features characterize nephrotic syndrome?
   1. Proteinuria
   2. Edema
   3. Hypoalbuminemia

4. Hyperlipidemia
   (a) 1, 2, and 3 are correct
   (b) 1 and 3 are correct
   (c) 4 is correct
   (d) all are correct

4. Clinical features that are characteristic of glomerular damage include all of the following *except*
   (a) edema.
   (b) hematuria.
   (c) proteinuria.
   (d) polyuria.

5. Which of the following disorders is characterized by cellular proliferation in Bowman's capsule to form cellular "crescents"?
   (a) Chronic glomerulonephritis
   (b) Membranous glomerulonephritis
   (c) Focal glomerulonephritis
   (d) Rapidly progressive glomerulonephritis

6. Eighty percent of patients who develop chronic glomerulonephritis previously had some type of glomerular disease. Which of the following disorders is implicated most frequently in the development of chronic glomerulonephritis?
   (a) IgA nephropathy
   (b) Membranous glomerulonephritis
   (c) Poststreptococcal glomerulonephritis
   (d) Rapidly progressive glomerulonephritis

7. When a patient has nephrotic syndrome, the microscopic examination of the urine sediment often reveals
   (a) granular casts.
   (b) leukocyte casts.
   (c) red blood cell casts.
   (d) waxy casts.

RENAL TUBULAR DISEASE

Renal tubular disease describes disorders that result from injury and damage to the tubules. It can also be caused by metabolic disorders, e.g., Fanconi syndrome, that damage the tubules.

Acute Tubular Necrosis

Acute tubular necrosis (ATN) is a kidney disorder involving damage to the renal tubular cells of the kidneys, which can lead to acute kidney failure. ATN is one of the most common causes of kidney failure in hospitalized patients. It is usually caused by lack of oxygen to the kidneys (ischemia of the kidneys). Ischemia can be caused by decreased blood flow due to cardiac failure, septic shock due to severe infection, massive hemorrhage, hypotension >30 minutes, transfusion reaction, disseminated intravascular coagulation, or trauma (crushing injuries or surgical procedures). It can also be due to the presence of toxic substances: medications (aminoglycoside antibiotics, amphotericin B, cyclosporine, ifosfamide), contrast dyes used in x-ray studies, or heavy metals.[29]

Symptoms

Acute tubular necrosis can lead to oliguria or anuria, generalized edema caused by fluid retention, nausea, vomiting, and decreased consciousness (coma, confusion, drowsiness, lethargy).

Laboratory Findings

Routine urinalysis reports indicate mild proteinuria, microscopic hematuria, renal tubular epithelial cells, and renal tubular epithelial casts. The pathognomonic findings are the presence of renal tubular epithelial cells and RTE casts. Hyaline, granular, waxy, and broad casts may also be found. ATN is also characterized by dilute urine (SG = ≤1.010), low osmolality (<400 mOsm/Kg), and high sodium (40–60 mEq/L).[30]

Treatment and Prognosis

ATN is reversible in most patients. The goal of treatment is to prevent complications leading to acute renal failure. The first step is identifying and treating the underlying cause of the problem. Restricting the intake of fluid and substances normally removed by the kidneys (protein, sodium, potassium) and medications helps control potassium levels and helps decrease fluid levels. Temporary dialysis can be ordered to remove excess waste and fluids.[31]

Patients with oliguric ATN have a worse prognosis than patients with nonoliguric ATN. This is probably due to more severe necrosis and a more significant electrolyte imbalance. A rapid increase in creatinine (>3 mg/dL) also indicates a poorer prognosis.[32]

Renal Tubular Acidosis

Renal tubular acidosis (RTA) is a class of disorders in which excretion of hydrogen ions or reabsorption of filtered bicarbonate (HCO_3^-) is impaired, leading to a chronic metabolic acidosis. **Type 1 distal RTA** refers to the point in the tubule where the defect occurs, which is the distal tubule. It may be inherited as a primary disorder or secondary to a systemic disease that affects many parts of the body. Type 1 is rare and occurs most often in adults. The common conditions associated with Type 1 are listed in Box 9-8. Many cause abnormal calcium deposits to build up in the kidney and impair distal tubule function. Untreated distal RTA causes growth retardation in children and progressive kidney and bone disease in adults.[33]

Type 2 proximal RTA is very rare and occurs as a result of impairment of reabsorption of HCO_3^- in the proximal tubules, producing a urine pH >7 if plasma HCO_3^- concentration is normal and a urine pH <5.5 if plasma HCO_3^- is already depleted. The most common cause of proximal RTA in children is Fanconi syndrome, which will be discussed in the next section. Other causes are cystinosis, hereditary fructose intolerance, and Wilson's disease. Medications such as ifosfamide (chemotherapy drug), acetazolamide, or outdated tetracycline can cause proximal RTA.[34]

Type 3 is rarely used as a classification because it is now thought to be a combination of Type 1 and Type 2.

Type 4 hyperkalemic renal tubular acidosis is caused by a generalized transport abnormality of the distal tubules. The transport of electrolytes, e.g., sodium, chloride, and potassium, that

---

BOX 9-8   Renal Tubular Acidosis

Type 1 Distal Renal Tubular Acidosis
- Autoimmune disease, e.g., Sjogren's syndrome, systemic lupus erythematosus
- Cirrhosis
- Drugs, e.g., amphotericin B, ifosfamide, and lithium
- Nephrocalcinosis
- Rejection of a transplanted kidney
- Chronic obstructive uropathy
- Sickle cell anemia
- Hyperthyroidism

Type 2 Proximal Renal Tubular Acidosis
- Fanconi syndrome
- Multiple myeloma (light chain nephropathy)
- Medications, e.g., acetazolamide, ifosfamide, outdated tetracycline
- Sjogren's syndrome
- Wilson's disease
- Cystinosis
- Inherited fructose intolerance

Type 4 Hyperkalemic Renal Tubular Acidosis
- Aldosterone deficiency
- Distal tubule unresponsive to aldosterone
- Diabetic nephropathy
- Chronic interstitial nephritis
- Medications
  - Angiotensin-converting enzyme inhibitor
  - Cyclosporine
  - Heparin
  - K^+-sparing diuretics, amiloride, eplerenone, spironolactone, triamterene
  - NSAID use
  - Pentamidine
  - Trimeoprin

---

normally occurs in the distal tubule is impaired. It is the most common cause of RTA. Type 4 occurs when serum levels of aldosterone are low or when the kidneys do not respond to it. Type 4 also occurs when the transport of electrolytes is impaired due to an inherited disorder or the use of drugs.[35] Box 9-8 lists the more common causes of Type 4 RTA.

Symptoms

Renal tubular acidosis is usually asymptomatic. Symptoms occasionally associated with Type 1 distal renal tubular acidosis are fatigue, impaired growth, confusion, nephrolithiasis, nephrocalcinosis, osteomalacia in adults, rickets in children, and muscle weakness. Type 2 proximal RTA patients exhibit bone pain and osteomalacia in adults and rickets in children. Symptoms may also include dehydration, fatigue, increased or irregular heartbeat, and muscle cramps.[36]

Laboratory Findings

The primary defect in Type 1 RTA is impaired hydrogen excretion, resulting in persistently high pH (>5.5) and systemic acidosis. Plasma HCO_3^- is usually <15 mEq/L and hypokalemia and hypercalciuria are characteristic of this disorder. Hypokalemia, if not treated, can lead to extreme weakness, irregular heartbeat, paralysis, and even death. Type 1 distal RTA is confirmed by a urine pH that remains >5.5 during systemic acidosis.[37]

Findings in Type 2 proximal RTA include low serum bicarbonate (12–20 mEq/L) and hypokalemia. The urine pH is >7.0 if plasma HCO_3^- is normal; <5.5 if plasma HCO_3^- is depleted (e.g., <15 mEq/L).

Type 4 RTA is associated with a plasma $HCO_3^- > 17$ mEq/L, hyperkalemia, and a pH < 5.5. Decreased aldosterone secretion in Type 4 RTA triggers Na reabsorption in exchange for K and hydrogen; therefore, there is reduced K^+ excretion causing hyperkalemia and reduced acid excretion explaining the acidic pH of the blood.

Treatment and Prognosis

The goal is to restore the pH to normal level and electrolyte balance. This will ultimately correct bone disorders and reduce the risk of calcium buildup in the kidneys and the formation of kidney stones. The underlying cause should be addressed if it can be identified.

Fanconi Syndrome

Fanconi syndrome can be due to defective genes, especially in children, or in adults it may be the result of kidney damage. Cystinosis is the most common cause of Fanconi syndrome in children. Other genetic disorders are fructose intolerance, galactosemia, and glycogen storage disease. Exposure to heavy metals and Wilson's disease are also associated with this syndrome in children. In adults medications, multiple myeloma, and kidney transplant can cause damage to the kidneys resulting in Fanconi syndrome.[38] See Box 9-9 for a list of the common causes.

BOX 9-9   Fanconi Syndrome

Children
- Cystinosis
- Fructose intolerance
- Galactosemia
- Glycogen Storage Disease
- Exposure to heavy metals, e.g., lead, mercury
- Wilson's disease

Adults
- Certain medications, e.g., azathioprine, cidofovir, gentamicin, tetracycline
- Multiple myeloma
- Kidney transplant
- Primary amyloidosis

Symptoms

Symptoms associated with Fanconi syndrome include polyuria as well as dehydration, bone pain, and weakness.

Laboratory Findings

Routine urinalysis indicates acidic urine and a positive glucose. The diagnosis is confirmed when high levels of glucose, bicarbonate, phosphates, uric acid, potassium, and sodium are detected in the urine.[39]

Treatment and Prognosis

Growth failure, osteomalacia in adults, and rickets in children are some of the complications associated with Fanconi syndrome. It cannot be cured, but it can be controlled and damage to the kidneys and bones prevented or minimized. Treatment begins with addressing the underlying cause and its symptoms. Bone disease is treated with phosphates and Vitamin D supplements. Low potassium levels can be increased by potassium supplements.[40]

The prognosis depends on the underlying disease. Kidney transplants may be required if a child with the disorder, especially caused by cystinosis, develops kidney failure.

INTERSTITIAL NEPHRITIS

Tubulointerstitial Nephritis

Tubulointerstitial nephritis describes a heterogeneous group of disorders that share similar features of tubular and interstitial (space or gap in the kidney outside of the structure of the nephron) injury. The etiology can be drugs including antibiotics, anticonvulsants, diuretics, NSAIDs, and miscellaneous; metabolic; and renal parenchymal infections. Over 95% of acute interstitial nephritis (AIN) are associated with an infection or allergic drug reaction. The most common causes are listed in Box 9-10.[41] Acute and chronic tubulointerstitial nephritis occurs as a result of the interaction of renal cells and inflammatory cells and their products.

BOX 9-10   Tubulointerstitial Nephritis

Drugs
- **Antibiotics**
  - β-Lactam antibiotics, e.g., methicillin
  - Isoniazid
  - Minocycline
  - Tetracycline
- **Anticonvulsants**
  - Carbamazepine
  - Phenobarbitol
  - Phenytoin
  - Valproate
- **Diuretics**
  - Furosemide
  - Thiazides
  - Triamterene

- **NSAIDS**
  - Ibuprofen
  - Indomethacin
  - Naproxen
- **Other**
  - Allopurinol
  - Captopril

Metabolic

Hypoxalaturia, ethylene glycol poisoning

Hyperuricemia

Renal Parenchymal Infection

- **Bacterial**
  - Brucella
  - Corynebacterium diphtheria
  - Salmonella species
  - Staphylococci
  - Streptococci

Fungal: Candida species

Parasitic: Toxoplasma gondii

Viral

- Cytomegalovirus
- Epstein-Barr virus
- Hepatitis C virus
- HIV
- Mumps

Immunologic

IgA nephropathy

Renal transplant rejection

Sarcoidosis

Wegener's granulomatosis

Neoplastic: Lymphoma, Myeloma

Symptoms

Symptoms and signs of acute tubular interstitial nephritis (ATIN) and chronic TIN (CTIN) are nonspecific and often absent unless symptoms and signs of renal failure develop. Drug-induced ATIN is characterized by fever and urticarial rash.

Laboratory Findings

Routine urinalysis reports sterile pyuria (WBCs but no bacteria present), including eosinophils; small to moderate proteinuria (<1 g/day). ATIN is characterized by signs of active kidney inflammation including RBCs, WBCs, and WBC casts, with no bacteria visible or on culture. Eosinophilia has a positive predictive value of 50% (i.e., the percentage of patients who test positive who have the disease) and a negative predictive value of up to 90% (the percentage of patients who

test negative who don't have the disease). The urinalysis findings in CTIN are similar except urinary RBCs and WBCs are uncommon.[42]

Prognosis and Treatment

In drug-induced ATIN renal function is usually restored within 6 to 8 weeks after the drug is discontinued. In other causes the damage may be reversible if the cause is identified and treated.

Treatment for both ATIN and CTIN is management of the cause. Corticosteroids, e.g., prednisone, may accelerate recovery in immunologically induced disease and sometimes drug-induced ATN.

Acute Pyelonephritis

Acute pyelonephritis is an infection of the upper urinary tract most often seen in women due to the shorter length of their urethra. It frequently results from an ascending infection in untreated cases of cystitis or lower urinary tract infections and doesn't cause permanent damage to the renal tubules. In more than 80% of cases the etiologic agent is *Escherichia coli.* Other bacteria associated with acute pyelonephritis are Proteus, Klebsiella, Enterobacter, *Staphylococcus saprophyticus*, Serratia, and Pseudomonas. **Vesicourethral reflux (VUR)**, the reflux of urine from the bladder back into the ureters, is the most common anatomic cause. Bacteria in the bladder are normally kept from entering the ureters, but in vesicourethral reflux they can enter the ureters and ascend to the kidney resulting in acute pyelonephritis. Although ascending infection is most common, hematogenous spread to the kidney from bacteria in the blood is also possible. Sources for infection by Gram-positive bacteria are IV drug abuse and endocarditis. Risk factors that can cause complicated acute pyelonephritis are reviewed in Box 9-11.[43]

BOX 9-11   Risk Factors for Complicated Acute Pyelonephritis

- Age: Infants and elderly
- Anatomic abnormality
  - Vesicourethral reflux
  - Polycystic kidney disease
  - Horseshoe kidney
- Immunosuppressed State
  - Diabetes mellitus
  - Sickle cell disease
  - Malignancy
  - HIV infection
  - Steroid use
  - Transplantation
  - Chemoradiation
- Pregnancy
- Obstruction
  - Calculi
  - Benign prostatic hypertrophy
  - Bladder neck obstruction

Symptoms

Symptoms of acute pyelonephritis may range from a mild illness to sepsis syndrome. Patients with acute pyelonephritis may complain of back, side, and groin pain; urgent, frequent urination; pain or burning during urination; fever; and nausea and vomiting.[44] It usually begins with an acute onset with urinary frequency and burning and lower back pain.

Laboratory Findings

Urinalysis and urine culture provide the clinically significant laboratory findings used to diagnose acute pyelonephritis. Pyuria (see Figure 9-3 ■) and bacteria are confirmed by leukocyte esterase and nitrite testing. White blood cell casts (see Figure 9-4 ■) and WBCs in clumps, although found in other conditions, are pathognomonic for acute pyelonephritis. Hematuria may also be present in patients with cystitis and pyelonephritis. Urine cultures are positive in 90% of cases, and specimens for culture should be obtained before beginning antibiotic therapy.[45] Box 9-12 summarizes the urinalysis findings in acute pyelonephritis.

Treatment and Prognosis

Most cases of acute pyelonephritis presenting with no nausea or vomiting are treated with oral antibiotic therapy. More seriously ill patients may be hospitalized with IV fluids and antibiotics until they can take the fluids and medications on their own.

In healthy, nonpregnant women with uncomplicated disease, the prognosis is excellent for full recovery and minimal damage to the kidney. In children the prognosis is good, but they should undergo a urologic evaluation after the first infection to rule out structural abnormalities, e.g., VUR.

Complications occur more often in patients with diabetes mellitus, chronic renal disease, AIDS, and renal transplant (especially the first three months). If a patient has one of the known complicating conditions, urologic examination should be performed to determine the status of the complicating condition and the status of the kidney.

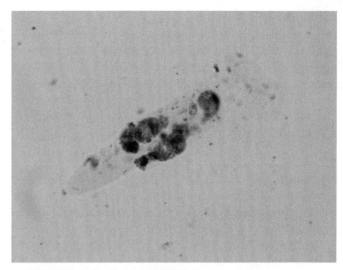

■ **FIGURE 9-4** Stained WBC Cast in Acute Pyelonephritis

Chronic Pyelonephritis

Chronic pyelonephritis is characterized by renal inflammation and fibrosis caused by recurrent or persistent renal infection, vesicourethral reflux, kidney stones, or other causes of urinary tract obstruction. It is associated with progressive renal scarring that can lead to end-stage renal disease. In 30–40% of children with symptomatic urinary tract infections (UTIs), vesicourethral reflux, if not corrected, is the cause. Chronic pyelonephritis occurs more often in infants and children (younger than 2 years) than in older children and adults.[46]

Symptoms

A history of recurrent infections of the renal tubules and interstitium is indicative of chronic pyelonephritis. Anemia and hypertension may be present in the later stages. Other symptoms that may be present are fatigue, itching, forgetfulness, fever, flank pain, pain on urination, nausea and vomiting, and failure to thrive in children.[47]

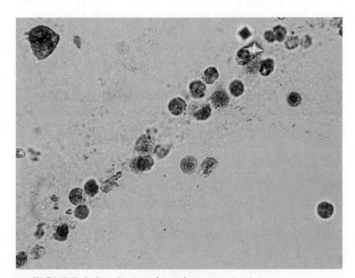

■ **FIGURE 9-3** Stained Leukocytes in Acute Pyelonephritis

BOX 9-12   Acute Pyelonephritis Urinalysis Findings

- *WBCs often in clumps
- *WBC casts
- Microscopic hematuria
- Granular, renal tubular, and waxy casts
- Bacteria variable
- Nitrite positive
- Leukocyte esterase positive
- Minimal to mild proteinuria (<1 g/day)
- Decreased specific gravity

*pathognomonic

Laboratory Findings

Urinalysis findings in the early stages of chronic pyelonephritis are comparable to those found in acute pyelonephritis, but as the disease progresses, the presence and number of granular, waxy, and broad casts increase and proteinuria and hematuria are also increased. The urine is less concentrated as the ability to concentrate urine is decreased. Hypokalemia and hyponatremia may also be complications of chronic pyelonephritis.[48]

Prognosis and Treatment

Antibiotic therapy is recommended for acute infections and antibiotic prophylaxis for the prevention of recurrent infections. Close monitoring of patients, especially children with vesicourethral reflux with no evidence of kidney damage, may resolve without surgery. Ingestion of cranberry juice has been shown in a number of studies to be effective as a prophylactic measure.

☑ CHECKPOINT 9-2

1. Most urinary tract infections are caused by
   - (a) yeast, e.g., Candida.
   - (b) Gram-negative rods.
   - (c) Gram-positive rods.
   - (d) Gram-positive cocci.

2. The most common cause of chronic pyelonephritis is
   - (a) cystitis.
   - (b) bacterial sepsis.
   - (c) drug-induced nephropathies.
   - (d) reflux nephropathies.

3. White cell casts are pathognomonic for which of the following renal diseases?
   - (a) Glomerulonephritis
   - (b) Pyelonephritis
   - (c) Cystitis
   - (d) Renal tubular acidosis

4. An inherited or acquired disorder associated with a high level of glucose, bicarbonate, phosphates uric acid, potassium, and sodium in the urine due to a defective tubular reabsorption is
   - (a) renal glucosuria.
   - (b) Fanconi syndrome.
   - (c) acute pyelonephritis.
   - (d) tubulointerstitial nephritis.

RENOVASCULAR RENAL DISEASE

Renovascular disease is a progressive condition leading to narrowing or blockage or renal arteries or veins. It is categorized into three disorders: renal artery occlusion, renal vein thrombosis, and renal artheroembolism. Renal artery occlusion is defined as blockage of one or both renal arteries. In renal vein thrombosis the renal veins that carry blood away from the kidneys are blocked. Renal artheroembolism occurs when there is a buildup of fatty material that blocks the renal arterioles.[49]

BOX 9-13   Risk Factors for Renovascular Disease[50]

- Age
- Female gender
- Artherosclerosis
- Hypertension, especially new onset in an older person
- Smoking
- High cholesterol
- Diabetes

Individuals who are at risk for other vascular diseases are also at risk for renovascular disease. Risk factors for renal vascular disease are listed in Box 9-13.

Symptoms are serious and vary with the cause of the condition. Renal artery occlusion and renal vein thrombosis may be asymptomatic if only one kidney is blocked. If both kidneys are partially affected and the occlusion occurred suddenly, back or side pain, blood in the urine, fever, nausea and vomiting, and anuria may be present. The complications of renovascular disease are listed in Box 9-14.

Cystitis

Cystitis is commonly known as a bladder infection or inflammation of the bladder. It is caused by a bacterial infection and is a lower urinary tract infection, as opposed to pyelonephritis, which is an upper urinary tract infection involving the kidneys. Bacteria, most commonly *Escherichia coli*, enter the urethra and ascend to the bladder. The bladder normally flushes out the bacteria upon urination, but in some cases bacteria can adhere to the wall of the urethra or bladder and multiply so fast that some bacteria remain in the bladder. Women are more prone to cystitis because their urethra is shorter and closer to the anus.

Less frequently, cystitis may also occur as a reaction to certain drugs, radiation therapy, potential irritants, e.g., feminine hygiene spray, spermicidal jellies, or long-term catheterization. It can also occur as a complication of another illness.[52]

Community-acquired cystitis occurs in patients outside of a hospital or nursing home. Hospital-acquired or nosocomial cystitis occurs in people in medical care facilities. Interstitial cystitis is a chronic, painful bladder inflammation that is difficult to diagnose and treat. See Box 9-15 for a list of the main types of cystitis.[53]

BOX 9-14   Complications of Renovascular Disease[51]

- Blood vessel damage
- Congestive heart failure
- Myocardial infarction
- Renal damage or failure
- Loss of vision
- Stroke

BOX 9-15 Types of Cystitis

Bacterial cystitis
- Hospital-acquired or nosocomial
- Community-acquired

Noninfectious cystitis
- Interstitial cystitis
- Drug-induced cystitis, e.g., chemotherapy drugs cyclophosphamide and ifosfamide
- Radiation cystitis
- Foreign-body cystitis, e.g., long-term catheterization
- Chemical cystitis
- Other conditions
  - Gynecologic cancers
  - Pelvic inflammatory disorders
  - Endometriosis
  - Lupus
  - Diverticulitis
  - Tuberculosis
  - Crohn's disease

Symptoms

Signs and symptoms include dysuria (burning or pain on urination), pressure in the lower abdomen, frequency of urination, and cloudy or bloody urine that may have a foul or strong odor.[54]

Laboratory Findings

A routine urinalysis will indicate the presence of leukocytes and bacteria. It can be differentiated from pyelonephritis by the absence of casts. Since casts are formed in the renal tubules, they will not be present in lower urinary tract infections. See Box 9-16 for the findings on the routine urinalysis.

Treatment and Prognosis

Cystitis caused by bacteria is generally treated with antibiotics. Treatment for noninfectious cystitis depends on the underlying cause. Antibiotics are usually prescribed for 3 days (women) and 7–14 days (men).

BOX 9-16 Typical Laboratory Findings in Cystitis

- Protein: small <0.5 mg/day
- Blood: positive usually small
- Leukocyte esterase: ±, usually positive
- Nitrite: ±, usually positive
- Increased WBCs
- Increased bacteria: variable small to large numbers
- Increased RBCs
- Increased transitional epithelium

Commonly used antibiotics include trimethoprim-sulfamethozole, Augmentin, doxycycline, and fluoroquinolones. Medications, e.g., phenazopyridine hydrochloride (Pyridium), may also be prescribed for the burning pain and urgent need to urinate.[55]

Most cases of cystitis are treated and resolved without complications.

MINI-CASE 9-3

Mary, a 22-year-old MLT student, performed a macroscopic urinalysis on her own urine as part of the macroscopic urinalysis laboratory. She had noted some dysuria, increased frequency, and urgency of urination. The program director recommended that she contact her physician for a complete routine urinalysis and possible culture and sensitivity.

Urinalysis
Macroscopic:

Day 1: Macroscopic performed at school

Day 2: Performed via Physician's Order

	Day 1	Day 2
Color:	Yellow	Yellow
Appearance:	Cloudy	Cloudy
Specific Gravity:	1.013	1.016
pH:	7.0	7.5
Glucose:	Neg	Neg
Bilirubin:	Neg	Neg
Ketones:	Neg	Neg
Blood:	Neg	Neg
Protein:	Neg	Neg
Urobilinogen:	Normal	Normal
Nitrite:	Positive	Positive
Leukocyte Esterase:	2+	2+

Microscopic:

	Day 2
WBCs:	25–40/HPF
RBCs:	0–3/HPF
Epithelial Cells:	Few Squamous/HPF
	Few Transitional/HPF
Casts:	Neg
Bacteria:	Moderate

Questions to Consider

1. Circle or highlight the abnormal or discrepant result(s).
2. Do the abnormal results indicate an upper or lower urinary tract infection? What single finding is most helpful in determining the source of the infection? Why?

3. What is the probable disease/condition?

4. Would you change your answer if either the leukocyte esterase or nitrite were negative and the microscopic remained the same? Explain why or why not.

5. Explain the presence of increased transitional epithelial cells in this condition.

6. What bacteria are most commonly identified in this condition?

7. What fruit juice is often recommended to reduce pyuria and bacteruria?

8. Why are patients instructed to increase their fluid intake?

9. Why are women more prone to this condition than men?

10. What conditions are associated with an increased incidence of this infection?

Acute Renal Failure

Acute renal failure (ARF), or acute kidney injury, is defined as an abrupt or rapid decline in renal filtration function marked by an increase in serum creatinine concentration or azotemia (an increase in blood urea nitrogen, BUN). ARF can be classified into three categories. Prerenal is described as an adaptive response to severe volume depletion or decreased renal blood flow and hypotension, with structurally intact nephrons. Intrinsic or renal ARF occurs in response to cytotoxic, ischemic, or inflammatory insults to the kidney leading to structural damage. Intrinsic ARF can result from any progressive glomerular, tubular, or vascular disease. Postrenal ARF is due to obstruction of urine flow, e.g., calculi or tumors. Box 9-17 lists common causes associated with the three categories of ARF.[56]

Symptoms

Signs and symptoms of ARF may include decreased urine output, edema, drowsiness, shortness of breath, fatigue, confusion, and nausea.

Laboratory Findings

A normal urinalysis may be present in prerenal or postrenal ARF; however, in postrenal ARF some cells might be present. RBCs are found in all renal forms of ARF. Red cell casts point to glomerulonephritis or vasculitis as the precipitating condition. Large numbers of WBCs and WBC casts suggest pyelonephritis or acute interstitial nephritis as the cause. The presence of large numbers of crystals may suggest uric acid, drugs or toxins as the source of the ARF.[57]

Treatment and Prognosis

Treatment of ARF begins with identifying the illness or injury that caused the damage to the kidneys and management based on the underlying reason. The next steps to control the complications that arise because of ARF include balancing fluids through diuretics, medications to control potassium levels, and dialysis to remove toxins from the blood.

BOX 9-17 Prerenal, Intrinsic, and Postrenal Causes of Acute Renal Failure

Prerenal ARF
- Volume depletion (decreased renal blood flow)
  - Renal losses (diuretics, polyuria)
  - GI losses
  - Hemorrhage
  - Pancreatitis
- Decreased cardiac output
  - Heart failure
  - Acute myocardial infarction
- Systemic vasodilation: caused by sepsis, anesthetics, drug overdose
- Septicemia
- Surgery
- Transfusion reaction

Intrinsic ARF
- Vascular: renal artery obstruction, e.g., thrombosis, transplant rejection
- Glomerular: Goodpasture syndrome, immune complex GN, e.g., lupus, postinfectious
- Tubular: rhabdomyolysis, seizures, ethylene glycol poisoning, medications, e.g., methotrexate
- Interstitial:
  - Drugs, e.g., penicillin, cephalosporins, NSAIDs, sulfonamides, allopurinol
  - Infection, e.g., pyelonephritis
  - Systemic disease: lupus, leukemia, lymphoma

Postrenal ARF
- Obstruction of the ureter
- Bladder neck obstruction: benign prostatic hypertrophy, cancer of the prostate
- Urethral obstruction: strictures, tumor

The prognosis for patients with ARF is directly related to the cause of renal failure and also to the duration of renal failure prior to diagnosis and intervention. Follow-up studies of survivors of ARF find from 1–64% are dialysis dependent, depending on the population, and 19–31% have chronic kidney disease.[58]

Chronic Kidney Disease

Chronic kidney disease (CKD) is defined as the gradual and usually permanent loss of kidney function over time, slowly usually months to years. The Kidney Disease Outcomes Quality Initiative (KDOQI) of the National Kidney Foundation (NKF) defines chronic kidney disease as either kidney damage or a decreased glomerular filtration rate (GFR) of less than 60 mL/min/1.73m^2 for three or more months. It is classified in five stages outlined in Table 9-1 ★.[59]

Stages 1–3 of chronic renal disease are usually asymptomatic, with signs and symptoms typically appearing in stages 4–5. The

★ **TABLE 9-1** Stages of Chronic Renal Disease

Stage	Description	GFR mL/min/1.73m²
1	Slight kidney damage with normal or increased GFR	>90
2	Mild decrease in kidney function	60–89
3	Moderate decrease in kidney function	30–59
4	Severe decrease in kidney function	15–29
5	Kidney failure	<15 or dialysis

etiology of chronic kidney disease includes diabetic nephropathy, hypertension, vascular disease, glomerular disease (primary or secondary), tubulointerstitial disease, and urinary tract obstruction.[60] See the previous sections in this chapter for a more detailed list of conditions under each category, e.g., glomerulonephritis.

Symptoms

Symptoms of chronic kidney disease are also associated with other diseases and may be the only signs until the more advanced stages. They include loss of appetite, headaches, itching, nausea, weight loss, nocturia, and edema. Other symptoms that may develop when kidney function deteriorates are shortness of breath due to fluid in the lungs, bone pain and fractures, excessive bruising or bleeding, excessive thirst, and vomiting, usually in the morning.[61] High blood pressure is almost always present in all stages of chronic kidney disease.

Laboratory Findings

The urinalysis may indicate proteinuria or other changes 6 months to 10 or more years before symptoms occur. Creatinine clearance is performed on a 24-hour urine and serum samples and is used to stage the progression of the disease. See Clinical Chemistry textbooks for more detailed descriptions, e.g., Sunheimer and Graves.[62]

Treatment and Prognosis

Treatment of CKD includes controlling blood pressure using medications if necessary, and changes in diet: limiting fluids, limiting salt or potassium, and low in fat and cholesterol. Controlling the disease that's causing the damage and extra calcium and Vitamin D are also recommended after consulting with the physician. When the disease progresses to renal failure, dialysis or kidney transplant may be required.

People are not diagnosed with chronic kidney disease until they have lost most of their kidney function. There is no cure for chronic kidney disease. If it is not treated, it usually worsens to end-stage renal disease. Lifelong treatment may help to control the symptoms of CKD.

Renal Lithiasis

Renal lithiasis is defined as calculi or stones in the kidneys. **Nephrolithiasis** is a common disease that is estimated to produce medical costs of $2.1 billion per year in the United States. Normally, crystals do not form or are so small that they pass through the urinary tract without incident (asymptomatic crystalluria); however, when conditions are such that the crystals grow larger and cannot be eliminated, kidney stones become problematic. Conditions that may be associated with kidney stones are (1) hyperparathyroidism associated with hypercalciuria (high calcium) and hypocitraturia (low citrate), (2) genetic alterations associated with hyperoxalia, (3) hypercystinuria, and (4) hypercalciuria.[63]

The most important environmental factor in stone formation is a low fluid intake, with the subsequent decreased urine production resulting in high concentrations of stone-forming solutes in the urine. Hypercalciuria is the most common abnormality. Magnesium and citrate are important inhibitors of stone formation in the urinary tract; therefore, decreased levels of magnesium and citrate predispose the patient to stone formation. Box 9-18 lists the four main types of renal calculi and the conditions associated with each.[64]

Symptoms

A kidney stone may not cause any signs or symptoms until it has moved into the ureter. Symptoms are severe pain in the side and back, pain that spreads to the lower abdomen and groin, dysuria, nausea and vomiting, persistent urge to urinate, and fever and chills if an infection is present.

Laboratory Findings

Chemistry profiles can detect excess uric acid or calcium as the source. Urinalysis and 24-hour urine collection can identify increased excretion of stone-forming minerals or too few stone-inhibiting substances, e.g., magnesium, citrate. The patient may be asked to strain his or her urine to catch any stones, and the stones may be analyzed to determine their composition, which will help in planning treatment to prevent the formation of future stones.[65]

BOX 9-18 Renal Calculi

- Calcium stones: 75%
  - Hyperparathyroidism
  - Increased intestinal absorption
  - Hyperuricosuria
  - Hyperoxaluria
  - Hypomagnesemia
- Struvite (magnesium ammonium phosphate) stones: 15%
  - Associated with chronic urinary tract infections
- Uric acid stones: 6%
  - High purine diets
  - Malignancy (e.g., rapid cell turnover)
  - Gout (25% of uric acid stones)
- Cystine stones: 2%
  - Intrinsic metabolic defect: defect in the renal tubular reabsorption of cystine, ornithine, lysine, and arginine

Treatment and Prognosis

Treatment, especially for small stones that don't require invasive action, is usually increasing fluid intake to 2 to 3 quarts (1.9 to 2.8 liters) a day to flush out the solutes and small stones in the urine. Mild pain relievers, e.g., ibuprofen (Advil, Motrin) or acetaminophen (Tylenol), may help alleviate the pain.

Hyperuricosuria associated with gout is treated with low purine diet and allopurinol. Hyperoxaluria is addressed with low oxalate diet and oxalate binders and hypomagnesemia with magnesium supplements.

For larger stones that cannot pass on their own or include bleeding and kidney damage, more invasive therapy may be required. Lithotripsy (using sound waves to create strong vibrations called shock waves) can break the stones into smaller pieces that can pass in the urine. Surgery, called percutaneous nephrolithotomy, may be required to remove large stones in the kidney.[66]

Approximately 80–85% of stones pass spontaneously with no intervention. Twenty percent of patients require hospitalization because of unrelenting pain, proximal UTI, or inability to pass the stone. The rate of recurrence for urinary stones is 50% within 5 years and 70% or higher within 10 years. Preventive measures may help to decrease the recurrence: increased hydration; diet low in oxalate-rich foods, salt, and animal protein; and caution with calcium supplements.

☑ CHECKPOINT 9-3

1. Where does community-acquired cystitis occur?
2. Which of the following urinalysis results would not be found in a patient with cystitis?
   (a) Blood: 1+
   (b) Nitrite: positive
   (c) WBC cell casts
   (d) WBCs: 20–30/HPF
3. Which of the following conditions is a cause of prerenal acute renal failure?
   (a) Goodpasture syndrome
   (b) Renal artery obstruction
   (c) Hemorrhage
   (d) Urethral obstruction
4. The most important environmental factor in kidney stone formation is:
   (a) low urine magnesium.
   (b) low fluid intake.
   (c) hypercalciuria.
   (d) high purine diet.

Key Points to Remember

- Renal diseases can be classified in four main categories: glomerular, tubular, interstitial, and renovascular. They can also be grouped as primary causes indicating a renal origin, or secondary due to a secondary disease or condition that affects other organs and the kidney secondarily.

- Glomerulonephritis is a sterile inflammatory process that is associated with damage and inflammation of the glomerulus by immune complexes (antigen–antibody). Acute glomerulonephritis is characterized by an acute onset of hematuria, proteinuria, and red blood cell casts. It is most often seen in children 1 to 2 weeks following a group A streptococcal infection (strep throat or a respiratory infection). It can also be caused by other bacteria or viruses, and noninfectious causes, e.g., multisystem diseases.

- Crescentic or rapidly progressive glomerulonephritis causes permanent damage to the glomeruli including crescent-shaped epithelial cells. Chronic glomerulonephritis is the end stage of persistent glomerular damage associated with irreversible loss of renal tissue and chronic renal failure. Rapidly progressive glomerulonephritis is the most common condition that progresses to chronic glomerulonephritis. Urinalysis findings include hematuria, heavy proteinuria, increased WBCs and renal tubular epithelial cells, glucosuria, and many types of casts including broad, granular, and waxy casts.

- Minimal change disease is the most common cause of nephrotic syndrome in children. Membranoproliferative glomerulonephritis is described as inflammation of the glomeruli caused by an abnormal immune response resulting in the activation of the complement cascade. Immune complex-mediated conditions, autoimmune diseases, chronic infections, and malignant neoplasms are associated with membranoproliferative glomerulonephritis.

- IgA nephropathy or Berger's disease is the most common type of glomerulonephritis caused by an increase in IgA following an infection of the respiratory, gastrointestinal, or urinary tract. Immune complexes deposit on the glomerular membrane, resulting in inflammation and eventual blockage of blood flow through the glomeruli.

- Diabetic nephropathy is a clinical syndrome characterized by persistent albuminuria confirmed on at least two occasions 3–6 months apart, progressive decline in the GFR, and hypertension. Screening and periodic checking levels of microalbumin are used to monitor the progression of the disease.

- Nephrotic syndrome is caused by changes in the permeability of the glomerular membrane allowing high molecular proteins and lipids into the glomerular filtrate resulting in damage to the glomeruli and tubules. The routine urinalysis will exhibit marked proteinuria, increased RBCs, urinary fat droplets (lipiduria), oval fat bodies, renal tubular cells and casts, especially renal tubular epithelial, waxy, and fatty casts.

- Renal tubular disease describes disorders that result from injury and damage to the renal tubules. Acute tubular necrosis involves damage to the tubular cells, which can lead to acute kidney failure. It is usually caused by ischemia (decreased blood flow) or lack to oxygen to the kidneys or the presence of toxic substances. Acute tubular necrosis can lead to oliguria or anuria, generalized edema, nausea, vomiting, and decreased consciousness.

- Renal tubular acidosis is a class of disorders in which excretion of hydrogen ions or reabsorption of filtered bicarbonate is impaired leading to a chronic metabolic acidosis. Type 4 hyperkalemic renal tubular acidosis, caused by a generalized transport abnormality of electrolytes, e.g., sodium, chloride, and potassium, occurs in the distal tubules.

- Fanconi syndrome can be due to defective genes, especially in children, or in adults it may be the result of kidney damage. In children cystinosis is the most common cause of Fanconi syndrome. In adults medications, multiple myeloma, and kidney transplants are associated with Fanconi syndrome. Routine urinalysis indicates acidic urine and a positive glucose.

- Tubulointerstitial nephritis describes a heterogeneous group of disorders that have similar features of tubular and interstitial injury. The etiology can be drugs, metabolic, and renal parenchymal infections. The routine urinalysis reports sterile pyuria (no bacteria) including eosinophils, and small to moderate proteinuria.

- Acute pyelonephritis is an infection of the kidneys or upper urinary tract from an ascending infection in untreated cases of cystitis. The most common anatomic cause is vesicourethral reflux. White blood cell casts, although found in other conditions, are pathognomonic for acute pyelonephritis.

- Chronic pyelonephritis is characterized by renal inflammation and fibrosis caused by recurrent or persistent infections, vesicourethral reflux, kidney stones, or other causes of urinary tract obstruction. Urinalysis findings are similar to those in acute pyelonephritis, but as the disease progresses, increased numbers of granular, waxy, and broad casts are present.

- Cystitis is caused by a bacterial infection, most commonly Escherichia coli, and is a lower urinary tract infection. A routine urinalysis will indicate leukocytes and bacteria, and it can be differentiated from pyelonephritis by the absence of casts, which are found only in upper urinary tract infections.

- Acute renal failure or acute kidney injury is defined as an abrupt or rapid decline in renal filtration function resulting in increased serum creatinine and BUN. ARF can be classified into three categories: prerenal, intrinsic or renal, and postrenal. Chronic kidney disease is the slow and usually permanent loss of kidney function over time, gradually over months to years. The Kidney Quality Outcomes Quality Initiative (KDOQI) of the National Kidney Foundation (NKF) defines chronic kidney disease as either kidney damage or a decreased glomerular filtration rate (GFR) of less than 60 mL/min/1.73m^2 for three or more months.

- Renal lithiasis is defined as calculi or stones in the kidneys. It can be associated with hyperparathyroidism, genetic alterations associated with hyperoxalia, hypercystinuria, and hypercalciuria. The most important environmental factor in stone formation is a low fluid intake. The four main types of renal calculi are (1) calcium stones: 75%; (2) struvite: 15%; uric acid: 6%; and cystine: 2%.

Review Questions

Level I

1. Acute glomerulonephritis usually follows an untreated infection with which of the following organisms? (Objective 2)

   A. Group A beta-hemolytic streptococci

   B. *Staphylococcus aureus*

   C. *Staphylococcus epidermidis*

   D. Group D streptococcus

2. A 10-year-old boy, two weeks after a bout with strep throat, begins to pass dark brown urine "like coffee." At this time low grade fever returns, the blood pressure rises to 150/110, and his eyelids are puffy. Microscopic examination of the urinary sediment is most likely to show which one of the following? (Objective 3)

   A. Hyaline casts and oval fat bodies

   B. Red blood cells and blood casts

   C. Granular and waxy casts

   D. White blood cells

   E. Urates

3. The following routine urinalysis results are obtained: pH: 5.0; glucose: negative; blood: small; ketone: negative; protein: 300 mg/dL; nitrite: negative; significant microscopic findings include: RBCs: 2–5/HPF, dysmorphic; casts: hemoglobin, granular. These findings are most consistent with a diagnosis of (Objective 3)

   A. acute cystitis.

   B. nephrotic syndrome.

   C. acute pyelonephritis.

   D. acute glomerulonephritis.

4. Antiglomerular basement membrane antibody is associated with (Objective 4)

   A. diabetic nephropathy.

   B. Goodpasture syndrome.

   C. IgA nephropathy.

   D. Wegener's granulomatosis.

5. Which of the following is characterized by the formation of cellular "crescents" in the Bowman's capsule? (Objective 4)

   A. Chronic glomerulonephritis

   B. Membranous glomerulonephritis

   C. Focal proliferative glomerulonephritis

   D. Rapidly progressive glomerulonephritis

6. Which of the following casts would more likely be found in chronic glomerulonephritis than with acute glomerulonephritis? (Objective 5)

   A. Hyaline cast

   B. WBC cast

   C. Waxy cast

   D. RBC cast

7. Which is the most common condition that leads to chronic glomerulonephritis? (Objective 5)

   A. Acute glomerulonephritis

   B. IgA nephropathy

   C. Rapidly progressive glomerulonephritis

   D. Membranoproliferative glomerulonephritis

8. The most common type of glomerulonephritis is (Objective 8)

   A. diabetic nephropathy.

   B. IgA nephropathy.

   C. minimal change disease.

   D. acute glomerulonephritis.

9. Occasional episodes of hematuria over a period of 20 years may be seen with (Objective 8)

   A. Wegener's granulomatosis.

   B. diabetic nephropathy.

   C. IgA nephropathy.

   D. membranoproliferative glomerulonephritis.

10. Which disease would be associated with the following urine profile? (Objective 10)

Appearance:	Pale, yellow, hazy
Urobilinogen:	0.1mg/dL
Glucose:	neg
Blood:	trace
Bilirubin:	neg
pH:	8.0
Leukocyte esterase:	pos
Ketone:	neg
S.G.:	1.012
Nitrite:	pos
Protein:	trace

   A. Acute pyelonephritis

   B. Cystitis

   C. Acute glomerulonephritis

   D. Nephrotic syndrome

11. The following are often observed in the examination of urine in pyelonephritis: (Objective 10)

   A. White cells in clumps

   B. Large numbers of bacteria

   C. Large numbers of RBCs

   D. Red cell casts

   E. a and b

12. Nephrotic syndrome is associated with all of the following EXCEPT (Objective 10)

   A. albuminuria.

   B. edema.

   C. hyperalbuminemia.

   D. hyperlipidemia.

   E. lipiduria.

13. Oval fat bodies, fatty casts, and free-floating fat droplets can be formed in the urine sediment during (Objective 10)

   A. nephrotic syndrome.

   B. acute tubular necrosis.

   C. acute interstitial nephritis.

   D. acute glomerulonephritis.

14. Which condition is associated with *massive* proteinuria? (Objective 10)

   A. Acute glomerulonephritis

   B. Chronic glomerulonephritis

   C. Nephrotic syndrome

   D. Acute pyelonephritis

15. The most common cause of Fanconi syndrome in children is (Objective 13)

   A. galactosemia.

   B. cystinosis.

   C. Wilson's disease.

   D. multiple myeloma.

16. Pyelonephritis follows an untreated infection with which of the following organisms? (Objective 15)

    A. Group A beta-hemolytic streptococci

    B. *Staphylococcus aureus*

    C. *Staphylococcus epidermidis*

    D. Coliform bacteria, i.e., *E. coli*, Proteus, Gram-negative rods

    E. Group D streptococcus

17. The most common cause of chronic pyelonephritis is (Objective 16)

    A. drug-induced nephropathies.

    B. cystitis.

    C. reflux nephropathy.

    D. membranous glomerulonephritis.

18. The presence of granular casts in urinary sediment may indicate any of these diseases EXCEPT (Objective 17)

    A. cystitis.

    B. glomerulonephritis.

    C. pyelonephritis.

    D. renal failure.

19. Renal failure would *not* be associated with which of the following? (Objective 18)

    A. Transfusion reaction

    B. Shock with a decreased blood pressure

    C. Urine with a high specific gravity

    D. Decreased GFR

20. Which of the following is a prerenal cause of acute renal failure? (Objective 18)

    A. Lupus erythematosus

    B. Benign prostatic hypertrophy

    C. Congestive heart failure

    D. Ethylene glycol poisoning

21. The most common type of kidney stone is (Objective 19)

    A. calcium.

    B. uric acid.

    C. cystine.

    D. struvite.

Level II

1. The most common type of renal tubular acidosis is (Objective 2)

    A. Type 1 Classical Distal RTA.

    B. Type 2 Proximal RTA.

    C. Type 3.

    D. Hyperkalemic RTA.

2. The five stages of chronic renal disease are based on the (Objective 3)

    A. renal blood flow.

    B. glomerular filtration rate.

    C. tubular reabsorption.

    D. tubular secretion.

3. Which of the following is not associated with acute tubular necrosis? (Objective 5)

    A. Transfusion reaction

    B. Antibiotics

    C. Cardiac failure

    D. Diabetes mellitus

4. Postrenal acute renal failure is associated with (Objective 4)

    A. acute interstitial nephritis.

    B. urethral obstruction by a tumor.

    C. Goodpasture syndrome.

    D. transfusion reaction.

5. Jane, a 45-year-old woman diagnosed with systemic lupus erythematosus, presents with hematuria, cloudy dark urine (cola or tea colored), edema, and hypertension.

    A. What is the probable diagnosis given the information given?

    B. Describe the cause of this condition.

Endnotes

1. Parmar M. *Acute Glomerulonephritis*. (2011). Medscape Reference. (www.emedicine.medscape.com/article/239278-overview) Accessed January 13, 2012.

2. Ibid.

3. Ibid.

4. Papanagnou D. *Emergent Management of Acute Glomerulonephritis*. (2011). Medscape Reference. www.emedicine.medscape.com/article/777272-overview. Accessed January 13, 2012.

5. Bhimma R. *Acute Poststreptococcal Glomerulonephritis*. (2011) Medscape Reference. www.emedicine.medscape.com/article/980685-overview. Accessed January 13, 2012.

6. Lohr JW. *Rapidly Progressive Glomerulonephritis*. (2011). www.emedicine.medscape.com/article/240457-overview. Accessed January 20, 2012.

7. Jennette JC. Rapidly progressive crescentic glomerulonephritis. *Kidney International* (2003) 63:1164–1177.

8. Parmar MS. *Crescentic Glomerulonephritis*. Medscape Reference. (2011). www.emedicine.medscape.com/article/239504-overview. Accessed January 20, 2012.

9. Salifu M O. *Chronic Glomerulonephritis*. (January 12, 2012) www.emedicine.medscape.com/article/239392-overview. Accessed January 16, 2012.

10. MD Guidelines. Glomerulonephritis, Chronic. www.mdguidelines.com/glomerulonephritis-chronic. Accessed January 17, 2012.

11. A.D.A.M. Medical Encyclopedia. Chronic Glomerulonephritis Overview. www.health.nytimes.com/health/guides/disease/chronic-glomerulonephritis/overview.html. Accessed January 18, 2012.

12. New York Times. *Chronic Glomerulonephritis Overview*. www.health.nttimes.com/health/guides/disease/chronic-glomerulonephritis/overview.html. Accessed January 18, 2012.

13. Mansur A. *Minimal Change Disease*. Medscape Reference. emedicine.medscape.com/article/243348-overview. Accessed January 30, 2012.

14. Ibid.

15. A.D.A.M. Medical Encyclopedia. *Minimal Change Disease*. www.ncbi.nlm.nih.gov/pubmedhealth/PMH0001526. Accessed January 30, 2012.

16. MedlinePlus. *Minimal Change Disease*. www.nlm.nih.gov/medlineplus/ency/article/000496.htm. Accessed January 30, 2012.

17. Kathuria P. *Membranoproliferative Glomerulonephritis*. www.emedicine.medscape.com/article/240056-overview. Accessed January 23, 2012.

18. Kathuria P. *Membranoproliferative Glomerulonephritis Workup*. www.emedicine.medscape.com/article/240056-workup. Accessed January 25, 2012.

19. A.D.A.M. Medical Encyclopedia. *Membranoproliferative GN*. www.ncbi.nlm.nih.gov/pubmedhealth/PMH0001507. Accessed January 23, 2012.

20. Kathuria P. *Membranoproliferative Glomerulonephritis*. www.emedicine.medscape.com/article/240056-overview. Accessed January 23, 2012.

21. A.D.A.M. Medical Encyclopedia. *IgA Nephropathy*. (2011). www.ncbi.nlm.nih.gov/pubmedhealth/PMH0001500. Accessed January 25, 2012.

22. IGNA. *Symptoms of IgAN*. The Foundation for IgA Nephropathy. (2008). www.igan.ca/id37.htm. Accessed January 25, 2012.

23. NIH. *IgA Nephropathy*. National Kidney and Urologic Diseases Information Clearinghouse. kidney.niddk.nih.gov/kudiseases/pubs/iganephropathy. Accessed January 26, 2012.

24. Bautuman V. *Diabetic Nephropathy*. (November 23, 2011) emedicine.medscape.com/article/238946-overview. Accessed January 25, 2012.

25. Cohen EP. *Nephrotic Syndrome*. emedicine.medscape.com/article/244631-overview. Accessed January 26, 2012.

26. NIH. *Nephrotic Syndrome*. MedlinePlus. www.nlm.nih.gov/medlineplus/ency/article/000490.htm. Accessed January 26, 2012.

27. NKUDIC. *Nephrotic Syndrome in Adults*. kidney.niddk.nih.gov/kudiseases/pubs/nephrotic. Accessed January 26, 2012.

28. Medscape. *Acute Tubular Necrosis*. emedicine.medscape.com/article/238064-overview. Accessed January 30, 2012.

29. Medical Clinic. *Acute Tubular Necrosis*. www.medical-clinic.org/diseases/acute-tubular-necrosis.html. Accessed February 2, 2012.

30. MedlinePlus. *Acute Tubular Necrosis*. www.nlm.nih.gov/medlineplus/ency/article/000512.htm. Accessed January 30, 2012.

31. Medscape. *Acute Tubular Necrosis*. emedicine.medscape.com/article/238064-overview. Accessed January 30, 2012.

32. NKUDIC. *Renal Tubular Acidosis*. kidney.niddk.nih.gov/kudiseases/pubs/tubularacidosis. Accessed February 2, 2012.

33. acidosis/overview.html. Accessed February 2, 2012.

34. Merkmanual. *Renal Tubular Acidosis (RTA)*. www.merckmanuals.com/professional/print/genitourinary_disorders/renal_transport. Accessed February 2, 2012.

35. NYtimes. *Proximal Renal Tubular Acidosis Overview*. health.nytimes.com/health/guides/disease/proximal-renal-tubular-acidosis/overview.html

36. Merkmanual. *Renal Tubular Acidosis (RTA)*. www.merckmanuals.com/professional/print/genitourinary_disorders/renal_transport

37. A.D.A.M. Medical Encyclopedia. *Fanconi Syndrome*. (www.ncbi.nlmnih.gov/pubmedhealth/PMH0001374/). Accessed February 2, 2012.

38. MerkManual. *Fanconi Syndrome*. www.merckmenuals.com/home/print/kidney_and_urinary-tract_disorders/tubular. Accessed February 2, 2012.

39. Ibid.

40. MerckManual. *Tubulointerstitial Nephritis*. www.marckmanuals.com/professional/print/genitourinary_disorders_tubulointerstitaildisease. Accessed February 2, 2012.

41. Ibid.

42. Ramarkrishnan, K. Diagnosis and treatment of acute pyelonephritis in adults. *American Family Physician* (2005, Mar 1) 71;5:933–942.

43. NIDDK. *Pyelonephritis (Kidney Infection) in Adults*. www.kidney.niddk.nih.gov/kudiseases/pubs/pyelonephritis. Accessed February 15, 2012.

44. Fulop T. *Acute Pyelonephritis*. Medscape Reference. emedicine.medscape.com/article/245559-overview. Accessed February 15, 2012.

45. Lohr JW. *Chronic Pyelonephritis*. Medscape Reference. emedicine.medscape.com/article/245464-overview. Accessed February 17, 2012.

46. RightDiagnosis. *Complications of Chronic Pyelonephritis*. www.rightdiagnosis.com/c/chronic_pyelonephritis/complic.htm. Accessed February 17, 2012.

47. Lohr JW. *Chronic Pyelonephritis*. Medscape Reference. www.emedicine.medscape.com/article/245464-overview. Accessed February 17, 2012.

48. Stanford Hospital and Clinics. *Renal Vascular Disease*. Accessed March 14, 2013.

49. Ibid.

50. Ibid.

51. Mayo Clinic. *Cystitis*. www.mayclinic.com/health/cystitis/DS00285. Accessed February 27, 2012.

52. Ibid.

53. NIH. *Cystitis-acute*. www.nlm.nih.gov/medlineplus/ency/article/000526.htm. Accessed February 27, 2012.

54. Mayo Clinic. *Cystitis*. www.mayclinic.com/health/cystitis/DS00285 Accessed February 27, 2012.

55. Workeneh BT. *Acute Renal Failure*. Medscape Reference. www.emedicine.medscape.com/article/243492-overview. Accessed February 27, 2012.

56. Dwinnell B. *Diagnostic Evaluation of the Patient with Acute Renal Failure*. www.kidneyatlas.org/book/adk1_12.pdf. Accessed February 29, 2012.

57. Workeneh BT. Acute Renal Failure. Medscape Reference. www.emedicine.medscape.com/article/243492-overview. Accessed February 27, 2012.

58. Emedicinehealth. *Chronic Kidney Disease*. www.emedicinehealth.com/script/main/art.asp?articlekey=58887. Accessed March 2, 2012.

59. Arora P. *Chronic Renal Disease*. emedicine.medscape.com/article/238798-overview. Accessed March 2, 2012.

60. MedlinePlus. *Chronic Kidney disease*. www.nlm.nih.gov/medlineplus/ency/article/000471.htm. Accessed March 2, 2012.

61. Sunheimer RL, Graves L. *Clinical Laboratory Chemistry*. Upper Saddle River, NJ: Pearson, 2011: 253–255.

62. Grases F. Renal lithiasis and nutrition. *Nutrition Journal* (2006, September) 5:23.

63. Wolf JS. *Nephrolithiasis*. Medscape Reference. emedicine.medscape.com/article/437096-overview. Accessed March 5, 2012.

64. Mayo Clinic Staff. *Kidney Stones*. www.mayoclinic.com/health/kidney-stones/DS00282. Accessed March 5, 2012.

65. Ibid.

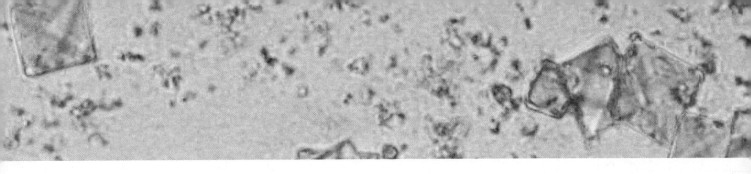

10 Cerebrospinal Fluid

Objectives

LEVEL I

1. Describe the location of anatomical structures of the brain, including subarachnoid space, ventricles, choroid plexus, arachnoid mater, and pituitary gland.
2. Describe the blood–brain barrier and identify three specific sites.
3. List the four types of spinal punctures or taps.
4. Identify the reasons to perform a spinal puncture.
5. Define the following terms: *meningitis, glycorrhachia, intrathecal,* and *subarachnoid hemorrhage.*
6. Identify the criteria used to distinguish a traumatic spinal tap from a subarachnoid hemorrhage.
7. Identify the unique protein present in CSF of many patients with multiple sclerosis.
8. Indicate which CSF specimen tube goes to chemistry, microbiology, and the laboratory that performs cell counts and differentials.
9. Define *xanthochromia.*
10. Calculate the total cell count if given a set of criteria for a Neubauer-type hemocytometer.
11. Discuss laboratory tests performed on CSF and associate them with diseases.
12. List specific diseases and conditions that may result in abnormal levels of protein, glucose, lactate/glutamine, oligoproteins, myelin basic protein, and CSF 14-3-3.
13. Calculate CSF/serum albumin index, CSF/serum IgG ratio, and CSF IgG index.

LEVEL II

1. Explain the technique used for obtaining CSF from a patient and indicate the reasons for performing the procedure properly.
2. Discuss the implications of abnormal laboratory tests in CSF-related disorders.

(continued)

Objectives *(continued)*

3. Describe the physical and microscopic findings from CSF analysis in both normal individuals and those with disease.

4. Interpret abnormal protein results in CSF specimens.

5. Explain the association of altered CSF distribution in the body to clinical conditions.

Key Terms

Blood–brain barrier
Cerebrospinal fluid (CSF)
Choroid plexus
Glycorrhachia
Hemocytometer

High-resolution electrophoresis
Intracranial pressure (ICP)
Intrathecal
Lumbar puncture
Meningitis

Neubauer hemocytometer
Oligoclonal proteins
Prion proteins
Spinal tap
Subarachnoid hemorrhage (SAH)

tau protein
Traumatic tap
Xanthochromia

A CASE IN POINT

Ben, a 21-year-old male is brought to the emergency department by his parents who states that he has "not been himself" for the past 18 hours. He is a college student who was home for the weekend complaining of headaches. The parents inform the physician that their son has no past medical history. They are not aware that he is taking any medication. History and physical findings per the physician are positive for headaches and altered mental status with a tactile fever during the past two days. Body temperature on examination is 38°C (104°F) orally; heart rate of 115 beats per minute, blood pressure 112/70, and a respiratory rate of 22 breaths per minute. His oxygen saturation is 97% on room air. His head and neck exhibited nuchal rigidity (i.e., resistance to flexion).

Results of a CT scan of the brain shows no mass, shift, bleeding, or edema. Opening pressure of a lumbar **spinal tap** is >190 mmH$_2$O (normal <180 mmH$_2$O). The laboratory test results are shown below.

Questions to Consider

1. What is the significance of a lower than normal CSF/serum glucose result?

2. Identify the abnormal findings in this patient's history and physical.

3. What are the patient's abnormal CSF analysis test results?

4. What is the most likely diagnosis?

Laboratory assessment of CSF:

Test	Result	Normal	Comments
Appearance	Cloudy	Clear	Indicates presence of WBCs, RBCs, bacteria, and protein
WBC/mm^3	26	<5	
Polymorphonuclear cells, mm^3	15	<1	
Glucose, mg/dL	30	40–70	
CSF/serum glucose	0.25	0.6–0.75	
Protein, Total, mg/dL	60	15–45	
Gram stain	Positive	None seen	

The brain weighs on average 1500 g and is suspended in **cerebrospinal fluid (CSF)**. The spinal column is also bathed within the fluid. This anatomical arrangement serves as protection for the brain and spinal column from potentially injurious blows or trauma and acute changes in venous pressure. In addition, the CSF provides the brain with buoyancy. The brain has a water content of approximately 80% and thus weighs only 50 g when suspended in CSF.[1] The maintenance of a relatively constant volume-pressure relationship of the CSF is critical and is discussed below in more detail. In addition, because the brain and spinal cord have no lymphatic channels, the CSF serves to remove the waste products of cerebral metabolism, including carbon dioxide, lactate, and hydrogen ions. The composition of CSF is maintained within narrow ranges; thus, the CSF along with intercellular fluid of the brain aids in the preservation of a stable chemical matrix for neurons and their myelinated fibers. The CSF also provides a medium for transporting hypothalamic releasing factors to the cells of the median eminence, which is located near the inferior boundary of the hypothalamus.

The average intracranial volume in an adult is 1700 mL; the volume of the brain is approximately 1300 mL, CSF volume ranges from 70–160 mL (average = 104 mL), and blood volume is approximately 150 mL. In addition, the spinal subarachnoid space consists of 10–70 mL of CSF. Thus in the average adult the CSF occupies less than 10% of the intracranial and intraspinal spaces. Refer to Figure 10-1 ■, the anatomical aspects of the brain, for details of structures and spaces.

FORMATION AND PHYSIOLOGY OF CSF

The **choroid plexuses** are a network of nerves, blood, and lymphatic vessels located in the floor of the ventricles of the brain and are the primary site of CSF formation. The average rate of CSF formation is approximately 20 ml/hour or 500 ml/day, and CSF as a whole is renewed four or five times daily.[2]

The walls of the plexuses are thin, which allows for passive diffusion of substances from the blood plasma in the extracellular space surrounding choroid cells. Each choriodal epithelial cell contains organelles capable of providing energy-dependent secretory functions, for example, active transport. Other areas of the brain contribute to the composition of CSF and include the subepidermal regions, the pia, and the meninges. Both electrolytes and glucose equilibrate with the CSF in all areas within the ventricles and subarachnoid spaces. Sodium transport at the apical surface of choroid plexus cells is facilitated by the Na^+-K^+ ion exchange pump using adenosine triphosphate (ATP) as an energy source. Transport of electrolytes from the plexuses into the ventricles occurs more easily than from plexus into the subarachnoid space.

The movement of water is just the opposite of electrolytes. Solubility in lipids is another factor that effects movement of drugs and metabolites between tissue and cells of the brain. Ionized compounds (e.g., hexoses and amino acids), which are relatively insoluble in lipids, enter CSF slowly unless they are impacted by a membrane transport system. The membrane transport system usually consists of a carrier protein or proteolipids that bind specifically to a compound, resulting in diffusion of that compound across a membrane that is ultimately released into CSF and intercellular fluid.

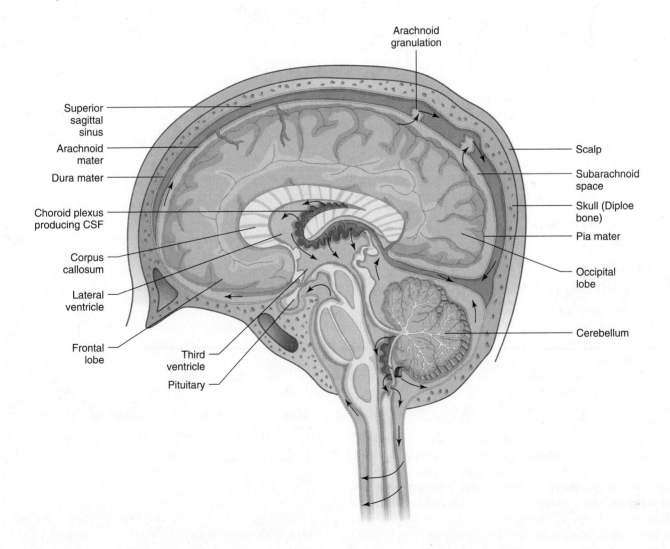

■ **FIGURE 10-1**   Anatomical Features of the Brain Illustrating the Location and Flow Pattern of Cerebrospinal Fluid

Blood–Brain Barrier

Movement of electrolytes, proteins, water, and carbon dioxide from blood into the CSF are facilitated by diffusion gradients. This movement is equivalent in either direction. The fluid constituents found in CSF are in dynamic equilibrium with the blood. This equilibrium exists between CSF located in the ventricles, subarachnoid space and intracellular fluid of the brain, spinal cord, and optic nerve. The **blood–brain barrier** refers to all of the interfaces between blood, brain, and CSF. Specific sites of the blood–brain barrier include (1) endothelium of the choroidal and brain capillaries, (2) plasma membrane and adventitia of these vessels, and (3) peri capillary foot processes of astrocytes. Large molecules such as albumin and substances carried by albumin (e.g., bilirubin and drugs) are unable to pass through the capillary endothelium and into CSF. CSF functions to facilitate the removal of various substances formed in the central nervous system (CNS) during its metabolic processes. These substances move into the CSF, pass into the bloodstream, and are subsequently transported elsewhere in the body.

Acid–Base Balance

Changes in acid-base balance that are manifested through alterations of pCO_2 and hydrogen ion concentration (pH) can affect **intracranial pressure (ICP)**, or the pressure inside the skull, and thus CSF pressure. ICP will be discussed in more detail in the following section. If an individual has a condition that causes retention of CO_2 (e.g., hypoventilation, respiratory acidosis, CNS trauma, tumors, and infections), his or her arterial blood pCO_2 will increase with a corresponding decrease in the pH of CSF. The acidification of CSF acts as a potent cerebral vasodilator, causing an increase in cerebral blood flow, which results in an increased ICP. Hyperventilation, which reduces pCO_2, can result in an increased blood pH and cerebral vascular resistance with a concomitant increase in CSF pressure. Reference ranges for CSF pH and pCO2 can be found in the Appendix H.

CEREBROSPINAL FLUID, PRESSURE, AND REMOVAL

The pressure created due to the presence of CSF in the spinal column and ventricles is assessed by monitoring ICP. A healthy adult in the recumbent (lying down) position normally has a CSF pressure of 50–180 mm H_2O (3.65–13.14 mmHg). As an adult moves from a recumbent position to a standing position, the weight of the column of CSF is added incrementally to the pressure in the lumbar subarachnoid space (lower back), and the ICP decreases. The ICP in an adult who is standing upright approaches zero mmHg.

The fundamental impact of many diseases and conditions associated with CNS is an elevation of ICP and alterations in CSF volume. Assessment of a patient with CNS abnormalities is facilitated by obtaining CSF by lumbar, cisternal, ventricular, or lateral cervical puncture. A **lumbar puncture** or spinal tap is commonly the preferred method of extracting CSF from a patient. The puncture is made between any two interspaces along the spinal column (e.g., Lumbar2 – Lumbar3, Lumbar3 – Lumbar 4 or Lumbar 5 – Sacral 1), and fluid is withdrawn. A *cisternal puncture* uses a needle that is inserted below the occipital bone (back of the skull). *Ventricular punctures* in the cranium are rarely performed but may be indicated in a patient with possible brain herniation. The procedure is performed in the operating room. A hole is drilled into the skull and a needle is inserted directly into one of the brain's ventricles. *Lateral cervical punctures* are made near the mastoid process between C1 and C2 vertebra. Finally, CSF can also be withdrawn using ventricular canulas or shunts where fluid can be withdrawn. This is a common procedure used in intensive care units. Detailed procedures for removal of CSF are described elsewhere.[3,4]

Prior to removal of CSF, an opening pressure measurement using a manometer is performed. A normal opening pressure for an adult is 70–180 mm H_2O under specified conditions. Normal pressure for infants and children is 10–100 mm H_2O. Obese individuals may produce pressures up to 250 mm H_2O.[5] Markedly elevated pressure measurements are diagnostic of intracranial hypertension due to meningitis, intracranial hemorrhage, or tumors.[6] Sampling protocols recommend that if a patient has an opening pressure >200 mm H_2O while relaxed, then no more than 2.0 mL of CSF should be withdrawn. Additional causes of variations in opening pressures are shown in Box 10-1.[7]

☑ CHECKPOINT 10-1

Why is it important to monitor opening pressures while removing CSF?

MINI-CASE 10-1

Bill is brought to the emergency department complaining of stiff neck and severe headache. The patient was febrile and "very tired" all of the time. He was not obese. The physician suspected that Bill has an infection, possibly something as serious as meningitis, so he requested a lumbar puncture. Bill was prepared by the nursing staff for a lumbar puncture. The intracranial pressure was 200 mmH$_2$O. Laboratory results for CSF tests includes: Leukocyte cell count, 25 cells/μL (normal = <5 μL) and CSF glucose test was 25 mg/dL (Reference Range = 50–80 mg/dL).

Question to Consider

1. What is the cause of the elevated intracranial pressure?

BOX 10-1   Causes of Elevated and Reduced CSF Opening Pressures

Increased pressure

Tenseness

Straining

Congestive heart failure (due to increased venous pressure)

Meningitis (expands CSF volume due to infection)

Superior vena cava syndrome (due to an increase in venous pressure)

Thrombosis of the venous sinuses (due to an increase in venous pressure)

Cerebral edema (brain swelling)

Mass lesions (increase pressure on brain)

Any conditions that inhibit CSF absorption

Cryptococcal meningitis (expanded CSF volume)

Decreased pressure

Spinal subarachnoid block

Dehydration

Circulatory collapse

CSF leakage

☑ CHECKPOINT 10-2

List four techniques used to remove CSF from a patient.

BOX 10-2 Diseases Detected by Laboratory Tests on CSF

Meningitis
  Bacterial
  Tuberculous
  Fungal
  Viral
Subarachnoid hemorrhage
Multiple sclerosis
Central nervous system syphilis
Infectious polyneuritis
Meningeal malignancy
Intracranial hemorrhage
Viral encephalitis
Subdural hematoma

CLINICAL SIGNIFICANCE OF CSF IN DISEASE

Spinal taps have been performed since the late 1800s to facilitate the assessment of patients with neurological-related conditions. Although not commonly used as a diagnostic tool, laboratory tests on CSF are useful when CSF test results are related to clinical findings. Several diseases that present with abnormal laboratory tests on CSF are shown in Box 10-2. Diagnostic usefulness in terms of sensitivity and specificity of laboratory tests on CSF obtained by lumbar puncture varies depending on clinical presentation of the patient and CSF assay performance.[8] Several specific diseases and conditions will be presented in this chapter and are commonly categorized as follows:

1. Meningeal infection
2. Subarachnoid hemorrhage
3. CNS malignancies
4. Demyelinating diseases
5. Others

Meningeal Infection

Meningitis is an inflammation of the meninges around the brain and/or spinal cord. It can be caused by bacteria (including spirochetes), fungi, mycobacteria, or viruses. Meningitis should be considered in any patient with a fever and stiff neck or neurologic symptoms. Patients with pre-existing infections or head trauma increase the likelihood of possible meningitis.

Aseptic meningitis is usually milder than bacterial meningitis and may be preceded by upper respiratory inflammation or pharyngitis. Viruses and drug-induced inflammations are common causes. Typical laboratory findings include a lymphocytic CSF, pleocytosis, and infections with enterovirus, herpes simplex virus, and human immunodeficiency virus (HIV).

Bacterial meningitis is considered a medical emergency and usually requires a lumbar puncture. Common laboratory findings from examination of CSF include cloudy or purulent CSF, increased polymorphonuclear cells, and low glucose levels.

There are additional laboratory procedures for examination of CSF, and their utilization depends upon the clinical presentation of the patient. Examples include India ink smears for crytococcus, latex agglutination antigen detection techniques, microscopic examination of CSF for acid-fast bacilli, polymerase chain reaction (PCR) techniques for herpes simplex virus (HSV) and enteroviruses, rapid plasma reagin (RPR), and Gram stain.

Subarachnoid Hemorrhage

Subarachnoid hemorrhage (SAH) is caused by the rupture of an arterial aneurysm with resulting bleeding into the CSF. Diagnosis of SAH can be made using a CT scan of the head and demonstration of blood in the sulci or fissures in the brain and cisternae or opening in the subarachnoid spaces within 24 hours of a crisis. If a situation occurs where the CT scan of the head is negative yet there is strong suspicion for SAH, then a lumbar puncture is requested to provide additional diagnostic information. The patient will typically present with a markedly elevated opening pressure. Cell counts are performed on tubes 1 and 4 (see section entitled "Specimen Collection, Handling, and Storage"). If the number of erythrocytes decreases dramatically from tube 1 and 4, traumatic lumbar puncture is more likely than SAH. A CSF specimen that appears bloody should be centrifuged and assessed for xanthrochromia (yellow color). Xanthrochromia is present when erythrocytes are lysed and indicates SAH rather than a traumatic tap. A **traumatic tap** is a term used to signify trauma from the needle causing bleeding into the lumbar space.

MINI-CASE 10-2

Lab technologist Susan received a bloody CSF specimen on a patient admitted to the Emergency Department. The doctor called the laboratory and requested a cell count on tubes 1 through 4 so that he could determine the cause of the bloody lumbar puncture. Susan centrifuged the CSF specimen, noted the color of the supernatant, and performed a cell count. The results are shown below:

Appearance after centrifugation: pale yellow

Cell counts

Tube #1	90,000 RBC/μL
Tube #2	85,000 RBC/μL
Tube #3	82,000 RBC/μL
Tube #4	75,000 RBC/μL

Questions to Consider

1. What are typical causes of bloody lumbar punctures?
2. Based on the lab results, what is the cause of the bloody lumbar puncture?
3. Why is the specimen xanthochromic?

Malignancy

With the advances made in neuroradiology and the risk of "coning" or movement of the brain matter due to herniation caused by elevated ICP, lumbar puncture is often not considered in early, untreated stages of the disease. However, in patients with malignancies that have spread to the meninges, examination of CSF (especially cytological) can be useful. The gross appearance of CSF in the presence of histologically confined malignancy is usually abnormal. In these patients the leukocyte count (especially monocytes) is elevated, CSF protein is slightly to markedly elevated, and glucose levels are normal to decreasing. CSF samples are submitted to cytology and histology laboratories to rule out central nervous system (CNS) involvement of leukemia, lymphoma, or patients with known primary cancers (e.g., breast, lung, or melanoma).

Leptomeningeal Metastases

CSF provides an important source of potential biomarkers for brain disorders. Proteomic techniques are being employed to identify and quantitate proteins in CSF.[9] Another procedure used to assess neoplasms (e.g., hematologic) is flow cytometric immunophenotyping (FCI) of CSF.[10] CSF cytological examinations are most useful in hematomalignancies. Leptomeningeal metastasis is a cancer that involves the pia mater and arachnoid membranes of the brain, but not the dura mater. Establishing a diagnosis of leptomeningeal metastases is challenging at times. Magnetic resonance imaging (MRI) techniques can be definitive in patients presenting with specific conditions but dubious in others. Demonstration of tumor cells in the CSF is definitive and often considered the gold standard.[11] Cytology examinations in these patients are not useful because only about 50% of patients produce positive results on the first lumbar puncture. Additional CSF abnormalities include increased protein and white blood cells.

Glycorrhachia is a term used to denote the presence of glucose in CSF. *Hypoglycorrhachia* is a decrease of glucose in CSF and is present in <25% of patients with leptomeningeal metastases.

☑ CHECKPOINT 10-3

T or F.   A patient's cell count on all four tubes containing CSF is higher than normal. These laboratory cell count results are consistent with subarachnoid hemorrhage.

Demyelinating Diseases

Multiple sclerosis (MS) is a demyelinating disease involving the white mater of the brain and spinal cord. It is prevalent in females more than males (2:1 ratio) and usually presents itself during young adulthood. Multiple sclerosis presents with a wide variety of signs and symptoms. Diagnosis of MS is determined from clinical observations and exclusion of all other disorders.

MS is described as a T cell-mediated autoimmune demyelinating disease that may be initiated by a virus infection.[12,13] The exact cause of MS is not known. No characteristic circulating autoantibodies have been noted in MS.

Oligoclonal Proteins

CSF examination in a clinical laboratory provides important information that supports a diagnosis of MS. Production of IgG increases abnormally within the CSF of MS patients. Determination of the IgG index and the IgG synthesis rate provides useful, albeit nonspecific, test results.[14] Discovery of **oligoclonal proteins** (i.e., O-bands or O-protein) in CSF samples is clinically useful because they are identified in >90% of patients with MS.

The presence of oligoclonal proteins in CSF is not diagnostically specific and may be detected in patients with neurosyphilis, CNS vasculitis, Lyme disease, Guillain-Barré syndrome, and Creutzfeldt-Jakob disease. Other laboratory findings in patients with MS include marginally elevated white blood cell counts, not to exceed 50 cells/μL (50×10^6/L), the presence of activated T-lymphocytes, possibly some plasma cells, normal glucose and normal lactate concentrations, increased protein concentrations (approximately 400 mg/dL), normal CSF/serum albumin ratios (70–80% cases), and IgG Index (Q_{IgG}) >0.7 in about 75% of patients.[15,16,17]

Diagnostic sensitivity of qualitative measurement of intrathecal production of Ig by isoelectric focusing (IEF) is greater than quantitative estimates of IgG indexes in 95–100% of the patients.[18,19] **Intrathecal** literally means "within the sheath," but in this context it refers to the introduction of IgG into the space under the arachnoid membrane that covers the brain and spinal cord. The clinical relevance of oligoclonal IgG proteins in the diagnostic workup of MS resides in both the origin of the proteins and banding patterns revealed by high resolution protein electrophoresis (HRE) as shown in Figure 10-2 ■. The concentration of IgG and IgM in CSF is restricted by the blood–brain barrier. Normally, the amounts of IgG and IgM found in CSF are 500 and 1000 times lower respectively than in serum. Immunoglobulins found in CSF originate from serum and intrathecal production

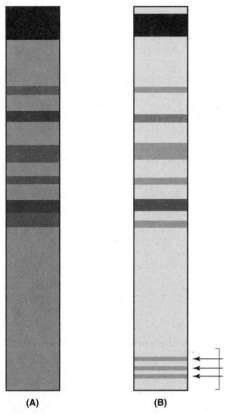

(A)   **(B)**

■ **FIGURE 10-2** Positive oligoclonal protein pattern in a spinal fluid sample using high-resolution electrophoresis (HRE). There are three bands present in CSF adjacent to the arrows but not serum.

(A) Serum, (B) CSF from same patient.

(i.e., immunoglobulin produced within the spinal canal or sheath). These findings are clinically significant.[20]

Normally, neither serum nor CSF contains oligoclonal proteins. Oligoclonal IgG proteins appear only in CSF and not in serum, and demonstrate an intrathecal Ig production that is commonly seen in patients with MS. Patients presenting with systemic inflammation combined with additional CNS involvement demonstrate IgG transudation of oligoclonal IgG from serum to CSF in combination with intrathecal IgG production. IEF of these samples reveal identical bands in serum and CSF plus additional bands in the CSF. This pattern may also appear in patients with MS with concomitant severe infection. Oligoclonal bands are also demonstrated in serum and CSF in patients with systemic immune activation.[21]

Guillain-Barré syndrome, although not strictly a demyelinating disease, is characterized by the presence of protein in CSF that often exceeds 200 mg/dL. In this syndrome, the body produces antibodies to the myelin sheath that surrounds peripheral cells, causing sensory and motor symptoms that usually start in the lower limbs. The weakness progresses over time and can involve the respiratory muscles, requiring ventilator support.

AIDS-Associated Disorders

The human immunodeficiency virus (HIV) can impact any portion of the CNS, including spinal cord, meninges, brain, peripheral nerves, and muscles. The most common AIDS-associated neurological

disorder is HIV encephalitis/AIDS dementia complex. This insidious disorder causes progressive memory loss, intellectual deterioration, behavioral changes, and motor deficits. Nonspecific laboratory findings in CSF include an increase in mononuclear cells, protein concentration, and demonstration of oligoclonal protein, as well as detection of viral nucleic acid using PCR techniques.

Inherited Disorders

Measurement of biochemical analytes or compounds in CSF is useful for assessing patients with various inherited metabolic disorders including inborn errors of amino acid metabolism (see Chapter 14). CSF lactate is elevated in conditions affecting the respiratory chain, when plasma lactates are normal or slightly increased. Examples of inherited disorders include deficiency of pyruvate dehydrogenase or cytochrome C oxidase. In this case, pyruvate is also elevated.[22] Other disorders include glycine encephalopathy where CSF glycine levels are high, 3-phosphoglycerate dehydrogenase deficiency characterized by low CSF serine levels, and organic acidemias with elevated CSF lactate.

Lyme Disease

Patients with Lyme disease can present with CNS involvement. The condition known as neuroborreliosis is caused by *Borrelia burgdorferi*. Spinal fluid analysis shows elevated CSF protein, numerous mononuclear cells, and a normal CSF glucose. Antibody tests to *Borrelia burgdorferi* in serum/CSF are used to confirm neuroborreliosis. Laboratory assays, for example, enzyme linked immunoabsorbant assay (ELISA) or immunofluorescent assay (IFA), are commonly used and borderline or positive results should be confirmed using Western blot techniques. CSF immunological assays to detect anti-*Borrelia burgdorferi* IgM provide a useful test to assess patients with suspected cases of Lyme disease. PCR techniques are very specific for detecting Borrelia DNA but lacks sensitivity at specific stages of the disease.

Sarcoidosis

A specific type of sarcoidosis, neurosarcoidosis, features the formation of granulomas in the CNS that represent an autoimmune response to CNS inflammation. Laboratory results of CSF analysis reveal a lymphocytosis, nonspecific elevation of protein, and negative cytology tests. These findings are used to differentiate neurosarcoidosis from infections affecting the CNS. Additional lab findings include elevated CSF levels of angiotensin-converting enzyme, lysozyme, and β_2-microglobulin.

☑ CHECKPOINT 10-4

Greater than 90% of patient with MS present with intrathecal production of which unique protein?

Dementia

Currently there are no clinically useful biomarkers for diagnosing Alzheimer's disease (AD) or differentiating AD from other dementias (e.g., vascular). There are candidate biomarkers, including the ratio of a phosphorylated form of a protein commonly used to identify

★ **TABLE 10-1** CSF Profiles in Disease

Disease	Appearance	Opening Pressure (mmH$_2$O)	WBCs (cells/μL)	RBCs (cells/μL)	Glucose (mg/dL)	Protein (g/dL)	Smear	Culture
Normal	Clear		<5 cells/	0	~50–70% of serum glucose	15–40	Neg	Neg
Bacterial meningitis	Cloudy	Inc	Inc (mainly PMNs)	0	Dec	Mod Inc	Pos	Pos
Fungal meningitis	N to cloudy	N to inc	N to Inc (Monos)	0	Dec	Inc	India ink pos	Pos
Tuberculosis meningitis	N to cloudy	Inc	N to Inc	0	Dec	Mod Inc	AFB Pos	Pos
Viral meningitis	Clear	Inc	Inc	0	N	N to Inc		
Subarachnoid hemorrhage	Bloody or xanthochromic	Inc	N to Inc	Inc	N	Inc	Neg	Neg
Brain tumor	N	Inc	0	0	N	Inc	Neg	Neg
Multiple sclerosis	N	N	N to sl inc	0	N	N or Inc	Neg	Neg
Guillain- Barré syndrome	N	N	0	0	N	Inc	Neg	Neg
Cerebral hemorrhage, trauma	Blood	N to Inc	Inc	Inc	N	Inc	NA	NA

* N = Normal, Inc = Increased, Dec = Decrease, Neg = Negative, Pos = Positive, NA = Not applicable

CSF (tau protein) to a protein known as β amyloid peptide-42.[23] CSF T-tau (total tau) is increased in AD and reflects neurofibrillary tangles but the increase overlaps with a wide number of other neurological diseases. Likewise, CSF levels of abnormally hyperphosphorylated P-tau are increased in AD but also overlap with other dementias. Many patients with AD have decreased concentrations of CSF β-amyloid-42 (Aβ42) but decreased Aβ42 concentrations also occur in patients experiencing other forms of neurological diseases and dementias. Efforts to increase diagnostic accuracy of laboratory tests have relied on measurement of combinations of these biomarkers with varied success.[24]

A summary of laboratory analysis of CSF relative to several diseases and conditions is presented in Table 10-1 ★. The table does not reflect all of the diseases discussed in this section.

Creutzfeldt-Jakob Disease

Creutzfeldt-Jakob disease (CJD) belongs to a group of fatal neurodegenerative diseases referred to as human transmissible spongiform encephalopathy, which features an accumulation of pathological **prion proteins** (PrP) in the CNS. Prion proteins comprise a prion, which is an infectious agent. The protein is typically "misfolded." Neuropathological studies are the only means of obtaining a definitive diagnosis; determining the clinical phenotypes is the best means of making the initial diagnosis as defined by WHO criteria.[25]

SPECIMEN COLLECTION, HANDLING, AND STORAGE

Specimen collection begins with a clinician penetrating the puncture site, attaching a manometer, and measuring the opening pressure. The clinician should look for normal oscillation in CSF pressure associated with pulse and respirations. The CSF will begin to exit the puncture site and should be allowed to drip into collection tubes. There should be a sufficient volume of specimen removed to enable all laboratory tests to be completed. Examples of tests that may be required include (1) cell count with differential; (2) protein and glucose concentrations;

(3) culture (bacterial, viral, mycobacterial fungal); (4) smears (e.g., Gram and acid-fast stains); (5) antigen tests; (6) PCR amplification of DNA or RNA of microorganism (e.g., herpes simples virus); (7) antibody levels against microorganism; (8) electrophoresis for gamma-globulin and oligoclonal protein; and (9) cytology procedures.

Specimen requirements vary from one laboratory to another, thus the clinician should be aware of the amount of CSF required for the necessary tests to ensure that a sufficient quantity of CSF is removed. Normally, up to 20 ml of CSF can be safely withdrawn from adults.

The CSF specimen is separated into three or four sterile plastic tubes. Glass tubes should not be used because cells may adhere to their surfaces, which will affect cell counts and differential. The tubes are each assigned a number for example, tube #1, tube #2, and so on. Tube #1 is for chemistry and immunology tests, tube #2 is for microbiology, and tube #3 for cell counts and differential. An additional tube may be necessary for cytological testing if, for example, a malignancy is suspected.

The protocol described above can be modified to meet specific requirements or situations. For example, if tube #1 contains a large amount of blood from a traumatic tap, it should not be used for protein measurements. Also, tube #1 should never be used for microbiology because it may be contaminated with skin bacteria.

CSF specimens should be delivered to the laboratory and processed quickly to reduce the amount of cellular degradation. Specimens for culture procedures should not be refrigerated because certain organisms may not survive the cold temperatures (e.g., *Haemophilus influenza* and *Neisseira meningitidis*).

PHYSICAL EXAMINATION

Spinal fluid specimens received in the laboratory should be inspected and assessed for alterations in physical appearance. Normal CSF is clear and colorless with a viscosity similar to water. See Figure 10-3 ■ for an of a normal appearing CSF specimen and a specimen showing xanthrochromia. Patient diseases involving brain and spinal column or patients injected with radiocontrast media usually present with abnormal-appearing CSF. Patient specimens may be cloudy or turbid, purulent (containing pus), or colored.

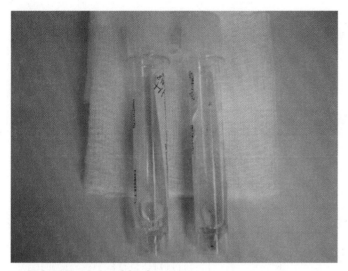

FIGURE 10-3 CSF Specimens

(A) Normal CSF is clear and colorless. (B) Xanthochromic with a RBC button at the bottom of the tube.

Color should be reported as colorless, pink, yellow, yellow-green, orange, or brown. Color variations are due to a variety of causes, as shown in Table 10-2 ★. A specific term associated with yellow colored CSF is **xanthochromia**. Each CSF specimen should be checked for discoloration by comparing the color of the CSF sample to water.

A question that often arises upon visual inspection of a CSF specimen is whether the appearance of the sample represents a traumatic tap or a pathologic hemorrhage? The following recommendations may be useful to make this determination:[26]

1. Set up all four tubes and inspect them for blood. A traumatic spinal tap will usually show evidence of blood in the first through third tube. A patient with a subarachnoid hemorrhage will present with a uniform intensity of blood throughout all four tubes.
2. A subarachnoid hemorrhage may also show xanthochromia, microscopic evidence of erythrophagocytosis, or hemosiderin-laden macrophages in the absence of a prior traumatic tap. Lysis of

★ **TABLE 10-2** Causes of Abnormal CSF Supernatant Colors

CSF Color	Cause(s)
Pink	Lysis of erythrocytes, hemoglobin breakdown products, presence of oxyhemoglobin due to delay of more than one hour without refrigeration before examination.
Pink-red	Blood present in CSF originating from a subarachnoid hemorrhage, intracerebral hemorrhage, cerebral infarct, or traumatic spinal tap
Yellow	Lysis of erythrocytes, hemoglobin breakdown products, hyperbilirubinemia, CSF protein concentration >150 mg/dL
Yellow-green	Hyperbilirubinemia due to the presence of biliverdin
Orange	Lysis of erythrocytes, hemoglobin breakdown products, hypervitaminosis A due to the presence of carotenoids
Red-orange	Rifampin therapy (a drug therapy for tuberculosis)
Brown	Meningeal metastatic melanoma

erythrocyte commences as early as 1–2 hours after a traumatic tap, therefore evaluation of a sample should be completed quickly to avoid false-positive results.

Cloudy specimens are typically due to an increase in the number of leukocytes or erythrocytes. Significantly bloody fluid due to a traumatic lumbar puncture contains a large number of erythrocytes.

Clotted specimens may result in false low cell counts due to entrapment of cells in the clot. Clot formation is usually due to the presence of fibrinogen. CSF specimens collected from a traumatic tap may form clots, whereas bloody CSF caused by intracranial hemorrhage does not contain a sufficient amount of fibrinogen to clot. Clots can form in CSF samples in patients diagnosed with meningitis, Froin[§] syndrome, and blockage of CSF circulation through the subarachnoid space. The mechanism involves damage to the blood–brain barrier which allows increased transport of protein and coagulation factors into the CSF.

Spinal fluid samples can be more viscous than normal due to a variety of causes, including metastatic mucin-producing adenocarcinoma, cryptococcal meningitis due to capsular polysaccharides, or withdrawing of liquid using a needle from the nucleus pulposus via penetration of the annulus fibrosis (fibrocartilage). These are anatomical structures of the spinal vertebrate.

The volume of spinal fluid withdrawn is relatively small and varies from 10–20 mL in adults. CSF yield for small children is approximately 8 mL. The specimens are usually separated into four tubes as outline earlier.

☑ CHECKPOINT 10-5

Why should tube #1 for spinal fluid analysis never be used for microbiology testing?

MICROSCOPIC PROCEDURES

The microscopic portion of CSF analysis consists of counting the number of cells, identifying cells, and reporting the findings to a clinician. Microscopic analysis of CSF can provide clinicians with significant information regarding the health of their patients. Several examples of microscopic findings and associated diseases or conditions are presented in Table 10-3 ★.

Total Cell Counts

Enumeration of the total number of WBCs and RBCs are performed either manually using a counting chamber or an automated flow cytometer. CSF specimens should be well mixed before counting. If the specimen is excessively bloody, it may required a dilution. In addition, CSF specimens with markedly elevated nucleated cell counts may require a dilution.

[§]Froin syndrome is described as an alteration in the spinal fluid that appears yellow and tends to coagulate spontaneously after withdraw due to high concentration of protein and albumin.

★ **TABLE 10-3** Cells Found in CSF of Adults with Disease

Type of Cells	Diseases
Lymphocytes	Meningitis (virtually all types)
	Degenerative disorders (most of the common ones)
	Sarcoidosis
	Parasitic infections
Neutrophils	Meningitis
	Bacterial
	Early viral
	Early tuberculous
	Early mycotic
	Cerebral abscess
	Following seizures
	Subarachnoid hemorrhage
	Intracerebral hemorrhage
	CNS infarction
	Metastatic tumors in contact with CSF
	Injection of contrast media and/or medications (e.g., methotrexate) into the subarachnoid space
Plasma cells	Acute viral infections
	Guillain-Barré syndrome
	Multiple sclerosis
	Parasite infections of the CNS
	Sarcoidosis
	Tuberculous meningitis
	Syphilitic meningoencephalitis
Monocytes	Viral meningitis
	Tuberculous meningitis
	Fungal meningitis
	Multiple sclerosis
Macrophages	Erythrocytes in spinal fluid
	Contrast media
Blast cells	Acute leukemia
Malignant cells	Metastatic carcinoma
	Primary CNS carcinoma

Manual Cell Counting

Counting cells manually using a counting chamber, also called a **hemocytometer**, is a commonly used technique. Two examples of counting chambers are the Fuchs-Rosenthal and the **Neubauer hemocytometer**, which is shown in Figure 10-4 ■. It consists of a thick glass microscopic slide with rectangular indentations that create a chamber with a specific dimension. This chamber is etched with a grid of perpendicular lines (grooves). The hemocytometer is designed so that the area bounded by the line is known as wells as the depth of the chamber. A precise count of the number of cells in a specific volume of fluid can be determined, and the number of cells in the fluid is derived by calculation.

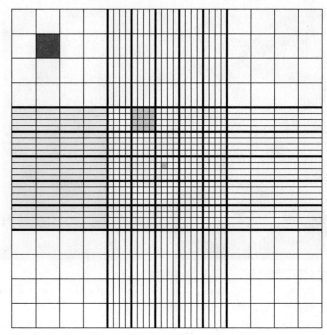

■ **FIGURE 10-4**   Improved Neubauer Hemocytometer
Yellow square = 1 mm², Red square = 0.0625 mm², Blue square = 0.04 mm² and Green square = 0.0025 mm².

Procedure

A CSF sample is introduced into the chamber using a transfer device such as a pipette and covered with a cover slip. Capillary action fills the chamber with sample. The glass cover slip must be free from any defects that may obscure the user's view. Size and placement of the cover slip is important. When the cover slip is placed correctly on the counting chamber, the central ruled area lies in the center of the rectangle to be filled with CSF. The counting chamber and cover slip form the boundaries of the volumetric chamber. The chamber dimensions vary with different types of hemocytometers. The Fuchs-Rosenthal chamber has a depth of 0.2 mm, a total sample volume of 3.6 μL (18 large squares times 0.2 μL/square). The Neubauer hemocytometer has two chambers; each chamber is divided into nine sections, and each section is divided into 16 squares that are 1 mm² with a depth of 0.1 mm. Once the hemocytometer has been "charged" with sample, the cells are counted using a microscope.

The ruled area of the hemocytometer (shown in Figure 10-4) consists of nine large squares with dimensions of 1 × 1 mm (1 mm²). These squares are subdivided in three ways; 0.25 mm × 0.25 mm (0.0625 mm²), 0.25 × 0.20 mm (0.05 mm²) and 0.20 × 0.20 mm (0.04 mm²). The middle 0.20 × 0.20 mm square is further subdivided into 0.05 × 0.05 mm (0.0025 mm²) squares. The raised edges of the hemocytometer support the cover slip, which is 0.1 mm off the marked grid. This creates a defined volume for each square. The dimensions and volumes are summarized in Table 10-4 ★.

Good microscopic technique must be used while preparing and counting cells using a hemocytometer. The chamber or an objective lens may be damaged if the user is not careful. A 40× high dry objective may be used to view the entire grid on standard hemocytometers with Neubauer rulings.

★ **TABLE 10-4** Dimensions and Volumes of a Hemocytometer

Dimension (mm)	Area (mm^2)	Volume (nL) at 0.1 mm Depth
1 × 1	1	100
0.25 × 0.25	0.0625	6.25
0.25 × 0.20	0.05	5
0.20 × 0.20	0.04	4
0.05 × 0.05	0.0025	0.25

Sample suspensions should be dilute enough so that the cells do not overlap each other on the grid, and they should be uniformly distributed. Prior to counting the cells, determine the magnification required to recognize the desired cell types. Select the squares to count; this is usually determined by the size and/or density of the cells. Systematically count the cells using a consistent pattern to minimize bias. If the sample was diluted prior to counting, remember to multiply your final count by the dilution factor.

Counting accuracy using manual techniques and hemocytometer depends on the following:

- Accurate mixing of the samples
- Number of chambers counted
- Number of cells counted

Errors in chamber counting are related to (1) technique, (2) uneven distribution of the cells in the chamber, and (3) misidentification of cells.

Erythrocyte counts have limited diagnostic value but are useful for determining a true CSF WBC or total protein in the presence of a traumatic puncture by correcting for leukocytes or protein introduced by the traumatic tap. For the best results, all counts and protein measurements should be made from the same tube. The calculation used to correct a WBC is shown in Equation 10-1.[27]

$$WBC_{corrected} = WBC_{observed} - WBC_{added}$$

Where

$$WBC_{added} = WBC_{blood} \times RBC_{CSF}/RBC_{blood}$$

and

$$WBC_{observed} = CSF \text{ leukocyte count}$$
$$WBC_{added} = \text{leukocytes added to CSF by traumatic tap}$$
$$WBC_{blood} = \text{peripheral blood leukocyte count}$$
$$RBC_{CSF} = CSF \text{ erythrocyte count}$$
$$RBC_{blood} = \text{peripheral blood erythrocyte count} \quad \textbf{(10-1)}$$

The formula to correct for added total protein (TP) is shown in Equation 10-2.[28]

CSF cell counting protocols may vary between laboratories. Once the number of cells is determined they must be reported in conventional units, μL or SI units, 10^6/L.

Automated Cell Counting

Several automated cell counters are currently available for body fluid analysis. Automated cell counters do have limitations. Analytical precision and accuracy may be compromised using automated cell counters because of the lower number of cells frequently encountered in patient CSF specimens. Specimens with high cell counts are suitable for most automated cell counters. Laboratory staff who are considering the purchase of an automated cell counter should exercise caution and follow the manufacturer's and CLSI guidelines (CLSI approved guideline H56-A) when implementing these systems.[29]

☑ CHECKPOINT 10-6

A staff technologist is required to perform a cell count on a CSF specimen. The sample requires a four-fold dilution prior to counting. The technologist counts the number of cells in five small squares, each square having an area of 0.04 mm^2 and a depth of 0.1 mm. A total of 25 cells were counted. What is the cell count per mm^3? Also convert the cell count per mm^3 to cells per milliliter.

DIFFERENTIAL COUNTS

Cerebrospinal fluid differential counts should not be performed using a counting chamber because of the low number of cells present. Both counting precision and identification of cells beyond granulocytes may be adversely affected. Direct smears prepared from CSF sediment should be avoided because of cell distortion and fragmentation.

Cytocentrifugation

The method that yields the most reliable differential counts requires preparation of a stained smear made from concentrated leukocytes. A popular technique for preparing leukocyte concentrates uses a cytocentrifuge, often referred to as a *cytospin* technique. A cytospin technique is fast, requires minimal training, and allows Wright's staining of air-dried cytospin preps. Preparation of cytospin slides for a cell differential is shown in Figure 10-5 ■. The process begins by assembling a sample chamber consisting of a slide clip, microscope slide, filter paper blotter, and cytofunnel disposable sample chamber. A small amount of CSF specimen and 20–30% albumin is pipetted into the cytofunnel. The albumin serves to increase cell yield and decrease cell distortion. Place the assembled sample chamber into the cytocentrifuge and begin centrifugation. While the specimen is centrifuged, the cells present in the CSF are forced into a monolayer within a small diameter circle on the slide. Fluid is absorbed by the filter paper blotter, resulting in a more concentrated area of cells. Once cytocentrifugation is complete, the slide is removed and stained with Wright-Giemsa.

$$TP \text{ added} = [TP_{serum} \times (1 - hematocrit)] \times RBC_{CSF}/RBC_{blood} \quad \textbf{(10-2)}$$

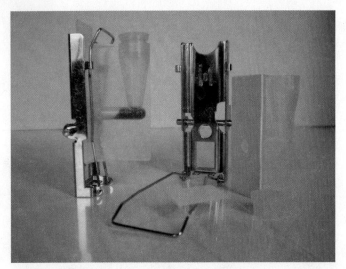

■ **FIGURE 10-5** Components used for Preparation of Cytospin Slides

Cell counting protocols vary with laboratories. It is advantageous to count at least 100 cells and determine the percentage of each specific cell. Fewer cells may be counted and the final result adjusted per laboratory protocol. Specific cell populations in adults vary with health and disease as shown in Table 10-3.

Cellular Components

The CSF of normal, healthy adults contains a small number of lymphocytes and monocytes in a relative ratio of 70:30. In neonates the ratio is reversed, and young children may present with approximately 80% monocytes.

Plasma cells are not normally present in CSF of adults but may appear in a variety of inflammatory and infectious conditions (see Table 10-3). Some patients may present with large and small lymphocytes, and there may be plasma cells in the CSF of patients with malignant brain tumors.

Eosinophils are rarely seen in the CSF of adults or children. However, eosinophilia can occur in a variety of CNS conditions, inflammatory responses, and parasitic invasion of the CNS, which is the most common cause worldwide. In endemic areas of the United States, the most common form of CSF eosinophilia is caused by *Coccidioides immitis*.

Monocytes are not diagnostically significant but are part of a "mixed cell reaction" that includes neutrophils, lymphocytes, and plasma cells. This cluster of cells is often seen in patients with meningitis of differing etiologies (e.g., bacterial, fungal). Macrophages with phagocytized erythrocytes appear 12 to 48 hours following a subarachnoid hemorrhage or traumatic tap. Also characteristic of subarachnoid hemorrhage is the presence of hemosiderin-laden macrophages (siderophages) that appear in CSF after 48 hours and may persist for weeks.

CHEMICAL TESTING

Reference values for chemical analytes in CSF are presented in Appendix H. These ranges should be used as guidelines and each laboratory should establish their own ranges for clinical use.

Proteins

The protein content of CSF, over 80%, originates from plasma by ultrafiltration and pinocytosis; the remainder is from intrathecal synthesis. Ventricular fluid contains a lower amount of protone than cisternal and lumbar. Refer to the Appendix H for reference intervals.

Spinal fluid protein levels may be elevated due to decreased resorption at the arachnoid villi, increased permeability of the blood brain barriers, an increased intrathecal synthesis of IgG, or a mechanical obstruction of CSF flow due to spinal blockage above the lumbar spinal tap site. Several examples of causes of increased lumbar CSF protein results are presented in Box 10-3.

Low CSF protein levels (<15 mg/dL), although not as common, can occur in both adults and children. It is normal for children between the ages of 6 months and 2 years to have subnormal CSF protein levels. Also adults with conditions resulting in an increase CSF turnover may present with lower CSF protein concentrations. Specific conditions that can result in subnormal CSF protein concentrations include (1) leakage of CSF due to trauma or lumbar puncture, (2) hyperthyroidism, (3) increased intracranial pressure, and (4) removal of large volumes of CSF.[30]

The presence of specific proteins in CSF has provided insight into the mechanisms of several diseases associated with the CNS. Furthermore, assays have been developed to identify and measure these proteins for use as (1) diagnostic tests, (2) a method to monitor disease progression, and (3) a means to assess the effects of therapy. Although the diagnostic utility of some of these proteins is very controversial, much research is still in progress to determine if routine measurement is warranted. Thus, measurement of many of these proteins is not provided by routine clinical chemistry laboratories. Several examples of these proteins and their associated diseases/conditions are shown in Table 10-5 ★ and a discussion of selected proteins will follow.[31]

BOX 10-3   Conditions Associated with Increased Levels of CSF Protein

CSF circulation defects
  Mechanical obstructions due to tumors, herniated disks, or abscesses
Toxic drug levels
  Ethanol, phenothiazines (Imiprimine), phenytoin (Dilantin)
Traumatic spinal tap
Increased blood-CSF permeability
  Meningitis (bacterial, viral, fungal, tuberculous)
  Subarachnoid hemorrhage
  Intracerebral hemorrhage
  Arachnoiditis following immunosuppressive drug therapy
  Endocrine disorders involving thyroid and parathyroid glands
Multiple sclerosis
Increased IgG synthesis (e.g., Guillain-Barré syndrome or lupus erythematosus)

★ **TABLE 10-5** CSF Proteins and Their Respective Diseases/Conditions

CSF Proteins	Diseases/Conditions
Myelin basic protein	Multiple sclerosis
Fibronectin	Lymphoblastic leukemia, AIDS, meningitis
C-reactive protein	Bacterial and viral meningitis
Protein 14-3-3	Creutzfeldt-Jakob disease
Alpha$_2$-macroglobulin	Subdural hemorrhage, bacterial meningitis
Beta$_2$-microglobulin	Leukemia/lymphoma
Bacterial amyloid and tau protein	Alzheimer disease
Transferrin	Otorrhea and rhinorrhea (CSF leakage from ear and nose)

★ **TABLE 10-6** Interpretive Guidelines for CSF/Serum Albumin Index

Cutoff Values	Interpretation
<9	Intact blood-brain barrier
9–14	Slight impairment
15–30	Moderate impairment
>30	Severe impairment

The integrity of the blood–brain barrier can be assessed by measuring chemical analytes in blood and CSF. Several of these measurements and their associated ratios and indexes are presented in the following text.

Albumin Index

Assessment of CNS IgG synthesis depends on an intact blood–brain barrier, otherwise false-positive results may occur. The albumin index is a reliable indicator of the integrity of the blood–brain barrier.[32] Abnormal values can be caused by several disorders that alter the blood–brain barrier, including Guillain-Barré syndrome, CNS systemic lupus erythematosus, obstruction of the CSF circulation, and cervical spondylosis. An elevated albumin index indicates compromised blood–brain barrier or contamination with blood thereby falsely elevating CSF IgG. The calculation shown in Equation 10-3 requires the measurement of both serum and CSF albumin concentrations.

$$\text{CSF/Serum albumin index} = \frac{\text{CSF albumin (mg/dL)}}{\text{Serum albumin (g/dL)}} \quad (10\text{-}3)$$

Interpretive guidelines for grading impairment of the blood–brain barrier are shown in Table 10-6 ★ (see also Appendix H).[33] The index is slightly higher in infants up to 6 months of age due to the immaturity of the blood–brain barrier. The index rises gradually after the age of 40 years. A traumatic tap adversely affects the index calculation and should not be used.

CSF/Serum IgG Ratio

An estimate of the amount of intrathecal synthesis of IgG can be determined by calculating a CSF/Serum IgG ratio as shown in Equation 10-4.

$$\text{CSF/Serum IgG ratio} = \frac{\text{CSF IgG (mg/dL)}}{\text{Serum IgG (g/dL)}} \quad (10\text{-}4)$$

The reference range for the ratio is 3.0–8.7.[34] An elevated index is evidence of increased intrathecal IgG synthesis or an increase in plasma IgG crossover due to a breakdown of the blood–brain barrier. Increased IgG due to plasma IgG crossover is corrected by including the contribution of albumin. The equations used to correct for plasma IgG crossover are shown below. Note the differences in the concentration units between the Equations 10-5 and 10-6.

A reference range should be established by each laboratory owing to the variability of measurements of each factor used in the calculation. An upper limit of 0.8 has been found to be acceptable or the reference range shown in Appendix H.[35]

IgG Synthesis Rate

Computation of the rate of CNS synthesis of IgG per day is useful for the assessment of patients with possible MS. The synthesis rate in MS patients is increased above normal in more than 90% of patients with MS and approximately 4% of patients who do not have MS. The sensitivity of this rate determination is similar to the IgG index.[36] The IgG synthesis rate is shown in Equation 10-7. The reference range for IgG synthesis rate is –9.9 to 3.3 mg/day.[37]

$$\text{CSF IgG index} = \frac{\text{CSF IgG (mg/dL)/Serum IgG (g/dL)}}{\text{CSF albumin (mg/dL)/Serum albumin (g/dL)}} \quad (10\text{-}5)$$

$$\text{CSF IgG index} = \frac{\text{CSF IgG (mg/dL)/Serum albumin (g/dL)}}{\text{Serum IgG (g/dL)/CSF albumin (mg/dL)}} \quad (10\text{-}6)$$

$$\text{IgG synthesis rate (mg/day)} = \left\{ \left(\left(\frac{[\text{IgG}_{csf}] - [\text{IgG}_{serum}]}{369} \right) - \left\{ \frac{[\text{Albumin}_{csf}] - [\text{Albumin}_{serum}]}{230} \right\} \right) \times \frac{0.43\,[\text{IgG}_{serum}]}{[\text{Albumin}_{serum}]} \right\} \times 5 \qquad (10\text{-}7)$$

Where:

369 = normal serum/CSF IgG ratio

230 = normal serum/CSF albumin ratio

0.43 = molecular weight ratio of IgG to albumin

5 = converts the result from concentration to a daily amount assuming normal daily production of CSF of 500 mL (i.e., 5.0 dL)

All protein units are in mg/dL.

CSF IgG–Albumin Ratio

Estimates of in situ CNS synthesis of IgG can be determined by calculating the CSF IgG–albumin ratio. Measurement of CSF IgG and albumin are substituted into the ratio shown in Equation 10-8.

$$\text{IgG–albumin ratio} = \frac{\text{IgG}_{CSF}\ (\text{mg/dL})}{\text{albumin}_{CSF}\ (\text{mg/dL})} \qquad (10\text{-}8)$$

If increased CSF IgG were the only serum proteins present in the CSF as a result of a defect in blood–brain barrier, then it would follow that there should be an increased amount of albumin, a CSF protein derived only from serum. Many cases of neurological diseases are characterized by increased permeability of the blood–brain barrier and thus an enhanced diffusion of IgG from serum to CSF. The CSF IgG–albumin reference interval is 0.09–0.25. This ratio is abnormal in approximately 80% of patients with MS and in about 18% of patients with other neurological diseases.[38]

Total CSF protein normal contains approximately 3–5% IgG, but in MS the percentage is nearly equivalent to that of plasma (15%–18%).[39] Diagnostic sensitivity of CSF IgG is 90% in patients with a confirmed diagnosis of MS, but the sensitivity is lower in patients with possible or suspected MS. This limitation decreases the clinical usefulness of the index as a diagnostic tool for MS.[40] The diagnostic specificity for multiple sclerosis is also decreased because increased intrathecal IgG synthesis occurs in many other inflammatory neurologic diseases.

☑ CHECKPOINT 10-7

Given the following laboratory results, select the appropriate calculated parameter to estimate the amount of intrathecal synthesis of IgG and correct for plasma IgG crossover. Also include an interpretation of the results.

Tests	Result	Reference Interval
CSF IgG (mg/dL)	8.0	0.9–5.7
CSF albumin (mg/dL)	6.0	10–30
Serum IgG (g/dL)	0.65	0.065–0.10
Serum albumin (g/dL)	3.0	3.5–5.0

Oligoclonal Proteins

Oligoclonal proteins represent a group of IgG proteins that are not normally found in CSF but are present in individuals under certain circumstances. These proteins separate from other proteins during electrophoresis procedures. An increase intrathecal synthesis of IgG can cause the appearance of oligoclonal proteins in CSF. Approximately 90% of cases of multiple sclerosis present with positive findings for oligoclonal proteins. Also, oligoclonal proteins can be present in other diseases of the CNS (e.g., chronic meningoencephalitis, Guillain-Barré syndrome, neurosyphilis, neuroborreliosis, and cryptococcal meningitis).

MS is characterized by patchy destruction of the surrounding myelin sheath of axons in the CNS. This directly affects conduction of nerve impulses. Beta-lymphocytes infiltrate the lesions and synthesize IgG and possibly other immunoglobulins. The immunoglobulins produced in the lesions appear in the CSF as a result of the close proximity of the CNS axons to CSF. Patients with MS may also test positive for the presence of oligoclonal light chains (kappa and lambda), which have been present in patients who test negative for CSF oligoclonal proteins.

The diagnosis of MS is made on the basis of established clinical criteria. There are no specific laboratory tests available, but detection of abnormalities in CSF does provide clinically useful information to support the diagnosis of MS. As stated above, these include elevations of IgG, IgG index, IgG synthesis rate, and detection of oligoclonal proteins in CSF using electrophoresis or IEF.

Glucose

Glucose in CSF is derived from blood glucose and is normally ~60% of the plasma value. Ideally, CSF glucose levels should be collected after a 4-hour fast and compared to plasma levels. The normal CSF/plasma glucose ratio varies from 0.3–0.9.

The clinically significant abnormality relating to CSF glucose levels is hypoglycorrhachia (see leptomeningeal metastases discussed earlier). CSF levels below 40 mg/dL or CSF/plasma glucose ratio below 0.3 is seen in patients with meningitis including bacterial, fungal, and tuberculous. Additional conditions in which CSF glucose levels are lower than normal are meningeal involvement by a malignant tumor, sarcoidosis, trichinosis, acute syphilitic meningitis, intrathecal administration of radioiodinated serum albumin, and subarachnoid hemorrhage.[41] Increased anaerobic glycolysis in brain tissue, leukocytosis, and impaired transport into the CSF may also result in hypoglycorrhachia. The presence of bacteria does not cause an appreciable decrease in CSF glucose levels because there is usually not a large enough population of bacteria. CSF glucose levels serve as useful tool for assessing patient recovery from meningitis because the levels normalize quicker than protein levels and cell counts.

Lactate

Lactate levels in CSF are not solely dependent upon plasma levels. Although their levels parallel one another, changes in the biochemical environment of CSF may alter lactate levels.

The cause of abnormally high CSF lactate is primarily anaerobic metabolism due to tissue hypoxia. Elevated levels of lactate in CSF are noted in cerebral vascular accidents, intracranial hemorrhage, epilepsy, bacterial meningitis, inborn errors of the electron transport system, and other conditions related to the CNS.[42]

Measurement of CSF lactate levels can be useful in differentiating viral meningitis from bacterial, mycoplasma, fungal, and tuberculous meningitis. Typically, patients with viral meningitis present with CSF lactate concentrations of <35 mg/dL, whereas in bacterial and fungal meningitis, CSF lactate will exceed 35 mg/dL.[43] Using 35 mg/dL for a cutoff value, the diagnostic sensitivity and specificity are about 80% and 90% respectively. The clinical usefulness of measuring CSF lactate is questionable because of the availability of more sensitive and specific diagnostic tests and the fact that the results of the microbiological cultures provide more definitive information. Persistently elevated levels of CSF lactate in patients suffering traumatic head injury are associated with a poor prognosis.[44]

Ammonia and Glutamine

Ammonia levels in CSF are approximately 30–50% of blood levels. Abnormally high CSF ammonia levels are seen in patients with hepatic encephalopathy, and their levels are proportional to severity of the condition. CSF ammonia is not routinely measured in a clinical laboratory nor is the result clinically useful because of the difficulties associated with obtaining reliable data and because hepatic encephalopathy is generally correlated with blood ammonia concentrations.

A more useful analyte to measure in a case of hepatic encephalopathy is CSF glutamine. Cerebral glutamine is synthesized from ammonia and glutamic acid and serves as a means to remove ammonia from CSF. Thus CSF glutamine levels reflect the concentration of brain ammonia. Reference interval and cut-off values are method dependent, therefore exercise caution when interpreting patient results. Moderately high values for CSF glutamine are seen hepatic encephalopathy, bacterial meningitis, carcinomatous meningitis, and patients with encephalopathy secondary to hypercapnia (high blood concentrations of carbon dioxide) and sepsis.[45,46]

Lactate Dehydrogenase

Brain tissue is rich in lactate dehydrogenase (LD) activity with a significant portion of electrophoretically fast-moving isoenzyme fractions LD_1 and LD_2. The total LD activity in adult CSF ranges from 20–40 U/L, depending upon method, and in neonates 60–70 U/L. Quantitative analysis of total LD activity is useful in differentiating a traumatic tap from intracranial hemorrhage because a recent traumatic tap with intact RBC does not significantly elevate the LD levels. LD activity is much higher in patients with bacterial meningitis than aseptic meningitis. It is also increased in cases of CNS leukemia, lymphoma, metastatic carcinoma, and subarachnoid hemorrhage.

Myelin Basic Protein

Myelin basic protein (MBP) has a molecular mass of 18.5 kDa and is a component of the myelin nerve sheath. It is released during demyelination due to neurological disorders such as MS. There is a positive correlation of MBP to CSF leukocyte counts, CSF/serum albumin ratio, and intrathecal synthesis.[47] Thus, MBP can serve as a useful biomarker for the following: (1) during acute MS exacerbation, (2) remission of MS, and (3) assessing the activity of demyelination. There are limitations to using MBP as a biomarker for assessment of CNS–related diseases. For example, the immunoassays available are limited because of the fragmentation of MBP *in vivo* by proteinases, which can cause a problem with antibody specificity. MBP is elevated in other conditions (e.g., Guillain-Barré syndrome, lupus, subacute sclerosis, pan encephalitis, and various brain tumors).[48]

Transthyretin

High resolution electrophoresis of CSF reveals two distinct differences compared to serum. CSF samples typically present a prominent transthyretin (prealbumin band) and two transferrin protein bands. Transthyretin was originally named prealbumin because of its electrophoretic mobility (i.e., before albumin thus toward the anode) and was renamed when it was discovered to be a carrier protein for thyroxine and triiodothyronine. Transthyretin is a relatively abundant protein because it is synthesized by the liver and choroid plexus. The second transferrin protein, β_2-transferrin, migrates more slowly than its serum equivalent due to cerebral neurominidase digestion of sialic acid residue.

Transferrin

Certain patients who have suffered head trauma experience leakage of CSF through their nose (rhinorrhea) or ears (otorrhea). This condition can progress to recurrent meningitis, which is a serious complication. Therefore, the clinician needs to determine whether the fluid is actually CSF or another body fluid originating from another source such as the nasal sinuses or inner ear. Measuring glucose or protein content of the fluid is not specific enough. Transferrin, an iron-binding glycoprotein synthesized primarily in the liver, consists of two isoforms. One isoform, β_1-transferrin, is present in all body fluids. The other β_2-transferrin is present only in the CNS and is produced in the CNS by the catalytic conversion of β_1-transferrin by neuraminidase. These isoforms can be separated and identified using immunofixation electrophoresis.

Beta Amyloid and Tau Protein

Currently, there are no acceptable or routinely used biomarkers for Alzheimer disease (AD). Diagnosis is derived from multiple factors outside the clinical laboratory. Pathologically, AD is characterized by the presence of neurofibrillary tangles and amyloid plaques. Studies have shown that measurement of two unique proteins—beta amyloid protein (βAP42) and phospho-tau protein (p-τ181p protein)—may provide clinicians with a useful tool, especially early in the course of the disease when patients are presymptomatic and are in the predementia phase. Biomarker βAP42 is an indicator of brain beta amyloid deposition, and CSF measurement of this protein would be expected to show it to be decreased. Biomarker **tau protein** is an indicator of neuronal injury or neurodegeneration, and CSF measurement of total tau and phosphorylated tau protein are expected to be elevated.[49,50]

CSF 14-3-3

A novel diagnostic test that measures CSF 14-3-3 protein has provided useful information to clinicians who are evaluating patients with suspected CJD. The origin of protein 14-3-3 begins with the discovery of two 30 kDa proteins detected by two-dimensional electrophoresis in CSF of patients with CJD. The proteins were designated as proteins 130 and 131. The presence of these proteins in CSF correlated well with high diagnostic sensitivities and specificities for CJD.[51] The methods required to measure proteins 130 and 131 were labor intensive and time consuming, thus efforts were undertaken to develop assays amenable to routine use in clinical laboratories. Refinements in two-dimensional electrophoresis amino acid sequencing techniques resulted in the discovery that proteins 130 and 131 matched the sequence of the human 14-3-3 proteins. Further experiments with 14-3-3 antibodies verified that CSF proteins 130 and 131 are 14-3-3 proteins.

Protein 14-3-3 is a reliable biomarker of rapid neuronal destruction and has been detected in the CSF of patients with several different neurological disorders. Diagnostic sensitivity for CJD of 81–90% and diagnostic specificity of 67–81% has been reported.[52] The lower diagnostic specificity value is due to the presence of increased levels of 14-3-3 in other conditions that result in acute neuronal damage (e.g., AD, malignancy, encephalitis).[53]

MINI-CASE 10-3

Samantha has completed protein electrophoresis on both serum and CSF for a 26-year-old female patient. Visual inspection of both protein separations revealed the following:

1. A distinct band in the CSF sample located in the prealbumin region. A similar band was not found in serum.

2. A distinct transferrin band in the CSF that is denser than a similar band in serum.

3. Four distinct bands in the gamma region of the CSF sample, but none in the serum sample.

Questions to Consider

1. What is the significance of a prealbumin and transferrin band?

2. What is the significance of the four bands found in the gamma region of the CSF sample but not seen in the serum sample?

3. What medical condition may present bands in the gamma region of the CSF sample but not the serum?

Multiple Markers

Improvements were made in diagnostic performance of laboratory tests for neurodegenerative disorders by using multiple biomarkers including biomarker S100b and the neuronal marker tau protein in isolation or in combination. A significant improvement in diagnostic specificity (91–98%) was shown by Chochan et al. when all three biomarkers were measured.[54] Coulthart et al. reported CSF tau showed better overall diagnostic accuracy (receiver operator curve range 0.931–0.961) than 14-3-3 or S100b.[55] They also concluded that combining tau with S100B could enhance medical interpretation in diagnosis and monitoring of CJD.

METHODS TO MEASURE CSF PROTEIN

Turbidimetric/Colorimetric

The low concentration of proteins in CSF limits the methods that can be used to reliably measure protein content. Quantitative analysis of total protein in CSF is routinely performed using turbidimetric methods. These assays are easy to perform and require no special instrumentation. Proteins are precipitated using trichloroacetic acid or sulfosalicylic acid and sodium sulfate. Precipitation assays for protein analysis depend on formation of a fine uniform, insoluble protein particulate, which scatters light while in suspension. A spectrophotometer is commonly used to measure the turbid solution. Limitations of turbidimetric assays include variations created due to temperature changes, variations due to changes in the albumin/globulin ratio, and large sample volumes required by several manual assays.

Reagents

Benzethonium chloride is widely used in automated turbidimetric assays. A small volume of CSF is added to sodium hydroxide, which denatures the protein and eliminates interference from magnesium ion. Benzethonium chloride is then added, producing a turbidity that is measured at ~500 nm. The assay is available as an endpoint or rate methodology. The analytical sensitivity is typically ~2 mg/dL.

Coomassie brilliant blue is a dye suitable for measurement of CSF protein and provides a sensitive method with some limitations. The sensitivity of the dye for albumin is significantly greater than globulin. Also, Coomassie brilliant blue produces a precipitate that may stick to the walls of the cuvet and result in significant carryover.[56]

Electrophoresis

Electrophoresis separation and identification of specific proteins in body fluids is a widely used technique in clinical laboratories. Separation methods designed for serum proteins are generally not adequate for CSF; therefore, adjustments must be made to the assay parameters. A term adopted to reflect these modifications and increase the detection of low concentrations of proteins in body fluids such as CSF is **high-resolution electrophoresis (HRE)**.

Serum versus High-Resolution Electrophoresis

The following is an example of the need for increased analytical sensitivity for separation of protein in CSF versus serum. These analytes were selected for this example because they will be used for clinical correlation later in this section. The total protein concentration in normal serum is 6.4–8.3 g/dL (64–83 g/L), whereas in CSF it is 15–45 mg/dL (150–450 mg/L). In normal adult serum the concentration of gamma globulins is 700–1600 mg/dL (7.0–16.0 g/L) and in CSF the range is 0.0–5.5 mg/dL (0.0–55 mg/L). Therefore, electrophoresis methods for separating proteins in CSF require modification that will ultimately lead to improved resolution, detection, and identification at low concentrations. The changes between serum and high-resolution CSF electrophoresis assays include adjustments to buffer pH, buffer ionic strength, power supply voltage, and current and migration times. Once the separation is complete, the proteins are made visible using a staining compound. Several stains are available that allow for increased sensitivity, especially in the gamma region and include acid violet, amido black, Coomassie brilliant blue, paragon violet, and silver nitrate. The stained separations are evaluated visually for pattern abnormalities. The visual observations can be complemented by densitometry to obtain semiquantitative values of the individual or combined protein fractions.

High-Resolution Electrophoresis and Oligoclonal Protein

High-resolution agarose electrophoresis of CSF is a technique aptly suited for the detection of a discrete population of IgG proteins, oligoclonal proteins in concentrated CSF samples. Oligoclonal proteins were discussed earlier in this chapter. The presence of two or more bands supports the diagnosis of MS.[57]

Coomassie brilliant blue or paragon violet stains are capable of resolving oligoclonal protein in only 5 μg of IgG.[58] Some manufacturers provide a silver stain with improved analytical sensitivities versus other stains, which can be used on unconcentrated CSF samples. It is advantageous for clinical laboratories to include serum samples in conjunction with CSF for electrophoresis to ensure that a polyclonal gammopathy associated with disease (e.g., lupus erythematosus, liver disease, or rheumatoid arthritis) is not present. The rational for assaying serum and CSF from each patient resides in the fact that these disorders may be accompanied by IgG diffusion into the CSF, yielding false positive results.

Immunofixation Electrophoresis

There are several advantages for using immunofixation electrophoresis (IFE) versus immunoelectrophoresis (IEP). IFE provides improved resolution of proteins, shorter migration times, and greater analytical sensitivity. This technique does not usually require concentrating CSF specimens. The procedure for separating proteins using IFE begins with the application of a sample into a depression formed within an agarose gel. The agarose gel is divided into several tracks. One track is treated with a chemical fixative solution to fix the proteins present in the specimen into the agarose and produce an electrophoresis reference pattern for the specimen. The remaining tracks are supplemented with specific antiglobulins that will react to their respective immunoglobulins, causing them to precipitate out. The gel is subjected to an electric field, and the proteins separate out based on their physical-chemical interactions with the gel. These fixed immunobands are rendered visible by adding an appropriate stain. Immunoglobulins can be identified by comparing their location to a reference sample.

Isoelectric Focusing Electrophoresis

Isoelectric focusing electrophoresis (IEF) reveals the presence of more proteins with better resolution than IFE. IEF is a separation technique for amphoteric compounds such as proteins that react as both an acid and a base. Specific proteins become "focused" in an area on the gel as they migrate in an electric field to a zone where the pH of the gel matches the proteins' isoelectric point (pI). At this point, the overall charge of the protein is zero as a result of an equal number of positive and negative charges, and migration is halted. The driving force for this separation technique is an electrical charge provided by a power supply. Resolution of specific proteins is sharp because the region associated with a given pH is very narrow.

A modification of IEF using IgG immunoblotting (IgG-IEF) provides a very sensitive method for detection of oligoclonal proteins.[59] This technique has shown a high positivity rate of 90% for patients with MS versus 60% for agarose electrophoresis.[60,61,62] An international consensus standard published in 2005 for the diagnosis of MS determined that IgG-IEF is the method of choice for qualitative detection of polyclonal IgG protein as evidenced of intrathecal synthesis of IgG.[63]

MICROBIOLOGY TESTS

Rapid assessment of patients with signs and symptoms of CNS involvement is paramount. Laboratory results of tests with fast turnaround times (i.e., CSF glucose, total protein, cell counts, and differentials) aid in the initial evaluation of patients, especially those with infections. A definitive diagnosis of most infections requires a Gram stain and culture.

Bacterial Meningitis

The causative agents of bacterial meningitis are group B streptococcus (neonates), *Neisseria meningitidis*, *Streptococcus pneumonia*, *Escherichia coli*, *Haemophilius influenza*, and other Gram-negative bacilli. The Gram stain remains a significant microscopic procedure for diagnosing CNS infection. Diagnostic sensitivity of Gram stain results varies with the type and concentration of the infectious organism in the CSF. Also, all smears and cultures should be performed on concentrated specimens because in some cases only a few organisms are present early in the course of the disease. Microbiology laboratories use a combination of techniques, including (1) culture-based procedures, (2) polymerase chain reactions (PCR) and 16S ribosomal RNA in CSF, and (3) latex agglutination bacterial antigen tests to identify organisms present in CSF.

Spirochetal Meningitis

Spirochetal meningitis is detected using a variety of laboratory tests including CSF protein, cell counts, serologic tests, and molecular DNA methods. They are clinically useful for detection of active cases of syphilis within the CNS (also termed *neurosyphilis*). The standard non-treponemal test performed on CSF is the Venereal Disease Research Laboratory (VDRL). Diagnostic specificity is high but diagnostic sensitivity is low (~50–60%). A better, albeit controversial, test for neurosyphilis is the treponemal antibody absorption test (FTA-ABS).[64] Diagnostic sensitivity and specificity are very high but false positives do occur. For a detailed interpretation of this test, see Davis et al.[65]

Viral Meningitis

Causative agents of viral meningitis include enteroviruses (echoviruses, coxsackie viruses, polio viruses) and arboviruses. A widely used laboratory test for patients with suspected viral meningitis is real-time polymerase chain reaction (RT-PCR), which is significantly more sensitive than cell cultures. The use of RT-PCR can result in decreased hospital stays and a reduction in unnecessary diagnostic and therapeutic interventions, thereby reducing health care costs.

Fungal Meningitis

Cases of fungal meningitis are evaluated using an India ink prep to locate and identify *Cryptococcus neoformans*, which is the most frequently isolated CSF fungal pathogen. CSF specimens stained with India ink (nigrosin stain) allow for the visualization of the *Cryptococcus* capsular halo. Positive India ink preps are seen in patients with multiple lumbar punctures and untreated HIV-infected patients. India ink preps have a low diagnostic sensitivity, thus a follow-up test that measures Cryptococci antigen using latex agglutination increases the sensitivity several fold should be available.

Tuberculous Meningitis

Tuberculous meningitis presents with consistent elevation of total protein in CSF and a predominance of lymphocytes. Acid-fast or fluorescent antibody stain techniques are time consuming, and their sensitivity is highly variable. Thus the Gram stain plays an important role in assessing patients with suspected tuberculous meningitis. PCR nucleic acid amplification techniques for *Mycobacterium tuberculosis* DNA sequence and DoT ELISA techniques are available for use in the clinical laboratory. These techniques provide increased sensitivity and specificity for diagnosis of tuberculous meningitis.

Key Points to Remember

- Determining the etiologic cause of alterations in CSF distribution is important in assessing CSF-related disorders.
- Many different diseases can display abnormalities in CSF. Therefore, examination of the CSF is an important laboratory function.
- Special collection techniques are invasive and associated with high risk of harm to patients.
- Appropriate laboratory examination of CSF involves both physical and microscopic findings.

- Chemical testing, especially proteins, of CSF and serum provide valuable information for assessing disease.
- Many of the assays performed in the clinical laboratory do not require a high degree of technology, but because some techniques are somewhat manual, skilled laboratory staff are required (e.g., Gram stains, cell counting, and cultures).

Review Questions

Level I

1. Which of the following is the primary site for CSF formation? (Objective 1)

   A. The lumbar region of the spine

   B. Bone marrow

   C. Choriod plexus

   D. Liver

2. The interface of the brain, spinal cord, and CSF is termed the (Objective 2)

   A. brain–spinal cord barrier.

   B. plasma–CSF barrier.

   C. brain–ventricle and blood barrier.

   D. blood–brain barrier.

3. Which of the following is a reason for monitoring opening pressures while removing CSF from a puncture site? (Objective 3)

   A. Abnormal values may signal the presence of a problem.

   B. Abnormal values indicate that the procedure is successful.

   C. Normal values indicate that the patient is at risk for neurogenic problems.

   D. It predicts the severity of head pain for the patient.

4. Lumbar, cisternal, and ventricle are all examples of which of the following? (Objective 3)

   A. Anatomical sites used to remove blood

   B. Anatomical sites used to remove CSF

   C. Anatomical sites used to measure a patient's barometric pressure

   D. Human pulse sites used to monitor opening pressures while removing CSF

5. Meningitis is an inflammation of the (Objective 5)

   A. lumbar region of the spinal column.

   B. meninges around the sacrum.

   C. meninges around the brain and spinal cord.

   D. meninges around the pituitary gland.

6. Oligoclonal protein is unique to which of the following disorders? (Objective 7)

   A. Multiple sclerosis

   B. Subarachnoid hemorrhage

   C. Heart disease

   D. Alzheimer disease

7. Which of the following terms literally means "within the sheath"? (Objective 1)

   A. Meninges

   B. Pituitary

   C. Choroid plexus

   D. Intrathecal

8. Which of the following test groups for CSF analysis are consistent with assessment of patients with CNS disorders? (Objective 11)

   A. Serum creatine kinase, lactate dehydrogenase, and lactate

   B. CSF cell count with differential, protein, glucose, culture, and Gram stain

   C. CSF cell count with differential, total bilirubin, aspartate aminotransferase, and alanine aminotransferase

   D. CSF oligoclonal protein by electrophoresis, prealbumin by electrophoresis, and transthyretin by electrophoresis

9. Xanthochromia is a term that describes (Objective 9)

   A. the blue–grey color of CSF.

   B. meningeal metastatic melanoma.

   C. the presence of xanthene compounds, for example, caffeine.

   D. the yellow color of the supernatant of a centrifuge CSF specimen.

10. The reason why tube #1 in a CSF specimen collection procedure should not be used for microbiology is (Objective 8)

    A. it may be contaminated with tumor cells.

    B. it may be contaminated with skin bacteria.

    C. it may contain red blood cells.

    D. it may be contain oligoclonal proteins.

11. Which of the following devices is used for CSF cell count? (Objective 10)

    A. A plain glass slide

    B. A refractometer

    C. A hemocytometer

    D. A hygrometer

12. A markedly high value (>30) for a CSF/serum albumin index indicates which of the following? (Objective 13)

    A. Intact blood–brain barrier

    B. Severe impairment of the blood–brain barrier

    C. Multiple sclerosis

    D. Viral meningitis

13. A CSF/serum IgG ratio is useful to determine which of the following? (Objective 13)

    A. Accurate cell count

    B. The level of xanthochromia

    C. Intrathecal synthesis of IgG

    D. The presence of oligoclonal proteins

14. Hypoglycorrhachia is defined as (Objective 5)

    A. increased CSF glucose concentration.

    B. decreased CSF glucose concentration.

    C. decreased CSF lactate concentration.

    D. decreased CSF protein concentration.

15. Which of the following diseases is usually characterized by elevated CSF lactate levels? (Objective 11)

    A. Bacterial meningitis

    B. Fungal meningitis

    C. Tuberculous meningitis

    D. Viral meningitis

16. CSF glutamine levels reflect the concentration of brain (Objective 11)

    A. ammonia.

    B. lactate.

    C. glucose.

    D. transthyretin.

17. Transthyretin is a protein found in CSF that migrates toward the anode in protein electrophoresis and is also referred to as (Objective 11)

    A. albumin.

    B. prealbumin.

    C. alpha1 antiglobulin.

    D. alpha 2 antiglobulin.

18. The presence of tau proteins in CSF may provide clinicians with a useful tool to assess patients with which of the following? (Objective 11)

    A. Multiple sclerosis

    B. Guillain-Barré syndrome

    C. The early course of Alzheimer disease

    D. The early course of Creutzfeldt-Jakob disease

19. Which of the following methods is acceptable for measuring total protein in CSF? (Objective 11)

    A. Mass spectrometer using deuterated isotopes (deuterium, hydrogen-2)

    B. Turbidimetric assay using benzethonium chloride

    C. Fluorescent assay using Coomassie brilliant blue

    D. High-performance liquid chromatography

20. Why is high-resolution electrophoresis (HRE) necessary to detect the presence of oligoclonal proteins in CSF? (Objective 11)

    A. HRE is more analytically sensitive than conventional electrophoresis methods.

    B. HRE is more analytically specific than conventional electrophoresis methods.

    C. HRE is more linear than conventional electrophoresis methods.

    D. HRE uses monoclonal antibodies, whereas conventional electrophoresis uses polyclonal antibodies.

Level II

1. Which of the following criteria is used to distinguish a traumatic lumbar puncture from a subarachnoid hemorrhage (SAH) if four tubes are drawn? (Objective 1)

    A. If the CSF specimen is clear and colorless in all tubes, then a traumatic lumbar puncture is more likely than SAH.

    B. If there is evidence of blood in tubes 1 through 3, traumatic lumbar puncture is more likely than SAH.

    C. If there is evidence of blood in tubes 1 through 4, traumatic lumbar puncture is more likely than SAH.

    D. If the number of white blood cells decreases dramatically from tubes 1 to 4, traumatic lumbar puncture is more likely than SAH.

2. Demonstration of tumor cells in the CSF is definitive for which of the following disorders? (Objective 2)

    A. Cerebral abscess

    B. Central nervous system infarction

    C. Viral meningitis

    D. Leptomeningeal metastasis

3. Which of the following describes a T-cell mediated autoimmune demyelinating disease that may be initiated by a viral infection? (Objective 2)

    A. Multiple sclerosis

    B. Guillain-Barré syndrome

    C. Viral meningitis

    D. Spirochetal meningitis

4. CSF from a normal, healthy adult contains which of the following? (Objective No. 3)

    A. Oligoclonal proteins

    B. No oligoclonal proteins

    C. Several variant forms of oligoclonal proteins

    D. The presence of tau proteins

5. Glass tubes should not be used for CSF collections because (Objective 1)

    A. antibodies will be neutralized upon contact with glass.

    B. glass tubes will turn the CSF specimen cloudy.

    C. cells may adhere to the surface and adversely affect the cell count and differential.

    D. the sodium in glass will degrade proteins in the specimen.

6. Which of the following interpretations is the most accurate assessment for a CSF specimen on a patient with three distinct bands in the gamma region of a high-resolution electrophoresis separation? (Objective 2)

    A. Positive for viral meningitis

    B. Negative for oligoclonal proteins

    C. Positive for oligoclonal proteins

    D. The patient has multiple sclerosis

7. Which of the following is the best interpretation of the CSF laboratory results on a 40-year-old male? (Objective 4)

Appearance	Clear
WBC	normal
RBC	normal
Glucose	(mg/dL) 0
Protein	(mg/dL) lumbar 50
Lactate	(mg/dL) 0
Smear	Negative (no bacteria seen)
Culture	N/A

    A. Bacterial meningitis

    B. Tuberculous meningitis

    C. Subarachnoid hemorrhage

    D. Multiple sclerosis

Endnotes

1. Ropper AH, Samuels MA. Chapter 30. Disturbances of Cerebrospinal Fluid and Its Circulation, Including Hydrocephalus, Pseudotumor Cerebri, and Low-Pressure Syndromes. In: Ropper AH, Samuels MA, eds. *Adams and Victor's Principles of Neurology*. 9th ed. New York: McGraw-Hill, 2009. http://www.accessmedicine.com/content.aspx?aID=3635067. (Accessed 3/6/2014)

2. Ropper AH, Samuels MA. Chapter 30. Disturbances of Cerebrospinal Fluid and Its Circulation, Including Hydrocephalus, Pseudotumor Cerebri, and Low-Pressure Syndromes. In: Ropper AH, Samuels MA, eds. *Adams and Victor's Principles of Neurology*. 9th ed. New York: McGraw-Hill, 2009. http://www.accessmedicine.com/content.aspx?aID=3635067. (Accessed 3/6/2014)

3. Fishman RA. *Cerebrospinal Fluid in Diseases of the Nervous System*. 2nd ed. Philadelphia: W.B. Saunders Company, 1992.

4. Ward E, Gushurst CA. Uses and techniques of pediatric lumbar puncture. *Am J Dis Child* (1992) 146:1160–1162.

5. Fishman RA. *Cerebrospinal Fluid in Diseases of the Nervous System*. 2nd ed. Philadelphia: W.B. Saunders Company, 1992.

6. Seehusen DA, Reeves MM, Fomin DA. Cerebrospinal fluid analysis. *Am Fam Physician* (2003) 68; 6:1103–1108.

7. Karcher DS, McPherson RA. Cerebrospinal, synovial, serous body fluids and alternative specimens. In: McPherson RA, Pincus MR, eds. *Henry's Clinical Diagnosis and Management by Laboratory Methods*, 22nd ed. Philadelphia: Elsevier Saunders (2011):480–490.

8. Marton KL, Gean AD. The diagnostic spinal tap. *Annals Internal Med* (1986) 104:880–885.

9. Hale, JE, Gelfanova, V, You JS, et al. Proteomics of cerebrospinal fluid: methods for sample processing. *Methods in molecular biol* (2008) 425:53–66.

10. Craig FE, Ohori NP, Gorrill TS, et al. Flow cytometric immunophenotyping of cerebrospinal fluid specimens. *Am J Clin Pathol* (2011) 135; 1:322–324.

11. DeAngelis LM, Wen PY. Chapter 379, Primary and metastatic tumors of the nervous system. In: Longo DL, Gauci AS, Kasper DL, Hauser SLO, Jameson JL, Loscalzo J, eds. *Harrison's Principles of Internal Medicine*. 18th ed. New York: McGraw-Hill, 2012. http://www.accessmedicine.comcontent. aspx?aID=9147519. Accessed March 6, 2014.

12. Kurtzke JF. Epidemiologic evidence for multiple sclerosis as an infection. *Clin microbial Rev* (1993) 6:382–427.

13. Miller SD, Vanderlugt CL, Begolka WS, et al. Persistent infection with Theiler's virus lead to CNS autoimmunity via epitope spreading. *Nat Med* (1997) 3:1133–1136.

14. Tourtellotte WW, Walsh MJ, Baumhefner RW, et al. The current status of multiple sclerosis intra-blood–brain-barrier IgG synthesis. *Ann NY Acad Sci.* (1984) 436:52–67.

15. McDonald WI, Compston A, Edan G, et al. Recommended diagnostic criteria for multiple sclerosis: guidelines from the international panel on the diagnosis of multiple sclerosis. *Ann Neurol.* (2001) 50:121–127.

16. Polman CH, Reingold SC, Edan G, et al. Diagnostic criteria for multiple sclerosis: 2005 revisions to the "McDonald Criteria." *Ann Neurol* (2005) 58: 840–846.

17. Reiber H. Flow rate of cerebrospinal fluid (CSF)—a concept common to normal blood-CSF barrier function and to dysfunction in neurological disease. *J Neurol Sci.* (1994) 122:189–203.

18. Tourtellotte WW, Walsh MJ, Baumhefner RW, et al. The current status of multiple sclerosis intra-blood–brain-barrier IgG synthesis. *Ann NY Acad Sci.* (1984) 436:52–67.

19. Reiber H. Flow rate of cerebrospinal fluid (CSF)—a concept common to normal blood-CSF barrier function and to dysfunction in neurological disease. *J Neurol Sci.* (1994) 122:189–203.

20. Tourtellotte WW, Potvin AR, Fleming JO, et al. Multiple sclerosis; measurement and validation of central nervous system IgG synthesis rate. *Neurology* (1980) 30:240–244.

21. Mehling M, Kuhle J, Regeniter A. 10 Most commonly asked questions about cerebrospinal fluid characteristics in demyelinating disorders of the central nervous system. *The Neurologist* (2008) 14; 1:60–65.

22. Hutchesson A, Preece MA, Gray G, et al. Measurement of lactate in cerebrospinal fluid in investigation of inherited metabolic disease. *Clin Chem* (1997) 43:158–161.

23. Mattsson N. CSF biomarkers in neurodegenerative disease. *Clin Chem Lab Med* (2011) 49; 3:345–352.

24. Blennow K, Hampel H, Weiner M, et al. Cerebrospinal fluid and plasma biomarkers in Alzheimer diseases. *Nat Rev Neurol* (2010) 6:131–144.

25. Chohan G, Pennington C, Mackenzie JM, et al. The role of cerebrospinal fluid 14-3-3 and other proteins in the diagnosis of sporadic Creutzfeldt-Jakob disease in the UK: a 10 year review. *J Neurol Neurosurg Psychiatry* (2010) 81:1243–1248.

26. Karcher DS, McPherson RA. Cerebrospinal, synovial, serous body fluids and alternative specimens. In: McPherson RA, Pincus MR, eds. *Henry's Clinical Diagnosis and Management by Laboratory Methods*, 22nd ed. Philadelphia: Elsevier Saunders (2011):480–490.

27. Karcher DS, McPherson RA. Cerebrospinal, synovial, serous body fluids and alternative specimens. In: McPherson RA, Pincus MR, eds. *Henry's Clinical Diagnosis and Management by Laboratory Methods*, 22nd ed. Philadelphia: Elsevier Saunders (2011):480–490.

28. Karcher DS, McPherson RA. Cerebrospinal, synovial, serous body fluids and alternative specimens. In: McPherson RA, Pincus MR, eds. *Henry's Clinical Diagnosis and Management by Laboratory Methods*, 22nd ed. Philadelphia: Elsevier Saunders (2011):480–490.

29. Clinical and Laboratory Standards Institute. *Body fluid analysis for cellular composition; Approved Guideline*. CLSI document H56-A. Wayne, PA: Clinical and Laboratory Standards Institute, 2006.

30. Fishman RA. *Cerebrospinal Fluid in Diseases of the Nervous System*. 2nd ed. Philadelphia: W.B. Saunders Company, 1992.

31. Karcher DS, McPherson RA. Cerebrospinal, synovial, serous body fluids and alternative specimens. In: McPherson RA, Pincus MR, eds. *Henry's Clinical Diagnosis and Management by Laboratory Methods*, 22nd ed. Philadelphia: Elsevier Saunders (2011):480–490.

32. Tourtellotte WW, Walsh MJ, Baumhefner RW, et al. The current status of multiple sclerosis intra-blood–brain-barrier IgG synthesis. *Ann NY Acad Sci.* (1984) 436:52–67.

33. Silverman LM, Christenson RH. Amino acids and proteins. In: Burtis CA, Ashwood ER, Eds. *Tietz textbook of clinical chemistry*. 2nd ed. Philadelphia: WB Saunders, 1994:625–626.

34. Tourtellotte WW, Staugaitis SM, Walsh MJ, et al. The basis of intra-blood–brain barrier IgG synthesis. *Ann Neurol* (1985):17–21.

35. Souverijn JHM, Smit WG, Peet R, et al. Intrathecal Ig synthesis: its detection by isoelectric focusing and IgG index. *J Neurol Sci* (1989) 93:211–212.

36. Silverman LM, Christenson RH. Amino acids and proteins. In: Burtis CA, Ashwood ER, Eds. *Tietz textbook of clinical chemistry*. 2nd ed. Philadelphia: WB Saunders, 1994:625–626.

37. Silverman LM, Christenson RH. Amino acids and proteins. In: Burtis CA, Ashwood ER, Eds. *Tietz textbook of clinical chemistry*. 2nd ed. Philadelphia: WB Saunders, 1994:625–626.

38. Harrington MG, Kennedy PGE. The clinical use of cerebrospinal fluid in demyelinating neurological diseases. *Postgra med J.* (1987) 63:735–740.

39. Hersey LA, Trotter JL. The use and abuse of the cerebrospinal fluid IgG profile in the adult: a practical evaluation. *Ann Neurol* (1980) 8:126–128.

40. Marton KL, Gean AD. The diagnostic spinal tap. *Annals Internal Med* (1986) 104:880–885.

41. Fishman RA. *Cerebrospinal Fluid in Diseases of the Nervous System*. 2nd ed. Philadelphia: W.B. Saunders Company, 1992.

42. Hutchesson A, Preece MA, Gray G, et al. Measurement of lactate in cerebrospinal fluid in investigation of inherited metabolic disease. *Clin Chem* (1997) 43:158–161.

43. Bailey EM, Domenico P, Cunha BA. Bacterial or viral meningitis? Measuring lactate in CSF can help you know quickly. *Postgrad Med* (1990) 88:217–218.

44. DeSalles AAF, Kontos HA, Becker DP, et al. Prognostic significance of ventricular CSF lactic acidosis in severe head injury. *J Neurosurg* (1986) 65:615–616.

45. Mizock BA, Rackow EC, Burke GS. Elevated cerebrospinal fluid glutamine in septic encephalopathy. *J Clin Gastroenterol* (1989) 11:362–363.

46. Wu AHB. *Tietz clinical guide to laboratory tests*. 4th ed. St. Louis MO: Saunders Elsevier, 1995.

47. Sellebjerg F, Christiansen M, Nielsen PM, et al. Cerebrospinal fluid measures of disease activity in patients with multiple sclerosis. *Mult Scler* (1998) 4:475–477.

48. Karcher DS, McPherson RA. Cerebrospinal, synovial, serous body fluids and alternative specimens. In: McPherson RA, Pincus MR, eds. *Henry's Clinical Diagnosis and Management by Laboratory Methods*, 22nd ed. Philadelphia: Elsevier Saunders (2011):480–490.

49. Jack CR Jr, Vemuri P, Wiste HJ, et al. Evidence for ordering of Alzheimer disease biomarkers. *Arch Neurol* (2011) 68;12:1526–1535.

50. Desikan RS, McEvoy LK, Thompson WK, et al. Amyloid β-associated clinical decline occurs only in the presence of elevated P-tau. *Arch Neurol* (2012):e1–e5. Accessed 3/6/14 from www.archeeurol.com

51. Harrington, MG, Merril CR, Asher DM, et al. Abnormal proteins in the cerebrospinal fluid of patient with Creutzfeldt-Jakob diseases. *N Engl J Med* (1986) 315:279–283.

52. Hsich G, Kenney K, Gibbs CL, et al. The 14-3-3 brain protein in cerebrospinal fluid as a marker for transmissible spongiform encephalopathies. *NEJM* (1996) 353;13:924–930.

53. Collins SJ, Sanchez-Juan P, Masters CL, et al. Determinants of diagnostic investigation sensitivities across the clinical spectrum of sporadic Creutzfeldt-Jakob disease. *Brain* (2006) 129:2278–2287.

54. Chohan G, Pennington C, Mackenzie JM, et al. The role of cerebrospinal fluid 14-3-3 and other proteins in the diagnosis of sporadic Creutzfeldt-Jakob disease in the UK: a 10 year review. *J Neurol Neurosurg Psychiatry* (2010) 81:1243–1248.

55. Coulthart MB, Jansen GH, Olsen E, et al. Diagnostic accuracy of cerebrospinal fluid protein markers for sporadic Creutzfeldt-Jakob disease in Canada: a 6-year prospective study. *BMC Neurology* (2011) 11:133–146.

56. van Wilgenbur MG, Werkman EM, van Gorkom, et al. Criticism of the use of Coomassie brilliant blue G-250 for the quantitative determination of proteins. *J Clin Chem Clin Biochem* (1981) 5:301–302.

57. Mehta PD. Diagnostic usefulness of cerebrospinal fluid in multiple sclerosis. *Crit Rev Clin Lab Sci.* (1991) 28:233–251.

58. van Wilgenbur MG, Werkman EM, van Gorkom, et al. Criticism of the use of Coomassie brilliant blue G-250 for the quantitative determination of proteins. *J Clin Chem Clin Biochem* (1981) 5:301–302.

59. Anderson M, Alvarez-Cermeno J, Bernardi G, et al. Cerebrospinal fluid in the diagnosis of multiple sclerosis: a consensus report. *J Neurol Neurosurg Psychiatry* (1994) 57:897–899.

60. Fortini AS, Sanders EL, Weinshenker BG, et al. Cerebrospinal fluid oligoclonal bands in the diagnosis of multiple sclerosis. *Am J Clin Pathol* (2003) 120:672–674.

61. Regeniter A, Kuhle J, Mehling M, et al. A modern approach to CSF analysis: pathophysiology, clinical application, proof of concept and laboratory reporting. *Clin Neuro and Neurosurgery* (2009) 111:313–318.

62. Pranzatelli MR, Slev PR, Tate ED, et al. Cerebrospinal fluid oligoclonal bands in childhood opsoclonus-myoclonus. *Ped Neurolgy* (2011) 45:27–33.

63. Freedman MS, Thompson EJ, Deisenhammer F, et al. Recommended standard of cerebrospinal fluid analysis in the diagnosis of multiple sclerosis: a consensus statement. *Arch Neurol* (2005) 63:865–869.

64. Davis LE, Schmitt, JW. Issues in cerebrospinal of cerebrospinal fluid tests for neurosyphilis. *Ann Neurol* (1989) 25:50–53.

65. Davis LE, Schmitt, JW. Issues in cerebrospinal of cerebrospinal fluid tests for neurosyphilis. *Ann Neurol* (1989) 25:50–53.

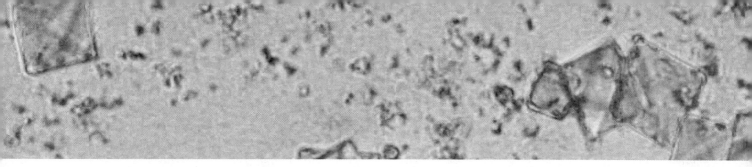

Serous Fluid

Objectives

LEVEL I

1. Describe in anatomical terms pleural cavity, pericardium and peritoneum.
2. Differentiate between a transudate and an exudate, including origin, appearance, and laboratory tests.
3. Differentiate between a chylous and pseudochylous exudate.
4. Explain the specimen collection options available for pleural fluid, pericardial fluid, and peritoneal fluid.
5. Discuss the findings of gross and microscopic examination of serous fluids.
6. Identify chemical and hematology tests available for serous fluid assessment.
7. Identify diseases associated with tissues and organs located in the chest and abdomen.

LEVEL II

1. Explain in anatomical terms the origin of serous fluids in the body.
2. Explain the techniques used for obtaining serous fluid specimens from patients and indicate any possible effects.
3. Discuss the diagnostic significance of paracentesis, pericardiocentesis, thoracentesis, and peritoneal lavage.
4. Describe the gross and microscopic findings from serous fluid samples.
5. Interpret abnormal gross and microscopic examination findings, chemical and hematology tests results.
6. Select proper laboratory tests for a given serous fluid sample and explain their response to disease.

Key terms

Ascites	Paracentesis	Peritoneum	Serous
Chylous effusion	Pericardial sac	Peritoneal cavity	Thoracentesis
Effusion	Pericardiocentesis	Pleural cavity	Transudate
Exudates	Pericardium	Pseudochylous effusion	

A CASE IN POINT

Armond, a 58-year-old male presents to the emergency department complaining of pain and bloating in his abdominal area. The patient has a history of hepatic cirrhosis associated with portal hypertension. Physical findings of the patient's abdominal region show bulging flanks when placed in the supine position. Also an area of tympany was discovered with shifting dullness. The ED physician requests an ultrasound, transjugular portal pressure measurement, and paracentesis. Results of the ultrasound confirmed the presence of fluid in the abdominal region. A measured difference between the pressure in the hepatic vein and portal vein was greater than 3 mm Hg. Approximately 45 mL of fluid was removed by paracentesis and sent to the laboratory for testing. Venous blood samples

were collected for serum chemistries including liver function tests (LFTs). Results of the LFTs confirmed the presence of cirrhosis. A unique measurement for assessment of serous fluid testing is the serum-ascites albumin gradient (SAAG). The result for the patient is 1.3 g/dL.

Questions to Consider

1. What is the term for accumulation of fluid in the abdominal area of the body?

2. What is the clinical significance of the elevated serum–ascites albumin gradient (SAAG)?

3. What are some additional laboratory tests that may be requested by the clinician to assess this patient?

Serous body fluids are fluids contained within the body that possess serum-like features whose consistency is more thin or watery, rather than thick or viscous. Serous fluids often move from one fluid compartment to another. A fluid compartment is a generic term applied to an anatomical area in the body where fluid accumulates. An example of a fluid compartment is the extracellular fluid compartment (ECF). Serous fluid acts like a lubricant and reduces friction caused by muscle movement. When serous fluid passes through a membrane, especially a capillary wall, and accumulates in a body cavity, it is called a **transudate**. Transudates typically have low protein concentrations and are clear, pale, and straw-colored in appearance. Transudates are not normally associated with infections. Serous fluid that contains a high concentration of protein or cells that accumulated in a body cavity as a result of increased capillary permeability is called an **exudate**. Typically, exudates are secondary to localized disorders such as infection or neoplasm. Exudates can be cloudy due to increased cellularity (leukocytes), red or pink from hemorrhage, green from purulence, or milky from increased lipid concentration. Two serous fluid samples with distinguishing laboratory results are shown in Figure 11-1 ■. Fluid A is an example of a transudate while fluid B is an exudate.

An **effusion** is the escape of fluid into a body part, for example, the pleural (lung) cavity. If blood escapes into the pleural cavity, the

term used is *hemothorax*; similarly, if air escapes, the term used is *pneumothorax*.

Turbid, milky, or bloody specimens should be centrifuged and the supernatant examined. If the supernatant is clear, the turbidity is usually due to cellular elements or debris. If the turbidity persists after centrifugation, a chylous or pseudochylous effusion is probable.

A **chylous effusion** is produced by leakage from a lymphatic duct (e.g., the thoracic duct) due to an obstruction, malignancy, or traumatic disruption. A creamy top layer of chylomicrons (large, low-density lipoprotein particles) may form in the specimen on standing as shown in Figure 11-2 ■.

A **pseudochylous effusion** can be milky or green, with a metallic sheen appearance. This forms gradually through the breakdown of cellular lipids in a long-standing effusion that commonly occurs in patients with tuberculosis or rheumatoid pleuritis. A few key features of chylous and pseudochylous are presented Table 11-1 ★.

CHECKPOINT 11-2

The creamy top layer of a chylous effusion contains a large amount of which lipoprotein? _____

ANATOMICAL LOCATIONS

Three anatomical locations are associated with serous fluids: the lungs (pleura), abdomen (peritoneum), and heart (pericardium). Each of these structures is located within a cavity or sac that is surrounded by tissues: pleural cavity, abdominal cavity, and **pericardial sac** (fibrous pericardium). A unique space exists between the tissue

☑ CHECKPOINT 11-1

A transudate differs from an exudate in that a transudate has a (high or low) total protein concentration and is usually (clearer or cloudier) than an exudate?

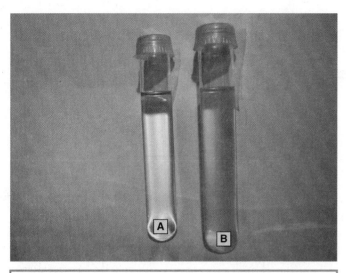

Component	(A) Transudate Fluid	Serum	(B) Exudate Fluid	Serum
Appearance	Clear, Yellow		Cloudy	
Specific gravity	1.008		1.020	
Absolute protein, mg/dL	0.9	6.0	3.9	6.4
Fluid protein to serum protein ratio	0.15		0.61	
Absolute LD, U/L	59	160	223	120
Fluid LD to serum LD ratio	0.02		1.86	
Glucose, mg/dL	116	104	161	185
Serum gluocse to fluid glucose ratio	0.89		1.15	

■ **FIGURE 11-1** Two Serous Fluids Samples with Distinguishing Laboratory Tests Results
(A) transudate, (B) exudate

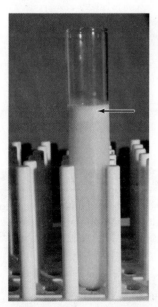

■ **FIGURE 11-2** Chylous Pleural Effusion with Milky-white Appearance and an Apparent Layer of Chylomicrons Floating on Top After Overnight Storage at 4°C (see arrow)

★ **TABLE 11-1** Descriptions of Chylous and Pseudochylous Effusions

Characteristic	Chylous	Pseudochylous
Onset	Acute	Gradual
Appearance	Milky-white	Milky
	Yellow to bloody	Greenish with metallic sheen
Microscopic	Primarily lymphocytes	Mixed cells
Triglycerides	Elevated	Low
Lipoprotein electrophoresis	Chylomicrons present	Chylomicrons absent

layers of each anatomical structure. The spaces are located between the outer layer of tissue for each structure and a layer of tissue integral to the body. An anatomical presentation of all the structures is shown in Figure 11-3 ■.

The **pleural cavity** is a closed space (similar to the inside of a balloon) within which the lung has grown. While the lung is growing into the space, the visceral pleura (a layer of pleura outside the balloon) begins to form. Another layer of cells, the parietal pleura, develops on the inner surface of the chest wall. It is thicker than the visceral pleura and is attached to the thorax (diaphragm, ribs, etc.) Pleural membranes are a single cell thick and, normally, only a very small amount of fluid is produced to fill the gap between the parietal and visceral layers of the pleura.

The **pericardium** is the fibroserous sac enclosing the heart and the roots of the great vessels. The pericardium and the heart are located in the middle of the thorax and consist of a parietal and visceral layer.

The fibroserous sac, more commonly referred to as the **pericardial sac**, has an external fibrous layer of the parietal pericardium and an internal serous layer of the parietal pericardium. The fibrous pericardium is dense collagenous tissue that joins the tunica externa of the great vessel and the tendon aspect of the diaphragm. The serous layer forms one of the inner surfaces of the fibrous pericardium. It also serves as the distal layer of the pericardial space. The other surface layer of the pericardial space is the visceral pericardium (also epicardium). The next layer, moving inward toward the cardiac chambers is the myocardium. The final layer that forms the internal surface of the heart chambers is the endocardium.

The **peritoneum** is a serous membrane that is comprised of a parietal peritoneum and visceral peritoneum. The parietal peritoneum lines the internal walls of the abdominal cavity, forming a closed sac known as the **peritoneal cavity**. In males, the peritoneal cavity is completely closed, whereas in females the peritoneal cavity has two openings where the uterine tubes, uterus, and vagina provide a passage to the outside. The parietal peritoneum lines the wall of the abdomen and forms a fused double layer of peritoneum surrounding the blood vessels, lymphatic system, and nerves leading to the abdominal organs. The double layer of peritoneum, called the mesentery, suspends the jejunum and ileum from the posterior abdominal wall. The visceral peritoneum surrounds the organs. The peritoneal membranes produce a serous fluid that lubricates the peritoneal surfaces, enabling the intraperitoneal organs to slide across one another with minimal friction.

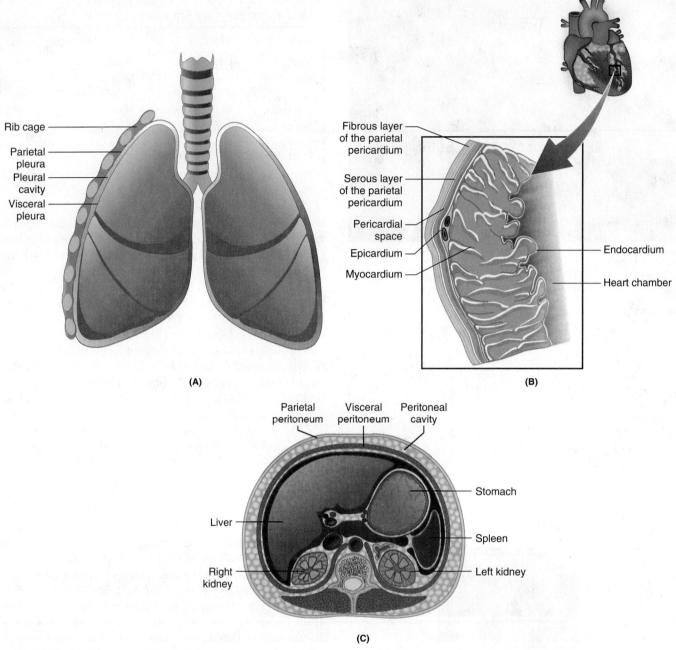

FIGURE 11-3 Serous Fluid Compartments
(A) Pleura, (B) Pericardium, and (C) Peritoneum.

SPECIMEN COLLECTION, HANDLING, AND STORAGE

Specimen collection for serous fluids often yields large volumes of fluid that can be separated into smaller volumes before transport to the laboratory. Specimens can also be separated into smaller volumes in the laboratory for storage and measurement at a later time. Specimens should be gently mixed during collection, before aliquotting, and before performing cell counts and differentials. Many procedures for serous fluid analysis require small volumes (e.g., ~ 1.0 mL.) but 5–8 ml is recommended to accommodate future requests for additional laboratory tests (e.g., flow cytometry). A list of tests with recommend specimen collection requirements is shown in Table 11-2 ★.[1]

☑ CHECKPOINT 11-3

What is the recommended anticoagulant to use for white blood cell counts and differential on serous fluids?

Specimen Processing

Specimen integrity must be maintained. Once a specimen is withdrawn from a patient, it is acceptable to transport at ambient temperature. The specimen should be delivered to the testing facility without delay. If there is a significant delay in transport, cell lysis, cellular degradation, and bacterial growth could occur that may affect the results.

★ **TABLE 11-2** Serous Fluid Specimen Requirements

Tests	Anticoagulant	Volume (mL)
Chemistries: 　Total protein 　Lactate dehydrogenase 　Glucose 　Amylase	None or heparin	8–10
Cell counts and differential	EDTA	5–8
Gram stain/bacterial culture	SPS None Anticoagulant without bactericidal or bacteriostatic effect	8–10
AFB culture	SPS None Anticoagulant without bactericidal or bacteriostatic effect	15–50
PAP stain/cell block	None Heparin EDTA	5–50

PAP = Papanicolaou, SPS = sodium polyanetholsulfonate, AFB = acid fast bacillus, EDTA = ethylenediaminetetraacetic acid

Specimen requiring cell counts and differential can be stored at 4–8°C for up to 24 hours.[2]

EXAMINATION OF SEROUS FLUIDS

Macroscopic examination of serous fluids includes color and clarity. Pathologic fluids may present with a variety of colors depending upon the etiology of the effusion. Transudates are straw-colored and clear. Other colors in various pathologies include red, brown, green, white, and black. Clarity is routinely described as clear, cloudy, or opalescent. A specimen may present as hyperviscous with a concomitant increase in total protein.

Cell counts on serous fluids can be performed manually using a hemocytometer chamber or an automated analyzer that has been properly calibrated and approved by regulatory agencies. Assessment of accuracy, precision, analytical sensitivity and specificity, reportable range, reference interval, and any other performance characteristic deemed necessary must be completed prior to implementation. Quality control must also be established and appropriate material used for each sample type. Laboratory staff can consult with their respective licensing agencies and the College of American Pathologists for guidelines.[3]

Refer to Chapter 10, Cerebrospinal Fluid, for microscopic procedures, information, and references to performing cells counts and differentials on serous fluid specimens. A dilution is not necessary if the fluid is clear. Bloody or cloudy fluid can be diluted using isotonic saline or other recommended fluids. All nucleated cells should be counted, because it is often difficult to accurately distinguish cell types in the chamber. Cell morphology requires the specimen to be stained prior to examination and identification. Wright's stain is commonly used in clinical laboratories. A variety of different types of cells may be seen in serous fluids. Examples include macrophages,

BOX 11-1 Chemistry Tests Available for Serous Fluid Evaluation

Total protein
Albumin
Glucose
Total bilirubin
Cholesterol
Triglycerides
Lipoprotein separation (chylomicrons)
Lactate dehydrogenase
Lactic acid
pH
C-reactive protein
Tumor markers (e.g., carcinoembryonic antigen, CA 15-3, CA 72-4)

leukocytes, mesothelial cells, and metastatic cells from solid tumors. Specific leukocytes cells include neutrophils, monocytes, lymphocytes, plasma cells, eosinophils, basophils, and immature granulocytes and blast cells. Serous fluid morphology is similar to blood or bone marrow but may present with increased degenerative changes. Stained preparation may also reveal bacteria or fungi.

Chemical tests are clinically useful and are routinely available in most laboratories. Most chemistry analyzers do not require any modification of their respective methods to perform serous fluid tests. Refer to the respective documentation for information relevant to the method and possible reference interval or interpretative comments. Several examples of chemistry tests that may be requested by a clinician are listed in Box 11-1. Specific discussion of chemistry tests used to evaluate serous fluids is found in their respective sections below.

PLEURAL FLUID
Pleural Effusions

The pleural cavity described above normally contains a thin layer of fluid that serves as a coupling system joining the lungs with the chest wall. A pleural effusion is present when there is an excess quantity of fluid in the pleural space. There are two mechanisms that lead to excess fluid: (1) excess formation and (2) decreased removal. Fluid normally enters the pleural space from the capillaries in the parietal pleura and is removed via the lymphatics in the parietal pleura. Body fluids also can enter the pleural space from the interstitial spaces of the lung via the visceral pleura or from the peritoneal cavity via small holes in the diaphragm. Normally, the lymphatic system has the capacity to absorb 20 times more fluid than is formed. Thus, a pleural effusion may develop when there is excess pleural fluid formation (e.g., from the interstitial spaces of the lung, the parietal pleura, or the peritoneal cavity) or when there is decreased fluid removal by the lymphatic system.

Diseases and conditions that may present with pleural effusion include left heart failure, pneumonia, malignancy (lung, breast, and lymphoma), pulmonary embolism, and viral diseases. Other less common but important conditions include hepatic cirrhosis, hepatic hydrothorax, pancreatitis, esophageal rupture, and lymphatic obstruction.

Diagnostic Approach

Patients who present with pleural effusion may be asymptomatic or exhibit signs and symptoms of respiratory distress. Dyspnea (shortness of breath) due to abnormal pulmonary mechanics can result when fluid accumulates in the lungs. Fluid volume can approach one liter. Pleurisy, which is an inflammation of the lining of the lungs and chest that leads to chest pain, may also occur. Assessment of vital signs is necessary, and the patient may present with a fever, hemodynamic instability, and hypoxemia. A chest examination can reveal decreased breath sounds and dullness to percussion.

Transduate and Exudate Pleural Effusions

The healthcare provider should evaluate the patient for congestive heart failure, malignancy, pneumonia, hepatic cirrhosis, venous thrombosis, and other causes of pleural effusion. The first step is to determine whether the effusion is a transudate or an exudate. Transudative pleural effusion occurs when systemic factors that influence the formation and absorption of pleural fluid are modified. Transudates occur typically when there is an imbalance between hydrostatic and oncotic pressure, so that fluid filtration exceeds reabsorption. In the United States, the leading causes of transudative pleural effusion are left-ventricular failure and cirrhosis. Exudative pleural effusions form from alterations in capillary permeability, which affects the formation and absorption of pleural fluid. The causes of exudative pleural effusions include viral infection, malignancy, pulmonary embolism, and bacterial pneumonia. Assessment and differentiation of pleural effusions at this stage are warranted because a finding of an exudative effusion typically requires additional diagnostic procedures to define the cause of the local disease.

Thoracentesis

The diagnostic criteria to differentiate both types of effusions are based upon the results of laboratory tests performed on pleural fluid obtained by thoracentesis. **Thoracentesis** is a technique that uses a needle and syringe to remove pleural fluid from the thoracic cavity. A pleural fluid collection is shown in Figure 11-4 ■. An effusion is

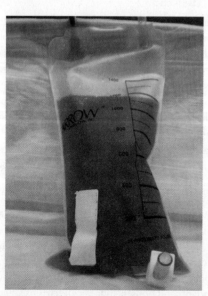

■ **FIGURE 11-4**   Pleural Fluid Specimen Collected in a Plastic Bag

---

BOX 11-2   Light's Criteria

1. Pleural fluid protein/serum protein 7 0.5
2. Pleural fluid LD/serum LD 7 0.6
3. Pleural fluid LD 6 0.67 of upper limit of normal for serum LD

deemed a transudate if NONE of Light's criteria is met whereas an exudate requires the present of ANY of Light's criteria (see Box 11-2).[4, 5] A patient with exudative pleural effusion requires additional laboratory tests, which are listed in Table 11-3 ★.[6]

☑ CHECKPOINT 11-4

Transudative pleural effusion usually occurs as a result of
_____.

Laboratory tests performed on pleural fluids provide clinicians with additional diagnostic information to support their assessment of a patient's condition. There are several diseases that are accompanied by development of pleural effusion. Examples of diseases and conditions with associated findings of pleural fluid analysis are presented in Table 11-4 ★ and Figures 11-5 ■ to 11-8 ■.[7]

☑ CHECKPOINT 11-5

What is the correct term for the removal of fluid from the pleural space? _____

★ **TABLE 11-3** Laboratory Tests and Results Used to Distinguish Pleural Fluid Transudates from Exudates

Laboratory Tests	Transudate	Exudate
Appearance	Clear yellow	Clear to turbid
Specific gravity	6 1.016	7 1.016
Absolute protein	6 3g/dL	7 3g/dL
Protein (pleural to serum ratio)	6 0.5	7 0.5
LDH (pleural to serum ratio)	6 0.6	7 0.6
*Absolute LDH	6 200 IU/L	7 200 IU/L
Glucose (serum to pleural ratio)	6 1.0	7 1.0
Fibrinogen (clot)	Negative	Positive
WBC (pleural)	Low	7 2500/mm³
Differential (pleural)		PMN early, monocytes later
(WBC, white blood count; PMN, polymorphonuclear)		
*More than two-thirds normal upper limit for serum.		

★ **TABLE 11-4** Diseases and Conditions and Associated Pleural Effusion Tests

Disease	Appearance	Protein (g/dL)	Glucose (mg/dL)	WBC And Differential ($10^3/\mu L$)	RBC (per μL)	Microscopic Exam	Culture	Comment
Hepatic cirrhosis	Serous	<3	Same as serum	<1000	<1000	Neg	Neg	Transudate develops as ascites moves across the diaphragm. Focus is on treatment of the ascites.
Congestive heart failure	Serous	<3	Same as serum	<1000	<10,000	Neg	Neg	Transudate, most common cause of pleural effusion.
Nephrotic syndrome	Serous	<3	Same as serum	<1000	<1000	Neg	Neg	Transudate, cause is low protein osmotic pressure.
Tuberculosis	Serous but may be bloody	>5.0	Same as serum	500 – 10,000, mostly monocytes	<10,000	May be pos for acid-fast bacilli	Mycobacterium tuberculosis	Exudate, PPD usually positive, pleural biopsy positive.
Empyema	Turbid to purulent	≥3	Less than serum	25,000 – 100,000	<5,000	Pos	Pos	Exudate, putrid odor suggestive of an anaerobic infection
Malignancy	Usually turbid, bloody	≥3	Same as serum	1,000–10,000	>100,000	Pos cytology in 50% of cases	Neg	Exudate

Ascites: accumulation of fluid in the peritoneal cavity
PPD: purified protein derivation
Neg: negative
Pos: positive

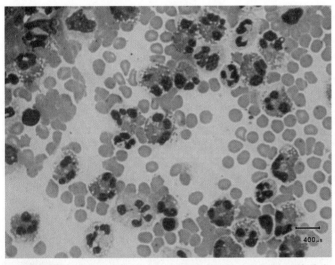

■ **FIGURE 11-5** Pleural Fluid with Numerous Eosinophils

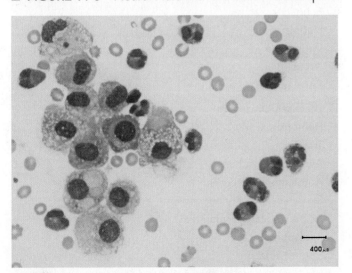

■ **FIGURE 11-6** Pleural Fluid Exudate with Eosinophils and Mesothelial Cells

MINI-CASE 11-1

Bernice required a thoracentesis to remove pleural fluid from her thoracic cavity. The sample was sent to the laboratory for analysis. The results are shown below:

Appearance	turbid
Protein (pleural to serum ratio)	0.7
Pleural fluid LD/serum LD	0.8
Absolute protein	4.0 g/dL
Glucose	10 mg/dL
White blood cell count	50,000 cells/μL
Red blood cell count	4,000 cells/μL

Questions to Consider

1. What type of effusion is represented by the data shown?
2. What condition does Bernice have?

PERICARDIAL FLUID

Pericarditis

Pericarditis is defined as an inflammation of the pericardium. There are several types and causes of pericarditis; a partial list is shown in Box 11-3.

Acute pericarditis is the most common pathologic process involving the pericardium. Acute pericarditis may result from viral or bacterial infections (including tuberculosis), collagen vascular disease (rheumatic fever), uremia, penetrating and nonpenetrating trauma, or myocardial infarction. There are four principal diagnostic features of acute pericarditis: (1) chest pain, (2) pericardial friction rub, (3) electrocardiogram changes, and (4) pericardial effusion.

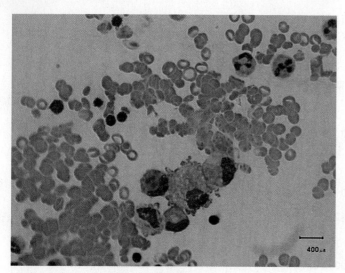

FIGURE 11-7   Pleural Fluid Transudate Showing a Macrophage that has Engulfed a Cell

Pericardial Effusions

The pericardial space normally contains approximately 10–15 mL of fluid, which is produced by a transudative process similar to pleural fluid. Pericardial effusions are usually caused by viral infection, and enterovirus is the usual etiologic agent. An expanded list of causes of pericardial effusion is shown in Box 11-4.

Pericardial effusions can develop as a result of pericarditis or an injury to the parietal pericardium. They can occur in the absence of pericarditis in clinical settings that include uremia, cardiac trauma, and malignancy. Clinical manifestations of pericardial effusion depend upon the amount of fluid retained. A large volume of fluid can lead to signs and symptoms, including dysphagia (difficulty swallowing), cough, dyspnea (shortness of breath), nausea, and a sense of abdominal fullness. Physical examination may reveal muffled heart sounds or lower lobe lung dullness upon percussion of the chest.

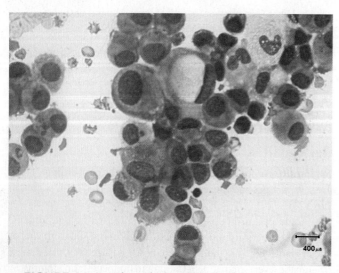

FIGURE 11-8   Pleural Fluid Exudate with a "Signet Ring" Cell

---

BOX 11-3   Classification of Pericarditis

Diagnostic classification
1. Acute pericarditis (<6 weeks)
2. Subacute pericarditis (6 weeks to 6 months)
3. Chronic pericarditis (>6 months)

Etiologic classification
1. Infectious pericarditis (e.g., viral, bacterial, fungal, tuberculous)
2. Noninfectious pericarditis (e.g., acute myocardial infarction, uremia, neoplasia)
3. Immune forms of pericarditis (e.g., rheumatic fever, collagen vascular disease)
4. Postcardiac injury (e.g., posttraumatic, postpericardiotomy)

Diagnostic Procedures

Diagnostic procedures may include chest radiography, echocardiography, cardiac magnetic resonance imaging, and computed tomography. Transthoracic echocardiography is the quickest and most accurate means of diagnosing and estimating the size of a pericardial effusion. Typically, the effusion appears as an echo-free space that can be observed during an echocardiogram procedure between the moving epicardium and the stationary pericardium.

BOX 11-4   Causes of Pericardial Effusions

General Causes
Bacteria
Virus
Tuberculosis
Fungi
Neoplasm
Lymphoma
Drugs
Renal failure

Diseases/Disorders
Hemorrhage
Trauma
Anticoagulant therapy
Autoimmune disorders
Systemic lupus erythematosus
Acute myocardial infarction
Radiation therapy
Hypothyroidism

Surgical pericardiotomy is a treatment for select pericardial diseases, including constrictive pericarditis. Postpericardiotomy syndrome is a common but nonspecific complication of cardiac surgery that may develop days to week following the initial injury. Clinical features include fever, pleuritic chest pain, and other signs of pleural, pericardial, and occasionally lung inflammation. Exudative pleural effusions develop in many of these cases. The effusion often contains a mixture of serous fluid and blood or may be completely hemorrhagic with a pH greater than 7.4 and a normal glucose level. There are no specific diagnostic tests for this syndrome but experts agree that it is an immune-mediated process.[8]

Specimen Collection

Removal of pericardial fluid is accomplished by pericardiotomy following limited thoracotomy or by **pericardiocentesis** (sterile needle aspiration). The amount of fluid present depends upon the extent of the effusion and any other event such as cardiac tamponade (fluid buildup in the pericardial sac). Examples of pericardial fluid samples collected in various containers are shown in Figure 11-9 ■.

Normal pericardial fluid is pale yellow and clear. A large effusion yielding several hundred milliliters can be caused by malignancy or uremia. Malignancy and infection typically produce a turbid effusion, while uremia produces an effusion that is usually clear and straw-colored. Bloody effusions obtained from pericardiocentesis may be a hemorrhagic effusion or inadvertent aspiration of blood from the heart. If the blood is from the heart, then the hematocrit will be similar to peripheral blood. Also blood from a cardiac puncture will clot, whereas a hemorrhagic effusion usually does not. Blood gas and pH measurements are also used to determine the origin of a bloody specimen. The blood gasses and pH from an inadvertent aspiration of blood from the heart will be similar to peripheral venous or arterial blood, whereas the pH and partial pressure of oxygen is lower and the partial pressure of carbon dioxide is higher in a hemorrhagic effusion.

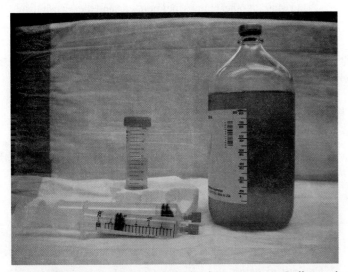

■ **FIGURE 11-9** Pericardial Fluid Specimens Collected in Various Containers

☑ **CHECKPOINT 11-6**

Bloody effusions obtained from pericardiocentesis may be due to _____.

Macroscopic and Microscopic Examination

Specimens received for analysis should be inspected for the presence of blood and other physical features such as consistency and clarity. Light's criteria for pericardial fluid have been shown to be a reliable tool for identifying pericardial exudates and transudate (see Box 11-1).[9] Routine testing should be limited to cell counts, glucose, total protein, lactate dehydrogenase (LD), bacterial culture, and cytology, if necessary.

Microscopic examination provides little diagnostic information but is necessary for white blood counts and differential. A measured hematocrit and red blood cell count supports the presence of a hemorrhagic effusion, but it is of limited value for diagnostic purposes. White cell counts exceeding $8,000/\mu L$ are consistent with bacterial, tuberculous, or malignant pericarditis but may also be low in these conditions, thus they are of limited value.

Cytological examination of malignant cells is warranted and not difficult to perform. A common finding in patients with malignant pericardial effusion is metastatic carcinoma of the lung and breast.

Chemical Testing

Testing chemical analytes in pericardial effusions has not been evaluated to the same level as the other body fluids. Pericardial effusions are similar to pleural effusions, but there is not enough clinical data to draw diagnostic parallels with assay results. The reader is directed to the reference cited for specific details on the diagnostic utility of common analytes measured in serous fluids.[10]

Microbiology Examination

Gram stain techniques for pericardial fluid specimens possess similar sensitivity as with other serous fluids. Clinically significant aerobic bacteria include *Staphylcoccus aureus*, *Streptococcus pneumonia*, *Streptococcus pyogenes*, and Gram-negative bacilli. Anaerobic bacterial infections of the pericardium are rare and difficult to isolate and identify due to technique-related issues; therefore, when a suspected case is discovered, proper technique is essential. Causative agents for anaerobic bacterial infections include *Bacteroides fragilis* group, Clostridium species, Fusobacterium species, and anaerobic Streptococci.

Isolation and identification of viral agents (e.g., coxsackie viruses and influenza virus) in pericardial effusion is difficult because the viruses are rarely isolated from pericardial fluid. Acute and convalescent sera antibody tests may provide the clinician with useful information.

Acid-fast stains and culture for tuberculous pericarditis have low sensitivity. A more sensitive technique is polymerase chain reaction (PCR). The specificity of PCR is also superior to acid-fast techniques.

MINI-CASE 11-2

Laboratory Technologist Marilyn received a fluid from a pericardiocentesis on Phillip, a patient in the intensive care unit. The specimen is bloody in appearance. Marilyn contacted the physician who performed the procedure immediately upon receiving the specimen to verify the integrity of the specimen. During the discussion the physician asked her if there was a test that could be performed that would determine if the aspiration was representative of blood from the heart or a hemorrhagic effusion. Marilyn acknowledged that there are tests available and the results are shown below:

Test	Patient Results	Reference Range for Peripheral blood
Hematocrit (%)	40	41–53
pH	7.36	7.38–7.44
pO$_2$ (mmHg)	90	83–108
pCO$_2$ (mmHg)	38	35–40
Ability to Clot	Clots	

Question to Consider

1. What is the source of the pericardial fluid?

PERITONEAL FLUID

Ascites

Ascites is the accumulation of fluid in the peritoneal cavity. If the fluid accumulation is not due to an inflammation, the term *ascites* is commonly used, whereas if the source of fluid is inflammatory, then the fluid is termed *peritoneal*. Typically, approximately 50 mL of fluid is present in this mesothelial-lined space. It is produced as an ultrafiltrate of plasma dependent on vascular permeability and on hydrostatic oncotic forces. The most common cause of ascites is advanced liver disease or cirrhosis. Other causes include malignancies (e.g., ovarian cancer, pancreatic cancer) and congestive heart failure. The predominant theory is that portal hypertension (increased pressure in the liver blood flow) is the main contributor for fluid production. The mechanism is thought to be an imbalance of pressure between the interior of blood vessels (high-pressure systems) and the exterior or the abdominal cavity (low-pressure space). An increase in hepatic portal blood pressure and a concomitant decrease in albumin may be responsible in forming the pressure gradient and resulting in abdominal ascites. There may be contributing factors to ascites that include salt and water retention. Circulating blood volume may be perceived as low by the pressure sensors in the kidneys because the formation of ascites may deplete some volume of blood. This signals the kidneys to reabsorb more salt and water to compensate for the volume loss.

Patients in congestive heart failure or advanced kidney failure develop increased pressure gradients due to generalized retention of fluid in the body. Obstruction of the portal vessel can cause increased pressure in the portal system in the absence of cirrhosis. For example, a tumor can develop that presses on the portal vessels from inside the abdominal cavity and result in increased pressure in the vessel.

☑ CHECKPOINT 11-7

Name two common causes of ascites.

Several additional causes of peritoneal effusions are presented in Box 11-5. Laboratory attempts to classify ascites as a transudate or an exudate are not as well defined as they are for pleural fluid. Thus Light's criteria are not commonly used.

Serum–Ascites Albumin Gradient

Ascites fluid specimens should be sent to the laboratory for measurements of albumin content. A blood specimen should accompany the ascites fluid for an albumin measurement and any additional chemistry (see below). These two albumin tests can be used to determine the serum–ascites albumin gradient (SAAG). SAAG is determined by subtracting the ascites albumin value from the serum albumin value. The SAAG represents the pressure within the hepatic sinusoids and correlates with the hepatic venous pressure gradient. Ascites caused by portal hypertension has a gradient of >1.1 g/dL and is a transudate, whereas ascites produced by other causes has a gradient of <1.1 g/dL and is classified as an exudate.[11,12]

Physical Features of Patients with Ascites

Patients with ascites present to their clinicians with physical features consistent with free fluid in the abdominal cavity. There are four signs characteristic of free fluid:

1. Bulging flanks in the supine position.
2. An area of tympany at the top of the abdominal curve caused by gas-filled, mobile intestines floating to the uppermost surface of fluid.
3. Shifting dullness produced by free fluid. This is assessed by percussing the level of dullness in the patient's flanks and then repositioning the patient and repeating the procedure. Dullness will be heard again.
4. Production of a fluid wave by tapping a flank sharply with one hand while the other receives the impulse against the opposite flank.

BOX 11-5   Causes of Peritoneal Effusions

Transudates

Congestive heart failure

Hepatic cirrhosis

Hypoproteinemia associated with nephrotic syndrome

Exudates

Infections

Neoplasms

Trauma

Bile peritonitis from a ruptured gall bladder

Chylous effusion

Damage to or obstruction of thoracic duct

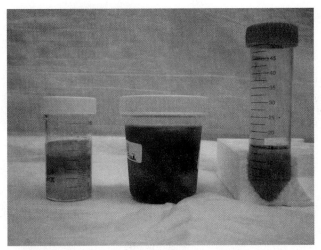

FIGURE 11-10 Three Ascites Fluid Specimens Collected from Three Different Patients and Transferred Into Sample Containers

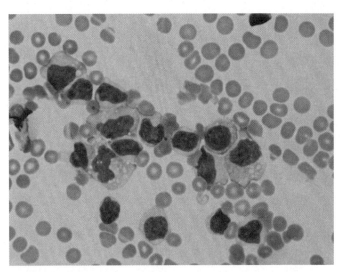

FIGURE 11-11 Peritoneal Fluid Showing Macrophages, Histiocytes, and Lymphocytes
There is also a moderate amount of proteinaceous debris present.

Specimen Collection

Paracentesis is the term used for the removal of ascites fluid from the abdominal cavity. It is a diagnostic procedure where approximately 30 mL of fluid is removed. Samples for cell counts should be place in EDTA-anticoagulated venipuncture tubes. Culture specimens should include blood culture bottles that have been inoculated at the bedside with at least 10 mL ascitic fluid. Representative samples of ascites fluid are shown in Figure 11-10 ■.

Peritoneal Lavage

Peritoneal lavage is a medical procedure to irrigate and remove fluid contained in the peritoneal cavity for the purpose of examining its contents. The procedure involves the insertion of a catheter through a small incision made in abdominal cavity. If less than 15 mL of gross blood can be aspirated, then a diagnostic peritoneal lavage can be performed. Typically, 1.0 L of saline or Ringer's solution is infused followed by removal of fluid by gravity drainage. A fluid volume of ~600 mL should be recovered to ensure reliable cell counts.[13] This procedure is currently limited to two medical situations: (1) rapid screening for significant abdominal hemorrhage and (2) evaluation of hollow viscous injuries. There are other applications for peritoneal lavage, such as for peritonitis or pancreatitis, that may provide the clinician with useful information. Once the fluid is obtained, it is sent to the clinical laboratory for analysis.

There are criteria for assessing peritoneal lavage fluid application to trauma. For example if the appearance of the fluid is bloody, the red blood cell count is >50,000–100,000/μL, the white blood cell count is >500/μL, and serum amylase is >110 U/L, then the cause of the excess fluid is most likely penetrating or blunt trauma. There are also criteria for assessing hollow organ injuries. The reader can refer to the references cited for further information on this topic.[14,15]

Gross Examination

Peritoneal fluid is normally clear and pale yellow. A turbid fluid indicates the presence of a bacterial infection. Bile-contaminated fluid is green or dark brown. Trauma, malignancy, and intestinal disorders typically present a blood-tinged specimen. A milky appearance to a peritoneal fluid may be due to a condition affecting the lymph vessels (e.g., blockage or trauma).

Microscopic Examination

Absolute neutrophil count and differential provides very useful information to the clinician evaluating patients presenting with ascites. The total leukocyte count is useful in distinguishing ascites due to uncomplicated cirrhosis from spontaneous bacterial peritonitis (SBP) caused by movement of bacteria from the intestine into the ascetic fluid. Several examples of cells and other materials present in peritoneal fluids are presented in Figures 11-11 ■ to 11-15 ■.

Patients with chronic inflammatory process associated with chronic peritoneal dialysis may have up to 10% eosinophils in their blood smears. Other conditions associated with elevated eosinophils are congestive heart failure, vasculitis, lymphoma, and ruptured hydatid cyst.

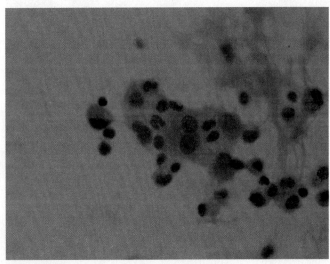

FIGURE 11-12 Ascites Fluid with Reactive Mesothelial Cells

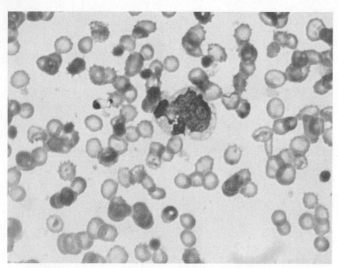

FIGURE 11-13   Malignant Cells with Anisonucleosis and Prominent Nucleoli

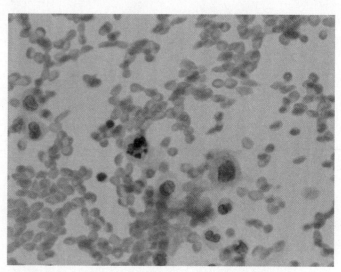

FIGURE 11-15   Ascites Fluid with Iron Stains Demonstrating Bloodladen Macrophages
This sample is from a patient with pelvic endometriosis.

In cases of malignant ascites, a cytological examination may be requested by the clinician. Peritoneal carcinomatosis accounts for approximately two-thirds of malignant effusions.

Chemical Testing

In addition to measuring serum and ascites albumin concentrations as described above, the clinician should consider measuring the following analytes for the purpose indicated:

- Measuring total protein can provide insight into assessment of bacterial peritonitis. In this infectious condition total protein concentrations are usually below 3.0 g/dL.

- Normally, peritoneal fluid amylase activity is similar to plasma levels. In patients with pancreas-related ascites, their peritoneal fluid amylase activity may present with levels up to three times that of serum.

- Alkaline phosphatase activity greater than 10 U/L in peritoneal lavage fluid are very useful in predicting hollow visceral injury in patients who would not otherwise undergo laparotomy.

- Lactate dehydrogenase activity is often increased in malignant effusion.

- Lactate and pH have been used to differentiate SBP from uncomplicated ascites.

Microbiology Examination

Primary peritonitis occurs at any age and is seen in children with nephrotic syndrome and in adults with cirrhosis. SBP occurs in individuals with ascites without secondary causes such as bowel perforations. Typically, the bacteria seen in SBP are normal intestinal flora, with *E. coli* being the predominant microbe. Inoculums placed in blood culture bottles at the bedside may improve the sensitivity, but about one-third of the infected patients will produce negative ascites fluid cultures.

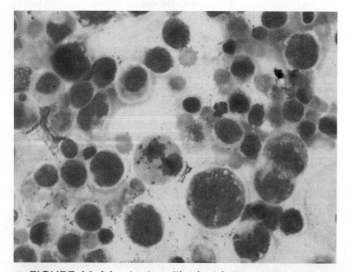

FIGURE 11-14   Ascites Fluid with Mitotic Figures

☑ CHECKPOINT 11-8

Using the laboratory data provided, determine what type of effusion (transudate or exudate) this patient has.

Serum albumin (mg/dL) = 4.0

Ascites albumin (mg/dL) = 3.8

MINI-CASE 11-3

Mason was admitted to the hospital complaining of pain in the upper left abdominal quadrant. His history, physical, electro-cardiogram, and serum cardiac troponin I, urea nitrogen, creatinine, were all unremarkable. A paracentesis was performed and the peritoneal fluid was sent to the laboratory. The results of the laboratory tests:

Serum albumin = 3.0 g/dL

Fluid albumin = 1.0 g/dL

Questions to Consider

1. Calculate the serum-ascites albumin gradient.

2. Is this an exudate or transudate? What is the rationale?

3. What is the most probable cause of the effusion?

Key Points to Remember

- Determination of the origin of fluid accumulation in body cavities (e.g., chest and abdomen) is most important for proper treatment of disorders.

- Proper selection of laboratory tests for body fluid analysis is essential for the diagnosis of diseases to organs located in and around these cavities.

- Correct test interpretation depends on proper specimen collection, valid gross and microscopic examination, and accurate chemical and hematology analysis.

- Identification and knowledge of diseases associated with serous fluid facilitates the correct correlation of laboratory tests to diseases.

Review Questions

Level I

1. Which of the following describes the primary purpose of serous fluids? (Objective 1)

   A. Lubricate serous membranes

   B. Lubricate muscles

   C. Remove biochemical waste products from the body

   D. Provide important cellular components for tissue maintenance

2. An effusion is defined as: (Objective 2)

   A. the movement of water against a concentration gradient.

   B. the movement of ions into cardiac muscle cells.

   C. the escape of fluid into a body cavity.

   D. the escape of fluid into the thoracic duct.

3. Leakage of fluid from a lymphatic duct (e.g., thoracic duct) due to an obstruction may result in developing which of the following? (Objective 1)

   A. Pericardial effusion

   B. Pneumonitis

C. Pseudochylous effusion

D. Chylous effusion

4. Which lipoprotein is most often found in chylous effusions? (Objective 3)

   A. Chylomicron

   B. High density lipoprotein

   C. Apo lipoprotein A

   D. Apo lipoprotein B

5. Serous fluid cell counts should be determined using (Objective 5)

   A. glass slide and cover slip.

   B. hemocytometer chamber.

   C. automated cell counter that has not been properly calibrated.

6. The pleural cavity is described anatomically as (Objective 1)

   A. the space occupied by the brain.

   B. a space that lies between the visceral and parietal pericardium.

C. a closed space (similar to the inside of a balloon) within which the lung has grown.

D. a space that lines the internal walls of the abdominal cavity.

7. Which of the following techniques is used to remove pleural fluid from a patient? (Objective 4)

A. Amniocentesis

B. Paracentesis

C. Pericardiocentesis

D. Thoracentesis

8. The total protein concentration of a pleural fluid exudate is (Objective 2)

A. equal to pleural fluid transudate.

B. lower than that found in transudates.

C. higher than pleural fluid transudate.

9. Another name for ascites is (Objective 2)

A. pericardial effusion.

B. peritoneal effusion.

C. transudate.

D. chylous.

10. Congestive heart failure is a common cause of (Objective 7)

A. pleural effusion.

B. peritonitis.

C. acute pericarditis.

D. ascites.

11. The determination of a serum–ascites albumin gradient is clinically useful for which of the following? (Objective 6)

A. Distinguishing acute peritonitis from chronic peritonitis

B. Distinguishing ascites caused by portal hypertension versus ascites caused by other means

C. Distinguishing chylous effusion from pseudochylous effusion

D. Determining the origin of a bloody sample obtained during a thoracentesis procedure

Level II

1. Light's criteria include which of the following determinations? (Objective 5)

A. Pleural fluid creatine kinase <0.67 of upper limit of normal for serum

B. Pleural fluid LD/serum LD >0.6

C. Pleural fluid albumin/serum protein >0.5

D. Pleural fluid protein/serum protein >0.5

2. A pleural fluid that meets ANY of Light's criteria is identified as (Objective 5)

A. pleurisy.

B. transudate.

C. exudate.

D. pseudochylous.

3. Which of the following tests is clinically useful for differentiating ascites due to bacterial peritonitis from cirrhosis? (Objective 5)

A. White blood differential

B. Absolute lymphocyte count

C. Total leukocyte count

D. Absolute neutrophil count

4. Which of following is the recommended measurement to determine if peritoneal fluid is a transudate or an exudate? (Objective 6)

A. Serum glucose to ascites fluid glucose

B. Serum–ascites albumin gradient

C. Total protein to albumin ratio

D. Serum lactate dehydrogenase to ascites fluid lactate dehydrogenase gradient

5. Production of peritoneal fluid is dependent upon (Objective 1)

A. development of intravascular ionic gradients.

B. vascular permeability and hydrostatic oncotic forces.

C. the ratio of serum total protein to peritoneal fluid total protein.

D. the ratio of oncotic pressure to osmotic pressure.

6. Which of the following can be a cause of bloody effusions obtained from pericardiocentesis? (Objective 3)

A. Inadvertent aspiration of blood from the heart

B. Hemolytic anemia

C. Renal failure

D. Bacterial endocarditis

7. A serum–ascites albumin gradient value of >1.1 indicates (Objective 5)

A. pericarditis.

B. peritonitis.

C. ascites caused by other means (i.e., not portal hypertension).

D. ascites caused by portal hypertension.

8. Laboratory testing of a peritoneal fluid specimen for albumin and serum albumin shows the following results: (Objective 5)

Serum albumin (mg/dL) = 3.8

Ascites albumin (mg/dL) = 3.7

Which of the following is the correct interpretation of these results?

A. Ascites is caused by portal hypertension.

B. Ascites is due to a condition other than portal hypertension.

C. Ascites is classified as a transudate.

D. A serum and ascites fluid lactate dehydrogenase is required to complete the calculation.

9. Sam's laboratory tests for a thoracentesis procedure performed while a patient in the hospital are: (Objective 5)

Pleural fluid protein/serum protein = 0.2

Pleural fluid LD/serum LD = 0.3

Appearance = clear yellow

Specific gravity = 1.007

Based on the laboratory results and according to Light's criteria, which of the following is the correct identification of his fluid type? (Objective 3)

A. Exudate effusion

B. Chylous effusion

C. Transudate effusion

D. Pseudochylous effusion

10. Samson was admitted to the local emergency department. He was unconscious and unable to respond. The physician noticed a bloated abdomen and performed a peritoneal lavage. Samples were sent to the laboratory and the results are: (Objective 5)

Red blood cell count = 60,000 cells/μL (markedly elevated)

White blood cell count = 700 cells/μL (elevated)

Serum amylase = 750 U/L (markedly elevated)

The specimen was bloody with slight turbidity.

Which of the following is a possible cause for the symptoms and laboratory results? (Objective 3)

A. Pericarditis

B. Tuberculosis

C. Acute myocardial infarction

D. Blunt trauma to the abdomen

Endnotes

1. Clinical and Laboratory Standards Institute (CLSI) body fluid analysis for cellular composition; Approved Guideline. CLSI document H56-A. Clinical Laboratory Standard Institute, 940 West Valley Road, Suite 1400, Wayne Pennsylvania 19087-1898 USA, 2006.

2. Clinical and Laboratory Standards Institute (CLSI) body fluid analysis for cellular composition; Approved Guideline. CLSI document H56-A. Clinical Laboratory Standard Institute, 940 West Valley Road, Suite 1400, Wayne Pennsylvania 19087-1898 USA, 2006.

3. College of American Pathologist. Commission on Laboratory Accreditation Program: hematology-coagulation checklist; 2004.

4. Light R, Macgregor M, Luchsigner P, et al. Pleural effusion: the diagnostic separation of transudate and exudates. *Ann Intern Med* (1977) 4:507–513.

5. Light RW. Clinical practice, pleural effusion. *N Engl J Med* (2002) 36;25:1971–1977.

6. Gomella, LG, Haist SA. Chapter 13, Bedside procedures. In: *Clinician's Pocket Reference*. 11th ed. Columbus, OH: McGraw-Hill, 2007.

7. Papadakis M, McPhee SJ, Rabow MW. *Current Medical Diagnosis and Treatment*. 52nd ed. Columbus, OH: McGraw-Hill, 2013.

8. LeWinter MW. Chapter 17: Pericardial diseases. In: Crawford MH. Ed. *Current Diagnosis and Treatment: Cardiology*. 3rd ed. Columbus, OH: McGraw-Hill, 2009.

9. Burgess LJ, Reuter H, Taljaard, JJ, et al. Role of biochemical tests in the diagnosis of large pericardial effusion. *Chest* (2002) 121;2:495–499.

10. Karcher DS, McPherson RA. Cerebrospinal, synovial, serous body fluids and alternative specimens. In McPherson RA, Pincus MR, eds. *Henry's Clinical Diagnosis and Management by Laboratory Methods*. 22nd ed. Philadelphia: Elsevier Saunders, 2011.

11. Runyou BA, Joefs JC. Ascitic fluid analysis in the differentiation of spontaneous bacterial peritonitis from gastrointestinal tract perforation into ascitic fluid. *Hepatology* (1984) 4;3:447–450.

12. Corey KE, Friedman LS. Chapter 43. Abdominal swelling and ascites. In: Longo DL, Fauci AS, Kasper DL, Hauser SL, Jameson JL, et al. *Harrison's Principles of Internal Medicine*. 18th ed. New York: McGraw-Hill, 2012. http://www.accessmedicine.com/content.aspx?aid=9113313. Accessed November 25, 2013.

13. Hemmila MR, Wahl W. Chapter 13: Management of the injured patient. In: Doherty GM. Ed. *Current Diagnosis and Treatment: Surgery*. 13th ed. Columbus, OH: McGraw-Hill, 2010.

14. Otomo Y, Henmi H, Mashiko K, et al. New diagnostic peritoneal lavage criteria for diagnosis of intestinal injury. *J Trauma* (1998) 44;6:991–997.

15. Fang JF, Chen RJ, Lin BC. Cell count ratio: new criterion of diagnostic peritoneal lavage for detection of hollow organ perforation. *J Trauma* (1998) 45;3:540–544.

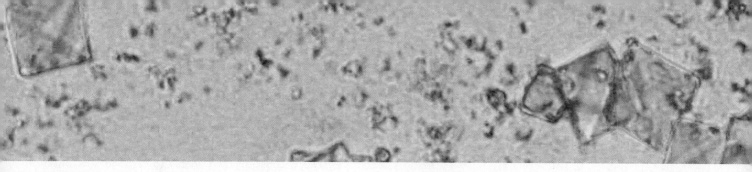

12

Synovial Fluid, Bronchoalveolar Lavage, and Sweat Testing

Objectives

LEVEL I

1. Describe in anatomical terms the key features of major joints in the human body.
2. Describe the physical appearance, cellular consistency, and chemical composition of synovial fluid.
3. Identify several different arthritis-like conditions.
4. Identify several preanalytical issues that must be recognized when collecting, handling, and storing synovial fluids.
5. Identify laboratory tests available for analysis of synovial fluid.
6. Explain the bronchoalveolar lavage procedure.
7. Identify the medical usefulness of bronchoalveolar lavage.
8. Explain the procedure for proper specimen collection, handling, and transport of bronchoalveolar lavage specimens.
9. Describe the characteristics of cystic fibrosis.
10. Identify tests suitable for measuring chloride in sweat.

LEVEL II

1. Explain in anatomical terms the origin of synovial fluid in the body.
2. Explain the techniques used for obtaining synovial fluid, bronchoalveolar lavage, and sweat specimens from patients.
3. Discuss the diagnostic significance of arthrocentesis, bronchoalveolar lavage, and sweat chloride collection.
4. Describe the gross and microscopic findings from an arthrocentesis, bronchoalveolar lavage, and sweat chloride collection.
5. Interpret abnormal gross and microscopic examination findings and chemical test results.
6. Select proper laboratory tests for a given body fluid sample.

Chapter Outline

Key Terms

Amperometry	Hemarthrosis	Lavage	Synovial joint
Arthritis	Hyaluronan	Podagra	Synoviocyte
Arthrocentesis	Hyperuricemia	Pseudogout	Tenosynovitis
Coulometric titration	Inflammasome	Ragocyte	Tophus
Gout	Iontophoresis	Synovial fluid	

A CASE IN POINT

Reginold, a 40-year-old Filipino male presents to the emergency department with extreme pain in the metatarsal-phalangeal (MTP) joint of the big toe (right foot). Inspection of the joint reveals it to be swollen, very tender to the touch, warm, with a dust red appearance. The "attack" was acute, sudden onset in nature. It also occurred around 2300 hours. The patient was febrile and admitted that he had drunk a significant amount of beer during the evening hours. Results of the joint fluid examination with microscopic, abnormal serum chemistries and abnormal white blood cell count are shown in the table below:

	Results (Conventional units/SI units)	Reference Interval (Conventional units/SI units)
Serum chemistries:		
Uric acid, mg/dL (μ mol/L)	8.8 (523)	3.5–7.2 (208–428)
(Method: Uricase)		
Ethanol, mg/dL (mmol/L)	180 (39.0)	<50 (<10.9)
(Method: Alcohol Dehydrogenase)		
White blood cell count: $\times 10^3/\mu L (\times 10^9/L)$	20.0 (20.0)	4.4–11.3 (4.4–11.3)

Joint fluid examination:

Positive identification of sodium urate crystals that appear within neutrophils. The crystals are shaped like needles and negatively birefringent.

Questions to Consider

1. What is Reginold's diagnosis?

2. Explain the clinical correlation of each abnormal laboratory finding with the patient's diagnosis.

3. What is the significance, if any, that the patient is Filipino?

4. What are the definitions of *tophus* and *Podagra*?

5. Why is the method of analysis indicated for serum uric acid?

SYNOVIAL FLUID

Anatomy

There are three types of joints in the human body: (1) fibrous, which are fixed; (2) cartilaginous, which are slightly movable; and (3) synovial, which are freely movable. The focus of this chapter will be on the synovial joints (e.g., the knee) because they yield a fluid that can provide useful information to a clinician relative to joint dysfunction. A diagram of the knee joint and significant anatomical features is shown in Figure 12-1 ■.

The inner lining of a **synovial joint** consists of the synovium (also termed synovial membrane), which is a thin layer located between the joint capsule and the joint cavity. The synovial membrane is divided into two layers—the outer layer (subintima) and the inner layer (intima). Specialized macrophages (macrophage-like synovial cells) and fibroblast-like **synoviocytes** make up the intima and are critical in maintaining the internal joint homeostasis. These cells are also the main source of hyaluronan and other glycoproteins, which are significant components of the synovial fluid. The bones are protected by cartilage, which is not covered by the synovial membrane. The whole joint and its synovial sac are contained within a tough connective tissue capsule. These joints may be single or double, the latter being divided into its two parts by an intervening disc, which is directly continuous with the capsule.

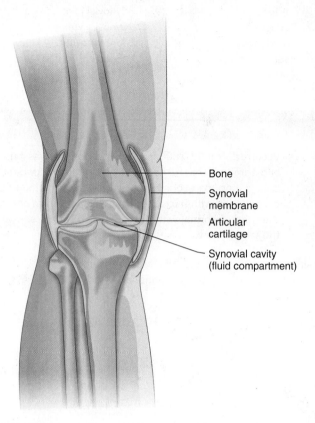

Bone

Synovial membrane

Articular cartilage

Synovial cavity (fluid compartment)

■ **FIGURE 12-1** Schematic Drawing of a Typical Knee Joint

Arthritis

Arthritis is any inflammatory process affecting a joint or joints that results in pain, swelling, and stiffness. Periarthritis is an inflammation around a joint, which can also be painful. The pain from a true articular process (i.e., pertaining to the joint) is usually present throughout the complete range of motion of a particular joint. The pain from periarthritis is usually evident at a single point of the range of motion, and it is confirmed by palpation in a specific area corresponding to a tendon, ligament, or bursa. Further examples

BOX 12-1 Several Examples of Distinguishing Features of Arthritis versus Periarthritis

Arthritis
Morning stiffness
Warmth
Erythema
Constitutional symptoms

Periarthritis
Bursitis
Tendinitis
Ligament strain
Soft tissue
Bone pathology

of the distinguishing features of arthritis versus periarthritis are shown in Box 12-1.

Table 12-1 ★ outlines several specific types of arthritis with both unique mechanisms of action and unique features. They are discussed further in the paragraphs that follow.

Gouty Arthritis

Gout is described as a crystal-induced synovitis of a heterogeneous nature. It is often familial and associated with abnormal amounts of urates in the body. Gout is characterized early on by a recurring acute arthritis and later by chronic deforming arthritis. Patients may present with **hyperuricemia**, which is characterized by elevated uric acid concentrations in blood due to overproduction or underexcretion of uric acid or sometimes a combination of both conditions. The disease is more common in Pacific Islanders (e.g., Filipinos and Samoans). Both primary and secondary causes of hyperuricemia are listed in Box 12-2. Alcohol ingestion can promote hyperuricemia by increasing urate production and decreasing renal excretion of uric acid. Last, hospitalized patients often experience episodes or attacks of gout that are precipitated by

★ **TABLE 12-1** General Features of Several Common Arthritis-like Diseases/Conditions

Diagnosis	Mechanism	Additional Features
Osteoarthritis	Degradation and degeneration of articular cartilage	Bone spurs; affects knee, hip
Gouty arthritis	Crystal-induced inflammation	Tophi*; acute attack followed by spontaneous resolution
Pseudogout	Crystal-induced inflammation	Acute or chronic attacks
Septic arthritis	Bacterial invasion	Sepsis, fever
Rheumatoid arthritis	Deposition of immune complexes	Extra-articular manifestations
Lyme disease	Bacterial invasion	Symptoms may not develop for weeks, months, or years
Viral arthritis	Infecting synovial tissue during systemic infections or by provoking an immunologic reaction	Vasculitis, autoantibodies
Reactive arthritis	Bacterial invasion	Typically follows GI or genitourinary infections

* A deposit of sodium biurate in tissues near a joint.

BOX 12-2 Causes of Primary and Secondary Hyperuricemia

Primary Hyperuricemia

A. Increased formation of purines
   1. Specific enzyme defects
   2. Idiopathic
B. Decreases elimination of uric acid by the kidneys (idiopathic)

Secondary Hyperuricemia

A. Increased catabolism of purine
   1. Chronic hemolytic anemia
   2. Cytotoxic drugs
   3. Myeloproliferative diseases
   4. Carcinoma
B. Decreased elimination of uric acid
   1. Intrinsic kidney disease
   2. Functional impairment of tubular transport
      a. Drug-induced (low-dose aspirin)
      b. Lactic acidosis
      c. Alcoholism
      d. Diabetic ketoacidosis
      e. Starvation
      f. Diabetes insipidus

changes in diet, fluid intake, or medications that either increase or decrease serum uric acid.

Primary gout occurs more frequently in males (~90%), usually over 30 years old, than in females where the onset typically appears after menopause. The principle feature is a lesion, the **tophus**, which is a nodular deposit of monosodium urate monohydrate crystals resulting in a foreign body reaction. Tophi are commonly found in cartilage, tendon, bone, periarticular and subcutaneous tissue, and the kidney. The acute inflammation of gout is thought to be due to the ingestion of uncoated urate crystals by monocytes and synoviocytes. Upon entry into the cells, the urate crystals are processed through Toll-like receptors and activated NALP3 (also known as cryopyrin) inflammasomes. An **inflammasome** is a multiprotein oligomer that is part of the body's innate immune system. It is responsible for activation of the inflammatory response. Toll-like receptors are part of the recognition process of invading structures, in this case, urate crystals. NALP-3 is a type of NOD-like receptor capable of "sensing" or detecting the presence of foreign substances. Once the immune system is activated, several types of chemotactic agents and cytokines are released to neutralize the foreign substances.[1,2]

☑ CHECKPOINT 12-1

All individuals with gouty arthritis have elevated serum uric acid levels. (T or F)

The exact relationship of hyperuricemia to gouty arthritis is still unknown since chronic hyperuricemia can occur in people who never develop gout or uric acid stones. Modulating uric acid levels, either increasing or decreasing, are important factors in precipitating acute gout. Uric acid kidney stone formation is present in 5–10% of patients with gouty arthritis. There is a strong likelihood of hyperuricemia with the development of kidney stones especially in patients with serum uric acid levels >13 mg/dL (SI units, >773 μmol/L). Chronic urate nephropathy is caused by deposits of monosodium urate crystals in the renal medulla and pyramids. Patients with acute gouty arthritis present with an acute attack, which is typically nocturnal. It may develop without any apparent precipitating cause, or it may follow sudden increases or decreases in serum uric acid levels. Several other causes include (1) alcohol excess (typically beer), (2) changes in medications that affect urate metabolism, and (3) in hospitalized patients, fasting before medical procedures. The most susceptible joint to attacks of gout is the metatarsal phalangeal (MTP) joint of the great toe (also referred to as **Podagra**), although other common sites include feet, ankles, knees, and the periarticular soft tissue in the arch of the foot. Progression of the infliction results in increased intensity of pain, swollen joints, and tenderness. Also the overlying skin is usually tense, warm, and red.[3] Fever is also a common manifestation of the condition.

Pseudogout is a type of arthritis characterized by an acute, painful swelling in one or more joints, typically the knees. Pseudogout is also referred to as calcium pyrophosphate deposition disease. The term *pseudogout* was used because of its similarities with gout. Both conditions are caused by crystal deposits in the tissue, although the crystals are different (see below).

The clinical laboratory serves an important role in providing clinicians with significant laboratory test information. Synovial fluid analysis includes serum uric acid levels, other appropriate ancillary chemistry tests (e.g., ethanol, electrolytes and lactate dehydrogenase), and complete blood count and differential. Microscopic examination of synovial fluid should be performed to detect the presence of crystals and perform a cell count and differential. Identification of monosodium urate crystals in joint fluid or material aspirated from a tophus can establish a diagnosis. The crystals may be extra- or intracellular, shaped like a needle, and are negatively birefringent when examined by polarized light microscopy.

☑ CHECKPOINT 12-2

What is the most common site of inflammation in patients with gouty arthritis?

Septic Arthritis

Septic arthritis is a potentially serious condition if not diagnosed in a timely manner. The bacterial infection and inflammatory response can destroy a joint within days. Septic arthritis is characterized as non-gonococcal or gonococcal. Causative agents of non-gonococcal septic arthritis include *Staphylococcus, Streptococcus,* and Gram-negative bacilli. Clinical features of non-gonococcal septic arthritis are joint pain, joint swelling, fever, chills, and rigor. Abnormal laboratory tests include elevated white blood cell counts and sedimentation rates.

Gonococcal arthritis is a common cause of septic arthritis in children and young adults. A typical clinical presentation of gonococcal septic arthritis is the presence of migratory* arthritis and **tenosynovitis**, which is described an inflammation of the fluid-filled sheath that surrounds a tendon prior to onset of pain and swelling of one or more septic joints. Synovial fluid cultures are often negative for *Neisseria gonorrhea*.

Viral Arthritis

A virus produces arthritis by infecting synovial tissue during systemic infection or by initiating an immunologic reaction that involves joints. Virus-associated arthritis is caused by several viral agents (e.g., Parvovirus, Rubella, Epstein-Barr, Hepatitis B and C, and HIV). In addition to the unique signs and symptoms associated with the specific viral agent, all affected patients will suffer with stiff and tender joints accompanied by swelling.

Lyme Disease

Patients with Lyme disease may not experience symptoms of arthritis for weeks, months, or years after primary stage I infection. Symptoms that eventually appear are often articular or periarticular asymmetric joint involvement.

Rheumatoid Arthritis

Rheumatoid arthritis is a progressive disease and typically involves several joints. Women appear to be affected more than men. Patients often complain of stiffness of the joints after prolonged periods of inactivity (morning stiffness). Synovitis may be evident upon examination of the phalanges, wrist, and other joints. Rheumatoid nodules may appear and are palpable. Laboratory tests for rheumatoid factor and anti-cycliccitrullinated peptides (CCP) are usually elevated in patients with rheumatoid arthritis.

Osteoarthritis

Osteoarthritis is characterized by deterioration of articular cartilage with subsequent findings of reactive new bone at the articular surface. The most commonly affected joints are the distal and proximal interphalangeal joints of the hands, hips, knees, and cervical and lumbar spine. This disease is more common in the elderly but may occur at any age, especially as sequelae to joint trauma and chronic inflammatory arthritis. Osteoarthritis affecting the spine may result in spinal stenosis, with aching or pain in the legs or buttocks on standing or walking.

Reactive Arthritis

Reactive arthritis (formerly known as Reiter syndrome) is an inflammatory-type arthritis that follows GI or genitourinary infection caused by organism including *Chlamydia trachomatis*, *Shigella flexneri*, *Campylobacter jejuni*, and *Yersinia enterocolitica*. The classic triad of Reiter syndrome is arthritis, urethritis, and conjunctivitis. Diagnostic testing involves the detection of causative microbes in stool and urine samples.

Specimen Collection and Handling

Analysis of synovial fluid and synovial tissue obtained from diseased joints provides valuable diagnostic information in specific clinical conditions. Many peripheral joints are readily accessible to sampling of both synovial fluid effusions and synovial tissue. The knee joint remains the most frequently sampled joint.

Specimen requirements for joint or synovial fluid analysis depend on the size of the joint and effusion. Routinely, 3–5 ml of fluid is enough to complete the analysis, but in cases where the joints are smaller, these volumes may not be present in the joints. In this situation, the clinician should consider establishing a new priority for testing, and the laboratory should not discard the specimen. There may be enough sample to provide valuable information, including a definitive diagnosis in a crystal-induced joint disease. Recommended specimen requirements for selected tests are shown in Table 12-2 ★.[4]

Some controversy exists regarding the use of lithium heparin and EDTA as an anticoagulant, because these substances produce crystalline material that can be confused with pathologic crystals.[5, 6] Others have used both without problems.[7] The use of oxalate should be avoided due the potential of forming calcium oxalate crystals.

> ☑ **CHECKPOINT 12-3**
>
> Which of the following microscopy techniques is used to determine whether crystals are positively or negatively birefringent?
> (a) Bright field microscopy
> (b) Fluorescent microscopy
> (c) Polarized light microscopy
> (d) Refractive light microscopy

Synovial Fluid Analysis

Normally, a small amount of synovial fluid is present in each joint, forming a thin interface between the surfaces of the articular cartilage that provides for friction-free movement of the surfaces. In larger joints, e.g., the knee, the volume of synovial fluid is between 2–3 mL. In addition, the intra-articular pressure (IAP) is typically subatmospheric, ranging from −2 to −4 mmHg.[8,9]

Synovial fluid is described as an ultrafiltrate of plasma to which proteins and proteoglycans (e.g., glycosylated mucoproteins) are added by fibroblast-like synoviocytes found in the lining layers.

Small molecular weight solutes (e.g., oxygen, carbon dioxide, lactate, urea, creatinine, and glucose) diffuse freely through the fenestrated endothelium of the synovium and exist at levels comparable to those of plasma. Synovial fluid total protein concentration is approximately 1.3 g/dL, and the individual plasma protein concentrations are inversely proportional to their molecular size. For example, small proteins such as albumin are present at approximately 50% of plasma levels, and large proteins—for example, fibrinogen, macroglobulins, and immunoglobulin—exist at low concentrations. A significant protein, **hyaluronan**, is a proteoglycan synthesized by synovial cells and secreted into synovial fluid. It is a highly polymerized protein and attains a molecular mass that exceeds one million Daltons. This gives

---

*Migratory arthritis is a problem characterized by an initial swelling in a joint that subsides in the original affected area only to reappear in another joint.

★ **TABLE 12-2** Synovial Fluid Specimen Requirements

Tests	Anticoagulant	Volume (mL)*	Comments
Chemistries:			
Total protein	None	2–3	
Glucose	Fluoride or none	2–3	8h fast preferred
CH50	None	2–3	Freeze if not tested immediately
C3,C4	None or EDTA	2–3	
Cell counts, Differential, Crystals, Inclusion	Heparin, EDTA	3–5	Mix specimens completely
Culture	SPS, none, or anticoagulant without bactericidal or bacteriostatic effect	3–5	Sterile tube required

SPS, sodium polyanetholsufonate
*Specimen requirements are determined by method and instrumentation.

synovial fluid its viscosity. It also serves to retain small molecules in the synovial fluid. Another glycoprotein, *lubricin*, functions as a principal lubricant fluid for articulated joints.[10]

☑ CHECKPOINT 12-4

Identify the protein that gives synovial fluid its viscosity.

Synovial Effusions

Synovial fluid is normally cleared through the synovial lymphatics through a process aided by joint movement. Accumulation of fluid in articulated joints occur as a result of several processes including septic disorders, non-inflammatory and inflammatory disorders. Also, **hemarthrosis** (bleeding into joint spaces) can result from both traumatic and non-traumatic conditions. The primary mechanism for the accumulation of joint effusion is an increase in synovial microvascular permeability. This anomaly allows plasma proteins to enter the synovium, especially larger proteins, which in turn increase osmotic pressure, the effects of which will be discussed later in the chapter. Leukocytes migrate through the endothelium via stimulation by chemokines and accumulate in the synovium. The synovial lymphatics cannot clear the influx of proteins, cells, and debris sufficiently, thereby overwhelming the synovial compartment.

Arthrocentesis

The removal of fluid from synovial joints is termed **arthrocentesis**. This technique can be performed in most ambulatory facilities equipped for sterile procedures. In the case of less accessible sites (e.g., hips) needle insertion procedures may require the use of imagining techniques such as fluoroscope or ultrasound to guide needle placement. Removal of synovial fluid may be complicated by the presence of debris such as rice bodies, which arise from detached ischemic synovial villi, hyperviscous fluid, and location of fluid into inaccessible sites.

Every sampling should be analyzed as quickly as possible upon completion of the arthrocentesis to avoid discordant results. Fluid cell counts and differentials are most susceptible to delays in analysis.

If the samples cannot be processed in a reasonable amount of time, they may be stored for a short period of time at 4°C. An aliquot of the sample should be placed in ethylenediaminetetraacetic acid (EDTA) to prevent clotting. Fluid specimens stored for 48 hours or longer should be reassessed for acceptability. A flow diagram presenting options for analyzing synovial fluids shown in Figure 12-2 ■.[11]

Gross Examinations

Characteristic features of synovial fluids are first observed as the fluid is being removed from the joint and deposited into a specimen container and onto slides. The typical appearance of a normal synovial fluid is shown in Figure 12-3 ■. For example, the viscosity of each specimen, which is primarily due to hyaluronan, is evidenced by the formation of a long string when a drop of fluid is expressed from the syringe needle. Normal fluid will form a string greater than 4 cm. Therefore, it is not necessary to make available more sophisticated methods to measure viscosity.[12] A loss of viscosity or "stringiness" that may be due to recruitment and activation of leukocytes into the synovial cavity and aid in digestion of hyaluronan can also be observed at this stage in the procedure. A large presence of rice bodies may result in a quick reduction of the flow of fluid in the syringe, thus necessitating possible manipulation of the syringe to another area within the joint.

Close inspection of synovial fluid as it is being aspirated and transferred into containers may provide preliminary diagnostic information. For example, fluids that are markedly purulent will be opaque due to very high cell counts. Fluids that are transparent to the degree where printed text can be read through it are typically representative of a non-inflammatory condition. Patients who present with rheumatoid arthritis (RA) commonly show signs of inflammation, and the fluid specimen appears cloudy and translucent. A patient with ochronosis (a syndrome associated with an accumulation of homogentisic acid in connective tissue) can have fluid samples with a speckled appearance, and particulate debris from joint prostheses may be visible on gross observation.

A bloody synovial fluid specimen is a concern, and the source of blood should be determined. Blood can appear in synovial fluid specimens because of a problem with the arthrocentesis procedure or as a result of trauma, tumors, pigmented villonodular synovitis, hemophilia RA, psoriatic arthritis, or anticoagulant therapy. The specimen

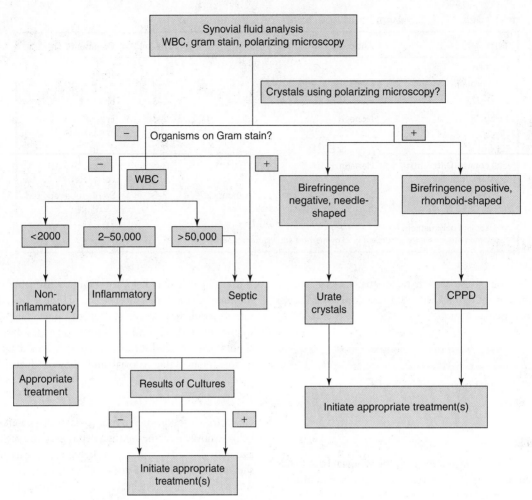

■ **FIGURE 12-2**   Basic Flow Diagram Illustrating a Simplified Algorithm for Analyzing Synovial Fluid Specimens

from a traumatic arthrocentesis may remain unmixed with synovial fluid that appears as reddish streaks in a yellow fluid. In hemarthrosis, the synovial fluid is typically a homogeneous mixture and does not form a clot.

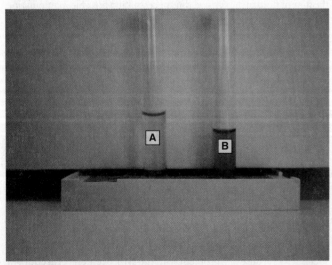

■ **FIGURE 12-3**   Synovial Fluid Specimen

(A) Clear, straw yellow color; (B) slight blood

Leukocyte counts, percent polymorphonuclear cells (PMN), physical appearance, crystals, and culture can provide the clinician with valuable diagnostic information regarding the cause of a synovial effusion. Characteristic features of synovial fluids in disease are presented in Table 12-3 ★. A normal synovial fluid specimen contains < 200 cells/μL and originates primarily from desquamated synovial lining cells. The cell counts shown in Table 12-4 ★ represent a broad-based classification of synovial fluid into five groups.[13,14] These cell ranges are useful to the clinician and aid in narrowing the differential diagnosis rather than characterizing inherent biological properties of the fluid.

☑ CHECKPOINT 12-5

A laboratory technologist receives a synovial fluid that is bloody in appearance. Identify two possible reasons for the presence of blood in a synovial fluid specimen.

Accumulation of synovial fluid in joints due to non-inflammatory causes includes mechanical manipulation, acromegaly, hyperparathyroidism, ochronosis, hemochromatosis, Wilson's disease, and Paget's disease. White blood cell counts for inflammatory-type arthritis range from 3–50 × 10^3/μL and occur due to a wide range

★ **TABLE 12-3** Synovial Fluid Test Results in Disease

	Appearance	Viscosity	Cells/μL	%PMNs	Crystals	Culture
Normal	Clear	High	<200	<10	Neg	Neg
Rheumatoid arthritis	Translucent	Low	1000–30,000	Variable	Neg	Neg
Psoriatic arthritis	Translucent	Low	2000–30,000	Variable	Neg	Neg
Gouty arthritis	Translucent to cloudy	Low	200–>30,000	>95%	Needle-shapes, negatively birefringent monosodium urate monohydrate crystal	Neg
Pseudogout	Translucent to cloudy	Low	500–40,000	>90%	Rhomboid, positively birefringent calcium pyrophosphate crystal	Neg
Bacterial arthritis	Cloudy	Variable	2000–40,000	>90%	Neg	Pos
PVNS	Hemorrhagic or brown	Low	NA	NA	Neg	Pos
Hemarthrosis	Hemorrhagic	Low	NA	NA	Neg	Neg

Neg = Negative, PMN = polymorphonuclear neutrophils, Pos = Positive, PVNS = pigmented villonodular synovitis

of joint disorders. Septic arthritis typically presents cell counts >40–50 × 10³/μL and requires microbiological testing. Patients who present with acute attacks of gout, pseudogout, active RA, reactive RA, and psoriatic arthritis often have cell counts in the range of 2–50 × 10³/μL.

Cytology

Examination and characterization of cells present in synovial fluid can provide the clinician with potentially useful information. The preparation of a wet mount of one drop of joint fluid aspiration is simple to perform. A drop of fluid is placed on a clean glass slide, which is then covered by cover slip and examined under low- and high-power light microscopy. This technique allows for the discovery of a wide variety of "objects," including cell clumps of fibrin, lipid droplets, crystals, cartilage, and synovium fragments. These "objects" may appear as amorphous material and be quickly dismissed as insignificant and go uncharacterized.

Correct identification of synovial fluid leukocytes is accomplished by staining a dry smear of the fluid. Proper phenotype and morphology of the leukocytes can then be determined under high power using oil immersion. Specific cells types are associated with causes of synovial fluid effusion and are shown in Table 12-5 ★.

Monocyte morphology varies from typical appearance in peripheral blood to an activated, enlarged form with a preponderance of cytoplasm and some vacuoles. Sometime during the activation process, the monocyte is called a histocyte.

A monocyte/histocyte that is observed to have ingested material is termed a *macrophage*. Typical macrophages are large with dense nuclear chromatin. The nucleus appears round or flattened against

★ **TABLE 12-4** Clinical Features of Synovial Fluid by Groups

Measure	Normal	Group I (Non-Inflammatory)	Group II (Inflammatory)	Group III (Septic)	Group IV (Crystal Induced)	Group V (Hemorrhagic)
Volume (mL)(knee)	<3.5	Typically >3.0	Typically >3.0	Typically >3.0	Typically >3.0	Typically >3.0
Clarity	Transparent	Transparent	Opaque	Purulent, opaque	Cloudy, turbid, or white opaque	Opaque
Viscosity	Normal	High	Variable	Low	Low	NA
Mucin clot	Firm	Firm	Variable	Friable	NA	NA
Color	Clear	Clear/Yellow	Yellow to white	Yellow to white	White	Red-brown or xanthochromic
WBC × 10³/μL	<0.2	<2.0	2000–75,000*	>100	0.5–200	50–10,000
PMN, %	<25	<25	≥50	≥90	<90	<50
Culture	Neg	Neg	Neg	Typically positive	Neg	Variable
Crystals present	No	No	No	No	Yes	No
RBCs present	No	No	No	No	No	Yes
Blood glucose minus synovial fluid glucose, mg/dL	0–10	0–10	0–40	20–100	0–80	0–20

*WBC will vary depending upon specific inflammatory condition present.

★ **TABLE 12-5** Predominant Cell Types Found in Synovial Fluid and Their Associated Conditions

Condition	Cell Type
Septic (>50 × 10³ cells/μL)	PMN cells
Viral arthritis	Monocytes
Lupus erythematosus	Monocytes
Other connective tissue diseases	Monocytes
Active RA	PMN cells
Reactive arthritis	PMN cells
Psoriatic arthritis	PMN cells
Acute attacks of crystal induced arthritis	PMN cells
Early RA (on occasion)	"Ragocytes"
Parasitic infections	Eosinophils
Hypereosinophilic syndrome	Eosinophils

one side of the cell. There is a large amount of cytoplasm, which is commonly vacuolated. Some vacuoles in the cytoplasm may coalesce to form a "signet ring" cell. Macrophages can ingest a variety of material, including erythrocytes (erythrophages), neutrophils (neutrophages), lipids (lipophages), crystals, and microorganisms.[15]

A unique finding in some patients with active RA is a significant number of cells called **ragocytes**, which are granulocytes containing phagocytized immune complexes. Neutrophils exist intact and present with necrobiotic alternations characteristic of apoptotic cells with single or multiple dense, hyperchromic, homogenous nuclear composition. In patients with disease (e.g., RA) the neutrophil may have dark cytoplasmic material consisting of immune complexes in wet preparations. The presence of ragocytes may indicate an unfavorable prognosis for patients with active RA.[16,17]

A second type of unusual cell, the Reiter's cell, is described as a cytophagocytic mononuclear cell that has phagocytized apoptotic PMN cells. It has been hypothesized that this occurrence represents a pathway by which autolysis and release of damaging mediators from apoptotic PMN cells are avoided.[18]

Other cell types that may appear in synovial fluid specimens include eosinophils, which are associated with parasitic infection, urticarial or hypereosinophilic syndrome. Many laboratories may also include the use a cytocentrifuge to examine synovial fluid. Unfortunately the cost of equipment, labor, and skill required to prepare specimens may prohibit most laboratories from utilizing this excellent technique.

Polarized Light Microscopy

The crystals commonly found in synovial fluid possess a unique physical property. They have two different indices of refraction and are said to be birefringent. Birefringence can be detected by polarized light microscopy. The principles underlying polarized light microscopy are discussed in Chapter 7.

The presence of crystals in synovial fluid is often used by clinicians to differentiate gout from pseudogout. If no crystals are found in a synovial fluid specimen, then the likelihood that a patient has septic arthritis increases. The patient may be admitted to a healthcare facility, followed by initiation of intravenous antibiotic therapy.

Crystal identification using a polarized light microscope requires the use of a slide and cover slip that are free of dust, talc, and other particulate material. Crystals present in the specimen rotate the light and appear as bright objects in a dark field. It should be noted that birefringent debris may be distributed throughout the slide and should not be mistaken for crystals.

Typically, the initial step in using a polarized light microscope to examine a wet preparation of synovial fluid is to place the first-order red compensator below the upper filter, which serves to block out green light. This will cause any birefringent objects in the specimen to appear as a bright yellow or blue color in the red field created by the first-order compensator. While rotating birefringent crystals in the field of view relative to the axis of the first order compensator, the color shifts from yellow to blue or vice versa. Crystals that are yellow when aligned parallel to the axis of the compensator are negatively birefringent, and those that are blue are positively birefringent. Refer to Figure 12-4 ■ for a view of the color patterns for monosodium urate and calcium pyrophosphate crystals.

Specific identification of crystals in synovial fluid is accomplished by meticulous examination of both morphology of the specimen and birefringence under both low and high power, using the techniques described above. Monosodium urate (MSU) crystals appear as negative birefringent, needle-shaped objects, several of which may be intracellular due to phagocytosis by leukocytes in synovial fluid. Monosodium urate crystals are shown in Figure 12-5 ■. The number of MSU crystals present is typically large during an acute attack of gout. Calcium pyrophosphate dihydrate (CPPD) crystals are smaller, rhomboid rods or rectangle-shaped crystals that are weakly positive birefringent with positive elongation (blue) when aligned with the compensator axis. These crystals are present in patients with attacks of pseudogout.

Synovial fluid may contain other crystals that signify the presence of a pathology or anatomical irritation. Hydroxyapatite or basic calcium phosphate is present within the joint and in periarticular sites, such as the shoulder area, and are associated with osteoarthritis.

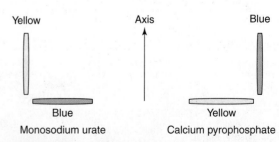

■ **FIGURE 12-4** Color Patterns of Monosodium Urate and Calcium Pyrophophate Crystals Produced at Both Parallel and Perpendicular Orientation to an Axis

☑ **CHECKPOINT 12-6**

Identify predominant cell types found in each of the following:

Septic arthritis (WBC > 50,000/μL) _____

Viral arthritis   _____

Gouty arthritis   _____

Early RA   _____

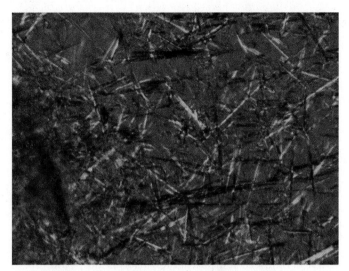

FIGURE 12-5 Monosodium Urate Crystals in Synovial Fluid

Hydroxyapatite crystals are not birefringent but may be detected by staining the fluid with alizarin red S and scanning for clumps of crystals under brightfield light microscopy.

Cholesterol crystals can appear in synovial fluid. They are characterized as flat, plate-like objects with notched corners. Lipid crystals have the appearance of a Maltese cross. These crystals can be strongly birefringent, either negative or positive. Corticosteroid crystals can be birefringent and appear similar to urate or CPPD crystals. The clinical significance of these crystals in synovial fluid remains uncertain, but it is unlikely that they are pathological in most cases.

Microbiology

Gram stain preparations should be included in arthrocentesis procedures as indicated in Figure 12-2.[19] Patients who present with septic or bacterial arthritis will show evidence of bacterial growth (i.e., positive Gram stain) in nearly 50% of cases.[20] Several different organisms can cause septic arthritis with Gram positive bacteria, for example *Staphylococci* and *Streptococci* being the most prevalent. Positive detection, identification, and initiation of antimicrobial therapies must be completed quickly because septic arthritis causes rapid destruction of the joint, has the ability to spread hematogenously to other areas, and is associated with significant mortality. Studies have shown that the sensitivity of a positive Gram stain approaches 100%, thus the positive predictive value for positive Gram stain is very high.[21] Furthermore, the gold standard for diagnosing septic arthritis is the bacterial culture, which has a diagnostic sensitivity of 75–95% and diagnostic specificity of 90% in cases of non-gonococcal septic arthritis.[22] Polymerase chain reaction (PCR) techniques are available for sensitive and specific detection of microorganism in synovial fluid and tissue, even in individuals who have negative cultures.[23]

Many bacteria can be detected using specific amplifying sequences in their ribosome RNA (16SrRNR). PCR has been shown to be a reliable technique for making the diagnosis of gonococcal arthritis.[24,25] It is also a highly sensitive and specific method of detecting tuberculous arthritis, although synovial tissue is a better specimen.[26,27] A virus is often the causative agent of acute infectious arthritis, and detection of viral DNA by nucleic acid amplification should be performed.

☑ CHECKPOINT 12-7

A laboratory technologist discovers the presence of calcium pyrophosphate dihyrate crystals in a synovial fluid. The technologist calls the findings to the clinician who states that the patient has gout. Does this microscopic finding support the clinician's assessment of the patient?

Biochemical Analysis

Measuring biochemical tests in synovial fluid provides supportive information or may add to the diagnostic impression of the clinician. Analytical specificity of some chemistry tests is problematic and therefore tends to limit their value.[28] Synovial fluid tests include glucose, total protein, and lactate dehydrogenase (LD), and the results should be compared to serum values. Additional tests include lactate, pH, uric acid, and hyaluronic acid. Patients with septic arthritis typically exhibit very low glucose, low pH, and high lactate, which indicate a switch by the body to anaerobic metabolism. Highly inflammatory synovial fluid in cases of RA will produce similar chemistry tests results, along with high protein and LD levels.

Mucin Clot Test

A mucin clot test is performed by adding acetic acid solution to synovial fluid, which will precipitate hyaluronan into the mucin clot. The precipitate is graded as good, fair, or poor. A fair to poor mucin clot test reflects dilutional depolymerization of hyaluronan. This is a nonspecific finding of several inflammatory types of arthritis.

Glucose

Synovial fluid glucose results ideally should be compared to the serum value and represent a fasting sample. This is not usually possible, though. The two glucose values are subtracted and the serum–synovial fluid differential is applied to clinical situations. A differential of <10 mg/dL is normal and is representative of many noninflammatory conditions. In septic arthritis, the differential may be from 20–60 mg/dL. *In vitro* glycolysis by a large number of leukocytes may falsely reduce synovial fluid glucose values unless tested within one hour of collection. Specimen stability is prolonged if the samples are drawn in a tube with sodium fluoride (NaF) an inhibitor of glycolysis.

Protein

Measuring synovial fluid proteins has little clinical significance due to non-specificity. Large proteins such as fibrinogen will enter the synovial space as the inflammation progresses. Spontaneous clot formation may occur in non-anticoagulated specimen tubes (fibrin clot test).

Enzymes

Lactate dehydrogenase is elevated in RA, gout, and infectious arthritis and may be due to the infiltration of leukocytes. Measurement of other enzymes (e.g., alkaline phosphatase, acid phosphatase, and aminoaspartate transaminase) has been studied, but none have provided clinically significant information and are not included in routine test menus.

Lactic Acid

Synovial fluid lactic acid levels are typically >30 mg/dL (S.I. units, 3.7 mmol/L) in patients with septic arthritis due to Gram positive cocci and Gram negative bacilli. Thus, quantitative analysis of synovial fluid lactate may provide the clinician with timely evidence of infection in specimens with negative Gram stains.

Uric Acid

Synovial fluid results normally parallel serum levels in patients with gout and other noninflammatory arthritic conditions. When correlating uric acid levels in body fluids, it is important to note the methods used for the analysis. The results produced are method dependent and may vary. Two methods are widely used in clinical laboratories: phosphotungstate and uricase. Synovial fluid urate levels may be significantly lower than in the paired serum in some inflammatory joint disorders other than gout.[29] Uric acid measurement in synovial fluid provides little clinical value in assessing patients with joint inflammation.

☑ CHECKPOINT 12-8

Arthur's synovial fluid glucose and lactic acid concentrations are elevated. Is this consistent with septic arthritis?

BRONCHOALVEOLAR LAVAGE

Bronchoalveolar lavage (BAL) is described as a bronchoscopy procedure that uses a flexible bronchoscope designed for retrieving cells and soluble substances from the fluid lining of the distal airways and alveolar units that contain immunologic components of the lungs.[30] The technique involves **lavage**, which is rinsing the organ with sterile saline. The procedure produces a specimen that is representative of endobronchial or transbronchial biopsy tissue and also cellular and immunologic components of vascular circulation. Specifically, BAL is a specimen that is part of a disease process or in close approximation to that disease. Examples of cells typically found in BAL are shown in Figure 12-6 ▪.

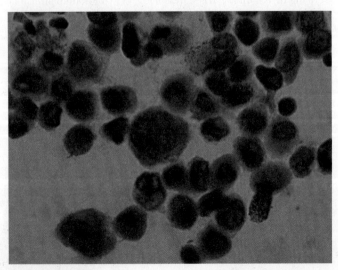

▪ **FIGURE 12-6**   Cells in a Bronchoalveolar Fluid Specimen

Aspiration and hemorrhage from BAL should be suspected in the presence of lipid and hemosiderin-laden macrophages, respectively, although lipid-laden macrophages can also be found in other conditions. Lavage fluids can be assessed for cell counts, surfactant proteins, and inflammatory mediators.[30] Transbronchial biopsy may have a role in diagnosing diffuse lung diseases such as sarcoidosis. This technique in children is limited to assessment of infection and rejection in transplant patients due to poor diagnostic yield in most conditions.[31]

Clinical Significance

The medical usefulness of BAL includes evaluating patients with interstitial lung disease, as well as infectious, noninfectious, immunologic, and malignant diseases. Several specific conditions are shown in Table 12-6 ★.[33,34,35]

Acute eosinophilic pneumonia is a rare disorder that is characterized by diffuse acute hypoxemic respiratory failure (AHRF) due to eosinophilic infiltrates in the lungs.[36] It is a form of acute respiratory distress syndrome and initiation of BAL with an estimation of the percentage of eosinophils is recommended.

A bedside bronchoscopy with BAL can be diagnostic for diffuse alveolar hemorrhage (DAH). It is common that the bronchoscopy will not produce fresh blood in the trachea and major bronchi. However, BAL usually produces a bloody specimen, which may deepen in red color as the lavage continues. A DAH can occur in the first week or two post-bone marrow transplantation, Goodpasture's syndrome, systemic lupus erythematous, and inhalation of crack cocaine.[37]

Bronchoalveolar lavage may be appropriate for patients with pulmonary alveolar proteinosis. Patients with this condition produce excess amounts of surfactant and fail to expel it. They typically present to their clinician with dyspnea and bilateral consolidation on the chest radiograph. A BAL may be indicated when the patient experiences worsening dyspnea and severe hypoxemia. The procedure may dictate that only one lung is lavaged at a time, giving the patient time to recover before the other lung is subjected to a lavage. It is a common practice that both lungs undergo BAL at the same time. In this case the clinician must ensure that the patient is being oxygenated effectively.[38]

Additional clinical disorders that may warrant BAL include Langerhans cell histiocytosis, alveolar hemorrhage, and dust exposure.

★ **TABLE 12-6** BAL Findings in Selected Conditions Associated with Interstitial Lung Disease

Condition	BAL Finding
Asbestos-related pulmonary disease	Dust particles, ferruginous bodies
Alveolar proteinosis	Milky effluent, foamy macrophages, and lipoproteinaceous intra-alveolar material
Eosinophilic lung disease	Eosinophils >25%
Diffuse alveolar damage, drug toxicity	Atypical hyperplastic type II pneumocytes
Opportunistic infections	Pneumocystis carinii, fungi, cytomegalovirus-transformed cells
Diffuse alveolar hemorrhage (DAH)	Red blood cells, hemosiderin-laden macrophages
Sarcoidosis	Lymphocytosis

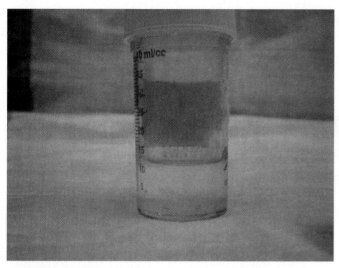

■ **FIGURE 12-7** Bronchoalveolar Lavage Fluid

BAL may also complement high-resolution computerized tomography (CT) and provides additional information in determining whether to proceed with a surgical biopsy.[39]

Specimen Collection, Handling, and Transport

The procedure required to obtain a specimen uses a fiberoptic bronchoscope that is wedged into a midsize segmental bronchus, and aliquots of sterile saline are instilled and aspirated into the alveolar spaces. This technique allows for aspiration of cells and organism in the alveoli distant to the bronchoscope. Approximately 100–300 mL of sterile saline administered in 20–50 mL aliquots is typically used to instill the fluid. Figure 12-7 ■ is an example of a BAL. The first aliquot should be discarded. The remaining aliquots may be processed separately or pooled for further analysis. Patients with diffuse lung disease will usually have the middle or lingular lobe used as the site for BAL.[40]

Removal of instilled solution should be performed with as little trauma as possible. The recovery of fluid is commonly in the range of 50–70%. Recoveries of less than 25% can occur in patients with chronic obstructive lung disease (COPD). Low recoveries should be documented on the appropriate forms being submitted to the laboratory.

Transport of BAL to the laboratory should be quick and specimens should be kept at room temperature. Analysis of cell number, viability, and differential count should be completed within three hours. Cellular features may begin to deteriorate after approximately 6 hours. Specimen that cannot be processed within 36 hours should be discarded.[41]

☑ CHECKPOINT 12-9

What are some examples of the clinical usefulness of BAL?

SWEAT

Chloride is the major extracellular anion, with median plasma and interstitial fluid concentrations of ~ 103 mmol/L. Chloride ions contribute the majority of the total inorganic anion concentration of ~ 154 mmol/L. Sodium plus chloride represents the majority of the

BOX 12-3 Elevated Sweat Electrolytes in Diseases/Conditions Other Than Cystic Fibrosis

Anorexia nervosa
Autonomic dysfunctions
Environmental deprivation
Glucose-6-phosphate dehydrogenase deficiency
Glycogen storage disease: type I
Hypogammaglobulinemia
Klinefelter's syndrome
Nephrogenic diabetes insipidus
Nephrosis
Protein calorie malnutrition
Pseudohypoaldosteronism
Psychosocial failure to thrive
Untreated adrenal insufficiency
Untreated hypothyroidism

SWEAT TESTING: SAMPLE COLLECTION AND QUANTITATIVE ANALYSIS: APPROVED GUIDELINE, 3rd ed, from The Clinical and Laboratory Standards Institute. Reproduced by permission of The Clinical and Laboratory Standards Institute.

osmotically active constituent of plasma. The chloride ion concentration in the intracellular fluid of erythrocytes is 45–55 mmol/L, and in the intracellular fluid of most other tissue cells, it is only ~ 1.0 mmol/L. Normal amounts of chloride in sweat are 5–35 mmol/L. Measuring chloride levels in sweat is useful in patients with cystic fibrosis (CF). Patients with this disease tend to lose an increased amount of chloride in their sweat.

Other diseases and conditions that may present with abnormal sweat electrolyte concentration are listed in Box 12-3.[42]

Cystic Fibrosis

The principal clinical utility for sweat testing, especially testing for chloride, is to evaluate patients with possible CF. Cystic fibrosis is characterized by abnormally viscous mucous secretions from the various exocrine glands of the body, including the pancreas, salivary glands, peribronchial glands, and sweat glands. Involvement of the intestinal glands may result in the presence of meconium ileus at birth. Approximately two-thirds of cases of CF are diagnosed before 1 year of age. Chronic lung disease and malabsorption resulting from pancreatic insufficiency are the major clinical problems of those who survive beyond infancy.

The diagnosis of CF is usually accomplished by utilization of a combination of clinical criteria and abnormal cystic fibrosis transmembrane conductance regulator (CFTR) gene functions documented by sweat tests, nasal potential difference (PD) measurement, and CFTR mutations analysis.[43]

Nasal Potential Difference Test

Cystic fibrosis is caused by abnormal physiologic events in sodium chloride transport that results from a defective CFTR protein. This protein serves as a chloride channel that controls the salt content in the fluid that covers the surface of the nose and lungs. Movement of sodium and chloride produces an electric PD across the airway lining. The mechanism is shown in Figure 12-8 ■. The PD developed

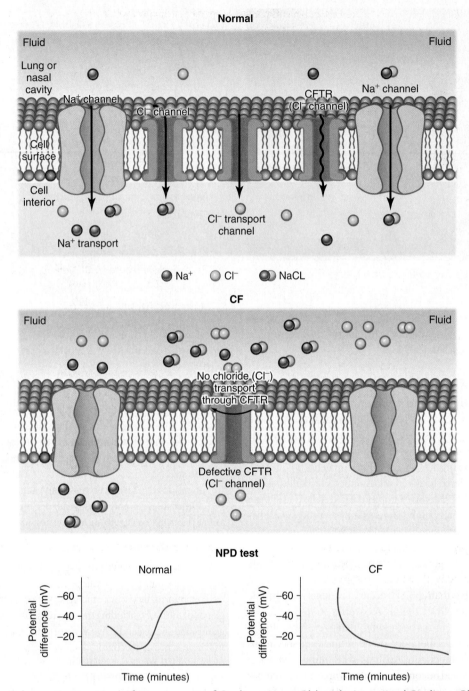

■ **FIGURE 12-8**   Schematic Drawing of Movement of Sodium Ions, Chloride Ions, and Sodium Chloride from the Cell Interior of Lung and Nasal Tissue to the Lung or Nasal Cavities Via Electrolyte Channels

The top drawing represents a normal distribution, and the middle drawing shows the effects of cystic fibrosis. The bottom left and right plots are the results of a NPD test for a normal patient (i.e., no cystic fibrosis) and a patient with cystic fibrosis.

within the nasal passage, or nasal potential difference (NPD), is measured by placing an electrode on the lining of the nose. The lining of the nose is rinsed in a series of solutions that contain different concentrations of salts. The electrolyte solutions are made to facilitate a predicable change in NPD. The patient's measured PD overtime is monitored. Because patients with CF either don't make CFTR chloride channels or have mutated forms of CFTR, the potentials across their nasal epithelium respond differently to the infusing of the various solutions. Three specific features of the NPD test distinguish patients who have CF from those who do not:

1. More negative baseline PD
2. A greater inhibition of NPD after addition of the solution containing amiloride
3. Small changes in NPD after rinsing with chloride-free solution and isoproterenol

The NPD test is not commercially available. Also, only a few CF centers nationally can perform the test.[44]

CFTR Mutation Analysis

DNA analysis of the most common mutations can identify CF mutations in >90% of affected patients. The basis for the test relies on the following genetic principle: All individuals carry two copies of the CFTR gene, one inherited from the father and one inherited from the mother. The CFTR gene is located on chromosome 7 and encodes a chloride channel of the same name that sits on the surface of specialized cells throughout the body. The criterion for a person to have CF is that they must have two abnormal copies—or mutations—of the CFTR gene. If an individual has only one mutation, he or she will not develop CF, but will be a "carrier." Carriers can pass this gene to their offspring, placing their children at risk for CF.

Nearly 1,000 CFTR mutations have been identified. In the Caucasian population, the most common mutation is call the ΔF508 mutation, which is found in approximately 70% of patients with CF. There are commercially available DNA tests whose accuracy depends on how many mutations are tested and the ethnic origin of the patients.[45]

Lung Disease

The major focuses of treatment modalities for CF are to promote clearance of secretions and control infections in the lungs, provide adequate nutrition, and prevent intestinal obstruction. Unfortunately, more that 95% of CF patients die of complications from lung infections. The reasons for these fatal outcomes include failure to maintain effective clearance of pulmonary secretions, inability of the body to reduce airway obstruction, and eventual onset of infection.

Gastrointestinal Disease

Patients with CF are required to maintain adequate nutrition. Many will need pancreatic enzyme replacement. Replacement of fat-soluble vitamins, particularly vitamins E and K, is often required. Hyperglycemia usually manifests itself in adults and requires insulin to regulate blood glucose concentrations. Patients may acquire acute distal intestinal obstruction and require medical intervention. Many patients will develop cholestasis liver disease or end-stage liver disease, which further complicates the overall medical situation of the patient.

☑ CHECKPOINT 12-10

Explain the association of CFTR protein and chloride channels.

Sweat Testing

Sweat Collection

There are two major steps involved in procuring a sweat sample: sweat stimulation and sweat collection. The first step requires a technique that will result in a sufficient amount of sweat produced by the patient. The technique routinely used is iontophoresis, which requires a cholinergic alkaloid compound, typically pilocarpine nitrate. **Iontophoresis** refers to the movement of small ions in an electric field. This movement is facilitated by pilocarpine, which stimulates sweat glands to produce sweat. The electric field is produced by the application of two electrodes, positive and negative, to the skin surface, which sends a small electrical current through the skin at the application site.

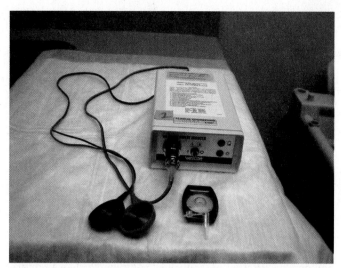

■ FIGURE 12-9   Items Required to Collect Sweat Samples from Patients that Includes a Power Source, Two Electrodes, a Macroduct Collection Device, and a Small Conical Sample Tube for Micro Volume of Sweat

The sweat produced can be collected using pre-weighed gauze or filter paper or into Macroduct coils. Whichever collection techniques are used, care must be taken to prevent evaporation and contamination of the specimen. A detailed procedure for stimulation and collection is provided in the reference cited.[46]

Patients should be at least 48 hours old before performing a sweat electrolyte measurement due to the variation in electrolyte levels.[47] The patient should be physiologically and nutritionally stable, well hydrated, not receiving mineral corticoids, and free of acute illness. The preferred site for specimen collection is the inner surface of the forearm, either left or right. Testing can be conducted on the patient upper leg if necessary. An example of items required to collect sweat samples from patients is shown in Figure 12-9 ■.

☑ CHECKPOINT 12-11

What type of compound is pilocarpine and why is it used in the sweat chloride procedure?

Qualitative Screening

Sweat testing using qualitative methods or screening tests may or may not measure the amount of sweat collected. Also, the results are typically reported as positive, negative, or borderline, but there are exceptions where some qualitatative devices may report actual chloride concentration. Patients with a positive or borderline result should have a quantitative measurement of chloride by coulometric titration, (e.g., a chloridometer) performed for confirmation of screening results. Screening tests may have a role in small facilities where test volumes are low. The Cystic Fibrosis Foundation (CFF) guidelines consider the following techniques not appropriate for sweat testing:[48,49]

1. Direct application of a chloride electrode to the patient's skin
2. Chloride precipitation reaction by placing a patch directly on the patient's skin

3. Measuring only potassium or sodium
4. Measuring osmolality
5. Conductivity testing including Sweat Check or Nanoduct (Wescor, Logan, UT)
6. Any other screening or qualitative tests

Note: CFF has approved the Wescor Macroduct Sweat-Check conductivity analyzer for screening at clinical sites, such as community hospitals, using the criterion that an individual having a sweat conductivity ≥50 mmol/L should be referred to an accredited cystic fibrosis (CF) care center for a quantitative sweat chloride test.[50]

Quantitative Analysis

Quantitative analysis of chloride in sweat is preferred over sodium because the former provides better discrimination in diagnosis.[51] Chloride in sweat can be measured using conductimetry and coulometric titration in tandem with amperometry (e.g., chloridometer) or manual titration using mercuric nitrate as a titrant to complex the chloride ion. If a laboratory considers an automated method using an ion selective electrode (ISE) to measure sweat sodium, potassium, or chloride, it must validate the assay for accuracy, precision, and lower limit of detection. For sweat chlorides, the lower limit of detection is typically 10 mmol/L. The functional upper limit for sweat chloride is typically 160 mmol/L.[52] This level is not physiologically possible. Therefore, if a patient's result exceeds this level, it will be due to either specimen contamination or analytical error.

Conductimetry

Electrolytic conductivity is a measure of the ability of a solution to carry an electrical current. Solutions of electrolytes conduct an electrical current by migration of ions under the influence of a potential gradient. The ions move at a rate that depends on their charge, size, the microscopic viscosity of the medium, and the magnitude of the electropotential gradient. This electrochemical principle can be applied to the measurement of chloride ion in sweat.

Conductimetry measurement of chloride in sweat correlates well with coulometric assays.[53,54] The decision limits for sweat conductivity have not been fully elucidated. According to the CFF, a patient with a sweat conductivity ≥50 mmol/L should be referred for a confirmatory (quantitative) sweat chloride test. Wescor, the manufacturer of the sweat conductivity analyzer, recommends that conductivity values up to 60 mmol/L can be considered normal and concentration >80 mmol/L are positive for CF.[55]

Coulometry

Laboratory application of coulometry includes the measurement of chloride ion in serum, plasma, CSF, and sweat samples by titration. A **coulometric titration** employs a titrant that is electrically generated by a constant electrical current. The active electrode process involves generation of silver ions, which are produced at the silver anode. The electrical current is carefully maintained at a constant and accurately known level by means of an amperostat. The amount of this current in amperes along with the time in seconds required to reach an end point yields the number of coulombs, which is proportional to the quantity of chloride involved in the electrolysis.

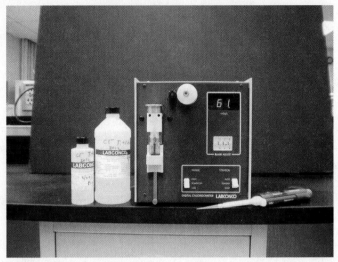

■ **FIGURE 12-10** A Chloridometer or Chloride Titrator. Displayed in the Figure are a Container of Reagent, 100 mEq/L Chloride Standard Solution, Pipette, and Reaction Vessel Filled with Reagent and 2.0 μL of a Sweat Sample

Amperometry

Amperometry is the measurement of the electrical current flow produced by an oxidation-reduction reaction. Amperometric methods have been used in clinical laboratories for decades. Several immobilized enzyme electrodes, including glucose, use this principle as well as PO_2 electrodes and chloride titrators.

The measurement of chloride in biological fluids involves the use of two electrochemical methods: coulometry and amperometry (both have been discussed above). The chloride titrator uses a pair of silver electrodes that serve as indicator electrodes. When all of the chloride ions have been complexed to silver and an excess of silver ions appear, an electrical current is generated that causes the coulometric generation of silver ions to cease. This represents the end-point of the titration. Figure 12-10 ■ shows a chloridometer with ancillary items.

Interpretation of Sweat Tests

The interpretive data shown in Table 12-7 ★ are provided as reliable guidelines for laboratories engaged in sweat testing or considering such testing.[56]

Sources of Errors in Sweat Testing

Errors in sweat testing may arise because of technical issues, unreliable methods, and errors in interpretation. Qualitative methods that do not quantitate sweat collected or do not have an established minimum sample volume or weight are subject to false-negative results because an adequate sweat rate cannot be ensured.

Sweat testing is subject to other potential sources of errors caused by evaporation of the specimen, contamination of the specimen, problems with electrodes and vessels, dilution issues, instrument miscalibration, failure to clean both sets of electrodes, problems with sample identification, and mistakes in reporting results. These problems occur more commonly in laboratories that do not perform many sweat test

★ **TABLE 12-7** CFF Guidelines for Interpretation of Sweat Tests

Concentration, mmol/L (mEq/L)	Interpretation
Sweat chloride	
≤6 months:	
≤29	CF is very unlikely
30–59	CF is possible
≥60	CF is likely to be diagnosed
>6 months:	
≤39	Very unlikely
40–59	CF possible
≥60	CF is likely to be diagnosed
Notes:	
1. All positive tests must be confirmed with a repeat sweat chloride test at a different time or another diagnostic test.	
2. Despite the availability of genetic testing, a quantitative pilocarpine iontophoresis sweat chloride test remains the gold standard for the diagnosis of CF.	
Sweat sodium (iontophoresis)	
Normal Child and Adult	40 mmol/L (mEq/L)
Cystic Fibrosis	70–190 mmol/L (mEq/L)

procedures. Problems with interpreting results are due to lack of knowledge about the methodology, failure to repeat borderline and positive results, failure to repeat negative test results when inconsistent with the clinical picture, and failure to repeat testing in patients diagnosed as CF who do not follow the expected clinical course. Patients who experience malnutrition, dehydration, eczema, and rash can have an increase in sweat electrolytes.[57]

Quality Assurance

Sweat chloride collection and measurement involves many manual techniques that require a high level of skill and knowledge. The measurement principles are electrochemical in nature that possesses inherent potentials for errors such as electrical drift and spikes. Each laboratory should initiate a quality assurance program that encompasses all aspects of the testing process including preanalytical, analytical, and postanalytical.

Preanalytical Phase

The Cystic Fibrosis Foundation recommends that duplicate testing from two body sites be performed, although for many laboratories this is not practical.[58] If duplicate testing is performed, the concentrations should agree within ± 5 mmol/L, although it is recommended that each laboratory establishes its limits of agreement. Stimulation and collection procedures should minimize the opportunity for evaporation and contamination of the sweat samples. The patient's skin at the site of collection should be free of infection or rash.

Analytical Phase

Two quality control samples should be assayed with each analytical run in accordance with the Clinical Laboratory Improvement Act of 1988 (CLIA, 1988).[59] The control levels should represent a negative and positive value. If sweat is collected on gauze or filter paper, the control material should be applied directly to the collection surface and eluted for analysis.

An important aspect of laboratory quality assurance is participation in an external quality control or proficiency program. The College of American Pathologists (CAP) offers a comprehensive sweat testing proficiency program.[60] The program provides several samples for analysis to the particpants. The survey participants provide measurements for chloride, sodium, and osmolality using collection techniques which includes, Macroduct coils, preweighed filter paper, and preweighed gauze. Sample measuring instruments included an automated electrolyte analyzer, digital chloridometer, and conductivity cell.

Postanalytical Phase

Interpretation of sweat tests results must be in association with the patient's clinical presentation by a physician knowledgeable about CF. There are many conditions other than CF that are associated with elevations in sweat electrolytes. Refer to Box 12-3 for some examples.

☑ CHECKPOINT 12-12

What is the reason why some laboratories tend to make more mistakes performing sweat testing than others?

Key Points to Remember

- The significant findings in a microscopic examination of synovial fluid for patients with gouty arthritis are the presence of needle-shaped, negatively birefringent sodium urate crystals.
- Elevated serum uric acid levels are a consistent finding in patients with gouty arthritis.
- Knowledge of the principles of polarized light microscopy is essential for microscopic examination of synovial fluid.
- Bronchoalveolar lavage is a sampling technique that is involved with a disease or in close approximation to that disease.

- The diagnosis of cystic fibrosis is usually accomplished by utilization of a combination of clinical criteria and abnormal cystic fibrosis transconductance regulator (CFTR) gene functions documented by sweat tests, nasal PD measurement, and CFTR mutations analysis. The most widely used quantitative method for sweat chloride testing is the chloridometer, which uses two electrochemical techniques, coulometry and amperometry.
- The techniques required to measure sweat in chloride require understanding of the sources of errors in sweat testing.

Review Questions

Level I

1. Synoviocytes are the main source of which of the following compounds? (Objective 1)

   A. Uric acid

   B. Hyaluronic acid

   C. Lactic acid

   D. Hemoglobin

2. Which of the following techniques is used to withdraw fluid from a synovial joint? (Objective 4)

   A. Iontophoresis

   B. Artericentesis

   C. Lavage

   D. Arthrocentesis

3. Which of the following crystals can be present in a patient with gouty arthritis? (Objective 2)

   A. Needle-shaped, negatively birefringent monosodium pyruvate

   B. Needle-shaped, negatively birefringent monosodium urate

   C. Rhomboid, positively birefringent calcium pyrophosphate

   D. Octagonal, sheet-like crystals

4. Why should powdered preparation of anticoagulants not be used in tubes for synovial fluid analysis? (Objective 4)

   A. They may interfere with cell counts.

   B. They may interfere with glucose tests.

   C. They may interfere with crystal examination.

   D. They may distort differential cell counts.

5. Synovial fluid hemarthrosis can result from which of the following? (Objective 4)

   A. A motor vehicle accident

   B. A spinal tap

   C. Leakage of fluid into the peritoneum

   D. Pilocarpine stimulation of the sweat glands

6. What is the color of the crystals that are shaped like needles and aligned perpendicular to the slow vibration of compensated polarized light? (Objective 2)

   A. Green

   B. Blue

   C. Violet

   D. Yellow

7. Which crystals are associated with pseudogout? (Objective 2)

   A. Calcium pyrophosphate

   B. Calcium sulfate

   C. Monosodium urate

   D. Monosodium phosphate

8. Lavage is a termed used to describe (Objective 6)

   A. the mixing of organ contents with an organic solvent.

   B. the flushing of an organ with antibiotics.

   C. the rinsing of an organ with sterile saline.

   D. weighing organs to determine total fluid content.

9. Which of the following procedures is used for bronchoalveolar lavage? (Objective 6)

   A. Endoscopy

   B. Fluoroscopy

   C. Colonoscopy

   D. Bronchoscopy

10. A bronchoalveolar lavage of a patient's lung that has a diffuse alveolar bleeding may reveal the presence of (Objective 6)

    A. red blood cells and hemosiderin-laden macrophages.

    B. eosinophils.

    C. dust particles.

    D. foamy macrophages.

11. Sweat testing is best used for which of the following: (Objective 10)

    A. Evaluating patients with lung carcinoma

    B. Evaluating patients with the flu

    C. Evaluating patient with possible cystic fibrosis

    D. Assessing patients with achlorhydria

12. What is the purpose of pilocarpine that is used in the collection of sweat? (Objective 10)

    A. Stimulate salivation

    B. Stimulate sweating

    C. Inhibit stimulation of chloride exiting the skin pores

    D. Stimulate gastrointestinal release of chloride

13. What two electrochemical techniques are used in a chloridometer? (Objective 10)

    A. Coulometry and potentiometry

    B. Amperometry and potentiometry

    C. Resistivity and conductimetry

    D. Coulometry and amperometry

Level II

1. The quality control results for both levels of chloride assayed on the chloridometer were −2.2 standard deviations from the mean. The technologist re-assayed the controls, and they were outside two standard deviations. Which of the following would be the most likely cause of the out of control situation? (Objective 5)

   A. The technologist used 100 μL pipettor instead of a 20 μL pipettor.

   B. The chloridometer miscalculated the concentrations of the controls.

   C. The technologist used serum-based controls instead of sweat-based controls.

   D. The technologist failed to clean the silver electrodes used for the coulometric generation of silver ions.

2. A clinician calls the laboratory and questions a sweat chloride result on a patient. The basis of the complaint was that the patient's sweat chloride was lower than anticipated. The clinical laboratory used the Macroduct sample collection system and a chloridometer to measure the concentration of chloride. Which of the following may have caused a spuriously low sweat chloride result? (Objective 5)

   A. The humidity in the room was higher than normal.

   B. An inadequate sweat rate was generated during the sweat collection procedure.

   C. The patient was sweating profusely before the procedure began.

   D. The sodium concentration was exceedingly high.

3. The laboratory director requests that the supervisor move her quantitative sweat chloride assay from the chloridometer to an automated chemistry analyzer. Which of the following tasks must be completed per the Cystic Fibrosis Committee before the automated assay is deemed acceptable for patient care testing? (Objective 6)

   A. Only perform a carryover study.

   B. Only update the linearity of the assay.

   C. The assay's analytical precision, accuracy, reportable range, and sensitivity must be determined.

   D. Only update the procedure manual.

4. A patient with suspected gouty arthritis was sent to an urgent care facility, and a serum uric acid was measured. The result was slightly abnormal. The urgent care physician suggested that the patient go to the arthritis clinic at the local hospital for further evaluation. A serum uric acid was determined by the hospital laboratory and the results were normal. What could account for the discordant serum uric acid results? (Objective 5)

   A. The two methods used different reagents

   B. High dose hook effect

   C. Different sample volumes

   D. Different venipuncture site cleansing compounds

5. A technologist examining a synovial fluid using a polarized light microscopy can see crystals but they are not yellow, blue, or any other color. What may be the problem? (Objective 4)

   A. The light intensity from the lamp was not high enough.

   B. The technologist was not using the proper objective.

   C. The technologist forgot to place the red compensator into position.

   D. The microscope prism monochromator was not aligned properly.

Endnotes

1. Hellmann DB, Imboden JB. Musculoskeletal & immunologic disorders. In: Papadakis MA, McPhee SJ, Rabow MD, eds. *Current Medical Diagnosis & Treatment*. 52nd ed. New York: McGraw Hill Companies, 2013.

2. Martinon F, Petrilli V, Mayor A, et al. Gout associated uric acid crystals activate the NALP3 inflammasome. *Nature* (2006) 440:237–241.

3. Hellmann DB, Imboden JB. Musculoskeletal & immunologic disorders. In: Papadakis MA, McPhee SJ, Rabow MD, eds. *Current Medical Diagnosis & Treatment*. 52nd ed. New York: McGraw Hill Companies, 2013.

4. Clinical and Laboratory Standards Institute (CLSI). *Body Fluid Analysis for Cellular Composition; Approved Guideline*. Wayne, PA.: Clinical and Laboratory Standards Institute; 2006. CLSI document H56-A.

5. McCarty DJ. Synovial fluid. In: Koopman WJ, ed. *Arthritis and Allied Conditions*. 14th ed. Philadelphia: Lippincott Williams and Wilkins, 2001: pp. 83–104.

6. Kjeldsberg C, Knight J. *Body fluids: Laboratory Examination of Amniotic, Cerebrospinal, Seminal, Serous and Synovial Fluids*. 3rd edition, Chicago: American Society of Clinical Pathology Press (ASCP), 1993.

7. Freemont AJ, Denton J, Chuck A, et al. Diagnostic value of synovial fluid microcopy: a reassessment and rationalization. *Ann Rheum Dis* (1991) 50:101–107.

8. Baxendale RH, Ferrell WR, Wood L. Intra-articular pressure during active and passive movement of normal and distended human knee. *J Physiol* (1985) 369:179–182.

9. Jayson MIV, Dixon A St. J. Intra-articular pressure in rheumatoid arthritis of the knee. III. Pressure changes during joint use. *Ann Rheum Dis* (1970) 29:401–408.

10. Swan DA, Slayer HS, Silver FH. The molecular structure of lubricating glycoprotein-I. The boundary lubricant for articular cartilage. *J Biol Chem* (1981) 256:5921–5925.

11. Clinical and Laboratory Standards Institute (CLSI). *Body Fluid Analysis for Cellular Composition; Approved Guideline*. Wayne, PA.: Clinical and Laboratory Standards Institute; 2006. CLSI document H56-A.

12. Clinical and Laboratory Standards Institute (CLSI). *Body Fluid Analysis for Cellular Composition; Approved Guideline*. Wayne, PA.: Clinical and Laboratory Standards Institute; 2006. CLSI document H56-A.

13. Clinical and Laboratory Standards Institute (CLSI). *Body Fluid Analysis for Cellular Composition; Approved Guideline*. Wayne, PA.: Clinical and Laboratory Standards Institute; 2006. CLSI document H56-A.

14. Kjeldsberg C, Knight J. *Body fluids: Laboratory Examination of Amniotic, Cerebrospinal, Seminal, Serous and Synovial Fluids*. 3rd edition, Chicago: American Society of Clinical Pathology Press (ASCP), 1993.

15. Clinical and Laboratory Standards Institute (CLSI). *Body Fluid Analysis for Cellular Composition; Approved Guideline*. Wayne, PA.: Clinical and Laboratory Standards Institute; 2006. CLSI document H56-A.

16. Clinical and Laboratory Standards Institute (CLSI). *Body Fluid Analysis for Cellular Composition; Approved Guideline.* Wayne, PA.: Clinical and Laboratory Standards Institute; 2006. CLSI document H56-A.

17. Davis MJ, Denton J, Freemont AJ, et al. Comparison of serial synovial fluid cytology in rheumatoid arthritis: delineation of subgroups with prognostic implications. *Ann Rheum Dis* (1988) 47:559–562.

18. Jones ST, Denton J, Holt PJ, et al. Possible clearance of effect PMN leukocytes from synovial fluid by cytophagocytic mononuclear cells: implications for pathogenesis and chronicity in inflammatory arthritis. *Ann Rheum Dis* (1993) 52:111–126.

19. El-Gabalawy HS. Synovial fluid analyses, synovial biopsy, and synovial pathology. In: Firestein: *Kelley's Textbook of Rheumatology.* 9th ed. Philadelphia: Elsevier Saunders, 2013.

20. Faraj AA, Omonbude OD, Godwin P. Gram staining in the diagnosis of acute septic arthritis. *Acta Orthop Belg* (2002) 68:388–391.

21. Shmerling RH. Synovial fluid analysis: a critical reappraisal. *Rheum Dis Clin North Am* (1994) 20:503–512.

22. Swan A, Amer H, Dieppe P. The value of synovial fluid assays in the diagnosis of joint disease: A literature survey. *Ann Rheum Dis* (2002) 61:493–498.

23. Jalava J, Skurnik M, Toivanen A, et al. Bacterial PCR in the diagnosis of joint infection. *Ann Rheum Dis* (2001) 60:287–289.

24. Muralidhar B, Rumore PM, Steiman CR. Use of the polymerase chain reaction to study arthritis due to *Neisseria gonorrhaeae. Arthritis Rheum* (1994) 37:710–717.

25. Liebling MR, Arkfeld DG, Michelini GA, et al. Identification of *Neisseria gonorrrhaeae* in synovial fluid using the polymerase chain reaction. *Arthritis Rheum* (1994) 37:702–709.

26. van der Heijden IM, Wilbrink B, Schouls LM, et al. Detection of mycobacteria in joint samples from patients with arthritis using a genus-specific polymerase chain reaction and sequence analysis. *Rheumatology (Oxford)* (1999) 38:547–553.

27. Titov AG, Vyshnevskaya EB, Mazurenko SI, et al. Use of polymerase chain reaction to diagnosis tuberculous arthritis from joint tissues and synovial fluid. *Arch Pathol Lab Med* (2004) 128:205–209.

28. Shmerling RH. Synovial fluid analysis: a critical reappraisal. *Rheum Dis Clin North Am* (1994) 20:503–512.

29. Beutler AM, Keenan GF, Soloway S, et al. Soluble urate in sera and synovial fluids from patients with different joint disorders. *Clin Exp Rheumatol* (1996) 14;3:249–254.

30. Reynolds HY. Use of bronchoalveolar lavage in humans. Past necessity and future imperative. *Lung* (2000) 178:271–293.

31. Federico MJ, Kerby GS, Deterding RR, et al. Respiratory tract & mediastinum. In: Papadakis MA, McPhee SJ, Rabow MD, eds. *Current Medical Diagnosis & Treatment.* 52nd ed. New York: McGraw Hill Companies, 2013.

32. Efrati O, Sadeh-Gornik U, Modan-Moses D, et al. Flexible bronchoscopy and bronchoalveolar lavage in pediatric patients with lung diseases. *Pediatr Crit Care Med* (2009) 10:80–84.

33. Costabel U, Guzman J. Bronchoalveolar lavage in interstitial lung disease. *Curr Opin Pulm Med* (2001) 7:255–261.

34. Rottoli P, Bargagli E. Is bronchoalveolar lavage obsolete in the diagnosis of interstitial lung disease? *Curr Opin Pulm Med* (2003) 9:418–425.

35. King TE. Interstitial lung disease. In: Longo DL, Fauci AS, Kasper DL. *Harrison's Principles of Internal Medicine.* 18th ed. New York: McGraw-Hill, 2012.

36. King TE. Interstitial lung disease. In: Longo DL, Fauci AS, Kasper DL. *Harrison's Principles of Internal Medicine.* 18th ed. New York: McGraw-Hill, 2012.

37. King TE. Interstitial lung disease. In: Longo DL, Fauci AS, Kasper DL. *Harrison's Principles of Internal Medicine.* 18th ed. New York: McGraw-Hill, 2012.

38. King TE. Interstitial lung disease. In: Longo DL, Fauci AS, Kasper DL. *Harrison's Principles of Internal Medicine.* 18th ed. New York: McGraw-Hill, 2012.

39. Lanken PN. Acute lung injury and the acute respiratory distress syndrome. In: Hall JB, Schmidt GA, Wood LD, eds. *Principles of Critical Care.* 3rd ed. New York: McGraw-Hill, 2005.

40. Clinical and Laboratory Standards Institute (CLSI). *Body Fluid Analysis for Cellular Composition; Approved Guideline.* Wayne, PA.: Clinical and Laboratory Standards Institute; 2006. CLSI document H56-A.

41. Clinical and Laboratory Standards Institute (CLSI). *Body Fluid Analysis for Cellular Composition; Approved Guideline.* Wayne, PA.: Clinical and Laboratory Standards Institute; 2006. CLSI document H56-A.

42. Clinical and Laboratory Standards Institute (CLSI). *Sweat testing: sample collection and quantitative analysis: approved guideline.* Wayne, PA: Clinical and Laboratory Standards Institute, 2000. CLSI document C34-A2.

43. Flume PA, Stenbit A. Making the diagnosis of cystic fibrosis. *Am J Med Sci* (2008) 335;1:51–54.

44. http://www.hopkinscf.org/main/whatiscf/diag_testnasal.html. Accessed March 10, 2014.

45. Guggino WB, Stanton BA. New insights into cystic fibrosis: molecular switches that regulate CFTR. *Nat Rev Mol Cell Biol* (2006) 7;6:426–436.

46. Clinical and Laboratory Standards Institute (CLSI). *Sweat testing: sample collection and quantitative analysis: approved guideline.* Wayne, PA: Clinical and Laboratory Standards Institute, 2000. CLSI document C34-A2.

47. Clinical and Laboratory Standards Institute (CLSI). *Sweat testing: sample collection and quantitative analysis: approved guideline.* Wayne, PA: Clinical and Laboratory Standards Institute, 2000. CLSI document C34-A2.

48. Cystic Fibrosis Foundation Center Committee. Sweat Testing Standard Memorandum, December 2006, Bethesda, Maryland.

49. LeGrys VA, Yankaskas JR, Quittell LM, et al. Diagnostic sweat testing: the cystic fibrosis foundation guidelines. *The J of Pediatrics* (2007):85–89.

50. CF Center Directors Update No. 1. Bethesda, MD: Cystic Fibrosis Foundation, 1990.

51. Gleeson M, Henry RL. Sweat sodium or chloride. *Clin Chem* (1991) 37;1:112.

52. Clinical and Laboratory Standards Institute (CLSI). *Sweat testing: sample collection and quantitative analysis: approved guideline.* Wayne, PA: Clinical and Laboratory Standards Institute, 2000. CLSI document C34-A2.

53. Tietz NW, Pruden EL. Siggaard Andersen O. Electrolytes. In Burtis CA, Ashwood ER, eds. *Tietz Textbook of Clinical Chemistry.* 2nd ed. Philadelphia: WB Saunders, 1994.

54. Lezana JL, Vargas MH, Karam-Bechara J, et al. Sweat conductivity and chloride titration for cystic fibrosis diagnosis in 3834 subjects. *J Cyst Fibros* (2003) 2:1–7.

55. http://www.wescor.com/biomedical/cysticfibrosis/sweatchek.html Accessed March 10, 2014.

56. Cystic Fibrosis Foundation Center Committee. Sweat Testing Standard Memorandum, December 2006, Bethesda, Maryland.

57. Rosenstein BJ, Cutting GR. The diagnosis of cystic fibrosis: A consensus statement. Cystic Fibrosis Foundation consensus panel. *J Pediatr* (1998) 132;4:589–595.

58. LeGrys VA, Yankaskas JR, Quittell LM, et al. Diagnostic sweat testing: the cystic fibrosis foundation guidelines. *The J of Pediatrics* (2007):85–89.

59. Health Care Financing Administration (42CFR part 493, et al) the Public Health Service, U.S. Department of Health and Human Services: Clinical Laboratory Improvements Amendments of 1988. Final Rule, *Federal Register* (1992) 57:7002–7288.

60. Comprehensive Sweat Analysis Set SW-B. Survey 2012 CAP, Chicago, IL: College of American Pathologists, 2012.

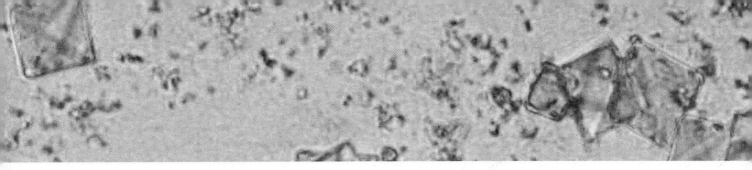

13

Semen, Pregnancy, and Amniotic Fluid

Objectives

LEVEL I

1. Describe the physical appearance, cellular consistency, and chemical composition of semen and amniotic fluid.
2. Identify several preanalytical issues that must be recognized when collecting, handling, and storing semen and amniotic fluid samples.
3. List several examples of laboratory tests performed on semen, amniotic fluid, and maternal serum that are used to assess patients in health and disease.
4. Discuss the techniques used to obtain specimens for semen and amniotic fluid analysis.
5. Predict the relative body fluid concentration of selected laboratory tests in disease.
6. Discuss issues associated with calibration and analyte specificity of hCG assays.
7. Define the following diseases/conditions/syndromes: gestational diabetes mellitus, neural tube defect, respiratory distress syndrome, erythroblastosis fetalis, preeclampsia, and Down syndrome.

LEVEL II

1. Explain the analytical principles for laboratory tests performed on semen and amniotic fluid.
2. Explain the clinical usefulness of laboratory tests available for semen, and amniotic fluid.
3. Discuss the impact of early prenatal testing on the mother and developing fetus and what may occur if these tests are not requested.
4. Interpret laboratory test results performed on semen and amniotic fluid obtained from adult males and females.
5. Correlate selected laboratory tests with fetal disorders.

Key Terms

Amnion	Erythroblastosis fetalis	Lamellar body	Surfactant
Amniocentesis	Fibronectin	Lecithin-sphingomyelin ratio	Triple test
Amniotic fluid	Gestational diabetes mellitus	Preeclampsia	Unconjugated estriol
Amniostat-FLM-PG	Hydramnios	Quad screen	
Down syndrome	Inhibin A	Sperm motility	

A CASE IN POINT

Sally, 24 years of age, went to her physician complaining of intermittent severe abdominal cramps and mild vaginal bleeding. A urine human chorionic gonadotropin (hCG) pregnancy test was performed in the doctor's office and the result was negative. Although the urine hCG was negative, her doctor was suspicious of her underlying condition and recommended that she go to the emergency department (ED) for further evaluation. The ED staff was able to estimate her gestational age to be 6 weeks based on her last missed period (LMP). A serum β-hCG test was requested and the result was 150 mU/mL. The reference interval for nonpregnant females is 0–5 mU/mL and for women at 6 weeks LMP typical concentrations of hCG are 10,000–80,000 mU/mL. An ultrasound was performed and revealed the possibility that an early gestational sac had formed in the uterus. Sally was discharged with a diagnosis of a threatened abortion.

Sally returned to the same ED seven days later with the same complaint: intermittent pain and mild vaginal bleeding. A serum β-hCG was requested and the result was 205 mU/mL. Women at 7 weeks LMP typically have concentrations of hCG between 90,000–500,000 mU/mL. An ultrasound revealed the presence of a gestation sac in the patient's right fallopian tube. No evidence of an intrauterine pregnancy was seen. The diagnosis was an unruptured ectopic pregnancy.

Questions to Consider

1. Why was the urine pregnancy test negative?
2. What other pathologies may present with similar signs, symptoms, and clinical findings?
3. Why are the β-hCG levels so low and how do they compare with β-hCG levels in a normally progressing intrauterine pregnancy (IUP)?
4. What are some treatment options available for Sally?

A spermatozoon unites with an ovum, and an embryo is created that resides in the amnion, *which contains liquor amnii.*

The approach to this chapter will be to move through this process, which involves participation of a male, a female, and eventually a fetus. The lives of a mother and fetus are intertwined, and the potential for harm to either or both is always present. The laboratory's role in health and disease for all participants will be discussed.

SEMEN

Semen analysis is used to evaluate reproductive dysfunction, particularly infertility, to select donors for therapeutic insemination, and to monitor the success of surgical procedures, such as varicocelectomy (excision of a portion of the scrotal sac) and vasectomy. Semen analysis consists of microscopic and macroscopic testing of seminal fluid.

Sample collection may involve obtaining both a semen and urine specimen. Patients need to follow the instructions provided by the clinician and laboratory staff to ensure the specimen collection is valid. There are specific specimen procurement procedures for different purposes. For example, the specimen requirements for assessing pathological disorders may be different than the requirements for assisted reproductive testing.

Macroscopic examination of seminal fluid should be performed after liquefaction of the specimen, which typically occurs within 20 minutes. The specimen should be thoroughly mixed and its viscosity recorded. The specimen volume must also be determined by weighing the collection cup before and after specimen collection. Specimen appearance should be noted and a pH measurement completed.

Microscopic examination of the specimen is required to determine sperm concentration, motility, and agglutination. The sample should be scanned for the presence of other cellular elements, such as polygonal cells of the urethral tract, and round cells, such as spermatogenic cells and leukocytes. Leukocytes can be counted using a hemocytometer. Sperm motility and velocity are assessed while the sample is on the hemocytometer.

Sperm motility is reported as the percentage of sperm that move. Forward movement is also noted and graded. A grade of 4 is given to sperm that present as rapidly moving in a straight line with little yaw and lateral movement. The lower grades indicate less active sperm activity and a grade of zero indicates that the sperm have no forward motion. Refer to Table 13-1 ★ for grading of sperm motility.

Sperm agglutination is also assessed for each sample. Agglutination occurs when motile sperm stick to each other in orientation

★ **TABLE 13-1** Sperm Motility

Grade	Description
0	Sperm not moving
1	Sperm moving with in-place motion (e.g., shaking or immobilized motion) with no forward progression.
2	Sperm moving with sluggish speed in a random direction
3	Sperm moving with reasonable speed in a linear direction
4	Sperm moving with fast speed in a linear direction

that is reproducible within a given specimen, for example, head-to-head, tail-to-tail orientation. Presentation of agglutination suggests an immunologic cause of infertility; therefore, it is important to document the occurrence.

Sperm morphology can indicate fertility. Typically, more than 50% of sperm in a specimen exhibit normal morphology. Specimens containing sperm with abnormal morphology usually have multiple defects. This occurrence can be estimated by determining the average number of defects per sperm and is designated as the *teratozoospermic index*. Several examples of microscopic findings are shown Figures 13-1 ■ to 13-4 ■.

Several immunologic tests are available to assess sperm viability. Sperm antibody binding to head or tail antigens is considered specific for immunologic infertility. Several antibodies are used, including IgG, IgA, and IgM. Current methodologies can detect sperm-bound antibodies by direct or indirect mixed agglutination reaction (MAR) tests for IgG and IgA, or by immunobead assays.

Patients that present with possible infertility based on their macroscopic and microscopic examination may have additional testing performed to further assess their condition. Several endocrine assays are available for this purpose and include testosterone, follicle stimulating hormone, and luteinizing hormone. These tests alone or in combination are useful for assessing a wide variety of male dysfunctions including infertility, ductal obstruction, gynecomastia, hypothalamic-pituitary disease, and tumors.

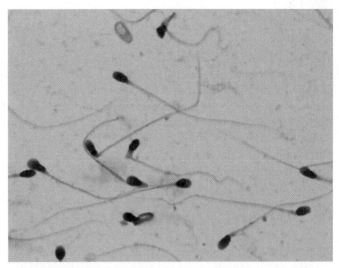

■ **FIGURE 13-2** Abnormal Spermatozoa with Elongated Heads

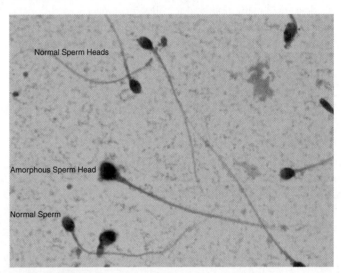

Normal Sperm Heads

Amorphous Sperm Head

Normal Sperm

■ **FIGURE 13-3** Amorphous Spermatozoa

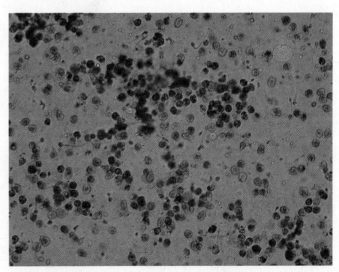

■ **FIGURE 13-4** Spermatozoa with Numerous Neutrophils Noting a Possible Seminal Infection

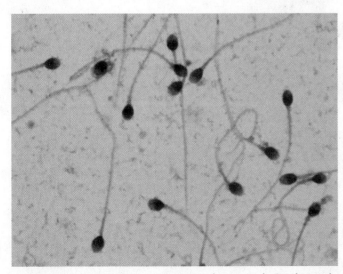

■ **FIGURE 13-1** Spermatozoa with Normal, Oval Heads

PREGNANCY
Placenta

The placenta and umbilical cord serve as a direct link between the mother and the fetus. The placenta grows throughout pregnancy and is usually delivered with the fetus at term. The connection is critical because it is a means by which the fetus is nourished, fetal waste is eliminated, and placental hormones are produced.

Hormones

Several hormones, both protein and sterols, are produced in the placenta and are shown in Figure 13-5 ■. The major hormones are chorionic gonadotropin (CG) also, human chorionic gonadotropin (hCG) and placental lactogen (PL) (also human chorionic somato-mammotropin (hCS). CG stimulates the ovary to produce progesterone, which, in turn, prevents menstruation, thereby protecting the pregnancy. CG will be discussed in detail later in this chapter. PL is a single polypeptide chain of 191 amino acids with two intermolecular disulfide bridges and a molecular mass of ~22 kilo Daltons (kDa). PL participates in many biological activities, including lactogenic, metabolic, somatotropic, luteotropic, erythropoietic, and aldosterone stimulating effects. Although PL has many functions, there is no apparent clinical reason to measure PL.

Maternal cholesterol is the precursor compound for steroid hormones, including placental progesterone and estrogen compounds.

The secretion of estrogens and progesterone throughout pregnancy ensures appropriate development of the endometrium, uterine growth, adequate uterine blood supply, and preparation of the uterus for labor. The measurement of most of these hormones is not considered necessary during pregnancy with the exception of estriol. Estimation of estriol, which is discussed in more detail later in the chapter, at 16 to 18 weeks gestational age is useful in predicting fetal trisomy 21 and 18.

Amniotic Fluid

Before the fetus develops, a non-restricting intrauterine environment develops. This environment exists only if it is part of the development of the fetus. The embryo resides within the amniotic cavity, which contains **amniotic fluid**. The **amnion**, which is the inner membrane in contact with the amniotic fluid, has a single layer of cuboidal cells lying on the basement membrane. These anatomic features are shown in Figure 13-6 ■. The functions of amniotic fluid include, (1) to protect the fetus; (2) to allow fetal movement and growth; (3) to maintain an even temperature; and (4) to participate in fetal biochemical homeostasis.[1] During the first half of the pregnancy, amniotic fluid volume seems to increase in association with growth of the fetus. The relative amounts of amniotic fluid volume for selected gestational ages are presented in Table 13-2 ★.[2] Coincidentally, the correlation between fetal weight and amniotic fluid is almost equivalent. Maternal serum analyte concentrations (e.g., sodium, creatinine, osmolality, and urea)

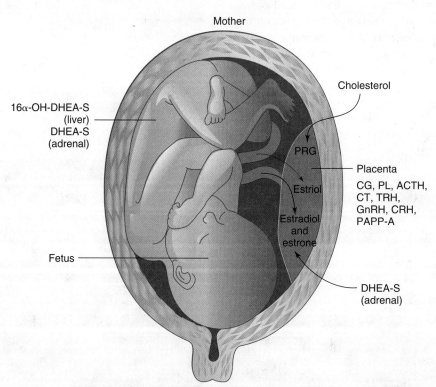

■ **FIGURE 13-5**   Original Distribution of Hormones and Proteins in Mother, Fetus, and Placenta. DHEA-S, Dehydroepiandrosterone Sulfate; PRG, Progesterone; CG, Chorionic Gonadotropin; PL, Placental Lactogen; ACTH, Adrenocorticotropic Hormone; CT, Chorionic Thyrotropin; TRH, Thyrotropin-releasing hormone; GnRH, Gonadotropin-Releasing Hormone; CRH, Corticotropin-Releasing Hormone; and PAPP-A, Pregnancy Associated Plasma Protein-A

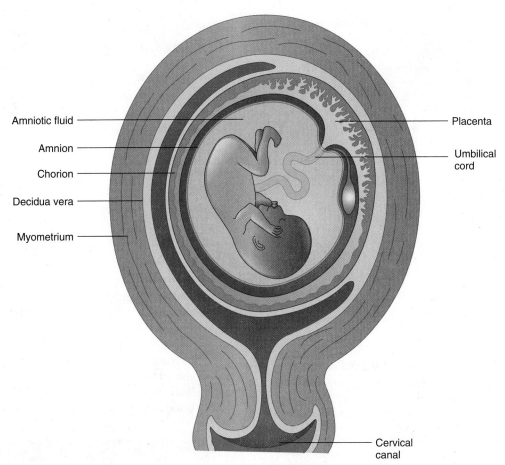

Amniotic fluid

Amnion

Chorion

Decidua vera

Myometrium

Placenta

Umbilical cord

Cervical canal

■ **FIGURE 13-6**   Schematic Drawing of Key Features of the Amniotic Cavity Environment Surrounding the Developing Fetus

are not very different than amniotic fluid. Thus, amniotic fluid is described as an ultrafiltrate of maternal serum.

Amniotic Fluid Formation

The principal source of amniotic fluid is fetal urination. In utero the fetal kidneys begin to make urine before the end of the first trimester, and production of urine increases until term. Results of numerous studies on amniotic fluid volume have shown that urine production rate appears to be 1000–1200 mL/day at term, thus indicating that the entire amniotic fluid volume is replaced more frequently than every 24 hours.[3]

A second key source of amniotic fluid is fetal lung liquid. The previous belief was that there was physical movement of amniotic fluid into the fetal lungs, but new studies reveal that this may not

be completely accurate. The prevailing thinking is that throughout gestation, the fetal lung produces fluid that exits the trachea and is either swallowed or leaves the mouth and enters the amniotic compartment.[4,5]

Another finding that supports the contribution of fetal lung liquid in amniotic fluid formation is the appearance of lung **surfactant** in amniotic fluid near term. Lung or pulmonary surfactant is a surface-active lipoprotein, typically a phospholipid, that is formed by alveolar cells. Surfactants function to reduce surface tension throughout the lungs, which allows the lung to inflate and deflate properly. In a normally developing fetus, fetal breathing movement provides a "to and fro" movement of amniotic fluid into and out of the trachea, upper lungs, and mouth. Amniotic fluid does move back and forth, but there is a net outward movement of fetal lung liquid into the amniotic fluid.[6]

It should be understood that the volume of amniotic fluid must be maintained at a normal and consistent volume. Fluid entering the fetus must be balanced with fluid leaving the fetus, otherwise the fetus will be compromised. Causes of variable amniotic fluid volume will be discussed later in this chapter.

Amniotic Fluid Removal

There are two mechanisms for the removal of amniotic fluid, and they are *fetal swallowing* and *intramembranous absorption*. The first, fetal swallowing, begins early in gestation. Several studies have

★ **TABLE 13-2**   Relative Volume of Amniotic Fluid at Selected Gestational Ages

Gestational Age	Amniotic Fluid Volume
12 weeks	35 mL
18 weeks	300 mL
30 weeks	800 mL
40 weeks	600 mL

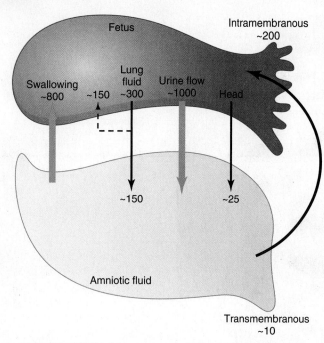

■ FIGURE 13-7 Movement of Fluid Through Fetal Blood, Fetus, and Amniotic Fluid. Arrows Represent Flow Movements and Rates with the Thicker Arrows Indicating Greater Flow Rates

Numbers are approximate flow of fluid in milliliters/day. Dashed arrow represents lung fluid that is swallowed directly after leaving the trachea. Intramembranous absorption is related to the movement of water and solutes between the amniotic compartment and fetal blood.

been conducted to investigate this mechanism of amniotic fluid removal.[7] A diagram of the movement of amniotic fluid is shown in Figure 13-7 ■.[8]

These studies revealed that fetal swallowing does occur, and fetal swallowing increases with advancing gestational age. An interesting fact was uncovered during these studies: Fetal swallowing alone could not account for the volume of fluid entering the amniotic sac and the volume of fluid leaving. Therefore, there must be one or more mechanisms present to remove amniotic fluid. The proposed mechanism is intramembranous absorption. It is a process involving the movement of water and solutes between the amniotic compartment and the fetal blood that circulates through the fetal surface of the placenta. A large osmotic gradient between amniotic fluid and fetal blood ensures a substantial driving force for the movement of amniotic fluid into the fetal blood. It is estimated that between 200–500 ml of amniotic fluid is removed via intramembranous absorption.[9,10,11]

Hydramnios

Hydramnios (*polyhydramnios*) is a condition characterized by an abnormal accumulation (typically ~2,000 mL) of amniotic fluid at term. Fetal and maternal conditions associated with polyhydramnios are shown in Box 13-1. Patient examination and ultrasound techniques can reveal the presence of polyhydramnios. Treatment modalities are usually tailored to the underlying cause.[12]

BOX 13-1 Fetal and Maternal Conditions Associated with Polyhydramnios

Fetal Conditions

Congenital anomalies

Aneuploidy, genetic conditions

Infections—parvovirus B19

Placental abnormalities

Maternal Conditions

Idiopathic

Poorly controlled diabetes mellitus

Fetal maternal hemorrhage

Oligohydramnios

Oligohydramnios is defined as less than ~300 mL of amniotic fluid. This typically develops when a chronically ill fetus swallows more fluid than normal.[13] Fetal and maternal causes of oligohydramnios are shown in Box 13-2. Patient assessment for oligohydramnios may include measurement of vaginal pH. Ultrasound and physical examination are also performed on each patient. Treatment of oligohydramnios includes a controversial technique referred to as amnioinfusion to reduce cardiac deceleration caused by low volume of amniotic fluid.

☑ CHECKPOINT 13-1

Define surfactant and indicate its clinical significance.

Specimen Collection and Handling

Amniocentesis is a procedure used to remove amniotic fluid. The patient has an ultrasound examination for orientation of the fetus and location of a pocket of amniotic fluid below the skin surface. With ultrasound guidance throughout the procedure, a 22-gauge needle is used to remove a volume of amniotic fluid (typically ~20 mL).[14]

BOX 13-2 Fetal and Maternal Conditions Associated with Oligohydramnios

Fetal Conditions

Failure of kidneys to develop

Obstructed uropathy

Spontaneous rupture of the membranes

Prolonged pregnancy

Maternal Conditions

Dehydration—hypovolemia

Hypertensive disorders

Uteroplacental insufficiency

Idiopathic

★ **TABLE 13-3** Indications for Amniocentesis

Indication	Week of Gestation
Assess preterm delivery	14–18
Chromosome abnormality	14–18
Neural tube defect	14–18
Gestational diabetes mellitus	20–32
Antibody screen for anti-Rh₀ (D)	20–32
Anemia (CBC)	20–32
Pulmonary immaturity	20–32
Repeat syphilis, HIV	36–delivery
Cervical culture for:	36–delivery
Neisseria gonorrhea	
Chlamydia trachomatis	

Amniotic fluid can be tested for biochemical substances (e.g., α-fetoprotein, lecithin and sphingomyelin) to be discussed later in the chapter. Other tests on amniotic fluid including cytologic, cytogenetic, and biochemical analysis for chromosomal disorders, HLA typing, and DNA probes may be clinically useful.

Amniocentesis can be performed at specific weeks of gestations to further evaluate patients with possible complications. Several examples are presented in Table 13-3 ★.

Gross Examination

Gross examination of amniotic fluid can reveal features that may indicate a fetal specimen should be scrutinized for color and consistency before and after centrifugation. Normal amniotic fluid is clear when removed at mid trimester. Discolored samples can reveal a disorder and examples of colors and their causes are shown in Table 13-4 ★.

Microscopic Examination

Cytology examination of amniotic fluid has limited clinical usefulness. Smears can be prepared using cytocentrifuge techniques. Cell staining is accomplished using eosin stain, Papanicolaou stains, Nile blue dye, or hematoxylin.

Microscopic examination provides useful information for the clinician in cases of possible ruptured membranes, chorioamnionitis, fetal maturity, determination of sex prenatally, and in the detection of neural tubal defects. Chorioamnionitis, which is an infection of the membrane that covers the fetus, is usually associated with

★ **TABLE 13-4** Amniotic Fluid Colors with Possible Causes

Color	Possible Causes
Colorless	Normal
Yellow	Erythroblastosis
Green (meconium)	Fetal hypoxia
Dark-red brown	Fetal death
Blood-tinged	Continuation of maternal blood
	Transplacental aspiration
	Recent intra-amniotic hemorrhage

polymorphonuclear leukocytes. This infection may follow premature rupture of membranes. A Gram stain procedure should be performed.

PRENATAL TESTS

The clinical laboratory provides a broad spectrum of laboratory tests during prenatal care of expectant mothers. These tests are designed to identify disorders that can be treated or prevented. A list of laboratory tests available in most hospital-based clinical pathology laboratories or as send outs to larger reference laboratories are presented in Box 13-3.

Several of these laboratory tests are routinely requested, whereas some tests are not considered by the clinician unless clinical information is presented during the patient history and/or physical examination. When a patient presents with signs and symptoms associated with a medical disorder any time during the pregnancy, appropriate action is taken, which includes requesting laboratory tests. Several examples of medical disorders and appropriate laboratory tests at specific times of gestation are shown in Figure 13-8 ■. Additional risk factors for diseases associated with pregnancy are listed in Box 13-4. All of these disorders are serious and have potential to do great harm to both mother and baby. The laboratory must be able to provide onsite laboratory testing or have access to quality laboratory tests that produce results in a timely manner.

Chorionic Gonadotropin

Chorionic gonadotropin (CG) measurements are useful for detecting pregnancy and associated abnormalities (e.g., molar and ectopic pregnancies), to screen for Down syndrome and trisomy 18, and to monitor patients with CG-producing tumors. There are many diverse types of measuring devices and assay methodologies designed to provide

BOX 13-3 Laboratory Tests Available for Routine Prenatal Care

Hematocrit
Hemoglobin
Blood type and Rh factor
Antibody screen
Pap smear screening
Glucose tolerance test
Fetal aneuploidy screening
Neural-tube defect screening
Cystic fibrosis screening
Urine protein
Urine culture
Rubella serology
Syphilis serology
Gonoccocal culture
Chlamydia culture
Hepatitis B serology
HIV serology
Group B streptococcus culture

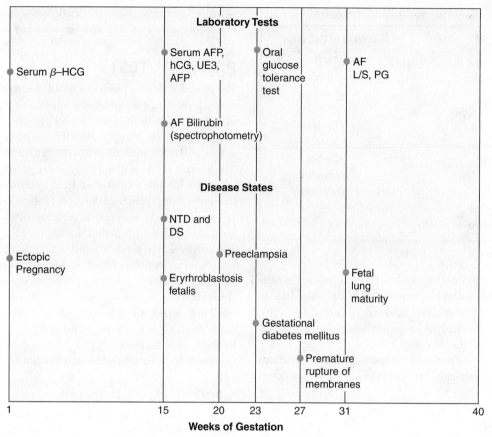

Laboratory Tests

Serum β–HCG

Serum AFP, hCG, UE3, AFP

Oral glucose tolerance test

AF L/S, PG

AF Bilirubin (spectrophotometry)

Disease States

NTD and DS

Preeclampsia

Ectopic Pregnancy

Eryrhroblastosis fetalis

Fetal lung maturity

Gestational diabetes mellitus

Premature rupture of membranes

Weeks of Gestation: 1   15   20   23   27   31   40

■ **FIGURE 13-8** Laboratory Tests that Provide Potentially Useful Clinical Information for Patients who Present With High Risk Disorders at Various Weeks of Gestation. β-hCG, Beta Human Chorionic Gonadotropin; AFP, Alpha-Fetoprotein; AF L/S, PG, Amniotic Fluid Lecithin/Sphingomyelin, Phosphatidylcholine; NTD, Neural Tube Defect and DS, Down Syndrome; UE3, unconjugated estriol.

both qualitative and quantitative determinations of CG in either urine or serum.

Chorionic gonadotropin is a glycoprotein with biological activity similar to luteinizing hormone (LH). Both hormones act via the plasma membrane LH-CG receptor. Although CG is produced almost exclusively in the placenta, it also is synthesized in fetal kidney. Fetal production of either β-subunit or intact hCG molecules also occurs in other fetal tissues described below.

Chemistry

The knowledge of CG chemistry has progressed significantly and impacted diagnostic testing methods along the way. For many decades the only compound that was associated with pregnancy was CG. In Box 13-5 the many forms of CG that may circulate in women and men are listed. The clinical implications and their impact on assays currently available are discussed below.

BOX 13-4   Risk Factors Identified in Early Pregnancy

Asthma

Cardiac diseases

Diabetes mellitus

Drug and alcohol use

Epilepsy

Family history of genetic problems (Down syndrome, phenylketonuria)

Hypertension

Deep vein thrombosis

Psychiatric illness

Pulmonary disease

Renal disease

BOX 13-5   Examples of Multiple Molecular Forms of Chorionic Gonadotropin

Intact hCG

Hyperglycosylated hCG (hCG-H)

Free beta subunit of CG (fCGβ)

Free alpha subunit of CG (fCGα)

Nicked free beta subunit of CG (fCGβn)

Core fragment of CGβ (CGβcf)

Chorionic gonadotropin is a glycoprotein with carbohydrate side chains that usually terminate with sialic acid. It has the highest carbohydrate content, approximately 30%, of any human hormone. The carbohydrate component, and especially the terminal sialic acid, protects the molecule from catabolism. Intact CG has a plasma half-life of 36 hours, whereas LH half-life is only 2 hours. CG is composed of two structurally different glycoprotein subunits, alpha (α) and beta (β). The carbohydrate composition changes as pregnancy progresses. In a normal pregnancy, after implantation the predominant form of CG is a large molecular mass form called hyperglycoslated CG (H-CG). As the pregnancy progresses, a 36–37kDa molecular mass form predominates. The alpha and beta subunits are structurally different than innate CG.[15]

Chorionic gonadotropin is structurally related to three other glycoprotein hormones, LH, follicle stimulating hormone (FSH) and thyroid stimulating hormone (TSH). The amino-acid sequence of the α-subunits of all four glycoproteins is identical. The uniqueness resides in the beta subunits, which share certain similarities, but distinctly different amino-acid sequences. This difference in sequences conveys the specificity of many immunoassays for hCG measurement.

Biosynthesis

Synthesis of both alpha and beta chains of CG is regulated separately. Alpha subunits of CG, LH, FSH, and TSH are regulated by a single gene located on chromosome 6. Seven separate genes on chromosome 19 encode the β-hCG and β-LH group; six genes code for β-hCG and one for β-LH. Both subunits are synthesized as large precursor compounds, which are then cleaved by endopeptidases. The intact form of CG is then assembled and rapidly released by exocytosis of secretory granules.[16]

Prior to the fifth week of pregnancy, CG is expressed in both syncytiotrophoblast cells and cytotrophoblast cells. The principal source of maternal serum CG is the syncytiotrophoblast cells. Separate messenger RNAs (mRNA) are transcribed from their respective genes, and the alpha and beta subunits are translated from their respective mRNA. During this time the amount of mRNA is greater than at term. This finding may be an important consideration when CG is used as a screening procedure to identify abnormally developing fetuses.

Serum and Urine CG Levels

The intact CG molecule is measurable in serum of pregnant women 7–9 days after the midcyle surge of LH that precedes ovulation. Therefore, CG enters maternal blood at the time of blastocyst implantation. Blood levels increase rapidly, doubling every two days, with maximal levels being attained at 8 to 10 weeks.[17]

Because CG circulates as multiple isoforms with variable cross-reactivity between commercial immunoassays, there is a large amount of variation in measured CG levels. The peak maternal blood levels in normal progressing pregnancies occur between the 60th and 80th days after menses. Plasma levels of hCG begin to decrease at about 10–12 weeks and reach their lowest levels by about 16 weeks. A typical progression of serum hCG levels and gestation age is presented in Figure 13-9 ■.

hCG levels in fetal blood follow a similar pattern to that of the mother. Plasma fetal concentrations are only about 3% of those in maternal plasma. Amniotic fluid hCG concentrations early in pregnancy are similar to that in maternal plasma. As the pregnancy progresses, hCG concentration in amniotic fluid decreases, and near term the levels are about 10–20% of those in maternal plasma.

Maternal urine is comprised of the same types of hCG degradation products as maternal plasma. The primary urinary form is the beta core fragment, which is a degradation product of hCG. The concentration of this fragment follows the same pattern as that in maternal plasma, peaking at approximately 10 weeks. Most beta subunit antibodies used in pregnancy tests react with both intact hCG (the major form) in the blood, with fragments of hCG (the major form) found in urine.

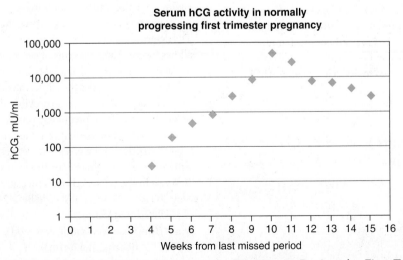

Serum hCG activity in normally progressing first trimester pregnancy

■ **FIGURE 13-9**   Serum hCG Activity in a Normal Progressing Pregnancy During the First Trimester

A key feature is the steep rise in hCG concentrations between the fourth and tenth weeks of gestation.

Qualitative CG Tests

Qualitative testing of CG was available decades before the quantitative immunoassays were approved by the Food and Drug Administration (FDA) for use in clinical laboratories. Qualitative assays are capable of detecting various forms of the CG molecule in both serum and urine. Testing platforms include point-of-care, over-the-counter (OTC) home tests and test kits designed for laboratory use. The analytical sensitivity and specificity of these assays are not comparable to the quantitative assays but have the advantage of ease of performance and interpretation.

Many OTC test kits provide a single test and use an enzyme immunometric or immunochromatographic method to measure urine CG. Detection limits (i.e., low-end sensitivity) vary considerably among assays with cut-off values set at between 25–50 mU/mL. False negative results are common and are usually due to difficulty by users in understanding the literature that accompanies the tests, or they may be due to the presence of hCG variants in the specimen. Some false positive results occur with these assays due to the presence of proteins, drugs, bacteria, erythrocytes, or leukocytes in urine specimens. Most qualitative tests will present with positive results on the day after the first missed menstrual period. A first-morning specimen is preferred because it is concentrated and contains a large amount of CG. The simplicity and speed with which the results are obtained make these tests very useful for affirmation of pregnancy, but they may miss the diagnosis of a very early or abnormal pregnancy.

Quantitative hCG Assays

Quantitative serum hCG assays provide the clinician with valuable information for assessing patients with a possible ongoing pregnancy or a high-risk pregnancy. Several analytical methods are commonly used and include the following:[18]

- Anti-CGβ: anti-CGβ sandwich immunoassay
- Anti-CGβ: anti-CGα sandwich immunoassay
- Anti-CGβ C terminal: anti-CGβ sandwich immunoassay
- Anti-CG: anti-CGβ sandwich immunoassay

Assay specificity varies considerably due to differences in antibody recognition of various forms of CG, nicked subunits, β-subunits, H-CG, and other fragments present in serum. Analytical sensitivity or detection levels are typically 1–2 mU/mL for most immunoassays. There are several key issues listed in Box 13-6 that should be addressed regarding immunoassays designed to detect and measure hCG.

BOX 13-6 Key Points Regarding Chorionic Gonadotropin Assays

Which specific form(s) are detected by the assay?

Assay limitations, interferences, and specificity

Detection limits

Specimen requirements

Source of calibration material

Material used as a standard reference for assay calibrators

Calibration of CG Assays

Calibration of CG assays is an integral function that requires full understanding and attention to details by the laboratory staff. The probability of producing discordant patient data between two different CG assays is greater if the source of calibrator is different for both assays. Therefore, laboratory staff should be knowledgeable of the source of standard reference material used for the preparation of calibrators. The World Health Organization (WHO) has produced standardized reference materials since 1938 when it released the first International Standard (1st IS). Several modifications have been made to the material throughout the years with notable improvements to purity and specificity. Most CG calibrators currently used in the United States are standardized against the 3rd IS, while some calibrators remain standardized with the 2nd IS.[19] There are differences in reactivity among the standard reference materials therefore results obtained from one method may not be the same (i.e., discordant) as from those of another method.

A fourth WHO international standard was released in 1999 that is essentially identical to the 3rd IS. Both contained about 5% nicked CG and other CG contaminants, and their purity has been questioned by the scientific community. An effort was undertaken to produce a highly purified CG material. This material was designated *reference reagent* (RR) and contained a mixture of CG, CGn, CGβ, CGβn, CGβcf, and CGα. The impact of using this reference reagent is currently under study.[20]

Specificity of CG Assays

Currently available CG assays have little or no cross reactivity with LH. Laboratories can test their CG assays for cross reactivity by measuring CG on post-menopausal women whose LH concentration is usually moderately elevated. CG assays should be designed so that low concentrations of CG are detected and false positive values caused by LH interference are minimized.

Clinical Significance

Quantitative β-hCG measurement may provide clinicians with clinically useful information on patients who present with early gestational vaginal bleeding and/or abdominal pain. These signs and symptoms are common in cases of ectopic pregnancy or spontaneous abortion. The determination of β-hCG concentrations and ultrasound findings allows for accurate diagnosis of several pregnancy-related disorders. Serial measurements of at least two serum β-hCG samplings is valuable because it provides the clinician with a second result that should increase significantly (refer to previous discussion of the sharp rise in hCG) during normal pregnancy versus a second result that increases less than 50% from the first result and is also significantly below the typical hCG level for a given week of gestation. For example, patients with an ectopic pregnancy or threatened abortion may show only a 10% rise in the second β-hCG measurement, and the result may be only 200 mU/mL when it should be >2,000 mU/mL.

Ultrasound techniques can reveal an intrauterine gestational sac when β-hCG concentrations exceed the "discriminating zone" value of ~1,200 mU/mL in a normal, single fetus pregnancy.[21] A patient who presents without an intrauterine gestational sac and unsuccessful doubling of serum β-hCG levels or the presence of an adnexal mass (e.g., outside the uterus) may have developed an ectopic pregnancy.

Treatment modalities for an unruptured ectopic pregnancy include intramuscular injection of methotrexate. Methotrexate is described as an anti-metabolite drug that interrupts all cycling processes by inhibiting DNA synthesis. Surgery is also an option but is more costly and presents with complications. A third possible course of action is termed "expectant management" with serial β-hCG measurement and ultrasound procedures performed until the ectopic pregnancy is resolved.

> ## ☑ CHECKPOINT 13-2
>
> Differentiate on a chemical basis the difference between the specificity of hCG and β-hCG assays.

Alpha-Fetoprotein

Alpha-Fetoprotein (AFP) is a glycoprotein that migrates in the alpha region of a protein electrophoresis separation procedure; its molecular weight is approximately 70 kDa. The gene responsible for AFP is located within q11-22 on chromosome 4. It is part of the family of genes that also codes for albumin and vitamin D-binding protein. The carbohydrate composition of AFP varies depending on the organ of synthesis, length of gestation, and source of the specimen.

Production of small amounts of AFP begins in the fetal yolk sac and then in large quantities by the fetal liver as the yolk sac degenerates. Minute amounts are also produced in the fetal gut and kidneys. The concentration of AFP in fetal serum is very high early in embryonic life and peaks in fetal serum at a level of approximately 3×10^6 ng/mL (3×10^6 μg/L) at about 9 weeks gestation. The concentration then decreases steadily to about 20,000 ng/mL (20,000 μg/L) at term.[22] Amniotic fluid concentrations of AFP follow a similar pattern of increasing and decreasing but to levels two or three orders of magnitude lower. In maternal serum the concentration of AFP is affected by several factors, including the rapid growth of the fetus, fetal-maternal transfer, the relatively constant size of the mother, the maternal clearance of the AFP, and variations of the volume of distribution in the mother relative to the mother's weight. In maternal serum, AFP is first detectable at about the 10th week of gestation. The relative concentrations of AFP in fetal/newborn blood, amniotic fluid, and maternal serum is presented as part of Table 13-5 ★.[23,24]

AFP Immunoassays

Several immunoassays developed for automated analyzers widely used in clinical laboratories are currently available to measure serum AFP. These immunoassays feature low detection limits and acceptable precision and specificity. The selection of calibration material for AFP assays dictates whether the results are reported in International Units/Liter (IU/L) or ng/mL (SI units = μg/L). There are two international standards (WHO Reference Preparation for AFP [72-225] and British Standard [72-227]) that are reported in IU. Most laboratories in the United States use calibrators other than the international standards, thus reporting their results as ng/mL. The relationship between ng and IU usually is given as 1.21 ng = 1 IU. There may be other factors that affect this unit relationship; thus the numerical value may not match the one shown.

★ **TABLE 13-5** Relative Concentrations of AFP in Fetal/Newborn Blood, Amniotic Fluid, and Maternal Serum. Concentration units: ng/mL (μg/L)

Weeks of Gestation	Fetal/Newborn Blood	Amniotic Fluid	Maternal Serum (median)
7	500,000	70,000	NA
9	3,000,000	30,000	NA
10	3,000,000	20,000	5
14	2,000,000	20,000	25.6
16	1,500,000	15,000	34.8
18	1,000,000	10,000	47.3
20	800,000	6,000	64.3
21	700,000	5,000	74.9

AFP in amniotic fluid can be measured using the same immunoassays that are available for maternal serum but may dilute the sample. AFP in amniotic fluid is less stable than in serum. Samples left at room temperature for prolonged periods can result in degradation of AFP.

Clinical Significance of AFP

Patients with elevated serum concentrations of AFP greater than two times the median should be investigated by ultrasound examination to rule out incorrectly estimated gestational age, multiple gestation, fetal death, or obvious anatomical malformations. Increased concentrations of AFP in maternal serum and amniotic fluid are associated with open neural tube defects, esophageal or duodenal atresia, fetal hepatic necrosis secondary to viral infection, and other conditions. Decreased concentrations of AFP are found in cases of Down syndrome (trisomy 21), fetal demise, molar pregnancy, and trisomy 18.

> ## ☑ CHECKPOINT 13-3
>
> Explain the origin of alphafetoprotein.

Unconjugated Estriol

Estriol is an estrogen with three hydroxyl groups (at positions 3, 16, 17). In blood, total estriol (TE$_3$) exists as unconjugated and conjugated. Normal concentrations in nonpregnant patients are very low. In pregnancy, blood levels of TE$_3$ increase steadily until term, and E$_3$ is the predominant estrogen present. Approximately 10% of TE$_3$ circulates as **unconjugated estriol** (uE$_3$) and because of its low solubility, the majority circulates as conjugates of glucuronic acid sulfate. Conjugation occurs in the maternal liver, making the hormone more soluble, and therefore, more able to be cleared via the kidney.

Estriol is produced in large concentration during the last trimester. Biosynthetic production requires three functional organs, including fetal adrenal glands, fetal liver, and placenta. An outline identifying the biosynthetic pathway of estriol is shown in Figure 13-10 ■.

The fetal adrenal cortex binds low density lipoprotein to attract cholesterol, which is converted to the steroid intermediates, pregnenolone sulfate and dehydroepiandrosterone sulfate (DHEAS). These intermediates enter into the fetal circulation en route to the fetal liver. In the fetal liver they are reconverted to 16α-OH-DHEAS, which then

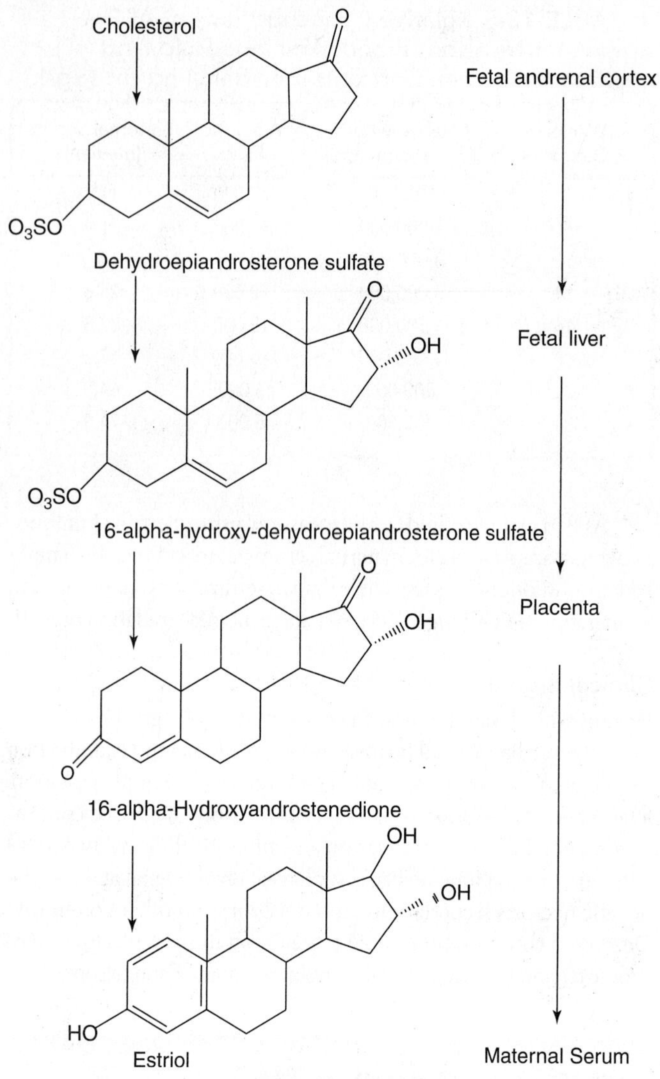

Cholesterol

O₃SO

Dehydroepiandrosterone sulfate

O₃SO

16-alpha-hydroxy-dehydroepiandrosterone sulfate

O

16-alpha-Hydroxyandrostenedione

HO

Estriol

Fetal andrenal cortex

Fetal liver

Placenta

Maternal Serum

■ **FIGURE 13-10** Biochemical Pathway for Estriol

passes into the fetal circulation. Last, the placenta synthesizes estriol from 16α-hydroxyandrostenedione.

Several immunoassays are available for quantifying both total TE_3 and uE_3 in serum and amniotic fluid. Circulating blood levels of uE_3 are very low compared to total TE_3, thus the immunoassays must be highly sensitive. In a normal progressing pregnancy, maternal serum level of uE_3 rises from a value of <10 ng/mL at about 22 weeks of gestation to <30 ng/mL at 40 weeks. (Note: Conversion to SI units, nMol/L = ng/mL × 3.47)

Clinical Significance of uE₃

Maternal serum uE_3 concentrations will be markedly decreased in variety of conditions that result in high-risk pregnancies involving diabetes, post maturity, preeclampsia, fetal growth retardation, intrauterine death, malnutrition, anemia, hypoplasia of fetal adrenal glands, and Down syndrome. Also, any disruption in the biosynthetic pathway illustrated in Figure 13-10 will result in low maternal levels of uE_3. Some examples include fetal anencephaly, placental sulfatase deficiency, fetal death, chromosome abnormalities, and molar pregnancies.

☑ CHECKPOINT 13-4

Explain the chemical and structural differences between total and unconjugated estriol.

Dimeric Inhibin A

Inhibins belong to the transforming growth factor β (TGFβ) super-family of proteins. Inhibins are heterodimeric structures that have two forms, hence dimeric, specifically **inhibin A** and B. Their structures consists of dimers of dissimilar subunits (α and β) linked by disulfide bridges. They function as part of a feedback mechanism that regulates FSH secretions in both males and females. The placenta produces a large quantity of inhibin A that suppresses nearly all FSH.

Inhibins are secreted by granulosa cells of the ovary and Sertoli cells located in the testes. Inhibin A and B are active in the human menstrual cycle. For example, inhibin A rises in the follicular phase of pregnancy, whereas inhibin B levels are maximal in the mid follicular phase, peak at ovulation, and then continue to decrease to basal level in the luteal phase.

Clinical Significance of Inhibin A

Dimeric inhibin A (DIA) is produced by the fetoplacental unit early in pregnancy. Serum maternal inhibin A levels peak at about 8–10 weeks gestation, decline to a minimum at 17 weeks of pregnancy, and then begin to slowly increase near term. Typical inhibin A levels of 175 ng/L (175 pg/mL) are seen in normal progressing pregnancies at 17 weeks gestation.

Several immunoassays are available to specifically detect and measure DIA. Highly specific and sensitive immunoassays are required to qualify for use as a screening test for Down syndrome. Maternal serum concentrations of DIA are elevated in cases involving Down syndrome. Inhibin A measurement is also useful for monitoring patients with ovarian (granulosa cell) cancers. DIA decreases significantly after surgical intervention and increases markedly in cases of recurrence.

MATERNAL DISORDERS

Gestational Diabetes Mellitus

The criteria relating to all aspects of diabetes are continually under close scrutiny, and any attempt by an author to provide in writing accurate information in a timely manner is nearly impossible. This is particularly true when attempting to define aspects of the disease or provide testing requirements and analytical concentrations indicating health or disease.

The American Diabetes Association (ADA) updated its position statement in 2011 and included the following modifications to its previous position statement from 1997. "Women with diabetes found at their initial prenatal visit should receive a diagnosis of overt gestational diabetes mellitus (GDM)."[25,26] The rationale is included in the discussion. The presence of GDM or overt DM carries a risk for the mother and baby. Prompt diagnosis and treatment of GDM may prevent maternal and fetal complications such as preeclampsia, fetal congenital malformation, fetal macrosomia (excessive birth weight), and fetal demise. The following protocol and glucose values reflect the most recent information proposed by the ADA. These protocols are still under consideration

BOX 13-7 Diagnostic Cut Points for Gestational Diabetes Mellitus

1. Perform a 75 g OGTT, with plasma glucose measurements performed after fasting and then at 1 and 2 hours post glucose challenge, at 24–28 weeks of gestation in women not previously diagnosed with overt diabetes mellitus.

2. The diagnosis of **gestational diabetes mellitus** is made when any of the following plasma glucose values are exceeded:

   - Fasting $\geq$92 mg/dL
   - 1 h $\geq$ 180 mg/dL
   - 2 h $\geq$ 153 mg/dL

by the American College of Obstetrics and Gynecology (ACOG).[27,28] All women not known to have diabetes should have a 75 g oral glucose tolerance test (OGTT) at 24–28 weeks gestation. The diagnostic cut points are shown in Box 13-7.

MINI-CASE 13-1

Samantha, a 29-year-old female, visited her physician as part of her prenatal care program. She was in her 25th week of gestation. The doctor suggested that Samantha complete a 2-hour oral glucose tolerance test. Samantha agreed and her laboratory results are shown below.

Fasting glucose:	108 mg/dL
1-hour glucose:	199 mg/dL
2-hour glucose:	165 mg/dL

Questions to Consider

1. According to the 2011 American Diabetes Association guidelines, does Samantha have gestational diabetes mellitus?

2. What is your rationale for the response that you provided?

☑ CHECKPOINT 13-5

Explain the current definition of gestational diabetes mellitus.

Preeclampsia

Preeclampsia (also termed toxemia of pregnancy) is a syndrome characterized by hypertension with systolic blood pressures >140 mmHg and diastolic blood pressures >90 mmHg with concomitant proteinuria >0.3 g/L in a 24-hour period (normally <140 mg/L). Additional findings in patients with preeclampsia are shown in Table 13-6 ★.

★ **TABLE 13-6** Laboratory Tests and Diagnostic Values in Mild-Moderate and Severe Preeclampsia. (LFT, liver function test; AST, aspartate aminotransferase; ALT, alanine aminotransferase; LD, lactate dehydrogenase)

Analytes	Mild-Moderate	Severe
Protein	0.3–5 g/24 h	> 5 g/24 h or catheterized urine with 4+ protein
Uric acid	> 4.5 mg/dL	> 4.5 mg/dL
Urinary output	> 30 mL/h	< 30 mL/h
LFTs: AST, ALT, LD	Normal	Elevated LFTs
Platelets	>100,000/μL	<100,000/μL
Hemoglobin	Normal	Elevated

Preeclampsia typically occurs at about 20 weeks gestation in women who have been normotensive before pregnancy. Several risk factors associated with preeclampsia exist and include first pregnancy, chronic hypertension, renal disease, obesity, and diabetes. This syndrome is serious with potential for harm to both mother and fetus. There are life-threatening manifestations that are a cause of maternal mortality, including eclampsia (defined as onset of grand mal seizure in women with preeclampsia, which may result in intracranial hemorrhage), and HELLP syndrome (**H**emolytic anemia, **E**levated **L**iver enzymes, **L**ow **P**latelet count).

The cause of preeclampsia is unknown, but there are pathophysiological abnormalities, for example trophoblastic invasion of the placenta, impaired uteroplacental flow, and interaction of chemicals that cause vasospasms that lead to diminished intravascular volume. Other factors include hematologic changes resulting in hemoconcentration, thrombocytopenia, and hemolysis. Hepatic dysfunction results in elevated serum transaminases (AST and ALT), LD, and bilirubin. The proteinuria seen in preeclampsia is a glomerular type, and the urine sediment may contain hyaline and finely granular casts. Serum creatinine, urea nitrogen, and uric acid are often elevated, depending upon the extent of damage to the kidneys.

Preterm Labor

Several biochemical markers have been evaluated for predicting preterm labor. In 1991, fetal **fibronectin** (fFN) measurements in cervical and vaginal secretions were proposed as a test to aid in predicting preterm delivery.[29]

Fetal fibronectin is an adhesive glycoprotein produced by fetal membranes and found in the choriodecidual junction amniotic fluid. The fetus contains a unique form of fibronectin, FDC-6, which was defined by a monoclonal antibody test. Fibronectin is responsible for the cellular adhesiveness of placenta and membranes of the decidua. Initiation of maternal labor results in disruption of the cellular adhesion between the placenta and the uterine wall, causing an increase in fetal fibronectin concentration in cervical and vaginal secretions. An fFN concentration of >50 ng/mL (50 μg/L) in these secretions during the second and third trimester in patients is interpreted as a high risk for preterm delivery.[30]

Patient assessment protocols exist for both asymptomatic and symptomatic presentations. In screening asymptomatic patients, testing should be performed between 24–30 weeks gestation. Women with an fFN result of >50 ng/mL are at a two- to fourfold higher risk for preterm delivery. For symptomatic patients (i.e., showing symptoms of preterm labor) experiencing regular uterine contraction, low back pain, lower abdomen cramping, vaginal bleeding, increased vaginal discharge, and a positive fFN test result, there is a greater likelihood for delivery before 34 weeks gestation or within the next seven days. A negative fFN result means that the patient can return safely home because she has only about 1% chance of delivery within one week.[31]

FETAL DISORDERS

Down Syndrome

Down syndrome is a serious disorder of autosomal chromosomes, occurring in 1 in 800 live births. The genetic origin is an extra copy of the long arm region q22.1 to q22.3 of chromosome 21. Down syndrome is characterized by severe mental retardation, hypotonia, congenital heart defects, and flat facial profile. Usually an affected child has three copies of chromosome 21 (i.e., trisomy 21). A small percentage (~5%) of cases are caused by translocations and 1% of causes are mosaics. The risk of having a pregnancy affected with Down syndrome increases slowly up to age 30 and then steadily increases as maternal age advances. The risk at 25 years of age is 1 in 1,000 and at age 40 it is 1 in 90.[32]

A common approach to screen mothers for Down syndrome in the United States is to perform laboratory tests that include uE_3, β-hCG, and AFP at 16–18 weeks gestation. This group of tests is often referred to as the **triple test**. Another option is to include a measurement of DIA, discussed previously, which would then make a quadruple testing panel also known as the **quad screen**. The quantitative results are derived from a single serum sample, and the results in mass units are converted to *multiple of the median* (MoM) for the appropriate week (or day) of gestation. MoM is a calculated value based on data from a reference population. The results are correlated with several other criteria and a final risk value is used as a basis upon which clinical decisions are derived.[33]

Neural Tube Defects

The neural tube in a developing embryo refers to the embryo's precursor structure to the central nervous system, which comprises the brain and spinal cord. Neural-tube defects (NTD) include spina bifida, anencephaly, cephalocele, and other spinal fusion abnormalities. This class of defects of neurulation (i.e. formation of the neural plate) occurs in 1.4–2 per 1,000 pregnancies and is the second most common class of birth defects after cardiac anomalies.[34] Approximately 95% of NTDs occur in the absence of known risk factors such as those shown in Box 13-8. Genetic causes present the largest group listed. Therefore, there is a need for routine screening.[35]

NTDs result from failure of the neural tube to close by the 27th day after conception. Anencephaly (i.e., congenital absence of the brain and cranial vault) is often present. Abnormalities of the caudal portion (i.e., toward the tail bone) of the neural tube, referred to as spina bifida, present as a lumbar (or cervical) meningomyelocele, with herniation of meninges, spinal cord and roots.[36] Several complications such as paralysis, muscle weakness, fecal and urinary incontinence, and intellectual impairment may be present depending upon the vertebral levels affected. Folic acid is a significant preventive agent for NTD. Several organizations are actively involved in supporting dietary supplements for women of childbearing ages. Some are listed in Box 13-9.[37]

> ## BOX 13-8 Some Risk Factors for Neural Tube Defects
>
> ### Genetic Causes
> Family history
> Syndromes with autosomal recessive inheritance
> Aneuploidy
> >   Trisomy 13
> >   Trisomy 18
> >   Triploidy
>
> ### Exposure to Certain Environmental Agents
> >   Medications
> >   Valproic acid
> >   Carbamazepine
> >   Coumadin
> >   Aminopterin
> >   Thalidomide
>
> ### Geographical Regions (factors such as ethnicity, diet, and other factors)
> >   United Kingdom
> >   India
> >   China
> >   Egypt
> >   Mexico
> >   Southern Appalachian United States

Erythroblastosis Fetalis

In 1953, Bevis demonstrated that elevated amniotic fluid bilirubin pigments correlate with the severity of Rh **erythroblastosis fetalis**, a hemolytic disease of the newborn marked by anemia, jaundice and enlargement of the spleen.[38] Since then amniotic fluid analysis has been a widely used test to predict fetal outcomes.

Liley Method

A method proposed by Liley has been accepted as a reliable means to assess severity of fetal disease. The principle of the method is based on the change (Δ) in optical density (OD) also known as absorbance at a wavelength of 450 nm of amniotic fluid.[39,40] This test is often referred to as delta (Δ) *OD450*.

A sample of amniotic fluid is placed into a spectrophotometer and a wavelength spectrum spanning from approximately 350 nm to 650 nm is determined. There are four principal wavelengths that are monitored and include 365, 410, 450, and 550 nm. The wavelengths correlate to light absorbing properties of specific compounds present in the sample. Absorbance of light by "background" compound(s) is apparent at 365 nm. Small absorbance (peaks) between 540 nm and 575 nm may be due to an artifact from hemolysis or fetal erythrocytes. A more striking peak at ~410 nm is due to oxyhemoglobin and is often referred to as the Soret Band. If the absorbance at 410 nm is great enough it could potentially interfere with any absorbance at 450 nm.

A scan of amniotic fluid in shown in Figure 13-11 ■. The ΔOD at 450 nm is calculated from the absorbance of each of the absorbing compounds identified above.

Liley's proposed three zones to delineate severity of disease in women at 27 weeks to term.

- Values in the high zone indicate severe disease
- Values in the mid zone require repeat measurements to determine a possible trend
- Values in the low zone indicate mild or no disease

Queenan Curve

The Liley method was clinically evaluated in pregnancies from 27 weeks to term. Several subsequent studies extended the Liley zones before 27 weeks but were not sufficiently investigated. Also additional challenges were made to the clinical usefulness of the Liley method.[41] Queenan et al. presented reliable data that showed amniotic fluid ΔOD_{450} analysis effectively predicts fetal conditions at 14 weeks (early second trimester) to term.[42]

Partial interpretation of Queenan's plot is shown in Figure 13-12 ■. Many clinical laboratories replaced the Liley method with Queenan's method because of its earlier prediction of possible hemolytic crisis.

- If a value falls in the intrauterine death risk zone or if the trend will carry the value there, the fetus is in jeopardy of dying in utero.
- If the value falls in the Rh-negative (unaffected) zone, the fetus can be presumed to be Rh negative (no erythroblastosis fetalis).
- If the value falls in the middle zones, additional values are necessary to indicate the condition of the fetus.

Fetal Lung Maturity

The maturing fetal lung produces a quantity of surface-active phospholipid compounds called surfactants. A surfactant tends to decrease surface tension within the alveolar space during inspiration that allows for continuous gas exchange without alveolar collapse during expiration. This type of phospholipid is produced by the type II pneumocytes in the form of lamellar bodies. A fetus that has a deficiency of surfactant can develop neonatal respiratory distress syndrome (RDS). This disorder results in hypoxia, acidemia, and vascular protein transudation into alveolar air spaces (hyaline membrane disease). Testing for fetal lung maturity (FLM) should be considered prior to scheduled delivery and at less than 39 weeks gestation.

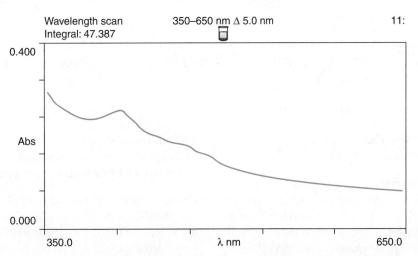

Wavelength scan   350–650 nm Δ 5.0 nm   11:
Integral: 47.387

■ **FIGURE 13-11** Absorbance Spectrum of Amniotic Fluid from a Patient with Possible Hemolytic Disease of the Newborn.

A Characteristic Increase in Absorbance Appears at 410 nm.

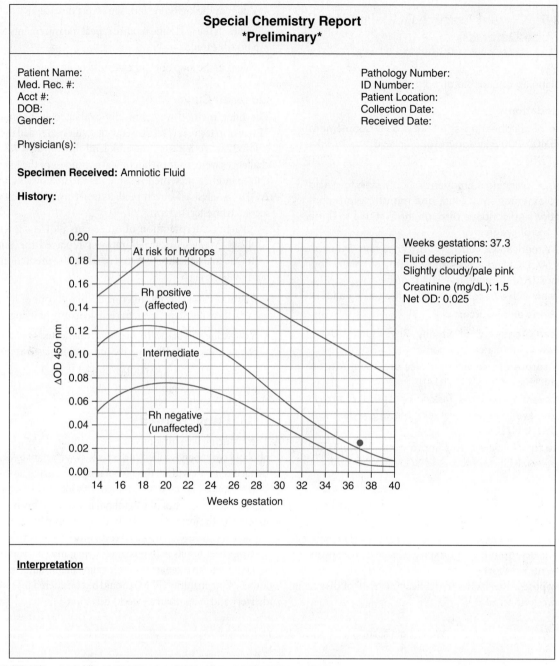

Special Chemistry Report
Preliminary

Patient Name:
Med. Rec. #:
Acct #:
DOB:
Gender:

Physician(s):

Specimen Received: Amniotic Fluid

History:

Pathology Number:
ID Number:
Patient Location:
Collection Date:
Received Date:

Weeks gestations: 37.3
Fluid description:
Slightly cloudy/pale pink
Creatinine (mg/dL): 1.5
Net OD: 0.025

Interpretation

■ **FIGURE 13-12** Modified Queenan Curve for ΔOD 450 nm Values
The calculated ΔOD 450 for this patient at 37 weeks is 0.025 which lies in the Rh positive (affected) zone.

Several tests on amniotic fluid for FLM are currently available. These tests are designed to (1) measure lamellar bodies directly or indirectly, (2) detect the type of surfactant present, or (3) measure the biophysical property of surfactant.

Lecithin/Sphingomyelin Ratio

The **lecithin/sphingomyelin (L/S) ratio** is one of the earliest tests to assess fetal pulmonary status.[43] This test estimates the ratio of the amount of lecithin to sphingomyelin in amniotic fluid. Normally, the concentration of sphingomyelin remains constant throughout the pregnancy, whereas the levels of lecithin continue to increase. The test procedure includes an extraction and purification step with solvents that separate out amniotic fluid surfactant lipids. The extract is applied

to a thin-layer silica gel and the lipids are separated using a thin-layer chromatography (TLC) procedure. The phospholipids are made visible with a dye and a densitometer is used to detect and quantify the lipids. L/S ratio >2.0 indicates fetal lung maturity, and a ratio <1.5 indicates that the fetal lungs are immature.

Phosphatidyl Glycerol by Thin Layer Chromatography

Phosphatidyl glycerol (PG) is a relatively minor lung phospholipid, but it is a potent surfactant with a greater hydrogen-binding capacity than lecithin and plays a role in stabilizing the surfactant lipoprotein complex. The PG TLC assay requires an organic extraction of phospholipids and subsequent application of the final solute onto a thin layer silica gel. The gel is immersed into a liquid mobile phase where the phospholipids are separated. The phospholipids are detected and measured using a densitometer. If PG is present, then the fetus presents with mature lungs, and if PG is absent, then the fetus presents with immature lungs.

Phosphatidyl Glycerol (Amniostat-FLM®-PG)

Amniostat-FLM®-PG (Irvine Scientific, Santa Anna, CA 92705) is an immunologic agglutination test for the detection of PG. PG in amniotic fluid is incorporated into lipid particles by adding amniotic fluid to optimize concentrations of lecithin and cholesterol in ethanol. A dilution with phosphate buffer is made, then the suspension is mixed with antibodies that react with the PG containing particle. The presence of PG in amniotic fluid is indicated by agglutination after background clearing. Results are reported as negative, low positive (0.5–2.0 μg/mL) or high-positive (2.0 μg/mL or greater). RDS rarely develops in an infant whose mother's Amniostat-FLM®-PG test result is a high-positive PG.

Combining the measurement %PG and determining the L/S ratio as a *lung panel* provides a useful tandem approach to assessing FLM. A % PG >1.0 of the total lipid present and an L/S >2.0 indicates that there is a high probability of the fetal lungs developing properly.

Lamellar Body Counts

Lamellar bodies are the storage form of surfactant released into amniotic fluid by fetal breathing movements. A lamellar body is approximately 0.2–2.0 μm in size and can be counted using a standard hematology cell counter to determine lamellar body count (LBC). The LBC has a slightly better specificity than the L/S ratio. A widely accepted cutoff value for LBC; with high negative predictive value for RDS is $\geq 50,000/\mu$L. Patients with LBCs $\leq 15,000/\mu$L are more likely to develop RDS.[44]

The LBC is a possible consideration to replace the discontinued Abbott TDxFLM II procedure. The reasons for the lack of acceptance of the Abbott method includes (1) lack of familiarity with the test, (2) a decreased demand for FLM testing, and (3) the fact that the LBC is a laboratory developed test. In 2010, Clinical Laboratory Standard Institute created a document to provide guidance for the use of automated cell counting to enumerate lamellar bodies in amniotic fluid.[45]

MINI-CASE 13-2

Bonny's physician has concerns that her fetus may be showing signs of respiratory distress and requests a "lung profile," which consists of determining lecithin/sphingomyelin ratio (L/S) and measuring the percent phosphatidylglycerol (PG) on amniotic fluid. Bonny agrees and the results of the test are shown below.

L/S ratio = 1.0

Phosphatidylglycerol = 0.3%

Question to Consider

1. What is the interpretation of these test results?

Key Points To Remember

- Semen analysis provides useful information to assess male reproductive dysfunction.
- Amniotic fluid is dynamic, with large-volume flows into and out of the amniotic compartment each day.
- Maternal serum and amniotic fluid testing provide a wealth of knowledge about the progress of a pregnancy.

- The clinical laboratory provides many medical useful tests on semen, amniotic fluid, and maternal blood that provides the physician with timely, reliable, and accurate results.

Review Questions

Level I

1. Gestational diabetes mellitus is currently defined as (Objective 7)

    A. diabetes that develops during pregnancy.

    B. diabetes that develops postpartum.

    C. diabetes that develops 6 months prior to becoming pregnant.

    D. diabetes that develops only in teenage pregnancies.

2. Unconjugated estriol is decreased in which of the following? (Objective 5)

    A. Preterm delivery

    B. Gestational diabetes mellitus

    C. Down syndrome

    D. Respiratory distress syndrome

3. Amniotic fluid is removed from a patient using which of the following procedures? (Objective 4)

    A. Thoracentesis

    B. Arthrocentesis

    C. Amniocentesis

    D. Brochoalveolar lavage

4. Surfactants in fetal lungs is described as (Objective 7)

    A. surface-active phospholipids.

    B. surface-active macromolecular proteins.

C. surface-active carbohydrates.

D. surface-active triglycerides.

5. Which of the following is a useful method to assist in predicting the severity of fetal disease especially erythroblastosis fetalis? (Objective 3)

A. 75 g oral glucose tolerance test

B. Measuring alpha-fetoprotein in serum and amniotic fluid

C. Measuring unconjugated estriol

D. Determine the change (i.e., delta) in optical density of an amniotic fluid sample at 450 nm

6. Sperm motility is evaluated on the basis of (Objective 1)

A. size.

B. speed.

C. concentration.

D. head-to-tail orientation.

7. Sperm viability can be assessed using which of the following techniques? (Objective 3)

A. Sperm antibody binding to head or tail antigen

B. Measuring the delta OD 450 nm

C. Immunoassay measurement of alpha-fetoprotein

D. Thin-layer chromatography separation of phospholipids

8. Sperm motility is graded from zero to 4. A grade of zero indicates (Objective 5)

A. sperm moving with fast speed in a linear direction.

B. sperm moving with reasonable speed in a linear direction.

C. sperm moving with in-place motion (e.g., shaking or immobilized motion) with no forward progression.

D. Sperm not moving

9. A significant rise in the delta OD450 measurement of amniotic fluid indicates the presence of which analyte? (Objective 5)

A. Glucose

B. Bilirubin

C. Sphingomyelin

D. Alpha-fetoprotein

10. The presence of a fetal neural tube opening may be detected by measuring (Objective 3)

A. lecithin and sphingomyelin.

B. unconjugated estriol.

C. alpha-fetoprotein.

D. dimeric inhibin A.

Level II

1. Marsha, a 28-year-old female who is pregnant has the following results for a 75 g oral glucose tolerance test: (Objective 4)

Fasting = 110 mg/dL
1 hr = 200 mg/dL
2 hr = 160 mg/dL

The most likely diagnosis is

A. hypoglycemia.

B. gestational diabetes mellitus.

C. Down syndrome.

D. diabetes insipidus.

2. The results of a lecithin/sphingomyelin ratio test for Donna; a 32-year-old pregnant female is 1.2. These results are suggestive for which of the following? (Objective 5)

A. The baby may have Down syndrome.

B. There is a high probability that the mother may experience preterm delivery.

C. The fetus's lungs are mature.

D. The fetus's lungs are immature.

3. The following statement is in reference to which chemistry analyte? (Objective 4)

"Blood levels increase rapidly, doubling every two days, with maximal levels being attained at 8 to 10 weeks."

A. Inhibin A

B. Plasma glucose

C. Human chorionic gonadotropin

D. Phosphatidyl glycerol

4. Brenda's prenatal testing results for phosphatidyl glycerol by Amniostat-FLM were highly positive. Which of the following is the best interpretation of this result? (Objective 5)

A. Respiratory distress syndrome (RDS) rarely develops in an infant from mothers with highly positive phosphatidyl glycerol by Amniostat-FLM.

B. Respiratory distress syndrome (RDS) is likely to develop in her fetus based on the results of the phosphatidyl glycerol by Amniostat-FLM.

C. She is mostly going to experience "preterm delivery."

D. Her baby will be born with Down syndrome.

5. Diane is a 28-year-old female who has an alpha-fetoprotein result 2.5 times normal at 14 weeks gestation. Which of the following statements is correct? (Objective 5)

A. Her baby will be born with Down syndrome.

B. She has gestational diabetes mellitus.

C. There is a possibility that her fetus has developed an open neural tube defect.

D. Her baby may deliver preterm.

6. The spectrophotometric technique used by Liley to detect the presence of bilirubin pigments is based on which of the following principles? (Objective 1)

   A. Measure the change in OD at 410 nm

   B. Measure the change in OD at 450 nm

   C. Measure the change in OD at 390 nm

   D. Measure the change in voltage at 30 seconds

7. Measuring fibronectin is clinically useful for assessing a patient for which of the following? (Objective 2)

   A. Down syndrome

   B. Erythroblastosis fetalis

   C. Respiratory distress syndrome

   D. Preterm labor

8. Failure to provide early prenatal testing for gestational diabetes mellitus in a patient who does develop the disease could result in which of the following? (Objective 3)

   A. A normal healthy baby

   B. Development of Down syndrome

   C. Development of preeclampsia, fetal congenital malformations, and fetal macrosomia

   D. Development of neural tube defects

9. Measurement of maternal serum unconjugated estriol is clinically useful for which of the following conditions or disease? (Objective 2)

   A. High-risk pregnancies involving fetal growth retardation, intrauterine death, and hypoplasia of fetal adrenal glands

   B. Maternal heart disease

   C. Erythroblastosis fetalis

   D. Hemolytic crisis in the mother

10. The quad test is clinically useful to assess which of the following? (Objective 2)

    A. Gestational diabetes mellitus

    B. Down syndrome

    C. Hemolytic disease of the newborn

    D. Possible pregnancy

Endnotes

1. Kjeldsberg CR, Knight JA. *Body Fluids.* 3rd ed. Chicago, IL: ASCP, 1993.

2. Kjeldsberg CR, Knight JA. *Body Fluids.* 3rd ed. Chicago, IL: ASCP, 1993.

3. Rabinowitz R, Peters MT, Vyas S, et al. Measurement of fetal urine production in normal pregnancy by real-time ultrasonography. *Am J Obstet Gynecol* (1989) 161:1264–1266.

4. Duenhoelter JH, Pritchard JA. Fetal repiration: Quantitative measurements of amniotic fluid inspired near term by human and rhesus fetuses. *Am J Obstet Gynecol* (1976) 125;3:306–309.

5. Seeds AE. Current concepts of amniotic fluid dynamics. *Am J Obstet Gynecol* (1980) 138;3:575–586.

6. Patrick J, Campbell K, Carmichael L, et al. Patterns of human fetal breathing during the last 10 weeks of pregnancy. *Obstet Gynecol* (1980) 56;1:24–30.

7. Pritchard JA. Deglutition by normal and anecephalic fetuses. *Obstet Gynecol* (1965) 25:289–297.

8. Gilbert WM, Moore TR, Brace RA. Amniotic fluid volume dynamics. *Fetal Med Rev* (1991) 3:89–90.

9. Gilbert WM, Brace RA. The missing link in amniotic fluid volume regulation: Intramembranous absorption. *Obstet Gynecol* (1989) 74:748–755.

10. Gilbert WM, Brace RA. Novel determination of filtration coefficient of ovine placenta and intramembranous pathway. *Am J Physiol* (1990) 259;6; Pt.2:R1281–R1285.

11. Jang PR, Brace RA. Amniotic fluid composition changes during urine drainage and tracheoesophageal occlusion in fetal sheep. *Am J Obstet Gynecol* (1992) 167:1732–1735.

12. Gilbert WM. Chapter 33, Amniotic fluid disorders. In: Gabbe SG, Niebyl JR, Galen HL, et.al. eds. *Gabbe: Obstetrics: Normal and problem pregnancy.* 6th ed. St. Louis, MO: Elsevier Saunders, 2012.

13. Gilbert WM. Chapter 33, Amniotic fluid disorders. In: Gabbe SG, Niebyl JR, Galen HL, et.al. eds. *Gabbe: Obstetrics: Normal and problem pregnancy.* 6th ed. St. Louis, MO: Elsevier Saunders, 2012.

14. Gilbert WM. Chapter 33, Amniotic fluid disorders. In: Gabbe SG, Niebyl JR, Galen HL, et.al. eds. *Gabbe: Obstetrics: Normal and problem pregnancy.* 6th ed. St. Louis, MO: Elsevier Saunders, 2012.

15. Cunningham FC, Leveno KJ, Bloom SL, et al. Chapter 15, Antepartum Assessment. In: Cunningham FC, Leveno KJ, Bloom SL, et al. eds. *Williams Obstetrics.* 23rd ed. New York: McGraw-Hill, 2010.

16. Cunningham FC, Leveno KJ, Bloom SL, et al. Chapter 15, Antepartum Assessment. In: Cunningham FC, Leveno KJ, Bloom SL, et al. eds. *Williams Obstetrics.* 23rd ed. New York: McGraw-Hill, 2010.

17. Goldstein DP, Kosasa TS. Chapter 3, The subunit radioimmunoassay for hCG-clinical application. In Taymor ML, Green TH, eds. *Progress in Gynecology.* Volume 6. New York: Grune and Stratton, 1975.

18. Cole LA, Kardana A. Discordant results in human chorionic gonadotropin assays. *Clin Chem* (1992) 38:262–270.

19. Ashwood ER, Knight GJ. Clinical chemistry of pregnancy. In Burtis CA, Ashwood ER, Bruns DE. Eds. *Tietz Textbook of Clinical Chemistry and Molecular Diagnostics.* 4th ed. St. Louis, MO: Elsevier Saunders, 2006.

20. Birken S, Berger P, Bidard JM, et al. Preparation and characterization of new WHO reference ranges for human chorionic gonadotropin and metabolites. *Clin Chem* (2003) 49:144–154.

21. Kadar N, Bohrer M, Kemmann E, et al. The discriminatory human chorionic gonadotropin zone for endovaginal sonography: a prospective, randomized study. *Fertil Steril* (1994) 61:1016–1020.

22. Gitlan D. Normal biology of alpha-fetoprotein. *Ann NY Acad Sci* (1975) 259:7–16.

23. Gitlan D. Normal biology of alpha-fetoprotein. *Ann NY Acad Sci* (1975) 259:7–16.

24. Wu AHB. *Tietz Clinical Guide to Laboratory Tests.* 4th ed. St. Louis, MO: Saunders Elsevier, 2006.

25. ADA. Report of the expert committee on the diagnosis and classification of diabetes mellitus. *Diabetes Care* (1997) 20:1183–1197.

26. ADA. Standard of medical care in diabetes-2011. *Diabetes Care* (2011) 34; suppl.1:s11–61.

27. ADA. Standard of medical care in diabetes-2011. *Diabetes Care* (2011) 34; suppl.1:s11–61.

28. Sacks DB, Arnold M. Bakris GL, et al. Guideline and recommendations for laboratory analysis in the diagnosis and management of diabetes mellitus. *Diabetes Care* (2011) 34;6: e61–e99.

29. Lockwood CJ, Senyei AS, Dische MR, et al. Fetal fibronectin in cervical and vaginal secretions as a predictor of preterm delivery. *N Engl J Med* (1991) 325:669–674.

30. Goldenberg RL, Mercer BM, Iams JD, et al. The preterm prediction study: patterns of cervicovaginal fetal fibronectin as predictors of spontaneous preterm delivery. *Am J Obstet Gynecol* (1997) 177:8–12.

31. Peaceman AM, Andres WW, Thorp JM, et al. Fetal fibronectin as a predictor of preterm birth in patients with symptoms: a multicenter trial. *Am J Obstet Gynecol* (1997) 177:13–18.

32. Hook EB, Cross PK, Schreinemachers DM. Chromosomal abnormality rates at amniocentesis and in live-born infants. *JAMA* (1983) 249;15:2034–2038.

33. Haddow JE, Palomaki GE, Knight GJ, et al. Second trimester screening for Down's syndrome using maternal serum dimeric inhibin A. *J Med Screen* (1998) 5:115–119.

34. American College of Obstetrician and Gynecologists. Neural tube defects. Practice bulletin No. 44, July 2003.

35. Cunningham FG, Leveno KJ, Bloom SL, et al. Chapter 13, Prenatal diagnosis and fetal therapy. In: Cunningham FG, Leveno KJ, Bloom SL, et al. eds. *Williams Obstetrics*. 23rd ed. New York: McGraw-Hill, 2010.

36. Cunningham FC, Leveno KJ, Bloom SL, et al. Chapter 13, Prenatal diagnosis and fetal therapy. In: Cunningham FC, Leveno KJ, Bloom SL, et al. eds. *Williams Obstetrics*. 23rd ed. New York: McGraw-Hill, 2010.

37. Esherick JS, Clark DS, Slater ED. CURRENT Practice guidline in primary care 2012: http://www.accessmedicine.com/guideline.aspx. Accessed March 11, 2014.

38. Bevis DCA. Composition of liquor amnii in hemolytic diseases of the newborn. *J Obstet Gynaecol Br Emp* (1953) 60:244–251.

39. Liley AW. Liquor amnii analysis in the management of the pregnancy complicated by rhesus sensitizaiton. *Am J Obstet Gynecol* (1961) 82;6:1359–1370.

40. Liley AW. Errors in the assessment of hemolytic disease from amniotic fluid. *Am J Obstet Gynecol* (1963) 86;4:485–494.

41. Nicolaides KH, Rodeck CH, Mibashan RS, et.al. Have Liley charts outlived their usefulness? *Am J Obstet Gynecol* (1986) 155:90–94.

42. Queenan JT, Tomai TP, Ural SH, et al. Deviation in amniotic fluid optical density at a wavelength of 450 nm of Rh-immunized pregnancies from 14–40 weeks gestation: a proposal for clinical management. *Am J Obstet and Gynecol* (1993) 168;5:1370–1376.

43. Gluck L. Biochemical development of the lung: clinical aspects of surfactant development, RDS and the intrauterine assessment of lung maturity. *Clin Obstet Gynecol* (1971) 14;3:710–721.

44. Wijnberger LD, Huisjes AJ, Voorbij HA, et al. The accuracy of lamella body count and lecithin/sphingomyelin ratio in the prediction of neonatal respiratory distress syndrome: a meta–analysis. *BJOG* (2001) 108:583–588.

45. CLSI. Assessment of fetal lung maturity by the lamellar body count; approved guidelines. Wayne, PA: CLSI; 2011. CLSI document C58-A.

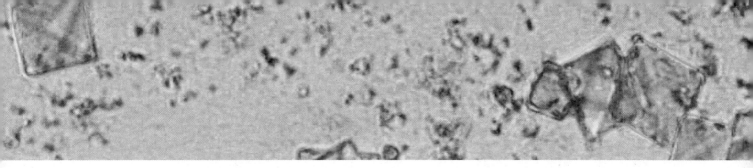

14 Metabolic Disorders

Objectives

LEVEL I

1. Discuss the importance of newborn screening procedures for metabolic diseases.
2. Explain the biochemical pathway leading to accumulation of metabolic products in patients with inborn errors of metabolism.
3. Discuss the advantages of tandem mass spectroscopy in newborn screening programs.
4. Identify the abnormal compounds present in urine for selected metabolic disorders.
5. Identify the characteristic odors of urine specimens in patients with metabolic disorders.
6. Identify enzyme defects for selected metabolic disorders.
7. Identify specimens used to test for amino acid disorders.
8. Discuss the clinical features of selected amino acid disorders.
9. Name the genetic disorders associated with select amino acid conditions.

LEVEL II

1. Correlate laboratory findings in metabolic disorders.
2. Discuss the genetic aspects of inborn errors of metabolism.
3. Discuss the importance of newborn screening programs for inborn errors of metabolism.
4. Identify diagnostic criteria for selected metabolic disorders.
5. Explain the significance of biochemical markers measured in metabolic disorders.
6. Discuss the significance of symptoms presented in metabolic disorders.
7. Describe treatment modalities for selected amino acid disorders.

Chapter Outline

Key Terms

Alkaptonuria
Alloisoleucine
Cerumen
Ectopia lentis

Essential amino acid
Failure to thrive
Homocystinuria
Inborn errors of metabolism

Maple syrup urine disease
Ochronosis
Phenylketonuria
Second-tier testing

Tandem mass spectrometry
Tyrosinemia

A CASE IN POINT

A 14-month-old female patient, Maria, is brought to her pediatrician's office because the mother was concerned about her development. She had a normal birth outside the United States. The mother stated that Maria is not achieving the normal milestones for a child her age. She mentioned the presence of an unusual odor in Maria's urine and lighter skin tones on areas of her face. She also noticed patches of lighter color hair on her head. On examination, the pediatrician noted that Maria showed evidence of muscle hypotonia and microcephaly. Urine and blood samples were collected for laboratory analysis. The nurse detected an unusual odor to the urine and described it as a "mousy" or "musty" odor.

The results of the laboratory tests are shown below:

Tests	Results	Reference Interval/Cutoff Value
Plasma phenylalanine, mg/dL (µMol/L)	10.0 (605)	0.38–1.14 (23–69)
Plasma tyrosine, mg/dL (µMol/L)	3.5 (193)	0.20–2.21 (11–122)
Phenylalanine/tyrosine ratio	2.8	<2.5

Questions to Consider

1. What is the most likely diagnosis?
2. What is the biochemical basis of the hypopigmented skin and hair?
3. What chemical compound can cause a urine to have a mousy or musty odor?
4. What is the clinical significance of each laboratory result for Maria?
5. Describe the biochemical events that occur when conversion of phenylalanine to tyrosine is inhibited.

A group of disorders affecting children very early in life are caused by single gene mutations that encode specific proteins. These mutations have the ability to modify primary protein structures, functions, and the amount of protein produced. Examples of proteins include enzyme catalyst, receptor proteins, transport proteins, and membrane components. These hereditary biochemical disorders are termed **inborn errors of metabolism** (IEM), or inherited metabolic disorders, and several examples are shown in Table 14-1 ★.

A compendium of human genes and phenotypes has been developed to provide detailed information about IEMs and hundreds of other Mendelian disorders. The source is Online Mendelian Inheritance in Man® (OMIM®), also available in printed format.[1]

All entries are given a six-digit OMIM number (No.), which is used as the identifier for a specific disorder and associated genes and phenotypes. The following is an example of the entry for maple syrup urine disease (MSUD). The OMIM No. is 248600 and the following information appears:

- Cytogenic location–1p212, 6q14.1, 7q31.1, 10q13.2
- Phenotype gene relationships
- Clinical synopsis

NEWBORN SCREENING

Screening of newborns for IEM was pursued in the early 1960s by Dr. Robert Guthrie in an effort to identify infants with phenylketonuria (PKU). This disorder, discussed in detail below, causes mental retardation unless treated with a phenylalanine-restricted diet before symptoms occur. Eventually, newborn screening was implemented as a public health program for PKU. Within a few years, other conditions for which early intervention can avoid mortality, morbidity, and disability were added.

Blood samples for analysis are collected on filter paper usually from a heel stick within 48–120 hours of age. The dried blood spot is sent to a newborn screening program where it is analyzed for biomarkers of diseases included in the screening panel.

In the 1990s **tandem mass spectrometry** or MS/MS coupled with either gas chromatography (GC) or high-pressure liquid chromatography (HPLC) was developed to become the principal analytical technique used in newborn screening of analytes in blood and urine. The superior analytical performance of MS/MS allows for testing a single dried blood spot called a "punch" for more than 60 amino acids and acylcarnitine with analyte-specific cutoff values. Tandem mass spectrometry is more sensitive, specific, precise, and accurate than other

★ **TABLE 14-1** Summary of Hereditary Disorders. (Online Mendelian Inheritance in Man® (OMIM®)

Name	OMIM No.	Enzyme Defect	Clinical Findings	Biochemical Markers
Alkaptonuria	203500	Homogentisic dioxygenase	Arthritis, ochronosis	Homogentisic acid
Homocystinuria	236200	Cystathionine beta synthase	Mental retardation, ectopia lentis, skeletal anomalies	Homocysteine and methionine
Homocystinuria	236270	Methionine synthase	Mental retardation, hypotonia, seizures, megaloblastic anemia	Homocysteine and methionine
Homocystinuria	236250	5,10-methylenetetrahydrofolate reductase	Mental retardation, gait and psychiatric abnormalities	Homocysteine and methionine
Maple Syrup Urine Disease	248600	Branched chain ketoacid dehydrogenase complex	Hypotonia, lethargy, seizures, coma	Branched chain amino acids and alloisoleucine
E_3 deficiency	246900	Dihydrolipoyl dehydrogenase (E_3)	Failure to thrive, hypotonia, developmental delay, seizures, coma	Branched chain amino acids, allo-isoleucine, lactic and pyruvic acids
Phenylketonuria (PKU)	261600	Phenylalanine hydroxylase	Mental retardation, fair complexion, and pigmentation	Phenylalanine, phenylpyruvate, 2-OH phenylacetic
Tyrosinemia type I	276700	Fumarylacetoacetase	Cirrhosis, hepatocellular carcinoma, renal disease, rickets	Tyrosine, succinylacetone, 4-OH phenyl pyruvate, 4-OH phenyl lactate
Tyrosinemia type II	276600	Tyrosine aminotransferase	Corneal ulcers, keratosis on palms and soles	Tyrosine 4-OH phenyl pyruvate, 4-OH phenyl lactate
Tyrosinemia type III	276710	4-hydroxyphenylpyruvate dioxygenase	Prematurity, possible mild developmental delay	Tyrosine, 4-OH phenyl pyruvate, 4-OH phenyl lactate

separation techniques (e.g., standalone GC and HPLC). Disorders detectable by tandem mass spectrometry are listed in Table 14-2 ★.

Newborn screening programs in the United States are typically maintained by the state health departments, and they determine which metabolic disorders should be screened for in each newborn. The testing menus of metabolic disorders are not uniform throughout the states due to differing opinions on which conditions to screen for and the slow response of laboratories to acquire tandem mass spectrometers.

☑ **CHECKPOINT 14-1**

What is the specimen of choice for newborn screening of inborn errors of metabolism?

In an effort to achieve a more uniform panel of screening tests, the American College of Medical Genetics (ACMG) in 2006 published recommendations that each newborn regardless of birthplace should be screened for at least 29 disorders listed in Table 14-3 ★. Tandem mass spectrometry is able to detect 20 conditions in a single dried blood spot punch, including IEM, inborn errors of fatty acid metabolism, and inborn errors of amino acid metabolism. Hemoglobin electrophoresis enables the detection of sickle cell disease and other hemoglobinopathies. There are also specific tests for biotinidase deficiency, cystic fibrosis, congenital adrenal hyperplasia, congenital hyperthyroidism, and galactosemia.[2]

In addition to the 29 disorders initially selected by ACMG, another 25 "secondary" disorders were included for testing. These represented disorders that are part of the differential diagnosis of the initial conditions. These secondary disorders are clinically significant, but no efficacious treatment is currently available.[3]

MS/MS provides a powerful tool for clinicians to use in their assessment of primarily children. Unfortunately, erroneous interpretation of the data provided occurs, and in some cases false positive results are produced. False positive results can cause significant stress, and even serious parent–child issues in some families.

SECOND-TIER TESTING

Second-tier testing is defined as a confirmatory test that is performed when primary screening tests, either by tandem mass spectrometry or another method, yield an equivocal result. Basically, there is overlap of the normal control range and the disease range, so there is poor specificity. The confirmatory test measures the disease specific analytes or an analyte profile.[4] The normal second-tier test result then overrules primary screening results; the second-tier test utilizes the same specimen so there is no additional patient contact necessary.

Following are two examples where second-tier testing is often performed. To clarify, these analytes have concentrations in the normal population that overlap with those in affected patients. The first example is testing for methionine, which is a nonspecific marker for both homocystinuria and remethylation defects. The second example involves the branched-chain amino acids, such as leucine, valine, and isoleucine, which are nonspecific markers for maple syrup urine disease and mostly elevated in patients that receive total parental nutrition. Second-tier testing is performed because it increases the specificity of the testing and the positive predictive value and reduces the false-positive rate, parental anxiety, and follow-up efforts and costs.

☑ **CHECKPOINT 14-2**

What is the purpose of second tier testing?

★ **TABLE 14-2** Disorders Detectable by Tandem Mass Spectrometry

Category	Disorders
Amino acidemias and urea cycle disorders	5-oxoprolinuria
	Argininemia
	Arginiosuccinic lyase deficiency (ASA)
	Carbamoylphosphate synthetase deficiency (CPS)
	Citrullinemia
	Hyperammonemia, hyperornithinemia, homocitrullinuria (HHH)
	Nonketotic hypergylcinemia
	Tyrosinemia type I
	Tyrosinemia type II
Organic academias	2-Methyl butyryl-CoA dehydrogenase deficiency (2MBDH deficiency)
	3-Methylcrontonyl-CoA carboxyl deficiency (3-MCC)
	3-Methylglutaconyl-CoA hydratase (3MGH deficiency)
	Glutaric Aciduria Type 1/Glutaryl-CoA dehydrogenase deficiency Type 1 (GA-1)
	Isobutyryl-CoA dehydrogenase deficiency
	Isovaleric acidemia/Isovaleryl-CoA dehydrogenase deficiency (IVA)
	Malonic aciduria
	Methylmalonic acidemia (MMA)
	Mitochondrial 3-acetoacetyl-CoA thiolase deficiency (β-KT or 3-ketothiolase)
	Multiple CoA carboxylase deficiency
	Proprionic acidemia/Propionyl-CoA carboxylase deficiency (PA)
Fatty acid oxidation disorders	2,4 Dienoyl-CoA reductase deficiency
	3-Hydroxy 3-methylglutaryl-CoA lyase deficiency (HMG)
	Carnitine/acylcarnitine translocase deficiency (CACT)
	Carnitine palmitoyl transferase deficiency Type I (CPT-I)
	Carnitine palmitoyl transferase deficiency Type II (CPT-II)
	Long-chain acyl-CoA dehydrogenase deficiency (LCAD)
	Long-chain hydroxy acyl-CoA dehydrogenase deficiency/3-Hydroxyacyl CoA dehydrogenase deficiency (LCHAD)
	Medium-chain acyl-CoA dehydrogenase deficiency (MCADD)
	Medium-chain 3-ketoacyl-CoA thiolase (MCKAT)
	Medium-chain hydroxy acyl-CoA dehydrogenase deficiency (MCHAD)
	Multiple acyl-CoA dehydrogenase deficiency (GA-II)
	Short-chain 3-ketoacyl-CoA thiolase/3-ketothiolase (SKAT)
	Short-chain acyl-CoA dehydrogenase deficiency (SCAD)
	Short-chain hydroxy acyl-CoA dehydrogenase deficiency (SCHAD)
	Trifunctional protein deficiency (TFP)
	Very long-chain acyl-CoA dehydrogenase deficiency (VLCAD)

★ **TABLE 14-3** American College of Medical Genetics (ACMG) Recommended Newborn Screening Disorders (Primary)

Category	Disorders
Disorders of organic-acid metabolism	Isovaleric acidemia
	Glutaric aciduria type I
	3-hydroxy-3-methylglutaric aciduria
	Multiple carboxylase deficiency
	Methylmalonic acidemia, mutase deficiency form
	3-methylcrotonyl-coA carboxylase deficiency
	Methylmalonic acidemia, cblA and cblB forms
	Propionic acidemia
	Beta-ketothiolase deficiency
Disorders of fatty acid metabolism	Medium-chain acyl-CoA dehydrogenase deficiency
	Very long-chain acyl-CoA dehydrogenase deficiency
	Long-chain 3-hydroxy acyl-Co A dehydrogenase deficiency
	Trifunctional protein deficiency
	Carnitine uptake defect
Disorders of amino-acid metabolism	Phenylketonuria
	Maple syrup urine disease
	Homocystinuria
	Citrullinemia
	Argininosuccinic acidemia
	Tyrosinemia type I
Hemoglobin-opathies	Sickle cell anemia
	Hemoglobin S-β-thalassemia
	Hemoglobin SC disease
Other disorders	Congenital hypothyroidism
	Biotinidase deficiency
	Congenital adrenal hyperplasia
	Galactosemia
	Hearing deficiency
	Cystic fibrosis

GENETIC METABOLIC DISEASES

Early detection of genetic metabolic diseases is essential for the welfare of the newborn. Caregivers should be vigilant for signs and symptoms postpartum and for years later because some disorders do not manifest themselves until later in life. In the newborn period, clinical findings may be nonspecific and similar to those of patients with sepsis. Also, a newborn who is severely ill should be evaluated for a possible IEM. Early symptoms of IEM include lethargy, poor feeding, convulsions, and vomiting. Knowledge of ethnic background is useful because some IEMs are more common in certain ethnicities (e.g., Tyrosinemia type I is more common in French Canadians of Quebec). Physical examination may reveal nonspecific findings—for example, hepatomegaly, which is common in some IEM. The presence of unusual odors in urine (e.g., mousy or musty odor in PKU and

★ **TABLE 14-4** Metabolic Diseases and Their Characteristic Urine Odors

Amino Acid Disorders	Urine Odor
Glutaric acidemia (type I)	Sweaty feet, acrid
Hawkinsinuria	Swimming pool
3-hydroxy-3-methylglutaric aciduria	Cat urine
Isovaleric acidemia	Sweaty feet, acrid
Maple syrup urine disease	Maple syrup
Hypermethioninemia	Boiled cabbage
Multiple carboxylase deficiency	Tomcat urine
Oasthouse urine disease	Hops-like
Phenylketonuria	Mousy or musty
Trimethylaminuria	Rotting fish
Tyrosinemia	Boiled cabbage, rancid butter

maple syrup in maple syrup urine disease) may also provide evidence of a possible IEM (see Table 14-4 ★).

Some patients develop signs and symptoms of genetic metabolic conditions months or years later in life. These children typically have mutations that affect a gene's function. The results may lead to mental retardation, motor deficits, delay in development, and convulsions. Some symptoms may be episodic, intermittent, acute, or chronic. Caregivers should suspect genetic disorders of metabolism in any child who presents with conditions listed in Box 14-1.[5]

Several treatment modalities are available and depend upon the time of presentation of a genetic metabolic condition. The following are examples of therapies that may improve the quality of life for patients suffering from these maladies:[6]

1. Special diets
2. Peritoneal dialysis or hemodialysis
3. Replacement of deficient metabolite
4. Replacement of deficient enzyme
5. Replacement of cofactor to facilitate the residual activity of a deficient or defective enzyme
6. Bone marrow transplant
7. Liver transplant

☑ **CHECKPOINT 14-3**

Why is early detection of inborn errors of metabolism important?

Alkaptonuria

Biochemistry and Etiology

The biochemical pathway of phenylalanine and tyrosine degradation is a precursor to the pathway shown in Figure 14-1 ■. Homogentisic acid (HGA) or 2, 5-dihydroxyphenylacetic acid, is cleaved to maleylacetoacetic acid by homogentisic acid oxidase (HGO). This enzyme serves to catalyze cleavage of the aromatic ring structure of HGA.[7] Individuals with **alkaptonuria** (OMIM No. 203500) are devoid of HGO activity in both liver and kidney tissue. HGA accumulates and undergoes renal excretion or is transformed to an ochronotic (dark colored) pigment within connective tissue. In some infants HGA is not present during the first days of life due to the absence of enzymatic activity of other enzymes in the biochemical pathway of tyrosine catabolism. Once HGA, a colorless compound, is excreted into urine, it gradually oxidizes to a dark-colored compound. The formation of the dark-colored compound is a result of exposure to air and its reaction in alkaline urine.

Alkaptonuria is inherited as an autosomal recessive trait. The incidence of the disease in the general population is about 1:250,000. The HGO gene maps to the q21-q23.60 region of chromosome 3.

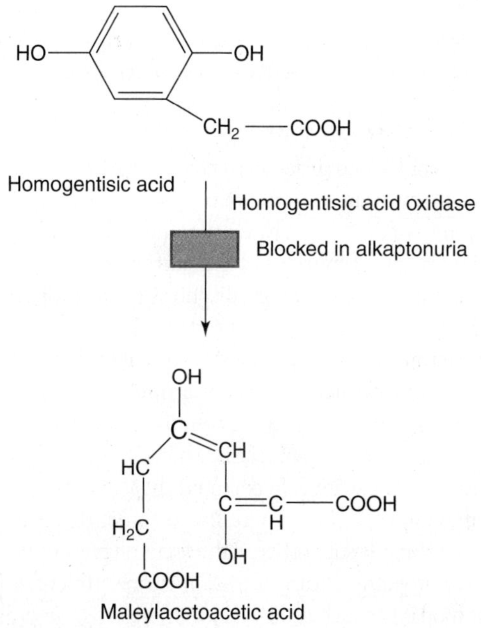

BOX 14-1   Clinical Manifestations That May Indicate Genetic Disorders of Metabolism

Delay in development

Motor deficit

Convulsions

Unusual odor

Unexplained mental retardation

Unexplained vomiting

Acidosis

Mental deterioration

Coma

Hepatomegaly

Renal stones

Muscle weakness

Cardiomyopathy

■ **FIGURE 14-1**   Metabolic Pathway of Homogentisic Acid

There are several multiple mutations whose clinical significance has not been completely evaluated.[8]

Clinical Features

The appearance of dark urine is not always the initial sign of HGO deficiency. The urine will discolor quicker when the pH is above 7.0 or when reducing substances, such as ascorbic acid, which normally protects HGA from oxidation, are not present in appropriate amounts. Early indications of HGO deficiencies are (1) family history, (2) discoloration of diapers after cleansing with an alkaline soap, (3) a more alkaline urine, (4) a positive finding with Benedict's solution, and (5) a negative glucose test using glucose oxidase.

Dark brown or black **cerumen**, a substance secreted by glands at the outer third of the ear canal, may be present in the first decade of a child's life. Another sign at this age is axillary skin pigmentation (greenish blue, blue, or brown) in glandular orifices. This may be associated with staining of underwear by sweat.[9]

Adults may present with **ochronosis**, which is a rare condition marked by dark pigmentation of the ligaments, cartilage, fibrous tissues, skin, and urine. The pigmentation is a result of an accumulation of oxidized HGA. A common physical finding is a grayish-blue discoloration of cartilage in the ears. It may also affect the sclera, cornea, and conjunctiva and eyelid skin. Other conditions that may be associated with ochronosis include cardiovascular disease, arthritis, coronary artery calcification, and intervertebral disk calcification. Ochronotic arthritis typically presents itself later in life, when degenerative joint disease develops.

Laboratory Findings

Detection of HGA in urine is a principal clinical finding in patients with alkaptonuria. Most patients do not have any other abnormal results for routine clinical laboratory tests. Normally, individuals do not excrete HGA, thus darkening of the urine on the addition of sodium hydroxide is presumptive evidence of alkaptonuria. Quantitative analysis of urine specimens for HGA is available using GC-MS. Patients with alkaptonuria typically excrete more than 2 g/day of HGA. Molecular analysis of the homogentisic acid oxidase gene is available but is not typically requested as follow-up testing.[10]

Diagnosis and Treatment

The diagnosis of alkaptonuria can be made at the time of urine discoloration, or it may await the onset of ochronosis in adulthood. There are other causes of darkened urine, including melaninuria, porphyria, myoglobinuria, bilirubinuria, and hematuria; therefore, they should be ruled out first before making a diagnosis of alkaptonuria. Ochronosis-like pigmentation of skin and cartilage has also been produced by (1) quinacrine administration for treatment of rheumatic disease; (2) antimalarial treatment; (3) amiodarone treatment for cardiac arrhythmias; (4) argyria, which is a condition due to treatment with silver compounds; and (5) chrysiasis, which is a dermatology condition due to treatment with gold compounds.

Alkaptonuria is a slow progressing disorder that is irreversible. Treatment is primarily supportive, with a focus on preventing the development of arthropathy, cardiac disease, and urinary tract disease. Other treatment modalities include avoidance of diets high in protein, phenylalanine, and tyrosine. Management options include genetic counseling, pain management with nonsteroidal anti-inflammatory agents,

physical therapy to increase range of motion, and regular follow-up visits. The disease is not incompatible with a normal life span, and oldest patient on record with Alkaptonuria lived to 99 years of age.[11]

☑ **CHECKPOINT 14-4**

What will be the color of urine from a patient with alkaptonuria and what causes the color formation?

Homocystinuria and Homocystinemia

The majority of homocysteine, an intermediate compound of methionine degradation, is remethylated to methionine. This reaction is catalyzed by the enzyme methionine synthase, which requires a metabolite of folic acid (5-methlytetrahydrofolate) as a methyl donor and a metabolite of vitamin B_{12} (methylcobalamin) as a cofactor (Figure 14-2 ■).[12] A small fraction of total homocysteine (and its dimer homocystine) exists in free form in plasma of normal individuals. The remainder is bound to proteins as mixed sulfides.

Currently, there are three forms of homocystinemia and homocystinuria:

- Homocystinuria due to cystathionine β-synthase (CBS) deficiency (classic homocystinuria)

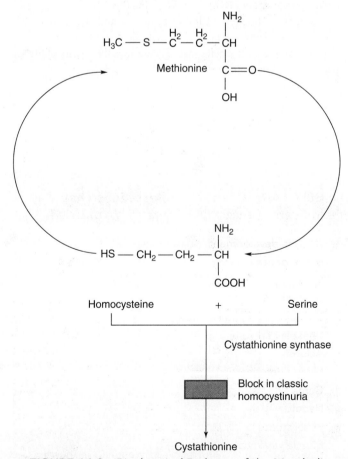

■ **FIGURE 14-2** Biochemical Pathway of the Metabolism of Methionine to Homocysteine

- Homocystinuria due to defect in methylcobalamin formation
- Homocystinuria due to deficiency of methylenetetrahydrofolate reductase (MTHFR)

Homocystinuria Due to CBS Deficiency (Classic Homocystinuria)

Biochemistry and Etiology

The incidence of homocystinuria (OMIM No. 236200) is estimated at 1:200,000–350,000 live births worldwide and is considered the second most treatable IEM after PKU. Homocystinuria results from an autosomal defect in the CBS gene on chromosome 21q22.3, which encodes for CBS. This enzyme is a pyridoxine-dependent hepatic enzyme that converts homocysteine to cystathionine, a precursor to cysteine. A deficiency of CBS results in an increase in homocysteine levels, and remethylation of this excess homocysteine leads to increased methionine levels.[13] A majority of patients have compound heterozygotes with over 92 different mutations discovered to date.

Some patients develop hyperhomocysteinemia that results in homocystinuria due to inherited disorders impairing the biological activation of cobalamin or acquired deficiency of that vitamin from methyltetrahydrofolate. This may lead to a biochemical form of homocystinuria.

Clinical Features

This is the most common inborn error of methionine metabolism and can affect multiple organs, including the skeletal, ocular, and vascular and central nervous systems. Most changes are progressive, although some manifest at earlier ages than others. Infants with this disorder are normal at birth. Clinical conditions during infancy are nonspecific and may include failure to thrive and delays in development. **Failure to thrive** describes children whose current weight or rate of weight gain is considerably lower than other children of comparable age and gender. Children begin to exhibit clinical manifestation of **ectopia lentis** (i.e., subluxation of the ocular lens) at about 3 years of age.[14] This condition causes severe myopia and iridodonesis (quivering of the iris). Later in life, patients may experience a variety of disorders such as astigmatism, glaucoma, cataracts, retinal detachment, and optic atrophy. Progressive forms of mental retardation are common. Some patients will develop psychiatric and behavioral disorders. Also, skeletal abnormalities resembling those of Marfan syndrome, characterized by irregular and unsteady gait, scoliosis pectus, osteoporosis, and thromboembolic episodes, can manifest themselves over time.

Laboratory Findings

Quantitative measurement of plasma reveals elevated levels of homocystine, total homocysteine and methionine, and detectable homocystine in the urine provide clinically useful information for the physician. Newborn screening tests performed in most states are available to detect elevated blood levels of methionine. Normal blood levels of methionine in vitamin B_6-responsive patients (see Box 14-2) during the newborn period should be further assessed. Another option available for newly diagnosed affected individuals is to perform a pyridoxine challenge test. Prenatal testing is available using cultured amniotic cells, chorionic villi, or DNA analysis.[15]

BOX 14-2 Summary of Vitamin B Complexes

Vitamin B_1	Thiamine
Vitamin B_2	Riboflavin
Vitamin B_3	Niacin
Vitamin B_6	Pyridoxine
Vitamin B_{12}	Cyanocobalamin

Diagnosis and Treatment

The diagnosis is usually made after 3 years of age, when the patient presents with ectopia lentis where the ocular lens is displaced in a downward direction (differentiating it from the upward displacement seen in Marfan syndrome).

Dietary intervention uses a methionine-restricted cystine-supplemented diet with the addition of folic acid and vitamin B_{12}. Some patients benefit from high-dose pyridoxine supplementation ($\sim$250 mg/day). Pyridoxine therapy tends to reduce the severity or incidence of thrombosis, seizures, and retardation and decrease mortality in responsive patients.[16]

☑ CHECKPOINT 14-5

Which amino acid is tested for in most newborn screening programs for homocystinuria?

Homocystinuria Due to Defect in Methylcobalamin Formation

Biochemistry and Etiology

Methylcobalamin is the cofactor for the enzyme methionine synthase, which catalyzes remethylation of homocystine to methionine (Figure 14-3 ■). This form of homocystinuria (OMIM No. 236270) is characterized by a reduction of methylcobalamin formation. There are at least five distinct defects in the intracellular metabolism of cobalamin, identified as *cblC*, *cblD*, *cblE*, *cblG*, and *cblF*.[17]

Clinical Features

The clinical features are similar in patients with any of the defects identified. Patients experience episodes of vomiting, lethargy, and hypotonia. They may eat poorly, and developmental delays can occur in the first few months of life.

Laboratory Findings

Patients with this condition may present with unique laboratory results, including megaloblastic anemia, homocystinuria, and hypomethioninemia. The presence of megaloblastic anemia differentiates these defects from homocystinuria due to methylenetetrahydrofolate reductase deficiency. The presence of hypomethioninemia differentiates both of these conditions from CBS deficiency.

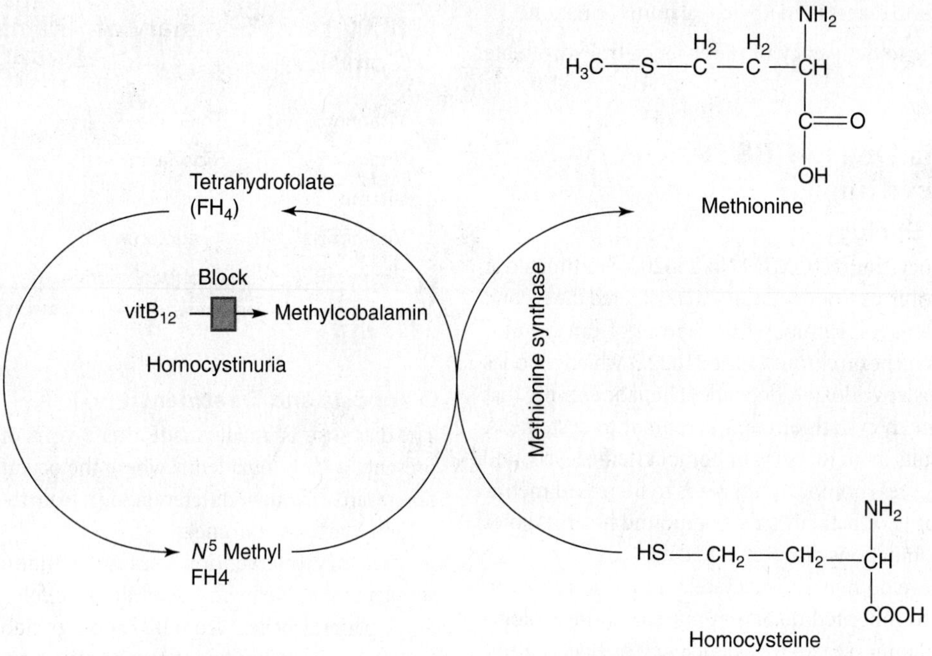

■ FIGURE 14-3   Remethylation of Homocysteine to Methionine with Methylcobalamin Used as a Cofactor

Diagnosis and Treatment

Diagnosis depends on a combination of laboratory tests, presenting symptoms, and conducting studies using specific complement proteins on cultured fibroblasts. Prenatal diagnosis is possible by initiating studies in amniotic cell cultures.

The principal therapy is supplementation with vitamin B_{12} in the form of hydroxycobalamin (1–2 mg/24hr) In most patients this treatment modality corrects the clinical and biochemical findings.

Homocystinuria Due to Deficiency of Methylenetetrahydrofolate Reductase

Biochemistry and Etiology

The enzyme methylenetetrahydrofolate reductase (MTHFR) reduces 5, 10-methylenetetrahydrofolate to form 5-methyltetrahydrofolate, which provides the methyl group required for remethylation of homocysteine to methionine (Figure 14-4 ■). This type of homocystinuria

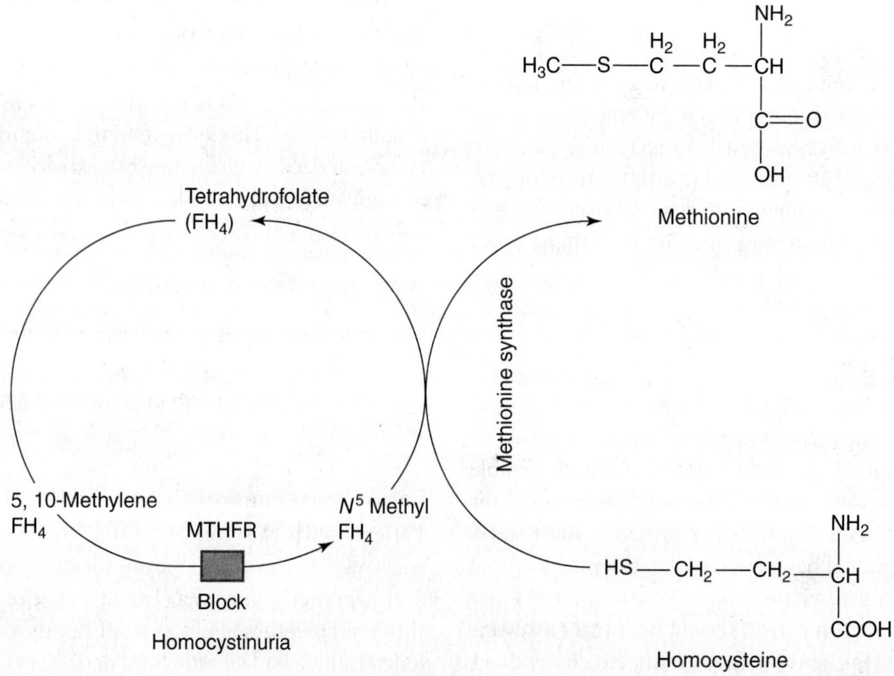

■ FIGURE 14-4   Remethylation of Homocysteine to Methionine with Methylenetetrahydrofolate Reductase Used as a Cofactor

(OMIM No. 236250) is inherited as an autosomal recessive trait. The gene for the enzyme has been located on chromosome 1p36.3, and several clinical disorders have been identified with genetic mutations.[18]

Clinical Features

Patients experience differing severity of symptoms, which may include apnea, seizure, microcephaly, muscle hypotonia, developmental delay, ataxia, and motor abnormalities. Some patients experience premature vascular disease or peripheral neuropathy.

Laboratory Findings

Plasma and urine tests typically show moderate homocystinemia and homocystinuria. The methionine concentration is low or low normal. This finding differentiates this condition from classic homocystinuria caused by CBS deficiency. Absence of megaloblastic anemia distinguishes these conditions from homocystinuria due to defect in methylcobalamin formation.

Diagnosis and Treatment

Diagnostic approaches used for this disorder include laboratory tests and enzyme assay in cultured fibroblast or leukocytes or by finding causal mutations in the MTHFR gene. Prenatal diagnosis is available by measuring MTHFR enzyme activity in cultured chorionic villi cells or amniotes, by gene linkage studies in families, or by DNA analysis of the mutations. Patients with a severe form of MTHFR deficiency are treated with a combination of folic acid, vitamin B_6, vitamin B_{12}, and methionine supplementation. Early administration of betaine has been tried and shown to be successful in reducing symptoms.[19]

MINI-CASE 14-1

Newborn baby Brian's tests results from a dried blood spot punch analyzed by tandem MS/MS are shown below:

Analyte	Result	Cutoff for Positive Newborn Screen
Methionine	90 μmol/L	>65 μmol/L

Follow up blood test:

Analyte	Result	Cutoff for Positive Newborn Screen
Homocysteine	200 μmol/L	>100 μmol/L

Questions to Consider

1. What condition does baby Brian most likely have based on the laboratory results?

2. What are the unique clinical feature(s) that may affect this infant if this condition is left undiagnosed and untreated?

Maple Syrup Urine Disease

Biochemistry and Etiology

Maple syrup urine disease (MSUD), also referred to as branched chain α-ketoacid (BCKA) deficiency, is an autosomal recessive disease caused by a deficiency in a subunit of the branched-chain alpha ketoacid dehydrogenase complex. This complex consists of thiamin (vitamin B_1) and pyrophosphate. The enzyme catalyzes the decarboxylation of three **essential amino acids**, leucine, isoleucine, and valine. These amino acids are essential because they cannot be produced by the body and must be obtained from food. Each branched chain amino acid (BCAA) has a nonpolar R-NH_2 group and is hydrophobic. The metabolic pathway of BCAAs is shown in Figure 14-5 ■.[20] The first reaction (reversible) is catalyzed by BCAA aminotransferase to produce branched ketoacid. In the second reaction, which is irreversible, the BCKAs are catalyzed by the enzyme branched-chain α-ketodehydrogenase (BCKDH). The results of this reaction are the production of CoA compounds that may enter various physiological cycles (e.g., urea cycle and tricarboxylic acid cycle).

BCKDH consists of three specific subunits or catalytic components identified as the branched chain α-ketoacid decarboxylase (E_1), the dihydrolipoyl transacylase (E_2), and the dihydrolipoyl dehydrogenase (E_3). The E_1 and E_2 components are specific to BCKDH.[21] The E_3 component is common among BCKDH, pyruvate dehydrogenase, and α-ketoglutarate dehydrogenases. The E_3 component functions to remove CO_2 from BCKA and then transfer the acyl moiety to E_2. This reaction requires thiamine pyrophosphate (TPP) as a cofactor. The E_1 component binding to TPP creates the ketoacid binding site for the release of CO_2 and consists of alpha and beta subunits. The $E_{1\alpha}$ subunit contains phosphates necessary for regulation of catalytic activity through interconversion of an active nonphosphorylated form to an inactive phosphate form of the BCKDH complex. The genes and chromosomes for catalytic components of branched-chain α-ketoacid enzymes are shown in Table 14-5 ★.

The prevalence of MSUD is 1:185,000 worldwide. In European and American Caucasians, it is 1:290,000 births; in a group of Mennonites in the United States, the incidence is 1:180. Individuals in this group are homozygous for a specific mutation (Y393N) in the $E_{1\alpha}$.

☑ CHECKPOINT 14-6

Identify the respective branched chain ketoacids of leucine, isoleucine, and valine.

There are four molecular phenotypes based on the affected locus of the BCKDH complex. Briefly, the phenotypes include (1) type IA, which is a mutation in the $E_{1\alpha}$ gene; (2) type IB, a mutation in the $E_{1\beta}$ gene; (3) type II, a mutation in the E_2 gene; and (4) type III, a mutation in the E_3 gene. There are more than 60 kinds of mutations reported in patients worldwide with MSUD. Medical discoveries focusing on the relationship between clinical phenotypes (discussed below) and

★ **TABLE 14-5** Genes and Chromosomes for Catalytic Components of Branched-Chain α-Ketoacid Enzymes

Gene	Chromosome
$E_{1\alpha}$	19q13.1–q13.2
$E_{1\beta}$	q14
E_2	1p31
E_3	7q31–32

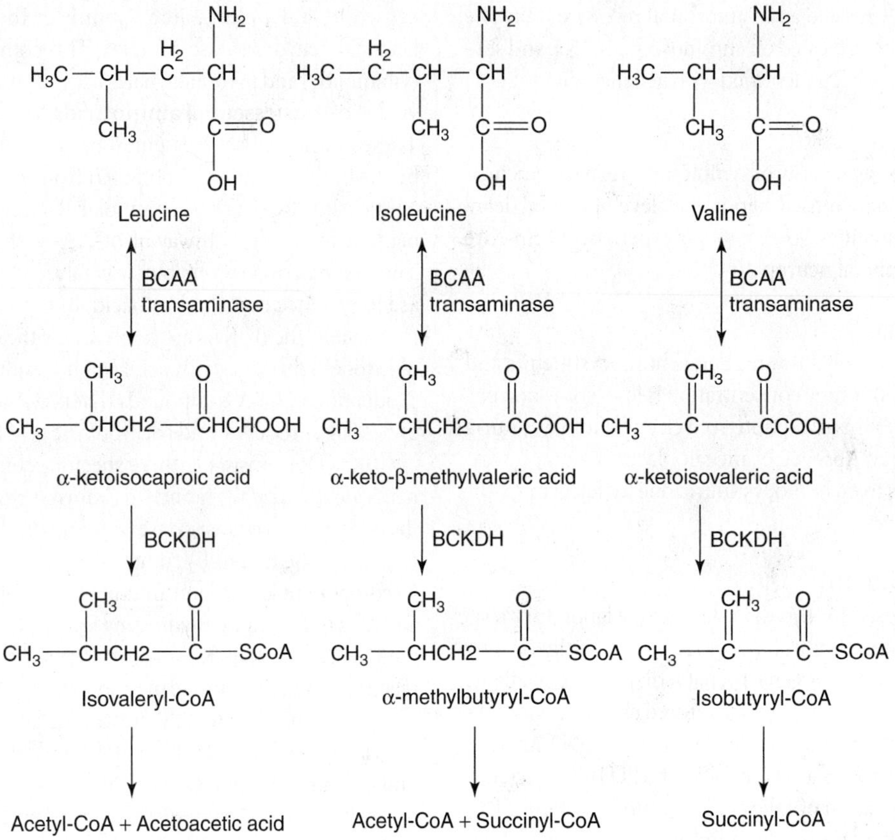

FIGURE 14-5   Metabolic Pathway of Branched-Chained Amino Acids

molecular phenotypes revealed that type 1A and 1B mutations had a tendency to cause the more severe classic phenotype of MSUD. A type II mutation has a tendency to cause the milder form of MSUD. Finally, all the thiamine-responsive forms are type II.[22]

The clinical phenotypes of MSUD, which will be discussed in more detailed below in the section "clinical features," include classic, intermediate, intermittent, thiamine responsive, and E₃ deficiency. The clinical and biochemical markers of these phenotypes are presented in Table 14-6 ★. Classic MSUD is the most common form of the disorder characterized by a <2% decarboxylation activity of the BCKDH complex. Mennonite patients with MSUD are included in this group.[23]

Clinical Features

The symptoms vary with age and genetic predisposition. The clinical features presented in Table 14-6 define the various clinical phenotypes.[24] Another method for presenting symptoms associated with MSUD is to identify them during stages of maturation. A newborn baby who is apparently normal and healthy may present with signs and symptoms of MSUD during first week of life. These signs and symptoms may include vomiting, lethargy, hypertonia, rigidity, severe opisthotonos (a spasm where the head and heels are bent backward and the body is bowed forward), seizures, general body sepsis, possible central nervous system infections, and hypoglycemia.

★ **TABLE 14-6** Clinical Phenotypes and Features of Maple Syrup Urine Disease

Clinical Phenotype	Clinical Features	Biochemical Marker(s)
Classic	Neonatal onset, poor feeding, vomiting, lethargy, hypotonia, seizures	Markedly increased alloisoleucine, branched-chain amino acids, and branched-chain ketoacids
Intermediate	Failure to thrive, developmental delay	Moderately elevated alloisoleucine, branched-chain amino acids, and branched-chain ketoacids
Intermittent	Normal early development; lethargy, ketoacidosis, semicoma	Normal amounts of branched-chain amino acid in patients who are asymptomatic
Thiamine responsive	Similar to intermediate or intermittent MSUD	Decreased branched-chain amino acids or branched-chain ketoacids with thiamin therapy
E₃ deficiency	Neonates are typically asymptomatic, failure to thrive, hypotonia, developmental delay, movement disorder	Moderately increased branched-chain amino acids and branched-chain ketoacids; slight increases in α-ketoglutarate and pyruvate

★ **TABLE 14-7** Several Forms of Hyperphenylalaninemia

Name	OMIM No.	Enzyme/Transport Defect	Gene/Chromosome	Clinical Features
Classic phenylketonuria (PKU)	261600	Phenylalanine hydroxylase	12q23.2	Mental retardation and hypopigmentation of skin and hair
Defect of biopterin cofactor biosynthesis, B	233910	Guanosine triphosphate cyclohydrolase I	14q22.2	Progressive mental retardation, seizures, muscle tone abnormalities
Defect of biopterin cofactor biosynthesis, A	261640	6-pyruvoyltetrahydropterin synthase	11q23.1	Progressive mental retardation, seizures, muscle tone abnormalities
Defect of biopterin cofactor biosynthesis, C	261630	Dihydropteridine reductase (DHPR)	4p15.32	Progressive mental retardation, spasticity, dystonia, myoclonus
Defect of biopterin cofactor biosynthesis, D	126090	Pterin-4α-carbinolamine dehydratase	10q22.1	Transient muscle tone abnormalities

Advanced stages also include neurovegetative (i.e., concerning the autonomic nervous system) deregulation with respiratory distress, bradycardia, hypothermia, infant encephalopathy, and central nervous dysfunction caused by leucine and its corresponding ketoacid. Some patients progress a year or more without symptoms but may develop them during adolescence or even adulthood. These include vomiting, ataxia, lethargy, and coma. There is also a form of chronic progressive MSUD that presents with persistent anorexia, chronic vomiting, failure to thrive, hypotonia, and osteoporosis.

Laboratory Findings

Patients with MSUD present with a characteristic sweet sugar odor to their urine, sweat, and ear wax. The odor is caused by the presence of elevated levels of ketoacids of leucine and isoleucine in these substances. There is a quick and easy urine screening test that could be used at the bedside to detect the presence of α-keto acids in patients with MSUD. The test uses an aliquot of a patient's urine sample mixed with a solution of 2, 4-dinitropenylhydrazine (DNPH). A positive test produces a yellow or chalky white precipitate. Positive results are also seen in patients with detectable amounts of phenylpyruvic acid (PKU), imidazole pyruvic acid (histidemia), and methionine (Oast-house syndrome).[25]

Alloisoleucine (allo-Ile) is a pathognomonic (i.e., indicative of disease) marker for MSUD. It is a transamination product of the keto acid of isoleucine.[26] Patients tend to show elevations of valine, isoleucine, and leucine. Newborn screening techniques include tandem MS/MS analysis of dried blood spot (punch). There are limitations with some mass spectroscopy assays—for example, a failure to differentiate between increased concentrations of the amino acids alloisoleucine, isoleucine, leucine, and hydroxyproline.

Another testing option available to pregnant patients is prenatal diagnostic testing using an enzyme assay in cultured amniocytes or chorionic villi and molecular analysis of the mutation(s) of genes.[27]

☑ CHECKPOINT 14-7

What compound is pathognomonic for maple syrup urine disease?

MINI-CASE 14-2

Newborn infant Joanne presents with the following clinical features during the first week of life:

- Refusal to feed
- Vomiting
- Lethargy

Joanne's urine has an odor that is described as sweet and smelling like maple sugar. Results of her newborn screening tests are shown below:

Analyte	Laboratory Results (mg/dL)	Cutoff for Positive Newborn Screen (mg/dL)
Leucine	6.6	<2.0
Alloisoleucine	6.8	<2.0
Valine	3.5	<2.0

Questions to Consider

1. What inborn error of metabolism does baby Joanne have?
2. What is the source of the maple syrup or sugar odor?

Diagnosis and Treatment

Diagnosis of MSUD often begins with the discovery of a peculiar odor of maple syrup found in the urine, sweat, and cerumen of the infant. A blood drop on a filter paper is submitted to a laboratory conducting newborn screening for amino acids. Patients with MSUD will show markedly elevated blood levels of leucine, isoleucine, valine, alloisoleucine, and lower concentrations of alanine. Urinary levels of leucine, isoleucine, valine, and their respective ketoacids are also elevated.[28]

The focus of treatment is to keep the concentration of toxic metabolites below pathologic concentrations while maintaining normal growth and development. In the acute stage it is necessary to hydrate and quickly remove BCAAs and their metabolites from tissues and body fluids. The techniques used to remove BCAAs may not be adequate enough; therefore, it is often necessary to initiate peritoneal dialysis or hemodialysis to complete the removal of toxins. Once patients are beyond the acute stage of MSUD, they require a diet low in BCAA. Patients with MSUD usually need to remain on a special diet for the rest of their lives.

Phenylketonuria

Biochemistry and Etiology

Phenylalanine is an essential amino acid. When excess phenylalanine is consumed in foodstuffs, it is converted to tyrosine by phenylalanine hydroxylase (PAH) and further degraded via a ketogenic pathway (Figure 14-6 ■).[29] A defect of PAH activity causes accumulation of phenylalanine, phenylketones, and phenylamines in body fluids. Elevated blood concentrations of phenylalanine are referred to as hyperphenylalaninemia. Several unique forms of hyperphenylalaninemia exist as listed in Table 14-7.[30] Deficiency of cofactor tetrahydrobiopterin (BH4) can also cause accumulation of phenylalanine in body fluids and in the brain (Figure 14-6).

All defects causing hyperphenylalaninemia are inherited as autosomal recessive traits. The incidence of **phenylketonuria** (PKU) in the United States is approximately 1:14,000 to 1:20,000 live births. For non-PKU hyperphenylalaninemia, the incidence is estimated at 1:15,000. PKU is more common in whites and Native Americans and less prevalence in blacks, Hispanics, and Asians.[31]

The gene for PAH resides on chromosome 12q23.2. There are several mutations that can cause disease in children. The majority of patients are compound heterozygotes for two different mutant alleles. The most common cause of BH4 deficiencies are 6-pyruvoyltertrahydropterin synthase (PTP synthase) mutations. The gene for PTP synthase resides on chromosome 11q23.1-23.3. Also the gene for dihydropteridine reductase is located on chromosome 4p15.32, and those of carbinolamine dehydratase and GTP cyclohydrolase are on 14q22.2.[32]

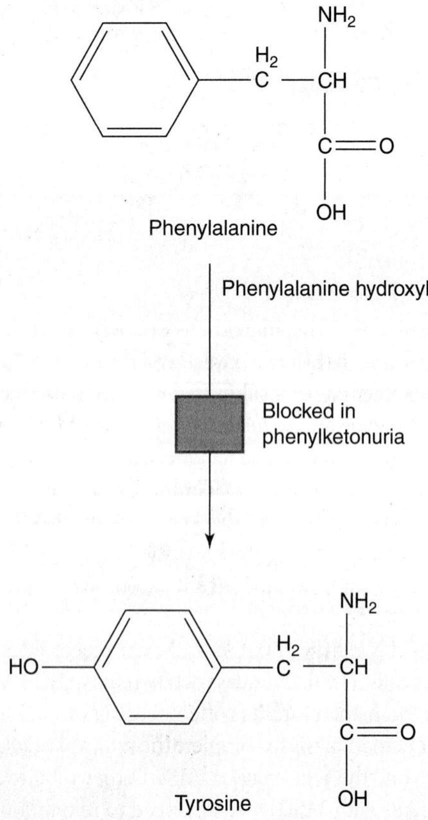

Phenylalanine

Phenylalanine hydroxylase

Blocked in phenylketonuria

Tyrosine

■ **FIGURE 14-6**   Metabolic Pathway of Phenylalanine

Clinical Features

The degree of hyperphenylalaninemia depends on the magnitude of enzyme deficiency and may vary from a high plasma concentration of >20 mg/dL or >1,200 μMol/L (reference interval = 1.2–3.4 mg/dL or 73–206 μMol/L) typical for the *Classic* form of PKU to mildly elevated level (2–6 mg/dL or 120–360 μMol/L).[33]

Infants with plasma phenylalanine levels >20 mg/dL, if untreated, usually develop signs and symptoms of classic PKU. The affected infant is normal at birth. Serious mental retardation develops gradually if the infant remains untreated. Some patients may experience severe vomiting, which presents as a possible early symptom. Hyperactivity, seizures, and other autistic-like behaviors may also be present in some patients. Children may not achieve the normal milestones at specific ages of development.

Infants with PKU have a lighter skin complexion, and some develop seborrhea or eczema that typically subsides with age. The hypopigmentation of skin and hair is based on the premise that phenylalanine is a competitive inhibitor of tyrosinase, a key enzyme in the pathway of melanin synthesis, which is reduced in PKU. These children develop an unpleasant odor of phenylacetic acid, which smells musty or mousy. The clinical features of classic PKU are rarely observed in those countries where neonatal screening programs for the detection of PKU are in effect.[34]

Laboratory Findings

Neonatal screening of dried blood on a filter paper by tandem MS/MS will reveal elevated levels of phenylalanine in patients with PKU. This method identifies all forms of hyperphenylalanine with a low false positive rate and a high degree of accuracy and precision. The number of false positives has been reduced by the inclusion of the phenylalanine/tyrosine molar ratio in the interpretation protocol. A ratio >2.5 supports the diagnosis of PKU. Plasma phenylalanine measurement is required to confirm the diagnosis of PKU.[35]

Diagnosis and Treatment

The clinical manifestations of PKU tend to develop gradually in the affected newborn infant. Therefore, newborn screening of dried blood samples using MS/MS within the first 12–48 hours of life is essential. Patients with a positive result from the screening test for hyperphenylalanine should have a confirmatory quantitative plasma measurement of phenylalanine performed. Another option, once a diagnosis of hyperphenylalaninemia is confirmed, is to initiate an assessment for biopterin metabolism to rule out biopterin deficiency as the cause of hyperphenylalaninemia.

Treatment modalities are designed to reduce phenylalanine levels in the plasma and brain. Dietary phenylalanine restrictions are usually initiated if blood phenylalanine levels are >6 mg/dL (360 μMol/L). Treatment consists of a special diet low in phenylalanine and supplemented with tyrosine, since tyrosine becomes an essential amino acid in phenylalanine hydroxylase deficiency.

☑ CHECKPOINT 14-8

What measurement and calculation tends to reduce the possibility of obtaining a false positive test for PKU?

Hyperphenylalaninemia Due to Deficiency of Cofactor BH4

Biochemistry and Etiology

Approximately 1–3% of infants with hyperphenylalaninemia have a defect associated with one of the enzymes required for production or recycling of cofactor BH4 (see Table 14-7). If these infants are misdiagnosed as having PKU, they may develop neurological symptoms despite adequate control of plasma phenylalanine. Patients with hyperphenylalaninemia due to BH4 deficiency may exhibit signs of neurological dysfunction due to deficiency of neurotransmitters dopamine or serotonin (Figure 14-7 ■). Four enzyme deficiencies are associated with formation of defective BH4 formation causing hyperphenylalaninemia (see Table 14-7).

Clinical Features

Patients with a deficiency of cofactor BH4 present with symptoms associated with diminished neurotransmitters (e.g., dopamine and serotonin). Neurologic symptoms include extrapyramidal signs with choreoathetotic or dystonic limb movement, axial and truncal hypotonia, hypokinesia, and feeding difficulties. Also seen is the possibility of seizures, mental retardation, hyper salivation, and swallowing difficulties.[36]

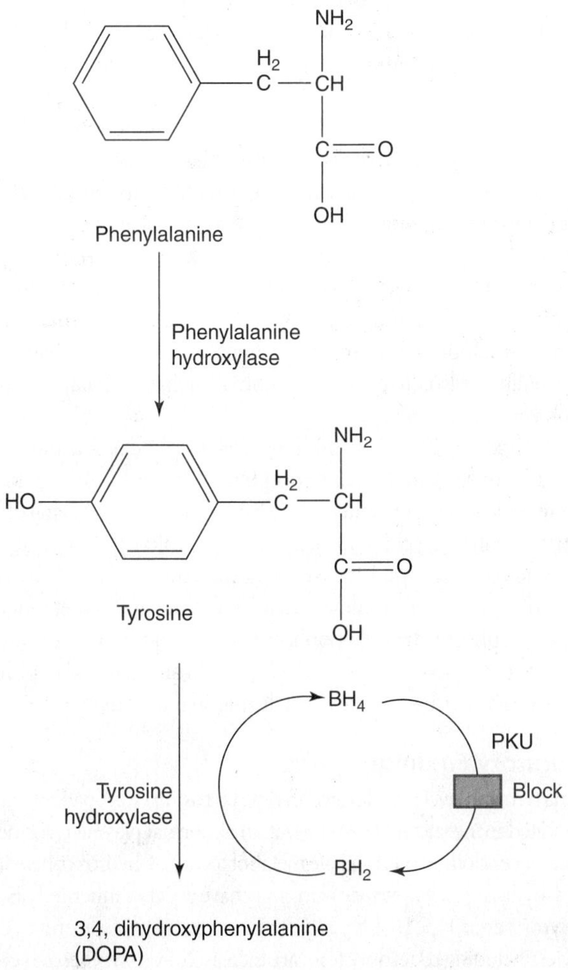

■ **FIGURE 14-7** Phenylalanine Metabolism Associated with BH4 Deficiency

Laboratory Findings

Newborn screening of dried blood filter paper samples is required. An infant's level of phenylalanine will be elevated. The distinguishing feature between PKU and deficient cofactor BH4 are the signs and symptoms of the neurotransmitter disorders. They are different for each disorder.

Additional studies can be initiated and include the following:

1. Measurement of neopterin and biopterin in urine
2. BH4 loading test
3. Performing laboratory tests for any of enzymes listed in Table 14-7

Diagnosis and Treatment

The diagnosis of cofactor BH4 is made based on the results of the newborn screening for phenylalanine. Assessment of symptoms associated with neurological function is also required. Further testing for the enzymes involved in their respective disorders provide information for the identification of the disorder. Genetic testing for mutations is also available but rarely necessary for establishing a diagnosis.

Treatment for hyperphenylalanine due to deficiency of cofactor BH4 is designed to correct for hyperphenylalanine and to correct the neurotransmitter deficiency in the central nervous system. Maintenance of acceptable plasma phenylalanine is accomplished by providing the patient with a diet low in phenylalanine and oral supplementation of BH4. Some patients may require lifelong supplementation with neurotransmitter precursors such as L-dopa and 5-hydroxytryptophan. This treatment modality aids in normalizing plasma levels of phenylalanine.[37]

> ☑ **CHECKPOINT 14-9**
>
> Identify two examples of neurotransmitting compounds that are associated with hyperphenylalaninemia due to deficiency of cofactor BH4.

Tyrosinemia

Biochemistry and Etiology

There are three types of **tyrosinemia** and their descriptions are outlined in Table 14-8 ★.[38] The skin is not involved in tyrosinemia type I and III but is involved in tyrosinemia type II. The metabolic pathway for tyrosinemia I, II, and III and their corresponding blockage points are shown in Figure 14-8 ■.[39]

The genetic forms of tyrosinemia are characterized by the accumulation of tyrosine in body fluids and tissue. Tyrosine is a semi-essential amino acid, derived from the liberation of tyrosine from hydrolysis of dietary or tissue proteins, or from the hydroxylation of the essential amino acid phenylalanine. It is the starting point for the synthesis of catecholamines (e.g. epinephrine and norepinephrine), thyroid hormones (e.g., thyroxine and triiodothyronine), and melanin.

Tyrosinemia is an autosomal recessive disease induced by a deficiency of enzymes related to a defect on chromosome bands. Tyrosinemia type I (tyrosinosis, hereditary tyrosinemia, hepatorenal tyrosinemia) specific chromosome bands are 15q25.1, which codes for the enzyme fumarylacetoacetic acid hydrolase. Tyrosinemia

★ **TABLE 14-8** Summary of Select Features of Three Types of Tyrosinemia

Name	OMIM No.	Enzyme/Transport Defect	Incidence	Significant Clinical Features	Principle Biomarkers
Tyrosinemia type I (hepatorenal)	276700	Fumarylacetoacetic acid hydrolase	<1:100,000	Cirrhosis, hepatocellular carcinomas, renal disease	Tyrosine, succinylacetone 4-OH-phenylpyruvate, 4-OH phenyllactate
Tyrosinemia Type II (oculocutaneous)	276600	Tyrosine α-ketoglutarate transaminase	<1:100,000	Corneal ulcers, keratosis on palms and soles	Tyrosine, 4-OH phenylpyruvate, 4-OH phenyllactate
Tyrosinemia type III	267610	4-hydroxyphenylpyruvate dioxygenase	<1:100,000	Prematurity, possible developmental delay	Tyrosine, 4-OH phenylpyruvate, 4-OH phenyllactate

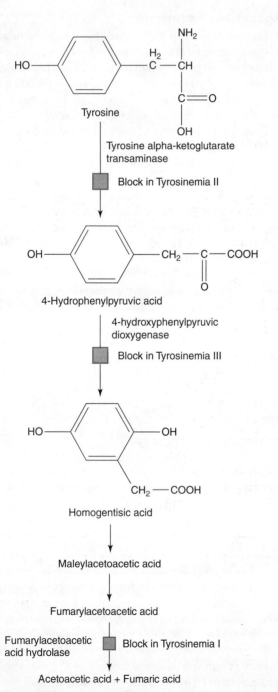

■ **FIGURE 14-8** Metabolic Pathway of Tyrosine Showing the Problematic Reactions for Tyrosinemia I, II and III

type II (Richner-Hanhart syndrome, oculocutaneous tyrosinemia) enzyme deficiency is tyrosine α-ketoglutarate transaminase, which gene maps to chromosome 16q22.2. The third tyrosinemia, type III (primary deficiency of 4-hydroxyphenylpyruvate dioxygenase) enzyme gene maps to 12q24.31. There are mutations to each gene for types I, II, and III, but their medical relevance has not been fully determined.[40]

Tyrosinemia Type I

Clinical Features

Infants born with tyrosinemia type I if left untreated appear normal at birth and usually present with symptoms between 2 and 6 month of age. They are rarely symptomatic in the first month and often appear healthy beyond the first year of life. The earlier the presentation of symptoms, the poorer is the prognosis. The 1-year mortality, which is about 60% in infants who develop symptoms before 2 months of age, decreases to 4% in infants who become symptomatic after 6 months of age.[41]

The hallmark for this disease is hepatic dysfunction. Findings in patients include fever, irritability, vomiting, hepatomegaly, jaundice, elevated levels of serum transaminases, and hypoglycemia. A characteristic odor resembling boiled cabbage may evolve due to increased amount of methionine (sulfur-containing amino acid) metabolites. Hepatic dysfunction can spontaneously resolve itself, but in some patients it may lead to liver failure and death. Other clinical manifestations include failure to thrive, hepatomegaly, and coagulation abnormalities. Also, cirrhosis and eventually hepatocellular carcinoma occurs with increasing age.[42]

Approximately 40% of children develop episodes of acute peripheral neuropathy resembling acute porphyria. Clinical features of this disorder include severe pain, often in the legs; hypertonic posturing of head and trunk; vomiting; paralytic ileus; marked weakness; and paralysis.[43]

Patients with type I tyrosinemia may develop renal disorders similar to Fanconi syndrome with a normal anion gap—metabolic acidosis, hyperphosphaturia, hypophosphatemia, and vitamin D-resistant rickets. These patients may also develop nephromegaly and nephrocalcinosis, which is usually discovered during an ultrasound examination.

Laboratory Findings

Plasma tyrosine levels are elevated in type I tyrosinemia. A patient without an elevated urine succinylacetone but an abnormal plasma tyrosine and the presence of other intermediate metabolites (e.g., 4-hydroxyphenyllactic acid, 4-hydroxyphenylpyruvic acid) may have another inherited disorder (e.g., tyrosinemia type II or type III). In untreated patients, liver-associated analytes, including α-fetoprotein, are increased, liver-synthesized coagulation factors are decreased, serum levels of transaminases are usually increased, and serum bilirubin is normal.

Diagnosis and Treatment

Diagnosis is based on the detection of elevated levels of succinylacetone in urine or blood. Neonatal screening for inborn errors performed on most infants for hypertyrosinemia detects only a minority of patients with tyrosinemia type I. Detection and identification of succinylacetone is included in many state protocols for newborn screening, provides a higher level of sensitivity and specificity than tyrosine, and is the preferable metabolite for screening. Clinicians should also attempt to differentiate tyrosinemia type I from other causes of hepatitis and hepatic failure in infants, including galactosemia, hereditary fructose intolerance, and neonatal iron storage disease.

Dietary restrictions on intake of phenylalanine and tyrosine can reduce but not halt the progression of the condition. A treatment regimen using nitisinone [2-(2-nitro-4-trifluoromethylbenzoyl)-1, 3-cyclohexaneione (NTBC)], which inhibits tyrosine degradation prevents episodes of acute hepatic and neurologic crises. Most patients will suffer some hepatic damage; therefore, they must be followed for development of cirrhosis or hepatocellular carcinoma.[44]

> ### ☑ CHECKPOINT 14-10
>
> Which organ is most affected in patients with tyrosinemia type I?

Tyrosinemia Type II

Clinical Features

This rare disorder presents with palmar and plantar hyperkeratosis, herpetiform corneal ulcers, and mental retardation. Ocular conditions include severe tearing, redness, pain, and photophobia. Tyrosine deposition in the cornea can create corneal lesions. Skin lesions typically develop later in life and are painful. Also nonpruritic hyperkeratotic plaques on the soles, palms, and fingertips may appear. Mental retardation occurs in <50% of patients and is usually mild to moderate.

Laboratory Findings

Untreated type II presents with markedly elevated plasma tyrosine levels (hypertyrosinemia). Levels typically exceed 20 mg/dL (1,100 μMol/L).[45] Patients may also have elevated 4-hydroxy phenylpyruvic acid and its metabolite in urine. Unlike tyrosinemia type I, liver and kidney function are normal.

Diagnosis and Treatment

Diagnosis of type tyrosinemia is assessed by assay of plasma tyrosine concentration in patients presenting with signs and symptoms of disease. Molecular diagnostic tests are available to determine genetic markers present.

A diet low in tyrosine and phenylalanine improves the biochemical abnormalities and can normalize the skin and eye symptoms. This treatment modality has been shown to prevent or lessen the degree of mental retardation, but the evidence is not conclusive.

Tyrosinemia Type III

Clinical Features

Very few cases of tyrosinemia III have been reported. Several were discovered while conducting amino acid chromatography for neurologic studies. The age of patients with type III has been from 1 to 17 months. These patients presented with developmental delay, seizures, intermittent ataxia, and self-destructive behavior. Liver and renal dysfunction are usually absent. Asymptomatic infants with 4-hydroxyphenylpyruvate dioxygenase (4-HPPD) deficiency have been discovered by neonatal screening for hypertyrosinemia.

Laboratory Findings

Patients will have elevated plasma tyrosine levels between 6–12 mg/dL (350–750 μMol/L).[46] Urine metabolites include 4-hydroxyphenylpuyruvic acid and its metabolite 4-hydroxyphenyllactic and 4-hydroxyphenylacetic acid. Genetics studies that focus on detecting mutations in the gene for 4-HPPD on chromosome 12q may be beneficial due to the rarity and issues with associated with measuring metabolites. A liver biopsy is also useful by demonstrating a low activity of 4-HPPD enzyme.

Diagnosis and Treatment

Diagnosis of patients suspected of having this disease depends on sustained moderate increases in plasma level of tyrosine and the presence in urine of 4-hydroxyphenyllactic and 4-hydroxyphenylacetic acids. The diagnosis can be supported with molecular diagnostic tests that demonstrate the presence of mutations in the gene for 4-HPPD on chromosome 12q.

Low levels of dietary tyrosine and phenylalanine are prophylactic for tyrosinemia type III given the possible association with neurologic abnormalities. Prophylactic administration of vitamin C, the cofactor for 4-HPPD has resulted in improved to patient health.

Key Points to Remember

- The affected infant is normal at birth and becomes symptomatic later in life.
- In general, the earlier the appearance of clinical symptoms, the more severe is the disease.
- Most of the disorders are inherited as autosomal recessive traits.

- Tandem mass spectrometry (MS/MS) is an accurate and sensitive technique for detecting metabolic products of inborn errors of metabolism.
- Newborn screening programs provide an opportunity for early detection of IEM, which allows for effective treatment modalities to be initiated sooner.

Review Questions

Level I

1. What is the defective enzyme in patients with alkaptonuria? (Objective 6)

   A. Cystathionine beta synthase

   B. Dihydrolipoyl dehydrogenase

   C. homogentisic acid oxidase

   D. Fumarylacetoacetic acid hydrolase

2. Patients with phenylketonuria (PKU) are deficient in which of the following enzymes? (Objective 6)

   A. Tyrosine α-ketoglutarate transaminase

   B. Phenylalanine hydroxylase

   C. Fumarylacetoacetic acid hydrolase

   D. Homogentisic dioxygenase

3. Urine of a newborn with Tyrosinemia may smell (Objective 5)

   A. like boiled cabbage.

   B. mousy.

   C. sweet.

   D. like vinegar.

4. Homocystinuria is caused by failure to metabolize (Objective 2)

   A. phenylalanine.

   B. valine.

   C. methionine.

   D. tyrosine.

5. The specimen of choice for newborn screening of inborn errors of metabolism is (Objective 7)

   A. plasma.

   B. serum.

   C. whole blood collected in a lithium heparin blood drawing tube.

   D. dried blood on a filter paper.

6. A mousy or musty odor in a newborn may indicate the presence of (Objective 5)

   A. phenylketonuria.

   B. homocystinuria.

   C. maple syrup urine disease.

   D. tyrosinemia type II.

7. Which of the following is a clinical feature of classic phenylketonuria (PKU)? (Objective 8)

   A. Congestive heart failure

   B. Mental retardation

   C. Keratosis on the soles

   D. Hepatocellular carcinoma

8. Which of the following provides the most sensitive screening technique for inborn errors of metabolism? (Objective 3)

   A. Absorbance spectroscopy

   B. Enzyme immunoassay

   C. Tandem mass spectrometry (MS/MS)

   D. Protein electrophoresis

9. Alkaptonuria, phenylketonuria, and homocystinuria are all (Objective 9)

   A. inherited as a dominant trait.

   B. conditions with no genetic foundation.

   C. inborn errors of carbohydrate metabolism.

   D. inherited as an autosomal recessive condition.

10. A deficiency of branched-chained alpha-ketoacids is associated with (Objective 4)

    A. maple syrup urine disease.

    B. tyrosinemia types I, II, and III.

    C. homocystinuria types I, II, and III.

    D. alkaptonuria.

Level II

1. A method for decreasing false positive results in newborn screening is (Objective 5)

   A. assess all patient samples in duplicate.

   B. second-tier testing.

   C. perform a double blind study.

   D. measure the analyte in blood and urine.

2. Dark brown or black cerumen is a finding for which of the following conditions? (Objective 1)

   A. Alkaptonuria

   B. Tyrosinemia type I

   C. E3 deficiency

   D. Argininemia

3. An adult patient with ochronosis will have which of the following features? (Objective 6)

   A. Grayish blue discoloration of the cartilage of the ears

   B. Urine that smells like boiled cabbage

   C. A deficiency of phenylalanine hydroxylase

   D. Hypopigmentation of skin

4. Which metabolic disorder is associated with ectopia lentis? (Objective 6)

   A. Tyrosinemia type III

   B. Homocystinuria

   C. E3 deficiency

   D. Isovaleric acidemia

5. A patient with laboratory findings that include megaloblastic anemia, homocystinuria, and hypomethioninemia suggest which of the following? (Objective 1)

   A. Tyrosinemia type I

   B. Classic phenylketonuria

   C. Propionic acidemia

   D. Homocystinuria due to defect in methylcobalamin formation

6. A treatment modality that includes administration of folic acid, vitamin B_6, and vitamin B_{12} is associated with which of the following? (Objective 7)

   A. Homocystinuria due to a deficiency of methylenetetrahydrofolate reductase

   B. Hyperphenylalaninemia

   C. Low blood levels of alloisoleucine

   D. Increased blood levels of succinylacetone

7. What is the source of the sweet, maple syrup odor present in a patient with maple syrup urine disease? (Objective 1)

   A. Tyrosine

   B. 4-hydroxyphenylpyruvic acid

   C. Ketoacids of leucine and isoleucine

   D. Methionine

8. Which of the following is pathognomonic marker for maple syrup urine disease? (Objective 5)

   A. Fumarylacetoacetic acid hydrolase

   B. 4-hydroxyphenyllactic acid

   C. Alloisoleucine

   D. Homocysteine

9. A positive newborn screening test result for succinylacetone in blood indicates the possible presence of (Objective 1)

   A. branched-chain ketoacidosis.

   B. tyrosinemia type I.

   C. hyperphenylalaninemia.

   D. dihydrolipoyl dehydrogenase deficiency.

10. An individual born with a defective gene that code for the enzyme phenylalanine hydroxylase will have which of the following? (Objective 2)

   A. Low concentrations of phenylalanine in blood

   B. High concentrations of phenylalanine in blood

   C. A normal concentration of phenylalanine in blood

   D. A high concentration of homogentisic acid in blood

Endnotes

1. http://www.ncbi.nlm.nih.gov/omim. Accessed March 16, 2014.
2. Rezvani I, Rezvani G. Chapter 78, An approach to inborn errors of metabolism. In: Kliegman RM ed. *Nelson Textbook of Pediatrics.* 19th ed. Philadelphia, PA: Elsevier Saunders, 2011.
3. Rezvani I, Rezvani G. Chapter 78, An approach to inborn errors of metabolism. In: Kliegman RM ed. *Nelson Textbook of Pediatrics.* 19th ed. Philadelphia, PA: Elsevier Saunders, 2011.
4. Oglesbee D, Sanders KA, Lacey JM, et al. Second-tier test for quantification of alloisoleucine and branched-chain amino acids in dried blood spots to improve newborn screening for maple syrup urine disease (MSUD). *Clin Chem* (2008) 54;3:542–549.
5. Rezvani I, Rezvani G. Chapter 78, An approach to inborn errors of metabolism. In: Kliegman RM ed. *Nelson Textbook of Pediatrics.* 19th ed. Philadelphia, PA: Elsevier Saunders, 2011.
6. Rezvani I, Rezvani G. Chapter 78, An approach to inborn errors of metabolism. In: Kliegman RM ed. *Nelson Textbook of Pediatrics.* 19th ed. Philadelphia, PA: Elsevier Saunders, 2011.
7. Rinaldo P, Hahn S, Matern D. Inborn errors of amino acid, organic acids, and fatty acid metabolism. In: Burtis CA, Ashwood ER, Bruns DE, eds. *Tietz Textbook of Clinical Chemistry and Molecular Diagnostics.* 4th ed. St. Louis, MO: Elsevier Saunders, 2006.
8. Itin PH. Chapter 131, Cutaneous changes in errors of amino acid metabolism. In: Goldsmith LA, Katz SI, Gilchrest B, et al. eds. *Fitzpatrick's Dermatology in General Medicine.* 8th ed. New York: McGraw Hill, 2012.
9. Itin PH. Chapter 131, Cutaneous changes in errors of amino acid metabolism. In: Goldsmith LA, Katz SI, Gilchrest B, et al. eds. *Fitzpatrick's Dermatology in General Medicine.* 8th ed. New York: McGraw Hill, 2012.

10. Itin PH. Chapter 131, Cutaneous changes in errors of amino acid metabolism. In: Goldsmith LA, Katz SI, Gilchrest B, et al. eds. *Fitzpatrick's Dermatology in General Medicine.* 8th ed. New York: McGraw Hill, 2012.

11. Itin PH. Chapter 131, Cutaneous changes in errors of amino acid metabolism. In: Goldsmith LA, Katz SI, Gilchrest B, et al. eds. *Fitzpatrick's Dermatology in General Medicine.* 8th ed. New York: McGraw Hill, 2012.

12. Rezvani I, Melvin JJ. Chapter 79, Defects in metabolism of amino acids. In: Kliegman RM ed. *Nelson Textbook of Pediatrics.* 19th ed. Philadelphia, PA: Elsevier Saunders, 2011.

13. Dyer JA. Chapter 137, Lipoid proteinosis and heritable disorders of connective tissue. In: Goldsmith LA, Katz SI, Gilchrest B, et al. eds. *Fitzpatrick's Dermatology in General Medicine.* 8th ed. New York: McGraw Hill, 2012.

14. Rezvani I, Melvin JJ. Chapter 79, Defects in metabolism of amino acids. In: Kliegman RM ed. *Nelson Textbook of Pediatrics.* 19th ed. Philadelphia, PA: Elsevier Saunders, 2011.

15. Rezvani I, Melvin JJ. Chapter 79, Defects in metabolism of amino acids. In: Kliegman RM ed. *Nelson Textbook of Pediatrics.* 19th ed. Philadelphia, PA: Elsevier Saunders, 2011.

16. Dyer JA. Chapter 137, Lipoid proteinosis and heritable disorders of connective tissue. In: Goldsmith LA, Katz SI, Gilchrest B, et al. eds. *Fitzpatrick's Dermatology in General Medicine.* 8th ed. New York: McGraw Hill, 2012.

17. Rezvani I, Melvin JJ. Chapter 79, Defects in metabolism of amino acids. In: Kliegman RM ed. *Nelson Textbook of Pediatrics.* 19th ed. Philadelphia, PA: Elsevier Saunders, 2011.

18. Rezvani I, Melvin JJ. Chapter 79, Defects in metabolism of amino acids. In: Kliegman RM ed. *Nelson Textbook of Pediatrics.* 19th ed. Philadelphia, PA: Elsevier Saunders, 2011.

19. Rezvani I, Melvin JJ. Chapter 79, Defects in metabolism of amino acids. In: Kliegman RM ed. *Nelson Textbook of Pediatrics.* 19th ed. Philadelphia, PA: Elsevier Saunders, 2011.

20. Rinaldo P, Hahn S, Matern D. Inborn errors of amino acid, organic acids, and fatty acid metabolism. In: Burtis CA, Ashwood ER, Bruns DE, eds. *Tietz Textbook of Clinical Chemistry and Molecular Diagnostics.* 4th ed. St. Louis, MO: Elsevier Saunders, 2006.

21. Rezvani I, Melvin JJ. Chapter 79, Defects in metabolism of amino acids. In: Kliegman RM ed. *Nelson Textbook of Pediatrics.* 19th ed. Philadelphia, PA: Elsevier Saunders, 2011.

22. Mitsubuchi H, Owada M, Endo F. Markers associated with inborn errors of metabolism of branched-chain amino acids and their relevance to upper levels of intake in healthy people: an implication from clinical and molecular investigations on maple syrup urine disease. *J Nutr* (2005) 135:1565S–1570S.

23. Mitsubuchi H, Owada M, Endo F. Markers associated with inborn errors of metabolism of branched-chain amino acids and their relevance to upper levels of intake in healthy people: an implication from clinical and molecular investigations on maple syrup urine disease. *J Nutr* (2005) 135:1565S–1570S.

24. Mitsubuchi H, Owada M, Endo F. Markers associated with inborn errors of metabolism of branched-chain amino acids and their relevance to upper levels of intake in healthy people: an implication from clinical and molecular investigations on maple syrup urine disease. *J Nutr* (2005) 135:1565S–1570S.

25. Holmes E, Foxall PJ, Spraul M, et al. 750 MHz 1H NMR spectroscopy characterization of the complex metabolic pattern of urine from patients with inborn errors of metabolism: 2-hydroxyglutaric aciduria and maple syrup urine disease. *J Pharm Biomed Anal* (1997) 15;11:1647–1659.

26. Oglesbee D, Sanders KA, Lacey JM, et al. Second-tier test for quantification of alloisoleucine and branched-chain amino acids in dried blood spots to improve newborn screening for maple syrup urine disease (MSUD). *Clin Chem* (2008) 54;3:542–549.

27. Chinsky J, Appel M, Almashanus S, et al. A nonsense mutation (R242X) in the branched-chain alpha – keto acid dehydrogenase E1 alpha subunit

28. Thomas JA, Van Hove J. Chapter 36, Inborn errors of metabolism. In Hay WW, Levin MJ, Deterding RR, eds. *Current Diagnosis and Treatment Pediatrics.* 21st ed. New York: McGraw-Hill, 2012.

29. Rezvani I, Melvin JJ. Chapter 79, Defects in metabolism of amino acids. In: Kliegman RM ed. *Nelson Textbook of Pediatrics.* 19th ed. Philadelphia, PA: Elsevier Saunders, 2011.

30. Rinaldo P, Hahn S, Matern D. Inborn errors of amino acid, organic acids, and fatty acid metabolism. In: Burtis CA, Ashwood ER, Bruns DE, eds. *Tietz Textbook of Clinical Chemistry and Molecular Diagnostics.* 4th ed. St. Louis, MO: Elsevier Saunders, 2006.

31. Rezvani I, Melvin JJ. Chapter 79, Defects in metabolism of amino acids. In: Kliegman RM ed. *Nelson Textbook of Pediatrics.* 19th ed. Philadelphia, PA: Elsevier Saunders, 2011.

32. Rezvani I, Melvin JJ. Chapter 79, Defects in metabolism of amino acids. In: Kliegman RM ed. *Nelson Textbook of Pediatrics.* 19th ed. Philadelphia, PA: Elsevier Saunders, 2011.

33. Wu AHB. *Tietz Clinical Guide to Laboratory Tests.* 4th ed. St. Louis, MO: Saunders Elsevier, 2006.

34. Longo N. Chapter 364, Inherited disorders of amino acid metabolism in adults. In: Long DL, Fauci AS, Kasper DL, et al. eds. *Harrison's Principles of Internal Medicine.* 18th ed. New York: McGraw-Hill, 2012

35. Longo N. Chapter 364, Inherited disorders of amino acid metabolism in adults. In: Long DL, Fauci AS, Kasper DL, et al. eds. *Harrison's Principles of Internal Medicine.* 18th ed. New York: McGraw-Hill, 2012

36. Rezvani I, Melvin JJ. Chapter 79, Defects in metabolism of amino acids. In: Kliegman RM ed. *Nelson Textbook of Pediatrics.* 19th ed. Philadelphia, PA: Elsevier Saunders, 2011.

37. Rezvani I, Melvin JJ. Chapter 79, Defects in metabolism of amino acids. In: Kliegman RM ed. *Nelson Textbook of Pediatrics.* 19th ed. Philadelphia, PA: Elsevier Saunders, 2011.

38. Rinaldo P, Hahn S, Matern D. Inborn errors of amino acid, organic acids, and fatty acid metabolism. In: Burtis CA, Ashwood ER, Bruns DE, eds. *Tietz Textbook of Clinical Chemistry and Molecular Diagnostics.* 4th ed. St. Louis, MO: Elsevier Saunders, 2006.

39. Rinaldo P, Hahn S, Matern D. Inborn errors of amino acid, organic acids, and fatty acid metabolism. In: Burtis CA, Ashwood ER, Bruns DE, eds. *Tietz Textbook of Clinical Chemistry and Molecular Diagnostics.* 4th ed. St. Louis, MO: Elsevier Saunders, 2006.

40. Rezvani I, Melvin JJ. Chapter 79, Defects in metabolism of amino acids. In: Kliegman RM ed. *Nelson Textbook of Pediatrics.* 19th ed. Philadelphia, PA: Elsevier Saunders, 2011.

41. Rezvani I, Melvin JJ. Chapter 79, Defects in metabolism of amino acids. In: Kliegman RM ed. *Nelson Textbook of Pediatrics.* 19th ed. Philadelphia, PA: Elsevier Saunders, 2011.

42. Itin PH. Chapter 131, Cutaneous changes in errors of amino acid metabolism. In: Goldsmith LA, Katz SI, Gilchrest B, et al. eds. *Fitzpatrick's Dermatology in General Medicine.* 8th ed. New York: McGraw Hill, 2012.

43. Oglesbee D, Sanders KA, Lacey JM, et al. Second-tier test for quantification of alloisoleucine and branched-chain amino acids in dried blood spots to improve newborn screening for maple syrup urine disease (MSUD). *Clin Chem* (2008) 54;3:542–549.

44. Rezvani I, Melvin JJ. Chapter 79, Defects in metabolism of amino acids. In: Kliegman RM ed. *Nelson Textbook of Pediatrics.* 19th ed. Philadelphia, PA: Elsevier Saunders, 2011.

45. Wu AHB. *Tietz Clinical Guide to Laboratory Tests.* 4th ed. St. Louis, MO: Saunders Elsevier, 2006.

46. Wu AHB. *Tietz Clinical Guide to Laboratory Tests.* 4th ed. St. Louis, MO: Saunders Elsevier, 2006.

gene (BCKDHA) as a cause of maple syrup disease. *Hum Mutat* (1998) 12;2:136–137.

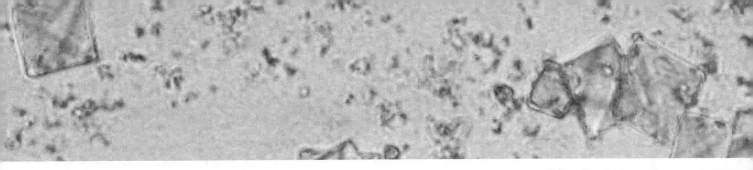

Fecal Analysis

Objectives

LEVEL I

1. Describe normal color, appearance, and consistency of feces.
2. Differentiate between osmotic and secretory diarrhea.
3. Identify proper collection procedures for random and timed stool collections.
4. Identify causes for alterations in stool colorization.
5. Describe significant clinical findings in microscopic examination of feces.
6. Identify clinically significant chemical tests performed on feces.

LEVEL II

1. Explain the proper procedures for collection, handling, and storage of stool samples.
2. Discuss the implication of abnormal chemical tests on stool samples.
3. Describe the physical and microscopic findings in stool samples in both normal and diseased individuals.
4. Interpret both qualitative and quantitative tests performed on stool samples.

Key Terms

Acute diarrhea
Chronic diarrhea
Chymotrypsin
Constipation

Diarrhea
Dysmotility
Elastase-1
Fecal osmotic gap

Inflammatory diarrhea
Malabsorption
Maldigestion
Occult blood

Osmotic diarrhea
Porphyrias
Secretory diarrhea
Steatorrhea

A CASE IN POINT

Ben is 72 years old and generally in good health. About 5 weeks ago, he developed a case of diarrhea that has made him tired and weak. He went to his physician who completed a history and physical examination. Ben revealed that he has been taking variable amounts of magnesium sulfate laxatives for several weeks because it made him feel better. Ben provided a stool sample that was sent to the clinical microscopy laboratory for analysis and the results are shown below:

Appearance/consistency: watery

Culture: negative

Fecal Osmotic gap: 185 mOsm/kg

Questions to Consider

1. Based on the results of the laboratory tests, what type of diarrhea does Ben have?

2. What is a possible cause of this type of diarrhea?

The gastrointestinal (GI) tract is comprised of the stomach, small and large intestines, pancreas, and gallbladder. They participate in the digestive process that commences with the ingestion of food and water and ends with the excretion of feces (Figure 15-1 ■).

ANATOMY OF THE GI TRACT

Food and fluids enter the body via the mouth and pass through what can be viewed as a 10-meter tube that ends with the anus. The foodstuff enters the stomach where chemicals begin the process of digestion.

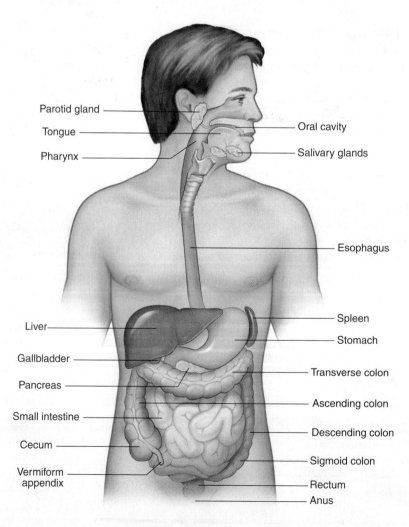

■ **FIGURE 15-1** Organs of the Alimentary Canal and Related Accessory Organs

The total quantity of fluid absorbed per day by the gut is approximately 9 L, which is composed of about 2 L oral intake, 1.5 L saliva, 2.5 L gastric juice, 0.4 L bile, 1.5 L pancreatic juice, and 1 L intestinal secretions. The small intestine absorbs about 90% of the weakly acidic digestive mixture.

Several GI hormones and other regulatory peptides are released by stimulatory factors. Digestion, absorption, and storage functions are stimulated or inhibited by these different hormones, producing a hormonal control mechanism to regulate the action of intestinal hormones and provide for secretion of bile acids, bicarbonate, and several enzymes involved in the digestion of food.

Carbohydrate, proteins, and lipids are broken down and absorbed. Nutrients, including vitamins and minerals, have been absorbed by the time food passes from the jejunum and ileum into the large intestine. In the large intestine, water is actively absorbed, electrolyte balance is regulated, and bacterial action commences. These processes result in the formation of feces.

DIARRHEA, MALABSORPTION, AND MALDIGESTION

The stomach, intestinal tract, and pancreas are functionally related, and symptoms such as diarrhea, malabsorption, or maldigestion may be associated with disease or disorders of any of these organs. **Malabsorption** is described as a pathologic state of impaired nutrient absorption in the GI tract. **Maldigestion** results from an intraluminal defect that leads to the incomplete breakdown of nutrients into their absorbable substrates. This chapter will focus on the conditions that require analysis of feces, and readers can expand their knowledge of other GI disorders through the cited references.

Diarrhea is described as the passage of abnormally liquid or unformed stools at an increased frequency. A stool weight of >200 g/day for adults on typical Western diets can be considered diarrhea. Diarrhea can be classified further as acute if lasting <2 weeks, persistent if 2–4 weeks, and chronic if >4 weeks in duration.[1]

There are two conditions usually associated with the passage of stool totaling <200 g/day that should be included in the overall assessment of a patient because diagnostic and therapeutic protocols differ. *Pseudodiarrhea* is described as frequent passage of small amounts of stool and is associated with rectal urgency (i.e., loss of regular bowel control), irritable bowel syndrome (IBS), and proctitis. *Fecal incontinence* is the involuntary discharge of rectal material that is usually caused by neuromuscular disorders or structural anorectal (anus plus rectum) problems. Pseudodiarrhea and fecal incontinence should be considered in patients presenting with symptoms of diarrhea.[2]

Acute Diarrhea

Most cases of **acute diarrhea** are caused by infectious agents and present with additional symptoms (e.g., vomiting, fever, and abdominal pain). A fewer number of cases are caused by medications, ingestion of toxins, and ischemia. A patient with acute diarrhea usually does not require medical intervention unless he or she has profuse diarrhea with dehydration, has a fever greater than 48 hours, has recently taken antibiotics, is experiencing severe abdominal pain during a new community outbreak, or is immune compromised.

Diagnosis of patients with severe acute infectious diarrhea relies on microbiologic analysis of stool samples. Testing strategies include procurement of cultures for bacterial and viral pathogens, direct examination for ova and parasites, and immunoassays for specific bacterial toxins (e.g., *Clostridium difficile*), viral antigens (rotavirus), and protozoan antigens (e.g., *Giardia*, *Entamoeba histolytica*). Advanced testing may include molecular diagnostic assays in stool for unique DNA sequence of select proteins.[3]

Chronic Diarrhea

Chronic diarrhea may require medical evaluation to determine the presence of an underlying pathology. Most causes of chronic diarrhea are noninfectious, unlike acute diarrhea. The causes of chronic diarrhea are typically classified by pathophysiological mechanisms as shown in Box 15-1,[4] although many diseases cause diarrhea by more than one mechanism.

BOX 15-1 Categories of Significant Causes of Chronic Diarrhea

Secretory Causes
Certain bacterial infections
Idiopathic secretory diarrhea
Exogenous stimulant laxatives
Chronic ethanol ingestion
Other toxins and drugs
Endogenous laxatives (e.g., dihydroxy bile acids)
Bowel resection, fistula (absorption) disease

Osmotic Causes
Osmotic laxatives (containing magnesium, phosphates, or sulfates)
Lactase and other disaccharide deficiencies
Nonabsorbable carbohydrates (e.g., lactulose, sorbitol, polyethylene glycol)
Steatorrheal causes
Intraluminal maldigestion (e.g., bariatric surgery, liver surgery, bacterial overgrowth, pancreatic exocrine insufficiency)
Mucosal malabsorption (e.g., Whipple's disease, infections, celiac sprue)
Postmucosal obstruction (lymphatic obstruction)

Inflammatory Causes
Lymphatic colitis
Immune-related mucosal disease
Crohn's disease
Chronic ulcerative colitis
Infections

Dysmotile Causes
Irritable bowel syndrome
Visceral neuromyopathies
Hyperthyroidism (hypermotility)
Drugs (i.e., prokinetic agents)

Factitial Causes
Munchausen syndrome
Eating disorders

Secretory Diarrhea

Secretory diarrhea is caused by derangement in fluid and electrolytes transport across intestinal mucosa. There is an increase in secretion of water and electrolytes that overwhelms the reabsorptive ability of the large intestine. Clinical presentation is characterized by production of a large volume of watery feces.

Osmotic Diarrhea

Osmotic diarrhea occurs when ingested, semi-absorbed, osmotically active solutes (e.g., sodium, potassium, and glucose) attract enough fluid into the lumen to exceed the reabsorptive capacity of the colon. The result is an increase in fecal water output proportional to the solute load. This type of diarrhea usually ends after fasting or discontinuation of the causative agent. Osmotic diarrhea is commonly caused by ingesting magnesium-containing antacids, health supplements, or laxatives and can present with a fecal osmotic gap of >50 mOsmol/kg (see discussion below).

Carbohydrate malabsorption due to defects in brush border disaccharidases and other enzymes can lead to osmotic diarrhea with a low stool pH. The presence of increased carbohydrate in stools results in an alteration of the osmotic pressure of unabsorbed sugars in the intestine that attracts fluids and electrolytes. A common cause of chronic diarrhea in adults is lactase deficiency. The dietary load of lactose determines the range of symptoms the patient may experience.

Steatorrhea

The term **steatorrhea** describes the presence of excess fat in stools. In quantitative terms, it represents an amount of stool fat that exceeds 7 g/day. In this condition of fat malabsorption, the stool sample appears greasy and has a foul smell. Patients often experience weight loss and nutritional deficiencies due to simultaneous malabsorption of amino acids and vitamins. There is also an increased fecal output caused by the osmotic effect of fatty acids. Steatorrhea often accompanies pancreatic insufficiency, intraluminal maldigestion, mucosal malabsorption, or post-mucosal lymphatic obstruction (Box 15-2).[5,6]

BOX 15-2   Steatorrheal Causes of Chronic Diarrhea

Intraluminal Maldigestion

- Results from pancreatic exocrine insufficiency due to chronic pancreatitis often a sequel of ethanol abuse
- Cystic fibrosis
- Pancreatic duct obstruction

Mucosal Malabsorption

- Associated with celiac disease, tropical sprue
- Whipple's disease

Post-mucosal Lymphatic Obstruction

- Due to congenital intestinal lymphangiectasis or to acquired lymphatic obstruction

---

Inflammatory Diarrhea

Inflammatory diarrhea is characterized by pain, fever, bleeding, or other signs and symptoms of inflammation. Diarrhea usually develops through exudation (i.e., movement of fluid and cells from blood vessels into tissues as a result of inflammation), fat malabsorption, fluid absorption, disrupted movement of electrolytes, hypersecretion, and hypermotility. Stool analysis of patients with inflammatory diarrhea will reveal the presence of leukocytes or leukocyte-derived protein. Middle-aged patients who present with signs and symptoms of chronic inflammatory diarrhea should be furthered evaluated to exclude a colorectal tumor.

Dysmotility

Dysmotility is a term that describes altered movement of feces. Increased motility or hypermotility is seen in inflammatory diarrhea, whereas slow motility describes **constipation**. Conditions that can cause hypermotility include hyperthyroidism, carcinoid syndrome and certain drugs (e.g., prostaglandins).

Irritable bowel syndrome (not to be confused with inflammatory bowel disease) is relatively common (~10% prevalence) in the United States and is characterized by altered intestinal and colonic motor and sensory responses to select stimuli. Common symptoms are decreased stool frequency at night, alternating with episodes of constipation and some abdominal pain that is resolved with defecation.

Factitial Diarrhea

Approximately 15% of unexplained causes of diarrhea are factitial (i.e., artificial or self-induced). Individuals with eating disorders or

---

☑ CHECKPOINT 15-1

Match the type of diarrhea with its key feature:

Types of diarrhea

_____Secretory

_____Osmotic

_____Steatorrhea

_____Inflammatory

_____Dysmotility

_____Factitial

Key features

A. Munchausen syndrome

B. Stool contains leukocytes and leukocyte-derived protein

C. Derangement in fluid and electrolytes

D. Excess fat in the stool

E. Caused by ingesting magnesium containing antacids or laxatives

F. Constipation

Munchausen syndrome (deception or self-injury) will self-administer laxatives alone or in combination with diuretics. These individuals typically develop hypotension and hypokalemia (low concentration of serum potassium).

SPECIMEN COLLECTION, HANDLING, AND STORAGE

Fecal specimen collection can be a challenge for patients. Patients should be properly instructed on specimen collection procedures and provided with a container for each collection. Stool collections should be made in a container such as a bed pan or a disposable container, followed by transferring the contents into an appropriate laboratory container. Patients should be instructed not to contaminate the specimen with toilet water, which may contain chemicals such as disinfectants or dyes. Containers that include preservatives for ova and parasites must not be used to collect specimen for other tests.

Qualitative tests (e.g., occult blood, microscopic examination for leukocytes, and fat) may require only a random stool specimen, which needs a glass or plastic container with a screw-cap, similar to a urine container. Small, flat wooden sticks (provided in kit tests) can be used for occult blood testing.

Some fecal analysis requires timed specimen collection, for example, 24- or 72-hour quantitative fecal fat tests or porphyrin analysis. For these timed collection procedures, the stool collection must be refrigerated during the entire collection. Because prolonged collection times can produce a large collection volume, the patient is often provided with a paint can or something similar to collect the sample. These larger containers are also useful to complete the emulsification of the feces prior to analysis. Laboratory staff should exercise caution when removing the paint can lid because gasses formed by the feces can increase the pressure in the can and cause the contents to explode out when the pressure is released. Note: Some reference laboratories will not accept paint cans or other collection containers greater than 500 mL (500 g). Also, specimens containing barium or charcoal may not be acceptable.

Specimen requirements for testing procedures requiring small amounts of feces such as occult blood may differ from larger collection test procedures. The sample should be from an excreted stool rather than from material obtained on the glove of a physician performing a rectal examination, because this invasive procedure can cause enough bleeding to produce a positive test result.

PHYSICAL EXAMINATON

Color

The normal brown color of feces is due to intestinal oxidation of stercobilinogen to urobilin. Alterations in the color of feces can be due to a number of causes as presented in Table 15-1 ★.[7] A pale color may indicate a blockage of the bile duct or ingestion of barium sulfate during an imaging procedure. Black- and red-colored feces can indicate GI bleeding or ingestion of certain medications or foods. Patients taking certain antibiotics may present with green-colored

★ **TABLE 15-1** Stool Color, Appearance, and Possible Etiologies

Color/Appearance	Etiology
Black	Iron therapy
	Charcoal
	Upper GI bleeding
	Antacids containing bismuth
Red	Beets and food coloring
	Lower GI bleeding
Pale yellow, gray	Bile duct obstruction
	Barium sulfate
Green	Biliverdin
	Oral antibiotic
	Green vegetable
Bulky/frothy	Bile duct obstruction
	Pancreatic disorders
Ribbon-like	Intestinal constriction
Mucus	Colitis
	Dysentery
	Constipation
	Cancer

feces. Certain foods and food coloring additives may also result in green-colored stool.

Appearance and Consistency

Stool specimens can present with altered appearance and consistency. For example, the feces may appear watery as in diarrhea or as small, hard stools as seen in cases of constipation. A stool sample that is slender or ribbon-like suggests an obstruction of the normal movement of feces through the intestine. Other examples are frothy feces due to biliary obstruction and steatorrhea and mucus-coated stools that are the result of colitis, dysentery, or excessive straining during elimination.

Mucus

Mucus observed in fresh stool specimens is considered abnormal and should be reported. The presence of translucent gelatinous mucus clinging to the surface of the formed stool may indicate spastic constipation or mucous colitis. Bloody mucus may suggest the presence of a tumor or inflammatory process in the rectal canal. Mucus can be present with ulcerative diverticulitis, intestinal tuberculosis, and bacillary dysentery.

Pus

Pus and mucus can be present in stools of patients with chronic ulcerative colitis and chronic bacillary dysentery. Typically, pus can be observed by microscopic examination. Patients with a localized abscess or fistula in association with the sigmoid colon, rectum, or anus also pass a large amount of pus.

☑ CHECKPOINT 15-2

Match the following physical features with their cause.

Physical features

_____ Pus

_____ Mucus

_____ Hard stool

_____ Pale white stool

_____ Black stool

_____ Red stool

_____ Green

Causes

A. lower GI bleeding

B. bile-duct obstruction

C. biliverdin

D. upper GI bleeding

E. chronic ulcerative colitis

F. tumor or inflammatory process in the rectal canal

G. constipation

MICROSCOPIC EXAMINATION

Fat

Fat in stool can be easily detected by microscopic examination of stained feces. Sudan III is commonly used, although Sudan IV or oil red O are acceptable. The procedure requires a small aliquot of stool suspension to be placed onto a glass slide and mixed with two drops of 95% ethanol. Then two drops of saturated ethanolic solution of Sudan III are added, with further mixing. A cover slip is placed onto the slide. A microscopic examination reveals the presence of different types of fats with examples shown in Box 15-3. Microscopic findings of more than 60 stained droplets of neutral fats per high power field are highly suggestive of steatorrhea (Figure 15-2 ■).

Contaminants such as mineral oil or castor oil may mimic neutral fats and can influence the droplet counts. At the completion of the procedure described above, a second aliquot of stool sample is placed onto a slide and several drops of 36% v/v acetic acid are added to the feces. The slide is heated by passing it through a flame until slight boiling occurs. This technique converts neutral fats and soaps to fatty acids and melts the fatty acids, causing them to form droplets that stain intensively with Sudan III. The slide is examined while warm for stained

BOX 15-3   Microscopic Findings of Different Types of Fats in Stool Samples

- Fatty acids present as lightly stained flakes or as needle-like crystals that do not stain (Caution: They are often missed.).

- Soaps are not stained but may appear as well-defined amorphous flakes or as rounded masses or coarse crystals.

- Neutral fats appear as large orange or red droplets.

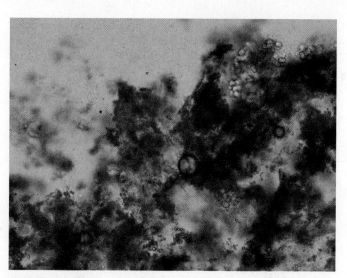

■ **FIGURE 15-2**   Fat Droplets in Stool Specimen

droplets. The presence of up to 100 stained droplets per high-power field is interpreted as normal. Patients with steatorrhea of pancreatic origin typically present with increased amounts of fatty acids and soaps.

Meat or Muscle Fibers

Microscopic examination for meat or muscle fiber is useful to screen for maldigestion and/or hypermotility. The procedure is similar to qualitative fecal fat. Mix an aliquot of stool on a slide with a solution of eosin in 10% ethanol; let stand for 3 minutes and examine for muscle fibers. The reviewer is encouraged to examine the whole area under the cover slip and count only regular fibers with clearly evident cross-striations. More than 10 fibers/high-power field is clinically significant.

Leukocytes

Abnormal leukocyte and cell count estimations are significant findings in patients with conditions that affect the intestinal mucosa (e.g., ulcerative colitis and bacterial dysentery). Low-power microscopic screening of a small aliquot of mucus or a drop of liquid stool mixed with two drops of methylene blue will allow for the estimation of the number of leukocytes and erythrocytes. The results of the microscopic screening can provide the clinician with information about whether the diarrhea is caused by bacterial pathogens (e.g., *Salmonella, Shigella,* or *Campylobacter*). Organisms that cause diarrhea by toxin production (e.g., *Staphylococcus aureus,* viruses, and parasites) do not result in the appearance of fecal leukocytes. The findings of a microscopic examination can be used to provide preliminary information for clinicians prior to receiving microbiology culture results. A manual differential count should be performed under high-power microscopy, with approximately 200 cells counted if possible. The examination should include only clearly identifiable mononuclear or polymorphonuclear cells, not macrophages or epithelial cells.

CHEMICAL TESTS

Enzymes

Enzymes play an important role in digestion and the pancreas is the source of several serine proteinases. Laboratory measurement of these enzymes provides clinicians with useful information related to specific disorders of the GI tract.

Trypsin

Trypsin is a serine proteinase originating in the acinar cells of the human pancreas. Spectrophotometric assays are available using p-toluene-sulfonyl-L-arginine methylester (TAME).[8] Inadequate trypsin secretion can lead to malabsorption and abdominal discomfort. Patients with pancreatic insufficiency will present with diminished levels ($<33 \mu$g trypsin/g stool).[9] In addition, children with cystic fibrosis typically have fecal trypsin levels of $<20 \mu$g trypsin/g stool. There are limitations to measuring trypsin in feces; for example, false negatives can occur due to intestinal degradation of trypsin and the presence of trypsin inhibitors. Also the proteolytic activity of bacterial enzymes can produce false positive results in specimens that have not been processed or tested for a prolonged period of time. Therefore, measurement of fecal chymotrypsin or elastase-1 can provide more reliable results.

Chymotrypsin

Chymotrypsin is a serine proteinase produced in the acinar cells of the pancreas. Chymotrypsin is more resistant to degradation in the intestine than trypsin. Thus it is the enzyme of choice for assay in feces. The clinical usefulness of measuring chymotrypsin in feces is to assess chronic pancreatic insufficiency, where fecal chymotrypsin levels are typically lower than normal. Low levels of fecal chymotrypsin are also seen in patients with cystic fibrosis and end-stage renal disease. Patients with diarrhea, lactose malabsorption, and irritable bowel syndrome may have falsely depressed fecal chymotrypsin levels.

Spectrophotometric assays using synthetic substrates are commercially available to measure fecal chymotrypsin. One commonly used reagent is succ-ala-pro-phe-4-nitroanailide, which produces a colored product that is measured at 405 nm.[10]

Elastase-1

Elastase-1 (E1) also belongs to the family of serine proteinases produced in the acinar cells of the pancreas. Quantitative stool analysis of E1 is the most reliable and sensitive noninvasive procedure for the diagnosis of chronic pancreatic insufficiency. Patients with chronic pancreatitis typically present with fecal E1 levels of $<200 \mu$g/g stool.[11] An enzyme linked immunoassay in a microplate sandwich format is commercially available to measure E1 concentration in stool samples.

> ### ☑ CHECKPOINT 15-3
>
> Ben's fecal chymotrypsin assay result was 5.0 U/g stool. What is his most likely diagnosis (Normal: 12 U/g stool)?

Chloride

The measurement of chloride ions in feces may be useful for the diagnosis of a rare congenital hypochloremic alkalosis with hyperchloridorrhea (increase excretion of chloride in stool). In this condition, the concentration of chloride in feces may reach 180 mmol/L, with very low amounts of chloride being found in urine. Patients with severe diarrhea can eliminate up to 500 mmol chloride/day.

Sodium and Potassium

Fecal sodium and potassium measurements are most useful in metabolic balance studies associated with nutritional and diet programs. Patients with diarrhea may eliminate over 60 mmol/day of sodium and potassium from their bodies. Measurement of sodium and potassium are also required to calculate the fecal osmotic gap (discussed below).

pH

Stool pH is not commonly determined in clinical laboratories. Normal stool pH is similar to the body, with a reference range of 7.0–7.5. Acidic stool pH occurs in malabsorption syndromes that allow for high rates of fermentation of undigested food by the gut bacteria. Other conditions that result in acidic stool pH include intestinal lactase deficiency, high lactose intake, decreased absorption of carbohydrates, and decreased fat absorption.[12] Conditions resulting in an alkaline pH include antibiotic use (due to impaired bacterial fermentation), inflammation of the colon, increased protein breakdown, and secretory diarrhea without food intake.

Fecal Osmotic (Osmolal) Gap

The normal osmolality of liquid stool is similar to that of serum (i.e., ~290 mOsm/kg). The actual contribution of electrolytes and nonelectrolytes to the total osmolality will vary depending on the cause of diarrhea. Estimation of **fecal osmotic gap** shown in Equation 15-1, expresses the difference between the theoretical normal osmolality and the contribution of sodium and potassium.

Measurement of fecal sodium and potassium on properly prepared samples does not pose any problems with current methods, whereas measuring total fecal osmolality is hindered due to false increases found in unrefrigerated samples. Therefore, the use of serum osmolality of 290 mOsm/kg has been recommended in equation 15-1 rather than a measurement of total fecal osmolality.[13]

Fecal osmotic gap provides a measurement of the contribution of electrolytes and non-electrolytes to the retention of water in the bowel and may assist in distinguishing between secretory and osmotic diarrhea. In patients with osmotic diarrhea, the unabsorbed solute leads to water retention and therefore makes a larger contribution than normal to fecal osmolality. Also, fecal concentration of sodium and potassium will be lower, resulting in a larger fecal osmotic gap. Conversely, in a patient with secretory diarrhea, it is the electrolytes that lead to water retention, and the fecal osmotic gap will be decreased. The fecal osmotic gap cutoff value used to distinguish osmotic from secretory diarrhea is 50 mOsm/kg. Thus patients with osmotic diarrhea

$$\text{Fecal osmotic gap} = 290 - [2(\text{fecal sodium} + \text{fecal potassium})] \qquad (15\text{-}1)$$

will have a fecal osmotic gap >50, and those with secretory diarrhea <50 mOsm/kg.

Measurement of Fecal Electrolytes and pH

Measurement of fecal electrolytes and pH usually require sample preparation to make it suitable for analysis. There are colorimetric assays and electrochemical devices available to measure fecal sodium, potassium, and chloride. A pH electrode is suitable to estimate fecal pH. Laboratory staff must consult the documentation of any FDA-approved assay or device for use with fecal samples.

☑ CHECKPOINT 15-4

Phyllis's laboratory results for fecal analysis are:

Sodium   10 meq/L

Potassium   15 meq/L

1. What is the fecal osmotic gap?
2. Which type of diarrhea is consistent with these laboratory results?

Porphyrins

A porphyrin is a ring structure with four pyrroles connected by methylene bridges. The entire structure is cyclic in nature with several side chains attached. A complete review of porphyrins can be found in most clinical chemistry and clinical laboratory chemistry textbooks. Porphyrin compounds are commonly present in feces and/or urine in a group of inherited and acquired disorders of heme biosynthesis referred to as **porphyrias**.[14]

Fecal analysis of metabolites associated with porphyrias is limited to the coproporphyrins, specifically I and III. High performance liquid chromatography (HPLC) can separate and quantitate individual porphyrins. When combined with measurement of total fecal porphyrins, it is a reliable means of distinguishing between acute intermittent porphyria (AIP) and hereditary coproporphyria (see Table 15-2 ★). Variegate porphyria may be diagnosed by measurement of fecal and urine metabolites. A ratio of fecal coproporphyrin III and coproporphyrin I is used to distinguish variegate porphyria from hereditary coproporphyria with interpretative information shown in Table 15-2.

Methods for detecting porphyrins include qualitative and quantitative assays. Fluorometry is a simple qualitative test to screen fecal samples for porphyrins. The test relies on the fluorescent properties of certain porphyrins. If porphyrins are present, the sample will fluoresce red-pink. This method lacks sensitivity and does not identify specific porphyrins. Results of this screening test are reported as positive or negative.[15]

"First-line" quantitative screening tests for porphyrins are available but do not identify individual porphyrins or isomers. Total porphyrin concentration can be determined in feces using a spectrophotometric or flurometric assays. The current method of choice is HPLC. This separation technique can isolate a specific fraction of porphyrins, detect them using spectrometry or fluorometry, and quantitate each fraction. Fluorometry is more sensitive than spectrophotometry and is the preferred technique.[16]

Occult Blood

Occult blood, or "hidden" blood can originate from bleeding in the upper GI tract, which produces black tarry stools, and bleeding in the lower GI tract, which is characterized by a large amount of blood in the stool. A normal individual loses 0.5–1.5 mL of blood into his or her GI tract daily due to normal shedding of epithelial cells. Any injury to the thin, one-cell-thick epithelial tissue may result in GI bleeding. Bleeding in excess of ~2.5 mL/150 g of stool is considered pathologically significant.

Colon cancer is a leading cause of cancer-related deaths in the United State, resulting in approximately 50,000 deaths annually. The most recent data reveals that nearly 143,600 new cases of colon cancer were diagnosed in 2012.[17] There is ample evidence that fecal occult blood testing (FOBT) is clinically useful in detecting these cancers at an earlier stage, potentially resulting in decreased mortality. The testing is relatively inexpensive, noninvasive, and may serve as a useful screening technique. The American Cancer Society guidelines for colorectal screening recommend annual FOBT and colonoscopy every 10 years, beginning at the age of 50 years in asymptomatic average risk individuals.[18]

Three types of tests available for FOBT are chemical (guaiac), immunochemical, and hemoporphyrin. Currently, the most widely used screening test is the guaiac-smear test (e.g., Hemoccult®, Beckman Coulter). Guaiac is a naturally occurring phenolic compound that is oxidized to quinone by hydrogen peroxidase, resulting in the formation of a blue color as shown in Figure 15-3 ■. The test is able to detect the pseudoperoxidase activity of heme as intact hemoglobin or as free heme. These tests are not specific to human hemoglobin, thus

---

★ **TABLE 15-2** Fecal Porphyrins and Porphyrias

Porphyrias	Feces	Urine
Variegate porphyria	Increased coproporphyrins and protoporphyrins (protoporphyrin exceeding coproporphyrin) and an coproporphyrin III/I ratio (<10)	Increased porphyrins and porphobilinogen
Hereditary porphyria	Increased coproporphyrin and coproporphyrin III/I ratio (>10)	Increased porphyrins and porphobilinogen
Acute intermittent porphyria	Noncontributory	Increased porphobilinogen and aminolevulinic acid
Porphyria cutanea tarda Erythropoietic protoporphyria	Noncontributory	Not applicable

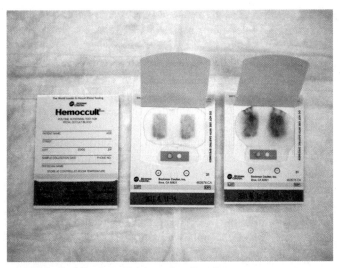

■ FIGURE 15-3 Fecal Occult Blood Test

(A) Hemocult® slide, unprepared. (B) Negative results for a patient's stool specimen indicated by the absence of a blue color around the stool sample. (C) Positive results for a patient's stool specimen indicated by the appearance of a blue color around the stool sample. Each slide contains a positive and negative control in the area of the orange rectangle.

hemoglobin from red meat, peroxidase from fruits and vegetables, and certain medications can lead to false-positive results (Box 15-4). The slide test will produce a positive result when at least 5–10 mL/day of blood is present in a stool sample.

The guaiac fecal occult blood test (gFOBT) usually requires stool samples from three consecutive stools. Two slides should be prepared for each stool sample. Each slide should be developed within 7 days of collection. Factors that may cause inaccurate results include bleeding gums or ingestion of large amounts of red meat before testing. Certain medications taken by the patient may also influence tests results. Drugs such as aspirin, anticoagulants, nonsteroidal anti-inflammatory drugs (e.g., ibuprofen), or colchicine can also cause erroneous results. A positive gFOBT should be followed up with diagnostic procedures designed to detect lesions within the GI tract such as sigmoidoscopy with barium enema or a colonoscopy, which currently is the preferred modality. A negative gFOBT does not rule out the possibility of a GI lesion in any patient presenting with signs and symptoms suggestive of colon cancer and should be further evaluated.

Another test methodology that provides several advantages over the gFOBT is the fecal immunochemical tests (FIT). These advantages are as follows:

- More sensitive
- More specific for blood
- Fewer false negatives
- Not affected by diet, animal hemoglobin, or human myoglobin
- Not affected by dietary peroxidase

The FIT are useful only for screening blood of the lower GI tract and are insensitive to upper GI bleeding because globin is destroyed in the small intestines. The assay principle is based on an antigen-antibody reaction with animal erythrocytes coated with antihuman globulin antibody. Samples demonstrating agglutination are interpreted as positive for occult human blood. FIT assay sensitivity is 50 μg hemoglobin/g feces.

Hemeporhyrin assays are not commonly used in hospital-based clinical laboratories, and they have a high false-positive rate. The assay is designed to detect porphyrins and intact heme using fluorescent spectroscopy. The assay can detect bleeding in upper GI esophagus, GI tract, and lower GI. Normal results are <2.0 mg total hemoglobin/g feces.

Fecal DNA testing using real-time polymerase chain reactions (PCR) has the potential to provide a very sensitive and specific test for detecting colorectal cancer and precancerous polyps. This test involves a single stool collection, which is then screened for DNA biomarkers. These DNA biomarkers shed continuously, remain stable in stool, and minute quantities are detectable. The assay is currently not approved by the FDA.

BOX 15-4   Sources of Errors in Fecal Occult Blood Testing

False Positives

Aspirin

Red meat

Horseradish

Raw broccoli, cauliflower, radishes, turnips

Melons

False negatives

Vitamin C >250 mg/day

Iron supplements containing vitamin C

MINI-CASE 15-1

Bill is 55 years old and reporting to his physician for an annual physical. At the completion of the examination, the doctor gave Bill a test kit for guaiac fecal occult blood. Bill took the kit home and completed the procedure and sent the kit back to the doctor's office. The results of the test were positive.

Questions to Consider

1. What does the positive test indicate?
2. What should the next course of action be for Bill?

☑ CHECKPOINT 15-5

Tests for the detection of occult blood are based on a reaction with which chemical compound?

APT for Swallowed Blood

APT-Downey test (APT) for fetal hemoglobin is used to determine whether blood found in the stool of neonates originated from maternal blood that was swallowed or is secondary to disease in the newborn. The APT is a qualitative test used to make this determination in bloody stool or vomitus from a newborn. The test is based on the premise that fetal hemoglobin is more resistant than adult hemoglobin to denaturation with an alkali. The procedure begins with a dilution of fecal sample with water that is then centrifuged. The supernatant, which should be pink, is then mixed with 1% sodium hydroxide. Fetal blood remains pink while maternal blood turns yellow-brown.[19]

Quantitative Fecal Fat

Quantitative fecal fat testing is used to assess fat malabsorption due to pancreatic insufficiency, hepatobiliary disorders, or intestinal disorders. The discussion on steatorrhea presented earlier in this chapter provided detailed information on the clinical aspects of this condition.

Estimation of the fat content in stool samples has been routinely conducted in clinical laboratories for many years. However, many clinical laboratories have abandoned the procedure due to low test volume, the use of several organic solvents for extraction, and issues related to specimen collection. Many hospital-based clinical laboratories send their quantitative fecal fat specimens to a reference laboratory.

There are several methods available to quantitate fat in stools including gravimetric, titrimetric, colorimetric, acid steatocrit, near infrared (NIR), and nuclear magnetic resonance (NMR), which is currently used by many reference laboratories.

All of the methods listed begin with a properly collected stool sample. Typically, a timed stool sample at 24, 48, or 72 hours is required, although random stool samples are acceptable. There are dietary fat requirements that must be met prior to initiation of the collection procedures. For example, a dietary fat intake of 50–150 g/day of long-chained triglycerides should be maintained for at least 2 days before and during the collection period. Proper containers should be supplied to the patient and can include paint cans or reference laboratory specimen containers.

Once the stool specimen is received by the laboratory, it must be processed according to the measuring technique available. Most methods require the stool sample to be homogenized using a homogenizer or food blender. Next the fats must be extracted from the mixture, which usually involves an array of organic solvents. At this juncture in the assay, the amount of fat in the sample is measured using any of the techniques previously listed. Each technique has strengths and weaknesses that are too numerous to discuss in this text. Patient results are typically reported in g/day (see Appendix L for reference ranges), although results maybe expressed as % of dry weight or % coefficient of fat absorption. The choice of units depends on the specific method used by the laboratory.

Carbohydrates

Carbohydrates in stool are typically associated with osmotic diarrhea discussed earlier in this chapter. This condition may be due to carbohydrate malabsorption or intolerance (i.e., maldigestion) and is assessed by measuring serum or urine sugars. Another option is to test feces for the presence of carbohydrates, especially reducing substance. The Clinitest tablet (Bayer HealthCare, Mishawaka, IN) using a copper reduction reaction is suitable for this test. Testing for fecal reducing substances can detect congenital disacchardase deficiency and enzyme deficiencies due to nonspecific mucosal dysfunction. An aliquot of a stool sample is emulsified in two parts water. The color produced by the sample is compared to a comparator (e.g., color chart). A result of 0.5 g/dL is considered presumptive evidence of carbohydrate intolerance.

Key Points to Remember

- Many different diseases can result in abnormalities in stool samples. Therefore, examination of stool samples is an important laboratory function.
- Special collection techniques are very important to ensure reliable laboratory results, and both patient and laboratory staff must follow instructions carefully.

- Appropriate laboratory examination of stool samples involves both physical and microscopic findings.
- Chemical testing of stool samples provides valuable information for assessing diseases, conditions and syndromes.

Review Questions

Level I

1. Steatorrhea is associated with (Objective 5)

    A. excess protein in stools.

    B. excess carbohydrates in stools.

    C. excess fats in stools.

    D. excess porphyrins in stools

2. A patient with a fecal osmotic gap of 100 mOsm/kg may have which type of diarrhea? (Objective 2)

    A. Secretory

    B. Osmotic

    C. Steatorrhea

    D. Acute

3. A person who consumes a large amount of beets may submit a stool sample that is what color? (Objective 4)

   A. Green

   B. Black

   C. Pale yellow

   D. Red

4. Which of the following laboratory results is consistent with chronic pancreatic insufficiency? (Objective 6)

   A. Decreased fecal chymotrypsin

   B. Increased fecal chymotrypsin

   C. Increased fecal trypsin

   D. Increased fecal elastase-1

5. What is the fecal osmotic gap for a patient whose fecal sodium is 50 meq/L and fecal potassium is 80 meq/L? (Objective 6)

   A. 10

   B. 30

   C. 60

   D. 290

Level II

1. A patient presents with the following results of porphyrin analysis: Increased coproporphyrin III/I ratio (>10)

   What type of porphyria does this patient have? (Objective 2)

   A. Hereditary porphyria

   B. Acute intermittent porphyria

   C. Variegate porphyria

   D. Porphyria cutanea tarda

2. Annual testing for fecal occult blood in men and women over the age of 50 has a high probability of detecting which of the following? (Objective 4)

   A. Ulcers

   B. Malabsorption syndromes

   C. Pancreatic insufficiency

   D. Colorectal cancer

3. What is the significance of a patient whose APT test remained pink after addition of sodium hydroxide? (Objective 4)

   A. Hemoglobin S is present.

   B. Fetal hemoglobin is present.

   C. Hemoglobin A1C is present.

   D. Vitamin C is present.

4. A laboratory technologist performs a microscopic procedure using Sudan IV to identify fats in a stool sample and discovered many small orange-red droplets. What type of fat is in that stool sample? (Objective 3)

   A. Cholesterol

   B. Soap

   C. Neutral fats

   D. Triglycerides

5. The APT test results for baby Allison stool sample is a yellow-brown color. What is the source of the blood? (Objective 4)

   A. Amniotic fluid

   B. Maternal

   C. Fetal

   D. Blood transfusion to the mother

Endnotes

1. Camilleri M, Murray JA. Chapter 40, Diarrhea and constipation In: Longo DL, Gauci AS, Kasper DL, Hauser SLO, Jameson JL, Loscalzo J, eds. *Harrison's Principles of Internal Medicine.* 18th ed. New York: McGraw-Hill, 2012. http://www.accessmedicine.com content.aspx? aID=9147519. Accessed March 17, 2014.

2. Camilleri M, Murray JA. Chapter 40, Diarrhea and constipation In: Longo DL, Gauci AS, Kasper DL, Hauser SLO, Jameson JL, Loscalzo J, eds. *Harrison's Principles of Internal Medicine.* 18th ed. New York: McGraw-Hill, 2012. http://www.accessmedicine.com content.aspx? aID=9147519. Accessed March 17, 2014.

3. Salwen MJ, Siddiqi HA, Gress FG, et al. Laboratory diagnosis of gastrointestinal and pancreatic disorders. In: McPherson RA, Pincus MR, eds. *Henry's Clinical Diagnosis and Management by Laboratory Methods,* 22nd ed. Philadelphia: Elsevier Saunders, 2011: 318–328.

4. Salwen MJ, Siddiqi HA, Gress FG, et al. Laboratory diagnosis of gastrointestinal and pancreatic disorders. In: McPherson RA, Pincus MR, eds. *Henry's Clinical Diagnosis and Management by Laboratory Methods,* 22nd ed. Philadelphia: Elsevier Saunders, 2011: 318–328.

5. Camilleri M, Murray JA. Chapter 40, Diarrhea and constipation In: Longo DL, Gauci AS, Kasper DL, Hauser SLO, Jameson JL, Loscalzo J, eds. *Harrison's Principles of Internal Medicine.* 18th ed. New York: McGraw-Hill, 2012. http://www.accessmedicine.com content.aspx? aID=9147519. Accessed March 17, 2014.

6. Salwen MJ, Siddiqi HA, Gress FG, et al. Laboratory diagnosis of gastrointestinal and pancreatic disorders. In: McPherson RA, Pincus MR, eds. *Henry's Clinical Diagnosis and Management by Laboratory Methods,* 22nd ed. Philadelphia: Elsevier Saunders, 2011: 318–328.

7. Strasinger SK, Di Lorenzo MS. *Urinalysis and body fluids.* 5th edition. Philadelphia: F.A. Davis, 2008.

8. Wu AHB. *Tietz Clinical Guide to Laboratory Tests.* 4th ed. St. Louis, MO: Saunders Elsevier, 2006.

9. Wu AHB. *Tietz Clinical Guide to Laboratory Tests.* 4th ed. St. Louis, MO: Saunders Elsevier, 2006.

10. Dockter G, Hoppe-Seyler F, Appel W, et al. Determination of chymotrypsin in stool by a new photometric method. *Clin Biochem* (1986) 19:329–332.

11. Wong RC, Steele RH, Reeves GE, et al. Antibody and genetic testing in coeliac disease. *Pathology* (2003) 35:285–304.

12. Wu AHB. *Tietz Clinical Guide to Laboratory Tests*. 4th ed. St. Louis, MO: Saunders Elsevier, 2006.

13. Duncan A, Robertson C, Russell RI. The fecal osmotic gap: technical aspects regarding its calculation. *J Lab Clin Med* (1992)119:359–363.

14. Sunheimer RL, Graves L. *Clinical Laboratory Chemistry*. Upper Saddle River, NJ: Pearson Education, 2011.

15. Deacon AC, Dip CB, Whatley SD, et al. Porphrins and disorders of porphyrin metabolism. In: Burtis CA, Ashwood ER, Bruns DE. Eds. *Tietz Textbook of Clinical Chemistry and Molecular Diagnostics*. 4th ed. St. Louis, MO: Elsevier Saunders, 2006.

16. Deacon AC, Dip CB, Whatley SD, et al. Porphrins and disorders of porphyrin metabolism. In: Burtis CA, Ashwood ER, Bruns DE. Eds. *Tietz Textbook of Clinical Chemistry and Molecular Diagnostics*. 4th ed. St. Louis, MO: Elsevier Saunders, 2006.

17. Siegel R, Naishadham D, Jemal A. Cancer Statistics, 2013. *CA Cancer J Clin* (2013) 63;1:11–30.

18. Smith RA, Cokkinides V, Eyre HJ. American cancer society guideline for the early detection of cancer, 2004. *CA Cancer J Clin* (2004) 54:41–52.

19. Gurizky RP, Rudnitsky G. Bloody neonatal diaper. *Ann Emerg Med* (1996) 27;5:662–664.

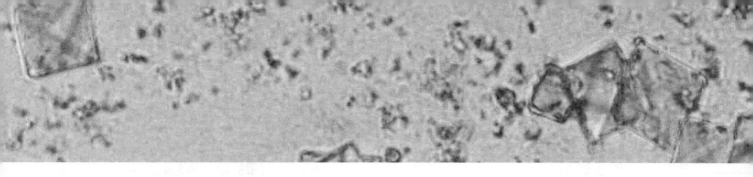

Appendix A: Answers to Mini-Cases

Chapter 1

Mini-Case 1-1

1. Allison failed to protect her eyes by wearing appropriate safety goggles.

Mini-Case 1-2

1. Jackie and Tonya did several things wrong.
   - They did not wear PPE, which should have included at least goggles, gloves, and lab coat.
   - They were handling a chemical that neither one of them was familiar with, yet they assumed they could pour it down the sink and flush it with water.
   - They were working is a small, confined space that may have been too hot and not well ventilated.

2. Solid picric acid is a strong oxidizer, flammable, and highly reactive in the wrong environment. It can become highly reactive and explosive when it comes into contact with certain heavy metals like lead (often found in sink drains). It is most dangerous when it has been dried out. Regular PPE would not have protected any exposed skin (e.g., face, ears, neck). The picric acid would have also reacted with the moisture and other chemicals on their skin and possibly on their clothing.

3. Several courses of action are appropriate for this situation:
   - Call the fire department.
   - Contact your institutional environmental health and safety staff.
   - Do not handle the material under any circumstances.

Mini-Case 1-3

1. Sam left a glass pipet in a glass volumetric flask which makes it much easier to tip over. He also left his lab coat unbuttoned which could result in the acid solution to splash onto his clothes. He was not wearing appropriate eyewear that would provide sufficient protection for his eyes. Sam pipetted a serum sample which is aqueous in nature into an acid. This could cause a moderately violent reaction resulting is splashing of acid.

2. Sam could use a chemical spill kit if one is available. He should also contact the laboratory safety group to assist with recommendations on the proper procedure to clean up the spill

Mini-Case 1-4

Nurse Denise should have yelled for a code silver, which is a commonly acceptable code signifying that a person has a weapon. The fact that a weapon was used elevated the severity of the situation from a simple upset intruder to an armed individual. The response for most hospitals is to include notification of local police officers and other special armed tactical response team units.

Chapter 2

Mini-Case 2-1

1. The calculated McNemar stat is 1.0 as shown by the solution below.

2. Janet can accept the null hypothesis.

Calculate the McNemar statistic using the following formula:

$$X^2 = \frac{[|O - E|]^2}{E} + \frac{[|O - E|]^2}{E}$$

where

O is the observed value

E is the expected value = total discordant data / 2

$$X^2 = \frac{[|1 - 2|]^2}{2} + \frac{[|3 - 2|]^2}{2}$$

$$X^2 = \frac{[|1|]^2}{2} + \frac{[|1|]^2}{2}$$

$$X^2 = \frac{1}{2} + \frac{1}{2}$$

$$X^2 = 0.5 + 0.5$$

$$X^2 = 1.0$$

The chi square value for one degree of freedom (from a table of chi squares) and $\alpha = 0.05$ is 3.84. The calculated McNemar statistic (X^2) is equal to 1.0. This is below the chi square critical value of 3.841 at 0.05 probabilities and 1 degree of freedom. The laboratory concludes that there is no difference between the two methods. Results on test kit 1 are not significantly different from results on test kit 2.

Mini-Case 2-2

1. A 2_{2s} Westgard rule violation indicated the presence of a systematic error. The typical course of action is to repeat the measurement using the same aliquot of quality control material.

2. The patient samples should be repeated once the quality control issue is resolved (i.e., the repeated value falls within two standard deviations).

Mini-Case 2-3

1. Possibly nothing. But mistakes are made when calibrating assays. For example, laboratory staff may assay the wrong lot number, mix the order of sampling, or fail to mix the calibrators sufficiently. In this scenario the measurement systems produced the wrong measured value for one of the calibrators.

2. Greg cannot continue running controls or patients specimens until the calibration is successful.

3. The typical course of action when a calibration fails is to rerun the calibration a second time.

Chapter 3

Mini-Case 3-1

1. An increase in blood flow is sensed by the macula dense in the juxtaglomerular apparatus, which responds to the increased blood pressure by decreasing the secretion of renin. Renin converts angiotensin to angiotensin I, which is converted to angiotensin II by the angiotensin-converting enzyme. Angiotensin II triggers the release of aldosterone.

2. Angiotensin II results in constriction of the afferent arteriole, dilation of the efferent arteriole, decreased secretion of aldosterone, decreased sodium reabsorption in the proximal convoluted tubule, and decreased release of antidiuretic hormone, which decreases water reabsorption in the collecting duct, all of which results in a decrease in blood pressure.

3. When the blood pressure returns to normal, the level of renin is gradually increased to keep the blood pressure in the "normal" range.

Chapter 4

Mini-Case 4-1

1. The most common problem associated with 24-hour or timed urine is timing and completeness of collection.

2. Yes, the omission of one urine can definitely affect the result of the creatinine clearance.

3. The laboratory scientist can stress the importance of the timing and completeness of collection by giving clear, concise oral directions as well as understandable written directions.

Mini-Case 4-2

1. Bilirubin decreases upon standing due to photo oxidation to biliverdin by exposure to light. Biliverdin does not react with the reagent strip reaction for bilirubin resulting in a falsely low or negative reaction.

2. Urobilinogen is oxidized to urobilin which does not react with the reagent strip reaction for urobilinogen.

Mini-Case 4-3

1. Improper storage and handling is one possible explanation. Glucose will decrease in an improperly stored specimen because of bacterial utilization/glycolysis.

2. Maximum time a specimen can sit unrefrigerated is 2 hours. The technologist can check the time collected and time it was delivered to the lab and how it was stored (room temperature or refrigerated).

Mini-Case 4-4

1. Oliguria is the term for decreased urine volume, usually a decrease in urine volume to < 400 mL/day.

2. Oliguria can be
   a. Prerenal: hemorrhaging, vomiting, diarrhea, hepatic failure, congestive heart failure, myocardial infarction.
   b. Renal: acute glomerulonephritis, toxemia of pregnancy, rapidly progressive glomerulonephritis, interstitial nephritis, connective tissue disorders, acute tubular necrosis.
   c. Postrenal: upper urinary tract obstruction, lower urinary tract obstruction

3. The physician would ask questions regarding the most common causes of dehydration:
   a. Have you had the flu lately, e.g., vomiting, diarrhea?
   b. Have you had any kidney infections, renal problems?
   c. Are you on any medications?
   d. How many glasses of water are you drinking daily?

4. A 24-hour urine collection would provide the physician an idea of the severity of the oliguria or if in fact the patient is oliguric.

Chapter 5

Mini-Case 5-1

1. The following are examples of possible causes of Jane's red urine :
   a. RBCs
   b. Hemoglobin

c. Porphyrins

d. Certain medications, e.g., phenytoin

e. Beets

2. Four causes of variations in color are:

a. Normal metabolic functions

b. Physical activity

c. Ingested material or diet

d. Pathological conditions/disease

Mini-Case 5-2

1. An amber color could indicate the presence of abnormal pigment bilirubin which is associated with hepatitis.

2. The amber color could also be due to dehydration. The urine pigment urochrome is diluted in less urine because the urine is very concentrated (high specific gravity).

3. The carotene pigment in carrots, nitrofurantoin and rifadin (antibiotics), pyridium, and serenium.

Mini-Case 5-3

1. Tom's urine is hypersthenuric.

2. Four common causes of hypersthenuric or concentrated urine are dehydration, gastrointestinal disorders (e.g., vomiting, diarrhea), heart failure, or shock.

3. Glucose and protein can be eliminated because reagent strip (RS) specific gravity measures only the ionic solutes, whereas glucose and protein are nonionic.

4. The results should be confirmed by performing the specific gravity with a refractometer.

Chapter 6

Mini-Case 6-1

1. The discrepant result is a positive reagent strip protein and a negative precipitation test.

2. Two possible explanations are 1) that highly buffered alkaline urine overrides the buffer and that the change in color is due to the pH indicating an acid pH and not the presence of protein; 2) because of improper technique allowing the strip to remain in the urine too long, which may leach out the buffer, again causing a color change due to pH and not protein.

Mini-Case 6-2

1. The abnormal or discrepant results are: glucose: negative and Clinitest: 2+.

2. a. non glucose-reducing substance

b. Interfering substance causing a false negative reagent strip reaction: Vitamin C, increased SG, or cold urine

c. Reagent strip defective or outdated

3. A newborn probably points to an inborn error of metabolism in this case a non-glucose reducing substance, galactose in galactosemia.

4. The technologist should check the quality control values, expiration date, and temperature of the urine.

5. Four possible complications are failure to thrive, cataracts, hepatic dysfunction, and extreme mental retardation.

6. Dietary restriction of galactose can reduce the complications.

Mini-Case 6-3

1. Ketone bodies are elevated in (1) starvation, malnutrition, (2) diet, eating disorders (anorexia nervosa, bulimia), (3) diabetes mellitus, (4) severe exercise, (5) exposure to cold, (6) frequent vomiting and digestive disturbances.

2. Acetone and acetoacetic acid are measured with the reagent strip. β-hydroxybutyric is not.

3. Starvation, malnutrition, eating disorders, severe exercise would result in a negative glucose and positive ketone.

4. The most likely explanation for the ketosis is anorexia nervosa, bulimia, or some type of eating disorder. Digestive disturbances, exposure to cold, and severe exercise would probably have been ruled out in the medical history.

Mini-Case 6-4

1. The abnormal or discrepant results are: Blood 1+; Protein: trace

2. Five possible explanations are: renal diseases (glomerulonephritis, pyelonephritis; cystitis); renal calculi; trauma; strenuous exercise; acute febrile episodes.

3. No the patient should not be overly concerned.

4. The most likely explanation is extreme physical exercise-the first practice of the season.

5. The physician would order a follow up urinalysis to confirm his/her diagnosis.

Chapter 7

Mini-Case 7-1

1. Objectives can become loose if used as a "handle" to maneuver the nosepiece when changing objectives.

2. The knurled ring on the nosepiece should be used to change objectives.

Chapter 8

Mini-Case 8-1

1. 12 mL of urine is the suggested volume for urinalysis.

2. The microscopic analysis may be performed on an uncentrifuged specimen per laboratory protocol.

3. A notification should be made clear on the report that evaluation was done on an uncentrifuged specimen so the physician can evaluate the results properly.

Mini-Case 8-2

1. Vaginal bleeding during menstruation and rectal bleeding.

2. It is customary to ask the patient at the time of the collection if she is having her menstrual period now.

Mini-Case 8-3

1. The structures indicated are the flagella on the Trichomonas vaginalis.

2. The tech must look for movement of the beating flagella to differentiate between WBC and Trichomonas.

Mini-Case 8-4

1. The cast may be a waxy cast due to the blunt ends. Further inspection with a high power objective would verify that possibility.

2. Low urine volume and urinary stasis causes casts to degrade within the renal tubule to form the waxy appearance of the cast.

3. Waxy casts may be an indication of end stage renal disease.

Chapter 9

Mini-Case 9-1

1. The urinalysis is indicative of acute glomerulonephritis (AGN). AGN onset is usually acute, and symptoms include fever, oliguria, malaise, edema, hematuria, and proteinuria.

2. Erythrocytes (RBCs) and RBC and hemoglobin casts are pathognomic of AGN. Erythrocytes and hemoglobin casts are indicative of a renal disease of glomerular origin.

3. The probable causative agent in this case is group A beta-hemolytic streptococci. Specific strains are nephritogenic, especially types 1, 4, and 12. AGN is caused by the formation of immune complexes, including antibodies and streptococcal antigens.

4. Other causes of AGN
   a. Other Gram positives: *Streptococcus viridians, Staphlycoccus aureus*
   b. Gram negatives: *Klebsiella pneumoniae, Salmonella typhus*
   c. Viruses
   d. Parasites
   e. Noninfectious, e.g., Systemic lupus erythematosus, Guillain-Barré syndrome

Mini-Case 9-2

1. Bonnie's urinalysis is consistent with nephrotic syndrome.

2. The basic defect is damage to the glomerular basement membrane in the renal nephron, which results in increased permeability of the glomerulus. The damage in some types of nephrotic syndrome is caused by deposits of immune complexes (antigen-antibody) in the basement membrane. Nephrotic syndrome is not actually a disease but a condition based on a combination of signs and symptoms.

3. Marked proteinuria and lipiduria (oval fat bodies and fatty casts) are hallmarks of nephrotic syndrome.

4. Secondary nephrotic syndrome may be associated with diabetes mellitus, systemic lupus erythematosus, viral infections (hepatitis B, hepatitis C, HIV), preeclampsia, and drugs of abuse.

Mini-Case 9-3

1. The abnormal macroscopic findings (Day 1/Day 2) are: Appearance: Cloudy/Cloudy; Nitrite: Pos/Pos; and Leukocyte Esterase: 2+/2+. Abnormal microscopic results (Day 2) are: WBCs: 25-40/HPF; Bacteria: Moderate. Discrepant Results: None.

2. The absence of casts indicates a lower urinary tract infection. Casts are the primary indicator of a renal problem because they are formed ONLY in the kidney, primarily in the distal convoluted tubule and collecting duct.

3. Mary has cystitis. Infections in the lower urinary tract, most commonly cystitis, are characterized by pyuria (increased WBCs) and the absence of casts (See Answer to Question 2).

4. No, it would not change the diagnosis, because false negative leukocyte esterase and nitrite results are possible.

False negative leukocyte esterase can be caused by:
   a. Low numbers of WBCs. Leukocyte esterase detects 10–25 WBCs/μL. The number of WBCs may be increased but not high enough to produce a positive result
   b. WBCs present which are not granulocytes and do not produce leukocyte esterase.
   c. Increased glucose, protein and specific gravity which decrease the sensitivity of the L.E. reaction and can result in a false negative result.

False negative nitrite reaction can be caused by:
   a. Infection by bacteria which do NOT reduce nitrate, i.e. gram positive
   b. Bacteria not being present in the bladder for a sufficient length of time to allow nitrate reduction. In urinary tract infections, frequency of urination may not allow sufficient time for nitrate reduction.
   c. A patient with a nitrate deficient diet not producing enough nitrate to result in a positive nitrite reaction.

5. Increased numbers of transitional epithelial cells are sloughed off from the renal calyces, renal pelvis, ureters, bladder and urethra (of males) during infection/ inflammation.

6. Cystitis is usually caused by fecal flora: Escherichia coli (75–95%), Klebsiella (5%), Proteus, Pseudomonas, etc. A colony count of 100,000 colony-forming units (CFU)/ml is usually considered diagnostic for an infection.

7. Cranberry juice reduces pyuria and bacteruria by reducing E. coli adherence to cells. The acidity of the juice also

sets up a less favorable environment for bacterial growth. Vitamin C supplements also acidify the urine.

8. Increased urine production will facilitate the excretion of bacteria from the bladder, because increased urine flow from the bladder helps to wash bacteria out of the bladder and urethra. Bacteria move up the urinary tract from the urethra (urethritis) to the bladder (cystitis) and if untreated to the kidney (pyelonephritis).

9. Women have shorter urethras providing the bacteria easier access to the bladder. Other reasons include: hormone levels appear to enhance adherence of the bacteria to the mucosa; bacteria may be "milked" up the urethra during sexual intercourse; and the lack of the antibacterial action of prostatic fluid.

10. Diabetes, calculi (kidney stones), prostatic hyperplasia, pregnancy, and catherization are associated with an increased incidence of cystitis. It is thought pregnant women are more prone to cystitis because of hormonal changes and possible changes in position of the kidney during pregnancy.

Chapter 10

Mini-Case 10-1

1. The elevated intracranial pressure is due to expansion of CSF due to an inflammation as a result of bacterial meningitis.

Mini-Case 10-2

1. Bloody lumbar puncture can be caused by trauma from the needle causing bleeding into the lumbar space and subarachnoid hemorrhage.

2. Subarachnoid hemorrhage: the pale pink color of the supernatant and consistent cell counts in all four tubes.

3. Xanthochromia is due to lysed red blood cells and hemoglobin breakdown products

Mini-Case 10-3

1. Prealbumin is often present in CSF but not serum. Also transferrin appears in higher concentration in CSF because of its small molecular size. It permits ultrafiltration from blood into CSF.

2. Intrathecal synthesis of IgG

3. Multiple sclerosis

Chapter 11

Mini-Case 11-1

1. Exudate

2. Empyema

Mini-Case 11-2

1. Inadvertent aspiration of blood from the heart

Mini-Case 11-3

1. $3.0 - 1.0 = 2.0$

2. Transudate because result of the serum-ascites albumin gradient is greater than 1.0.

3. Liver disorder

Chapter 12 contains no minicases

Chapter 13

Mini-Case 13-1

1. Yes

2. Because at 25 weeks gestation the ADA uses the following glucose values for the 2-hr oral glucose tolerance test:
   - Fasting ≥93 mg/dL
   - 1 h ≥180 mg/dL
   - 2 h ≥153 mg/dL

Mini-Case 13-2

1. The indications for the fetus based on the "lung profile" are that the fetal lungs are immature and the fetus may have respiratory distress syndrome (RDS).

Chapter 14

Mini-Case 14-1

1. Classic form of homocystinuria

2. Ectopia lentis

Mini-Case 14-2

1. Maple syrup urine disease

2. Ketoacids of leucine and isoleucine

Chapter 15

Mini-Case 15-1

1. The positive test result for the fecal occult blood may indicate the presence of blood in the stool. There are potential interferences with the test and issues with specificity.

2. Therefore, the patient should be encouraged to follow up with a colonoscopy procedure that has the potential to reveal the presence of polyps or other growths in the intestines.

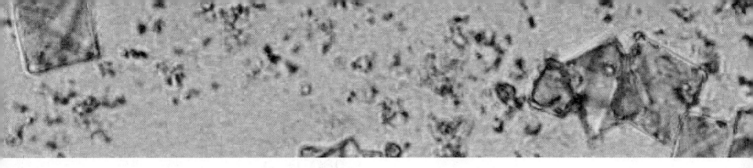

Appendix B: Answers to Checkpoints

Chapter 1

Checkpoint 1-1

CFR 1910.1030

Checkpoint 1-2

Universal precautions

Checkpoint 1-3

False. It not acceptable to wear any footwear that exposes the toes.

Checkpoint 1-4

Gloves with reduced protein content (e.g., latex-, powder-. or cornstarch-free gloves) may prevent the allergy-like symptoms.

Checkpoint 1-5

Do not use water with this chemical.

Checkpoint 1-6

1. Do not store chemicals in alphabetical order.

2. The mixture of acetic acid and ammonium nitrate will ignite, especially if the acid is concentrated.

Checkpoint 1-7

Dry chemical fire extinguishers are used for fire class A, B, and C.

Checkpoint 1-8

Recommendations:

1. Remove the staff technologist from that work area.

2. Have the staff technologist examined by a physician.

3. Contact someone who can perform a decibel test over an 8-hour period in the laboratory to determine the time weighted average (TWA). If the TWA is greater than 85 decibels/8 hours, the laboratory should initiate a plan to reduce the overall noise level in the laboratory.

Chapter 2

Checkpoint 2-1

• Mean	179.95
• Standard deviation	1.05
• Variance	1.10
• Percentage coefficient of variation	0.58
• Median	180.0
• Mode	180.0
• Range	178–182

Checkpoint 2-2

- Linear regression by least squares, including slope and intercept

Linear regression equation	$y = -0.67 + 1.01X$
Slope	1.01
Intercept	−0.67

- Correlation coefficient   0.992

Checkpoint 2-3

Out of Control Day:

Day 2	1_{3s}	Level I	Random error: reanalyze control sample
Day 4	1_{2s}	Level II	Random error: "Warning rule" and/or reanalyze control sample
Day 5	2_{2s}	Level II	Systematic error: reanalyze control sample and/or troubleshoot
Day 8	1_{3s}	Level I	Random error: reanalyze control sample

Checkpoint 2-4

Quality control material cannot be used as a replacement for calibrators because the values of the mean and standard deviation for control material are determined by measurement using the specific method and analyzer located in the laboratory. The value for a calibrator is determined by a definitive method with a high degree of accuracy.

Checkpoint 2-5

a. chemistries measured on the strip (e.g., glucose, protein, bilirubin, urobilinogen, pH, blood, ketones, nitrite, and leukocytes)

b. specific gravity

c. flow cytometry

Chapter 3

Checkpoint 3-1

1. c

2. a. 2
   b. 5
   c. 3
   d. 4
   e. 1
   f. 6

3. a

Checkpoint 3-2

1. a

2. d

3. d

4. c

Chapter 4

Checkpoint 4-1

1. c

2. c

3. pH   increase
   Glucose   decrease
   Bilirubin   decrease
   Ketones   decrease
   Nitrite   increase

4. The most common method of preservation is *refrigeration*.

Checkpoint 4-2

1. c

2. a

3. b

4. b

Chapter 5

Checkpoint 5-1

1. a

2. b

3. b

4. a

Checkpoint 5-2

1. b

2. c

Checkpoint 5-3

1. b

2. 1.012

3. Three variables affecting specific gravity are of those listed below:
   a. Wavelength of light used
   b. Size and number of particles
   c. Concentration of solution
   d. Temperature of the solution

Chapter 6

Checkpoint 6-1

1. c and d

2. c

3. b

4. c

Checkpoint 6-2

1. a

2. Low levels of glucose may be detected by the reagent strip, but not the Clinitest.

3. d

4. d

5. Fat

6. People with diabetes mellitus do not have the insulin to absorb glucose for energy; therefore, they utilize fats as the secondary source of energy. The human body can only metabolize so much fat and therefore an incomplete metabolism of fat results in excess ketone formation.

7. c

Checkpoint 6-3

1. b
2. c
3. b, liver
4. d
5. Improper storage and handling
6. b

Checkpoint 6-4

1. a
2. c
3. c
4. Lysed leukocytes will release leukocyte esterase and give a positive reaction.

Chapter 7

Checkpoint 7-1

1. d
2. b
3. b
4. c

Checkpoint 7-2

1. b
2. a
3. a
4. b

Chapter 8

Checkpoint 8-1

1. c
2. b
3. c
4. c
5. True

Checkpoint 8-2

1. c
2. b
3. a
4. b
5. c

Checkpoint 8-3

1. a
2. d
3. c
4. c
5. d

Chapter 9

Checkpoint 9-1

1. a
2. a
3. d
4. d
5. d
6. d
7. d

Checkpoint 9-2

1. b
2. d
3. b
4. b

Checkpoint 9-3

1. Community-acquired cystitis is a bladder infection outside of a hospital or nursing home.
2. c
3. c
4. a

Chapter 10

Checkpoint 10-1

Monitoring opening pressures can serve as a guide to estimate the amount of CSF that can be safely removed. Also, an abnormal opening pressure can signal or reveal the presence of an abnormality.

Checkpoint 10-2

Lumbar puncture
Cisternal puncture
Lateral cervical puncture
Ventricle puncture

Checkpoint 10-3

T

Checkpoint 10-4

Oligoclonal protein

Checkpoint 10-5

It may be contaminated with skin bacteria.

Checkpoint 10-6

The total volume of each square is $(0.04 \times 0.1) = 0.004$ mm^3. The total volume for five squares is 5×0.004 mm$^3 = 0.02$ mm^3. A total of 25 cells were counted in a volume of 0.02 mm^3, yielding $25/(0.02) = 1250$ cell/mm^3. Next, the sample was originally diluted four-fold, therefore multiply your total cell count (1250) by $4 = 5000$ cells/mm^3. To convert to cells per milliliter, multiply $(5000) \times 1000 = 5,000,000$ (5.0×10^6) per mL.

Checkpoint 10-7

CSF IgG index (Equation 10.5)

$$\text{CSF IgG index} = \frac{\text{CSF IgG (mg/dL)/Serum IgG (g/dL)}}{\text{CSF albumin (mg/dL)/Serum albumin (g/dL)}}$$

$$\text{CSF IgG index} = \frac{8/0.65}{6/3} = \frac{12.3}{2} = 6.15$$

Interpretation: This patient has experienced an increase in intrathecal synthesis of IgG or an increase in IgG crossover from the breakdown of the blood-brain barrier.

Chapter 11

Checkpoint 11-1

low, clearer

Checkpoint 11-2

chylomicrons

Checkpoint 11-3

EDTA

Checkpoint 11-4

imbalance between hydrostatic and oncotic pressure

Checkpoint 11-5

Thoracentesis

Checkpoint 11-6

A hemorrhagic effusion or inadvertent aspiration of blood from the heart

Checkpoint 11-7

Any two of the following: liver diseases, cirrhosis of the liver, malignancies (ovarian and pancreatic), congestive heart failure

Checkpoint 11-8

Exudate

Chapter 12

Checkpoint 12-1

False

Checkpoint 12-2

Metatarsal phalangeal (MTP) joint of the great toe.

Checkpoint 12-3

C

Checkpoint 12-4.

Hyaluronan

Checkpoint 12-5

A bloody synovial fluid may be due to a bloody tap from an arthrocentesis or a clinically significant condition such as trauma, tumors, hemophilia RA, pigmented villonodular synovitis, or anticoagulant therapy.

Checkpoint 12-6

Polymorphonuclear cells
Monocytes
Polymorphonuclear cells
Occasionally "ragocytes"

Checkpoint 12-7

No. If the patient truly has gout, then the synovial fluid should contain monosodium urate crystals. Calcium pyrophosphate dihydrate crystals are typically found in patients with pseudogout.

Checkpoint 12-8

Yes

Checkpoint 12-9

The clinical usefulness of this diagnostic procedure includes patients with interstitial lung disease of an infectious, non-infectious, immunologic, or malignant nature.

Checkpoint 12-10

The CFTR protein serves as a chloride channel that controls the salt content in fluid that covers the surface of nasal and lung tissues.

Checkpoint 12-11

Pilocarpine is a cholinergic alkaloid that serves to stimulate the sweat glands to produce sweat.

Checkpoint 12-12

The reason why some laboratories commit more errors than others may be due to the low volume or number of sweat tests performed. Labs that only perform a few sweat measurements per year are prone to make more procedural errors.

Chapter 13

13.1 A surfactant is surface-active lipoprotein, typically phospholipids that are formed by alveolar cells. This finding provides evidence for the outward flow of lung liquid.

13.2 A β-hCG assay uses antibodies that specifically recognize the beta subunit of hCG and not the alpha subunit. Assays for hCG use antibodies that recognize both alpha and beta subunits.

13.3 Production of small amounts of AFP begins in the fetal yolk sac and then in large quantities by the fetal liver as the yolk sac degenerates. Minute amounts are also produced in the fetal gut and kidneys. The concentration of AFP in fetal serum is very high early in embryonic life and peaks in fetal serum at a level of approximately 3 million ng/mL (3 million μg/L) at about 9 weeks gestation. The concentration then decreases steadily to about 20,000 ng/mL (20,000 μg/L) at term.

13.4 Total estriol is comprised of both conjugated and unconjugated forms. The conjugated form is bound to protein while the free form is not.

13.5 "Women with diabetes found at their initial prenatal visit should receive a diagnosis of overt diabetes mellitus not gestational diabetes mellitus."

Chapter 14

Checkpoint 14-1

Drop of blood on a filter paper (punch)

Checkpoint 14-2

To reduce the number of false positive results originating from newborn mass screening tests such as tandem MS/MS

Checkpoint 14-3

Early detection of inborn errors of metabolism is important so that treatment modalities can be initiated to prevent the disease from worsening.

Checkpoint 14-4

Brown or black due to oxidation of homogentisic acid

Checkpoint 14-5

Methionine

Checkpoint 14-6

Leucine – α-ketoisocaproic acid

Isoleucine – α-keto-β-methylvaleric acid

Valine – α-ketoisovaleric acid

Checkpoint 14-7

Alloisoleucine (allo-Ile)

Checkpoint 14-8

phenylalanine/tyrosine molar ratio

Checkpoint 14-9

dopamine and serotonin

Checkpoint 14-10

liver

Chapter 15

Checkpoint 15-1

Secretory	C
Osmotic	E
Steatorrhea	D
Inflammatory	B
Dysmotility	F
Factitial	A

Checkpoint 15-2

Pus	E
Mucus	E, F, G

Hard stool	G
Pale yellow stool	B
Black stool	D
Red	A
Green	C

Checkpoint 15-3

chronic pancreatic insufficiency

Checkpoint 15-4

1. 240 mOsm/kg and

2. Is consistent with osmotic-type diarrhea

Checkpoint 15-5

pseudoperoxidase

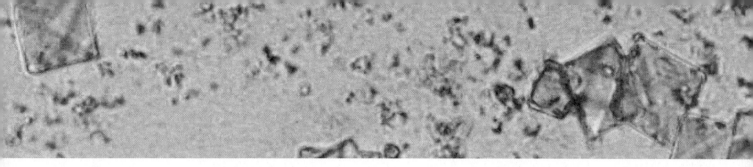

Appendix C: Answers to Review Questions

Chapter 1

Level I

1. B
2. D
3. C
4. B
5. C
6. A
7. B
8. D

Level II

1. C
2. A
3. A
4. C
5. B
6. C
7. D
8. A
9. B
10. B
11. C
12. D

Chapter 2

Level I

1. A
2. C
3. C
4. A
5. C
6. D
7. B
8. C

Level II

1. C
2. A
3. C
4. B
5. D
6. C
7. B
8. B
9. D
10. B
11. C

Chapter 3

Level I

1. B
2. D
3. B
4. C
5. B
6. C
7. A
8. D

9. A
10. A
11. B
12. A
13. C
14. A
15. C
16. B

Level II

1. B
2. C
3. C
4. D

5. Dolores is a diabetic and her serum glucose is out of control. The renal threshold for glucose is 160–180 mg/dL. When her serum glucose exceeds the renal threshold, the excess glucose is not reabsorbed and is excreted in the urine.

6. John would be dehydrated from running a marathon in warm temperatures. The secretion of antidiuretic hormone would be increased, which would decrease urine volume and increase plasma volume. An increase in antidiuretic hormone renders the walls of the distal convoluted tubule and collecting duct permeable to water; therefore, the urine volume is decreased and water reabsorption is increased.

Chapter 4

Level I

1. C
2. A
3. C
4. C
5. C
6. B
7. D
8. B
9. C
10. B
11. B
12. B
13. B
14. D

15. B
16. B
17. C

Level II

1. C
2. B
3. A

4. a. Increased urine production is called polyuria.
b. Jane's condition is probably diabetes mellitus.

Chapter 5

Level I

1. B
2. A
3. D
4. D
5. D
6. C
7. D
8. D
9. B
10. B
11. A
12. B
13. A
14. A
15. A
16. C

Level II

1. B
2. B
3. A
4. C

5. Two solutes that can cause an elevated refractometer specific gravity are glucose and protein. One gram of protein will elevate the SG by 0.003, and one gram of glucose will elevate the SG by 0.004. The reagent strip, however, does not measure nonionic solute, therefore protein and glucose will not affect the SG. The student should review the urinalysis findings for elevated protein and or glucose.

Chapter 6

1. C
2. B
3. B
4. C
5. A
6. B
7. A
8. B
9. B
10. A
11. B
12. A
13. B
14. D
15. C
16. B
17. D
18. B
19. C
20. C
21. D
22. D
23. C
24. C
25. A
26. B
27. B
28. D
29. D
30. D

Level II

1. C
2. C
3. B
4. C
5. A positive urine glucose with a normal plasma glucose, well below the renal threshold (160–180 mg/dL) indicates the renal reabsorption of glucose by the renal tubules has been compromised, "renal glycosuria" or a defect in tubular reabsorption of glucose. Fanconi's syndrome is an example of a condition characterized by a defective tubular reabsorption of glucose.

   a. Ictotest detects 0.05–0.1 mg/dL. Low levels of bilirubin may result in a strongly positive Ictotest and a negative or weaker reagent strip bilirubin.

   b. Bilirubin is rapidly destroyed when exposed to light, with bilirubin oxidized to biliverdin, which yields a negative reaction. The urine had been exposed to light for four hours, leading to oxidation of some of the bilirubin.

Chapter 7

Level I

1. D
2. B
3. C
4. A
5. C
6. A
7. B
8. B

Level II

1. C
2. B
3. A
4. D
5. D
6. A

Chapter 8

Level I

1. A
2. A
3. B
4. B
5. D
6. C
7. A
8. C

9. D

10. C

11. B

12. A

13. D

14. C

15. D

16. A

17. B

18. D

19. D

20. C

Level II

1. B

2. A

3. D

4. C

5. B

6. B

Chapter 9

Level I

1. A

2. B

3. D

4. B

5. D

6. C

7. C

8. B

9. C

10. A

11. E

12. C

13. A

14. C

15. B

16. D

17. C

18. A

19. C

20. C

21. A

Level II

1. D

2. B

3. D

4. B

5. a. Jane's most likely has membranoproliferative glomeru-lonephritis (MPGN).

   b. Membranoproliferative glomerulonephritis is an in-flammation of the glomeruli by an abnormal immune response. Immune complex-mediated conditions, au-toimmune diseases, chronic infections and malignant neoplasms are associated with MPGN.

Chapter 10

Level I

1. C

2. D

3. A

4. B

5. C

6. A

7. D

8. B

9. D

10. B

11. C

12. B

13. C

14. B

15. D

16. A

17. B

18. C

19. B

20. A

Level II

1. B
2. D
3. A
4. B
5. C
6. C
7. D

Chapter 11

Level I

1. A
2. C
3. D
4. A
5. B
6. C
7. D
8. C
9. B
10. A
11. B

Level II

1. B
2. C
3. C
4. B
5. B
6. A
7. D
8. B
9. C
10. D

Chapter 12

Level I

1. B
2. D

3. B
4. C
5. A
6. B
7. A
8. C
9. D
10. A
11. C
12. B
13. D

Level II

1. D
2. B
3. C
4. A
5. C

Chapter 13

Level I

1. A
2. C
3. C
4. A
5. D
6. B
7. A
8. D
9. B
10. C

Level II

1. B
2. D
3. C
4. A
5. C

Chapter 14

Level I

1. C
2. B
3. A
4. C
5. D
6. A
7. B
8. C
9. D
10. A

Level II

1. B
2. A
3. A
4. B
5. D
6. A

7. C
8. C
9. B
10. B

Chapter 15

Level I

1. C
2. B
3. D
4. A
5. B

Level II

1. A
2. D
3. B
4. C
5. B

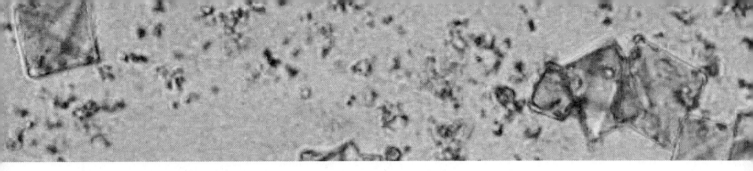

Appendix D: Answers to Case in Point

Chapter 1

1. For concentrated hydrochloric acid:

   Fire/flammability, Red diamond – 0

   Health hazard, Blue diamond – 3

   Reactivity, Yellow diamond – 2

   Special/specific hazard, White diamond – corrosive

2. The physical appearance of the chemical is described as clear and liquid and the color is yellow.

3. The laboratory staff should find the SDS for the chemical either in the laboratory or from an online source.

4. The following information is significant.

   Potential health effects:

   Inhalation: May be harmful if inhaled. Material is extremely destructive to the tissue of the mucous membrane and upper respiratory tract.

   Skin: May be harmful if absorbed through skin. Causes skin burns.

   Eyes: Causes eye burns.

   Ingestion: May be harmful if swallowed. Causes burns.

5. Handling HCL: Wear protective eyewear, lab coat and acid resistance gloves. Use a proper carrier to transport the acid.

   Use of HCL: Remember to carefully pour acid into water.

   Disposal: Handle as hazardous waste; send to an RCRA approved facility; do not pour down the sink; contact the institutions environmental health and safety department.

Chapter 2

1. There are several troubleshooting strategies applicable to this situation. Here is one approach to this problem.
   - Repeat testing
   - Check sample integrity
   - Check to make sure you have the right specimen
   - Check for previous results on the same patient

2. Verify that the calibration was performed and was acceptable

3. Verify that the quality control was acceptable.

4. Check to see if there were any electrical power interruptions.

Chapter 3

1. Paul's creatinine clearance is

$$CrCl = \frac{U \times V}{P} = \frac{120 \text{ mg/dL} \times \frac{1850 \text{ mL/24 h}}{1440 \text{ min/24 h}}}{6.5 \text{ mg/dL}} = 24 \text{mL/min}$$

2. Creatinine clearance measures the glomerular filtration rate. (The rate at which a creatinine is excreted by the kidneys in relation to the concentration of the same substance in the plasma usually expressed and mL/min.)

   The glomerulus is the part of the nephron which is responsible for the GFR.

3. Paul has a decreased GFR.

4. Most labs routinely report as estimated GFR using an estimating or prediction equation based on the serum creatinine, age, gender and ethnicity.

5. If Paul's body surface area is smaller than 1.73 m^2 his corrected CrCl would be higher than the calculated.

Chapter 4

1. No, it is not acceptable because it was over 2 hours old and was not refrigerated. When it arrived, it was room temperature.

2. The maximum time allowable before testing without preservation, e.g., refrigeration is 2 hours.

3. Urine specimens can be refrigerated up to 24 hours.

4. a. Clarity/Appearance: darkens/modified
   b. Glucose: decreases
   c. Urobilinogen: decreases
   d. Nitrite: increases

Chapter 5

1. An amber urine can be a sign of dehydration or any of the following causes:

   Bilirubin*

   Carrots/Vitamin A

   Acriflavine

   Nitrofurantoin

   Rifadin (rifampin)

   Coumadin (warfarin)

   Pyridium (phenazopyridine)

   Serenium (ethoxazene)

   *Pathologic

2. Bilirubin in the urine is a sign of liver disease, possibly hepatitis. The other causes are not pathologic. Vitamin A can be from a multivitamin and the remaining are medications that the patient may be taking.

3. Hazy urine can result from
   a. *WBCs
   b. *RBCs
   c. Squamous epithelial cells
   d. *Bacteria
   e. *Non squamous epithelial cells
   f. *Lipids
   g. Semen
   h. Mucus
   i. *Lymph fluids
   j. * Normal crystals
   k. *Abnormal crystals
   l. *Yeast
   m. Fecal material
   n. Extraneous contamination (talcum powder, x-ray contrast media)

   *pathologic

4. Mary's specific gravity would be hypersthenuric, which is a specific gravity over 1.010. Explanations for hypersthenuric urine are three of any of the following: dehydration, diarrhea, excessive sweating, vomiting, water restriction, glucosuria, congestive heart failure, liver disease, and nephrosis. Conditions resulting in decreased blood flow to the kidneys and decreased glomerular filtrate which results in the total dissolved solutes being excreted in lower urine volume.

Chapter 6

1. The abnormal results are: Glucose: 4+ (Clinitest: 3000 mg/dL); Ketones: 2+ (Acetest: 2+)

2. Glucosuria and ketonuria are most commonly associated with Type I Insulin-Dependent Diabetes Mellitus patients in diabetic ketoacidosis (DKA). The elevated serum glucose is further evidence of DM.

3. The fruity odor is caused by the ketones (acetone) in Heidi's breath.

4. Reagent strip glucose is more sensitive to glucose (i.e., Chemstrip: detects 40 mg/dL) than Clinitest, which detects 250 mg/dL reducing substances including glucose. Therefore, you would expect the reagent strip reaction to be higher than Clinitest.

5. The pass-through phenomenon in the Clinitest reaction is observed in urines with high levels of reducing substances (glucose) when the color goes rapidly from blue to orange (4+) and returns to a blue-green or greenish brown color. The pass-through phenomenon occurs because of reoxidation of the cuprous oxide to cupric oxide due to the presence of high levels of reducing substances. The caramelization (burning) of the sugar also contributes to the brownish color.

6. If the technologist does not monitor the reaction it would be reported as a lower than the actual value (i.e., 1+) or neg. If a pass-through effect is noted the Clinitest is repeated using the 2-drop method instead of the normal 5-drop.

7. The reagent strip glucose reaction is glucose oxidase/peroxidase, which is specific for glucose. Glucose oxidase will not react with other carbohydrates, i.e., galactose, lactose, fructose, and pentose, which could be clinically significant.

   The Clinitest or copper reduction method will react with ANY reducing substance, any substance which can reduce cupric (II) to cuprous (I) ions. It is nonspecific and will be positive with any reducing sugar (except for sucrose which is non reducing) as well as uric acid, creatinine, homogentisic acid, ascorbic acid, chloroform and formaldehyde.

8. The ketone reagent strip and Acetest reactions detect only diacetic acid and acetone. β-hydroxybutyric acid is not measured by any method currently used in the laboratory.

9. At this point Heidi is not exhibiting any signs of renal damage/diabetic nephropathy because the protein is negative.

10. Microalbuminuria provides any early indication of early nephropathy. Diabetics should be screened yearly for proteinuria. If protein is negative, microalbumin should be ordered to best detect, prevent, and treat early nephropathy. Microalbuminuria will occur in 20 to 30% of Type 1 when they are diagnosed, or Type 2 diabetics within 10 to 15 years of diagnosis, even in well-controlled diabetics.

Chapter 7

1. Refer to Box 7-1. It is important to focus up and away from the specimen that has been placed on the stage to avoid damaging the objective or the slide containing the specimen. Once the specimen has been focused using the 10× and 40× objectives, a drop of oil is placed on the slide before putting the 100× objective in place. Light intensity is increased when the next higher objective is put in place.

2. Clean the microscope objectives using lens paper and lens cleaner to prevent oil and dust from building up causing poor illumination and stray "non-specimen" objects to appear in the field. Clean the eyepieces to remove loose dirt, mascara, and eye secretions that may be present.

Chapter 8

1. The reagent strip indicates 1+ blood, while the microscopic report states >100 RBC/HPF.

2. Diabetes

3. Red blood cells and yeast are present.

4. Yeast does not produce nitrite and would not show a positive result.

5. Counting non-budding yeast as red blood cells will falsely increase the red cell count. In addition, the number of cells per field will increase due to evaporation of the specimen when exposed to the heat of the microscope lamp over time.

Chapter 9

1. The abnormal macroscopic findings are: Appearance: Cloudy; Protein: 1+ (30 mg/dL) (SSA: 1+); Blood: 1+; Nitrite: pos; Leukocyte Esterase: 2+. The abnormal microscopic findings are: WBCs: 40-60/HPF (2-4 clumps/HPF); Casts: 3-6 WBC/LPF, 0-2 Granular/LPF; 0-1 Bacterial/LPF. Discrepant results: none.

2. The presence of renal epithelial cells and casts are consistent with an upper urinary tract infection. Renal epithelial cells line various parts of the nephron and indicate a renal origin. They are usually reported as renal tubular epithelial, but they can be divided into convoluted renal tubular cells from the proximal and distal convoluted tubules or collecting duct cells from the collecting ducts. Rare renal epithelial cells indicate only normal sloughing off and replacement of old cells, but in greater numbers they may point to more significant damage to the tubules and collecting ducts. Casts are also only formed in the renal tubules (distal convoluted tubule and collecting duct); therefore their presence signifies renal involvement.

3. The urinalysis results are indicative of acute pyelonephritis. Acute pyelonephritis is characterized by mild proteinuria (<1 g/d); leukocyte esterase +/±; nitrite: +/±; increased WBCs; bacteria; WBC, granular, renal cell and waxy casts; RBCs; and renal epithelial cells. Chronic pyelonephritis is differentiated by moderate proteinuria (<2.5 g/d); leukocyte esterase ±; increased WBCs; granular, waxy and broad casts; and few WBC and renal cell casts. The history of recurrent infections is the hallmark of chronic pyelonephritis.

4. Pyuria is associated with neutrophils (polymorphonuclear neutrophils- PMNs).

5. Leukocyte casts are pathognomonic of this disease although they may be found in other conditions. The WBCs that form WBC casts can be from the glomeruli or tubules. If they are glomerular in origin (glomerulonephritis), red cells casts would also be present and in larger numbers than leukocyte casts. A tubular source (pyelonephritis) would have bacteria along with the leukocyte casts. Mary's urinalysis and related information point to a tubular source, i.e., pyelonephritis.

6. Two mechanisms leading to acute pyelonephritis are: (1) ascending pyelonephritis: bacteria moving up the urinary tract, i.e. cystitis (bladder), to the kidney; (2) hematogenous pyelonephritis: bacteria in the circulatory tract settling in the kidney.

7. Reflex testing would include a urine culture and sensitivity. *Escherichia coli* is the most common pathogen, although Proteus, Klebsiella, Enterobacter, and Pseudomonas are also frequently identified causes of pyelonephritis.

8. The treatment is a suitable antibiotic. The most frequently used antibiotics are furadantin, amoxicillin, cephalosporins, sulfisoxazole/trimethoprim, and sulfa drugs for 10 to 14 days. Patients must be cautioned to complete the entire course of antibiotics even if the symptoms have subsided and they are feeling better.

9. Pyelonephritis is most often caused by untreated cystitis when the bacteria continue to migrate up the urinary tract through the ureters and finally to the kidney (pyelonephritis). Catherization, diabetes mellitus, pregnancy, and urinary obstruction increases the risk for acute pyelonephritis. Other conditions that are risk factors for pyelonephritis are cancer or AIDS (immunocompromised patients), recurrent cystitis, benign prostate hyperplasia, and structural abnormalities (vesicourethral reflux—persistent backflow of the urine from the bladder into the ureters).

10. Most patients with acute pyelonephritis recover without complications. Complications can include recurrence of pyelonephritis (chronic pyelonephritis), sepsis, and in rare cases acute renal failure. Acute pyelonephritis should be treated carefully and completely, especially in elderly patients who are more likely to have severe cases and recurrent infections.

Chapter 10

1. The CSF/serum glucose ratio corrects for hyperglycemia that may mask a relative decrease in the CSF glucose concentration. The CSF glucose concentration is low when the CSF/serum glucose ratio is <0.6. A CSF/serum glucose ratio <0.4 is highly suggestive of bacterial meningitis but may also be seen in other conditions, including, tuberculosis, fungal and carcinamatous meningitis.

2. Altered mental status, persistent headaches, fever, fast heart rate or tachycardia, hyperventilation, and nuchal rigidity.

3. Abnormal findings include all of the tests shown.

4. This patient has bacterial meningitis. Meningitis is the inflammation of the meninges around the brain and/or spinal cord. Etiologic agents include viral, bacterial, or noninfectious causes such as medications. Meningitis should be considered in a patient presenting with fever and stiff neck or neurologic symptoms. Bacterial meningitis is a medical emergency. Thus, therapy should not be delayed for diagnostic test results because prognosis depends on rapid initiation of antimicrobial treatment. Diagnosis of bacterial meningitis requires a lumbar puncture with measurement

of opening pressure, examination of CSF protein, glucose, and cell count with differential and Gram stain with culture. It is advisable to include blood cultures.

The hallmark abnormalities in bacterial meningitis are (1) elevated number of polymorphonuclear cells, (2) decreased glucose concentration, (3) increased protein concentration, and (4) increased opening pressure. The result of a Gram stain will be positive in most cases and subsequent CSF bacterial cultures will be positive.

Chapter 11

1. Ascites results from increased accumulation of peritoneal fluid by transudation of fluid from the surface of the liver as a result of increased portal venous pressure (portal hypertension).

2. The serum-ascites albumin gradient, defined as the serum albumin concentration minus the ascitic fluid albumin concentration, is commonly considered as the most reliable method to differentiate peritoneal transudate from exudates. Ascites caused by portal hypertension has a gradient of at least 1.1 g/dL, whereas ascites produced by other causes has a gradient less than 1.1 g/dL (exudate).

3. Additional tests include gross appearance, cell count and differential, cytology, and culture for bacteria and mycobacteria.

Chapter 12

1. Gouty arthritis

2. Ethanol can promote hyperuricemia

   Serum uric acid is typically elevated in patients with this disease.

   Elevated WBC is typically elevated in patients with this disease.

   Microscopic examination reveals the presence of sodium urate crystals that appear within neutrophils, are shaped like needles, and are negatively birefringent in this disease.

3. The disease is more common in Pacific Islanders (e.g., Filipinos).

4. *Tophus* is the lesion that is present in patients with this disease.

   Podagra is a term associated with the metatarsal phalangeal joint of the great toe.

5. Reference intervals or ranges for serum uric acid are method dependent.

Chapter 13

1. False negative results may be due to difficulty by users in understanding the literature that accompanies the tests or false negatives can occur with specimens containing hCG variants.

2. • Appendicitis
   • Inflammatory bowel disease
   • Ovarian pathology
   • Cyst
   • Pelvic inflammatory disease
   • Endometriosis
   • Urinary tract infections (UTIs)

3. Patients with an ectopic pregnancy or threatened abortion may show only a moderate rise in the serum β-hCG measurement, for example, less than 1,000 mU/mL when it should be >2,000 mU/mL.

Chapter 14

1. Phenylketonuria (Classic)

2. Phenylalanine is a competitive inhibitor of tyrosinase, a key enzyme in the pathway of melanin synthesis, and accounts for the hypopigmentation of hair and skin.

3. The mousy odor of urine is due to the presence of an accumulation of the metabolic product phenylacetate.

4. Diagnosis of PKU depends upon the plasma levels of phenylalanine and tyrosine. The addition of a phenylalanine/tyrosine molar ratio reduces the chances of obtaining a false positive result and arriving at an incorrect diagnosis.

5. Under normal conditions phenylalanine is converted to tyrosine in the presence of phenylalanine hydroxylase (PAH). In patients with PKU, the enzyme activity of PAH is reduced significantly, thereby increasing the concentrations of phenylalanine and its by-products in body fluids.

Chapter 15

1. Ben has osmotic type diarrhea

2. Ben did not tell the physician that he was taking four times the amount of laxative than he should have because he was not sure what amount he should be taking. Also it made him feel good so he thought it would not cause any harm. Unfortunately, a large amount of laxative could lead to a significant case of osmotic diarrhea.

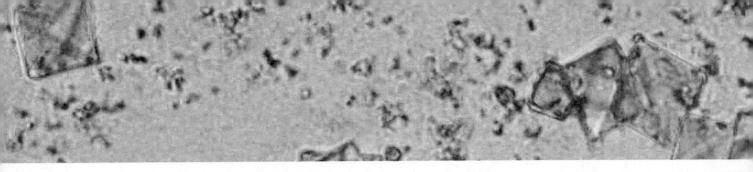

Appendix E

Nomogram for the Determination of Body Surface Area of Children and Adults

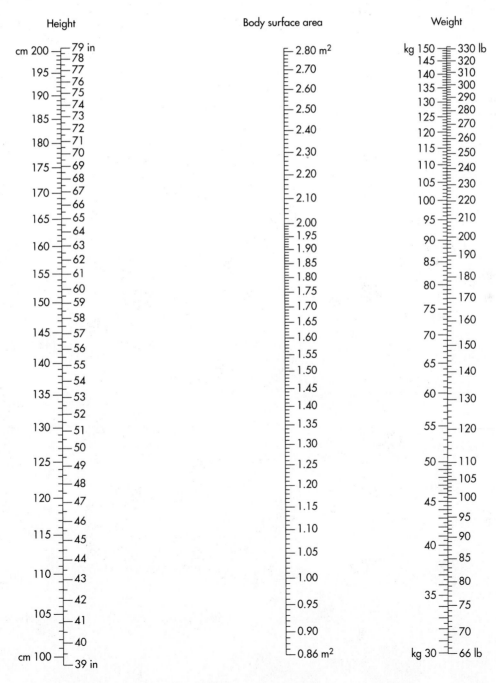

Height	Body surface area	Weight
cm 200 — 79 in	— 2.80 m²	kg 150 — 330 lb
78		145 — 320
195 — 77	— 2.70	140 — 310
76		135 — 300
190 — 75	— 2.60	130 — 290
74		— 280
185 — 73	— 2.50	125 — 270
72	— 2.40	120 — 260
180 — 71		115 — 250
70	— 2.30	
175 — 69	— 2.20	110 — 240
68		105 — 230
170 — 67	— 2.10	100 — 220
66		
165 — 65	— 2.00	95 — 210
64	— 1.95	90 — 200
160 — 63	— 1.90	
62	— 1.85	85 — 190
155 — 61	— 1.80	— 180
60	— 1.75	80 —
150 — 59	— 1.70	75 — 170
58	— 1.65	— 160
145 — 57	— 1.60	70 —
56	— 1.55	— 150
140 — 55	— 1.50	65 —
54		— 140
135 — 53	— 1.45	60 —
52	— 1.40	— 130
130 — 51	— 1.35	55 —
50	— 1.30	— 120
125 — 49	— 1.25	50 — 110
48	— 1.20	— 105
120 — 47	— 1.15	45 — 100
46	— 1.10	— 95
115 — 45		— 90
44	— 1.05	40 —
110 — 43	— 1.00	— 85
42		— 80
— 0.95	35 —	
105 — 41		— 75
— 0.90	— 70	
40		
cm 100 — 39 in	— 0.86 m²	kg 30 — 66 lb

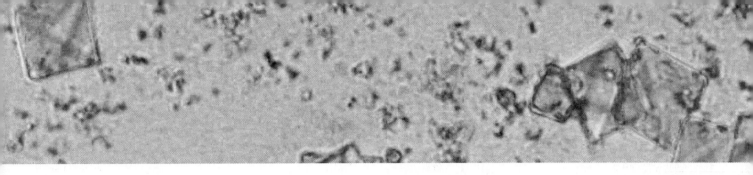

Appendix F

Chapter 6: Urine Reference Ranges and Cutoff Values

Component	Type of Specimen	Conventional Units	SI Units
Acetoacetic acid	Random	Negative	Negative
Acetone	Random	Negative	Negative
Albumin, mg/day(g/day)	24 hr	15–150	0.015–0.150
Alkapton bodies	random	Negative	Negative
Ammonia nitrogen, mEq/day (mmol/day)	24 hr	20–70	20–70
Amylase, U/L (μKat/L)	24 hr	170–2000	2.89–34.0
Ascorbic acid, mg/day (μmol/day)	24 hr	>50	>284
Bence Jones protein	Random	Negative	Negative
Bilirubin, qualitative	Random	Negative	Negative
Blood, occult	Random	Negative	Negative
Calcium, quantitative, mg/day (mmol/day)	24 hr		
	Average diet ·	100–300	2.5–7.50
	Low-calcium diet	50–150	1.25–3.75
	High-calcium diet	240–300	6.0–7.5
Chloride, mEq/day (mmol/day)	24 hr	110–250	110–250
Creatinine, mg/kg/day (μmol/kg/day)	24 hr	M: 14–26	M: 124–230
		F: 11–20	F: 97–177
Estriol (E3), μg/day(nmol/day)	24 hr	M: 1.0–11.0	M: 3.5–38.2
		F: 0–15.0	F: 0–52
Fat, qualitative	Random	Negative	Negative
Glucose, qualitative	Random		
Glucose, quantitative, mg/dL (mmol/L)	24 hr	M: 1–42	M: 0.055–2.33
		F: 0–33	F: 0–18.3
Copper reducing substances, g/day (g/day)	Random	0.5–1.5	0.1–1.5
Magnesium, mEq/day (mmol/day)	24 hr	6.0–10.0	3.0–5.0
Mucin, mg/day(mg/day)	24 hr	100–150	100–150
Myoglobin mg/day (μmol/day)	24 hr	14–40	41–117
Osmolality, mOm/kg, H2O(mmol/Kg)	Random	500–800	500–800
pH	Random	4.6–8.0	4.6-8.0
Phosphorus, mg/dL (mmol/day)	24 hr	M: 5–189	M: 1.6–61
		F: 7–148	F: 2.3–48
Potassium, mEq/day (mmol/day)	24 hr	40–80	40–80
Protein, qualitative	Random	Negative	Negative

Component	Type of Specimen	Conventional Units	SI Units
Sodium, mEq/day (mmol/day)	24 hr	75–200	75–200
Specific gravity	Random	1.002–1.030	1.002–1.030
Urea nitrogen, g/day(mol/day)	24 hr	12–20	0.43–0.71
Uric acid, mg/day(mmoL/day)	24 hr (average diet)	250–750	1.48–4.43
Urobilinogen, mg/day (μmol/day)	24 hr	0.05–2.5	0.1–4.2
Uroporphyrins, quantitative, μg/day(nmol/day)	24 hr	10–30	12–36
Volume, total, ml/day(L/day)	24 hr	600–1600	0.6–1.6

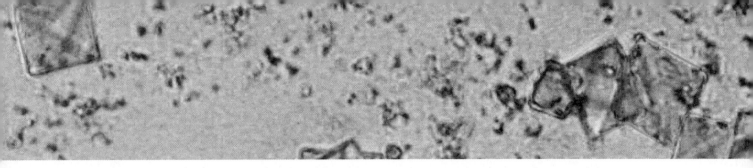

Appendix G

Chapter 8: Reference Table: Enumeration of Microscopic Elements

Element	Reference value	Magnification	Clinical Significance
Red blood cells	3–5 cells	High-power field (HPF)	Increased numbers may indicate glomerulonephritis, trauma, acute tubular necrosis, or lower urinary tract disease.
White blood cells	Less than 5	HPF	Infection or inflammation of the urinary tract.
CASTS			
Hyaline	Less than 2	LPF	Increased numbers due to exercise, dehydration, renal disease.
Granular	Rare	LPF	Extreme stress, strenuous exercise; may appear with glomerular or renal diseases.
Waxy	None seen	LPF	Chronic renal disease, tubular degeneration.
EPITHELIAL CELLS			
Squamous	Few	Low power field (LPF)	May be seen in increased number in female specimens.
Renal tubular	Rare, few	LPF	Increased numbers may indicate tubular damage.
Transitional	Few	LPF	Increased numbers due to catheterization; may be due to carcinoma.
MICROORGANISMS			
Bacteria	None seen		Bacteria present may be due to collection and subsequent timing of examination.
Yeast	None seen		May be contaminant from skin, female genital tract or air bubbles.

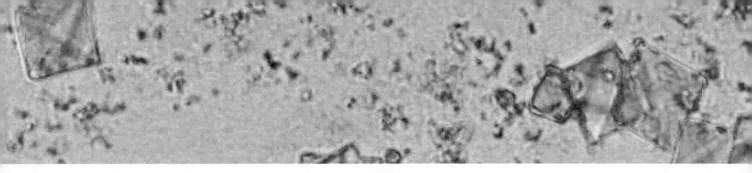

Appendix H

Chapter 10: Reference Ranges for CSF and Serum or Whole Blood

Analyte/Parameter (Conventional Units/SI Units)	CSF	Serum or whole blood
Electrolytes		
Sodium, meq/L (mmol/L)	135–150 (135–150)	136–145 (136–145)
Potassium meq/L (mmol/L)	2.6–3.0 (2.6–3.0)	3.5–4.5 (3.5–4.5)
Chloride meq/L (mmol/L)	115–130 (115–130)	98–107 (98–107)
Carbon dioxide meq/L (mmol/L)	20–25 (20–25)	23–29 (23–29)
Calcium, mg/dL (mmol/L)	4.2–5.4 (1.0–1.4)	8.6–10.0 (2.15–2.5)
Phosphorus, mg/dL (mmol/L)	1.2–2.0 (0.4–0.7)	2.3–4.7 (0.74–1.52)
Magnesium, mg/dL (mmol/L)	2.9–3.6 (1.2–1.5)	1.6–2.6 (0.66–1.07)
Lactate, mg/dL (mmol/L)	10–22 (1.1–2.4)	4.5–19.8 (0.5–2.2)
Osmolality, mOsm/L (mmol/L)	280–300 (280–300)	280–301 (280–301)
Metabolics		
Ammonia, μg/dL (mmol/L)	10–35 (5.9–20.5)	19–60 (11–35)
Creatinine, mg/dL (μmol/L)	0.6–1.2 (45–92)	0.62–1.10 (55–96)
Glucose, mg/dL (mmol/L)	40–80 (2.8–4.4)	74–106 (4.1–5.9)
Glutamine, mg/dL (mmol/L)	5–20 (0.3–1.4)	5.9–10.4 (0.4–0.68)
Iron, μg/dL (μmol/L)	1–2 (0.2–0.4)	65–175 (11.6–31.3)
Total lipids, mg/dL (g/L)	1–2 (0.01–0.02)	400–800 (4–8)
Urea Nitrogen, mg/dL (mmol/L)	6–16 (2.0–5.7)	6–20 (2.1–7.1)
Urate, mg/dL (μmol/L)	0.5–3.0 (30–180)	4.4–7.6 (262–452)
Lactate dehydrogenase, U/L	<20	140–280
pH		
Lumbar	7.28–7.32	
Cisternal	7.32–7.34	
pCO2		
Lumbar, mmHg (kPa)	44–50 (5.85–6.65)	N/A
Cisternal, mmHg (kPa)	40–46 (5.32–6.12)	N/A
Proteins		
Total protein, mg/dL (g/L):		
Lumbar	15–45 (0.15–0.45)	N/A
Cisternal	15–25 (0.15–0.25)	N/A
Ventricular	6–15 (0.06–0.15)	N/A
Prealbumin, %	1–7	0.2
Albumin,%,	49–73	56–65
α1-globulin, %	3–7	2.5–5.0
α2-globulin, %	6–13	7–13
β-globulin ($\beta_1$plus tau), %	9–19	8–14

Analyte/Parameter (Conventional Units/SI Units)	CSF	Serum or whole blood
γ-globulin, %	3–12	12–22
IgG, mg/dL (g/L)	0.9–5.7 (0.009–0.057)	650–1600 (6.5–16.0)
IgG index	0.29–0.59	N/A
CSF IgG synthesis rate (mg/day)	−9.9 − +3.3	
CSF IgG-albumin ratio	0.09–0.25	
Albumin index	0.0–9.0	
O-bands	<bands not present in matched serum samples>	
Myelin basic protein, ng/mL (μg/L)	<2.5 (<2.5)	N/A
Cell counts		
WBC, $10^3/\mu L$ (10^9/L)	<5 (<5)	4.4–11 (4.4–11.3)
RBC, $10^6/\mu L$ (10^{12}/L)	0	M: 4.5–5.9 (4.5–5.9) F: 4.5–5.1 (4.5–5.1)
Differential		
Lymphocytes, (%)	60–70	34
Monocytes, (%)	30–50	4
Neutrophils, (%)	0	56
Others		
CSF pressure, mmH2O(mmHg)	50–180 (3.65–13.14)	
CSF volume, mL	~150	

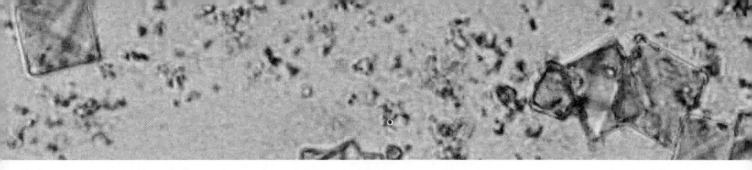

Appendix I

Chapter 12: Synovial Fluid Reference Values

	Conventional Units	SI units
Leukocytes, $\times 10^3/\mu L$ ($\times 10^9/L$)	<15.0	<15.0
Differential (WBC)		
PMNs, %	<25	<0.25
Lymphocytes, %	<75	<0.75
Monocytes, %	<70	<0.70
Synoviocytes, %	0–12	0–0.12
Erythrocytes $\times 10^6/\mu L$ ($\times 10^{12}/L$)	<20	<20
Glucose (blood/synovial fluid difference)	<10	<0.55
Hyaluronate, g/dL (g/L)	0.30–0.41	3.0–4.1
Lactate, mg/dL (mmol/L)	<25	<2.8
Protein, g/dL (g/L)	1–3	10–30
Uric acid (uricase method), mg/dL ($\mu Mol/L$)	M: 3.5–7.2	M: 208–428
	F: 2.6–6.0	F: 155–357
Fibrin clot	Absent	
Mucin clot	Abundant	
Viscosity	High	
Volume, mL (L)	<3.5	<0.0035

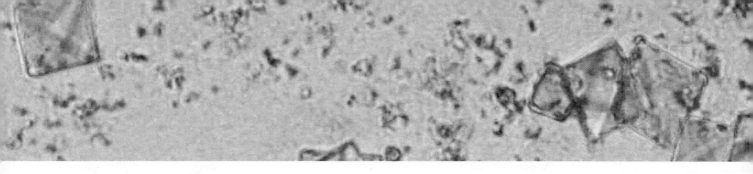

Appendix J

Chapter 13: Reference Values for Amniotic Fluid Components

(The reference values shown in this table represent fetus/newborn at term)

Component	Conventional units	SI Units
Appearance	Clear or slightly opalescent	
Volume	500–1400	0.50–1.4
Analytes		
Albumin, g/dL (g/L)	0.19	1.9
Alpha-fetoprotein, mg/L (g/L)	<30	<0.030
Bilirubin, total, mg/dL (µmol/L)	<0.025	<0.41
Chloride, mEq/L (mmol/L)	Typically 1–3 lower than serum	Typically 1–3 lower than serum
Creatinine, mg/dL (µmol/L)	1.8–4.0	159–354
Glucose, mg/dL (mmol/L)	<10	<0.56
Estriol, µg/dL (nmol/L)	<60	>2081
Lecithin: Sphingomyelin ratio	>2:1	>2:1
Osmolality, mOsm/Kg H2O (mmol/Kg)	230–270	230–270
Phosphatidylglycerol (chromatography) mg/dL	Present	
Phosphatidylglycerol (AmnioStat-FLM, mg/dL)	Low-positive: >0.5	
	High-positive: >20	
	Negative: <0.5	
pCO2, mmHg (kPa)	42–55	5.6–7.3
pH	6.91–7.43	6.91–7.43
Protein, total, g/dL (g/L)	0.15–0.35	1.5–3.5
Sodium, mEq/L (mmol/L)	7–10 lower than serum	7–10 lower than serum
Urea Nitrogen, mg/dL (mmol/L)	28.9–41.7	4.81–6.94
Uric acid, mg/dL (µmol/L)	7.67–12.13	456–721

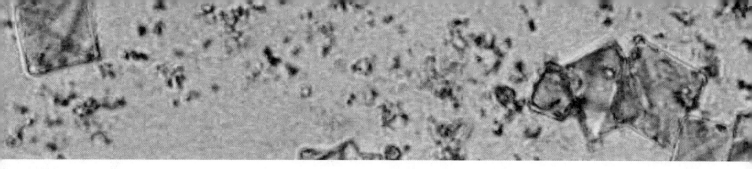

Appendix K

Chapter 14: Reference Ranges and Cutoff Values for Amino Acids

References

1. Sehlub J, Jacques PF, Rosenberg IH, et al. Serum total homocysteine concentrations in the Third National Health and Nutrition Survey (1991–1994): Population reference ranges and contribution of vitamin status to high serum concentrations. *Ann Intern Med* (1999) 131:331–339.

2. Chace DH, Hillman SL, Millington DS, et al. Rapid diagnosis of maple syrup urine disease in blood spots from newborns by tandem mass spectrometry. *Clin Chem* (1995) 41:62–68.

3. Schulze A, Lindner M, Kohlmoller D, et al. Expanded newborn screening for inborn errors of metabolism by electrospray ionization-tandem mass spectrometry: results, outcome, and implications. *Pediatrics* (2003) 111:1399–1406.

4. Chace DH, Sherwin JE, Hillman SL, et al. Use of phenylalanine to tyrosine ratio determined by tandem mass spectrometry to improve newborn screening for phenylketonuria of early discharge specimens collected in the first 24 hours. *Clin Chem* (1998) 44:2405–2409.

5. Chace DH, Hillman SL, Millington DS, et al. Rapid diagnosis homocystinuria and other hypermethionemias from newborn's blood spots by tandem mass spectrometry. *Clin Chem* (1996) 42:349–355.

Analyte	Specimen	Age	Mg/dL	μMol/L
Homocysteine[1]:	Plasma	Age dependent		
Male (adult)				≤11.4
Female (adult)				≤10.4
Homogentisic acid	Plasma	Neonate	Non detected	Non detected
Isoleucine[2]	Dried blood	Neonate	1.98 ± 0.61	151 ± 47
Leucine[3]	Dried blood	Neonate	1.98 ± 0.61	151 ± 47
Phenylalanine[4]	Dried blood	Neonate	<2.0	<120
Phenylalanine/tyrosine			2.5	
Tyrosine[4]	Dried blood	Neonate	0.65–3.77	36.0–208
Valine[5]	Dried blood	Neonate	1.53 ± 0.68	131 ± 58

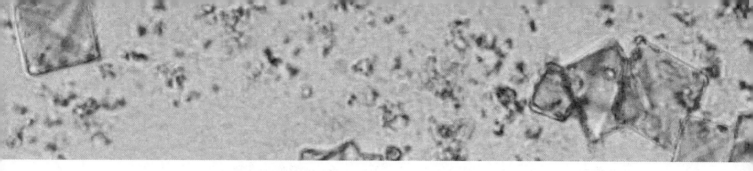

Appendix L

Chapter 15: Reference Ranges and Cutoff Values for Stool Analysis

Component	Conventional Units	SI Units
Alpha-1-antitrypsin, mg/dL (mg/L)	>54	>540
Amount, g/24hr (kg/24hr)	100–200	0.1–0.2
Chloride[1], mEq/24hr (mmol/24hr)	2.5–4.2	2.5–4.2
Chymotrypsin[2], U/g stool (U/g stool)	12	12
(lower reference limit)		
Coproporphyrins[3] I, μg/24hr (nmol/24hr)	<500	<756
Coproporphyrins[3] III, μg/24hr (nmol/24hr)	<400	<612
Elastase-1, μg/g stool (μg/g stool)	200	200
(lower reference limit)		
Fat, g/24hr (g/24hr)	<4	<4
Fatty acids, g/24hr (mmol/24hr)	0–6	0–21
Leukocytes	None	None
Nitrogen, g/24hr (mmol/24hr)	<2.5	<178
pH		
Adults	7.0–7.5	7.0–7.5
Newborn	5.0–7.0	5.0–7.0
Potassium[4], mEq/24hr (mmol/24hr)	13–23	13–23
Occult blood	Negative	Negative
Osmolality, mOsm/Kg H2O (mmol/Kg)	280–325	280–325
Osmol Gap:		
Secretory Diarrhea	<50	<50
Osmotic Diarrhea	>50	>50
Porphyrins, total[5], mmol/g dry weight	<200	N/A
Sodium[6], mEq/24hr (mmol/24hr)	5.8–9.8	5.8–9.8
Trypsin[7], μg/g stool		N/A
Child and adult	40–760	
Pancreatic insufficiency	0–33	
Fibrocystic child	<20	
Urobilinogen, mg/24hr (μmol/24hr)	50–300	85–510
Uroporphyrins[3] I, μg/24hr (nmol/24hr)	<120	<144
Uroporphyrins[3] III, μg/24hr (nmol/24hr)	<50	<60

References

1. Wallace J. *Interpretation of diagnostic tests.* 7th ed. Philadelphia, PA: Lippincott Williams & Wilkins; 2000.

2. Melzi d'Eril GV, Polinie, Morattie R, et.al. Proposed reference values for fecal chymotrypsin as measured photometrically. *Clin Chem* 1985;31:1088–1089.

3. Mayo Medical Laboratories: Test Catalog, Rochester, MN, 2005. Mayo Medical Laboratories.

4. Cuprilli R, Sopranzi N, Colaperi O, et al. Salt-losing diarrhea in idiopathic proctocolitis. *Scand J Gastroenterol*, 1979;13:331–335.

5. Lockwood WH, Poulos V, Rossi E, et al. Rapid procedure for fecal porphyrin assay. *Clin Chem* 1985;31;1163–1167.

6. Wallach J. *Interpretation of diagnostic tests.* 5th ed. Boston, MA: Little, Brown and Company; 1992.

7. Burtis CA, Ashwood ER. *Tietz textbook of clinical chemistry.* 2nd ed. Philadelphia, PA: WB Saunders; 1994.

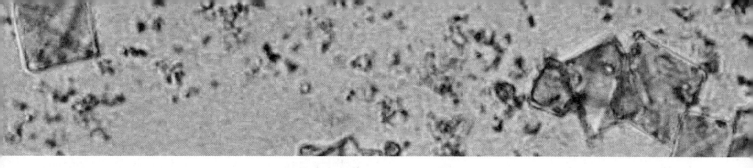

Glossary

24-hour specimen   A collection of all of the urine produced in 24 hours to measure the exact concentration of a urine chemical or analyte.

Abbé condenser   A condenser having two simple lenses that are not corrected for spherical or chromatic aberration. This type of condenser is found on most inexpensive microscopes.

Accuracy   Closeness of the agreement between the measured values of an analyte to its "true" value.

Acetoacetic acid   A ketone body formed when fats are incompletely metabolized. It is found in urine in abnormal amounts in uncontrolled diabetes mellitus and eating disorders, e.g., anorexia, starvation.

Acetest   A confirmatory test for ketones in tablet form. The tablet contains sodium nitroprusside, glycine, disodium phosphate, and lactose.

Acetone   A ketone body formed when fats are incompletely metabolized. It is found in urine in abnormal amounts in uncontrolled diabetes mellitus and eating disorders, e.g. anorexia, starvation.

Achromatic   An engraved notation on objective lenses indicating correction for image distortion due to color or chromatic aberration.

Active transport   The process by which a cell membrane moves molecules against a concentration or electrochemical gradient using a carrier protein and requiring energy.

Acute diarrhea   Diarrhea characterized by sudden onset.

Acute glomerulonephritis   A sterile (not bacterial) inflammatory process that affects the glomerulus or a group of nephrotic conditions characterized by damage and inflammation of the glomeruli. It is characterized by the sudden onset of hematuria, proteinuria, and red blood cell casts.

Acute pyelonephritis   An infection of the upper urinary tract that frequently results from an ascending infection in untreated cases of cystitis or lower urinary tract infections.

Acute renal failure   An abrupt or rapid decline in renal filtration function marked by an increase in serum creatinine concentration or azotemia (an increase in blood urea nitrogen-BUN).

Acute tubular necrosis   A kidney disorder involving damage to the renal tubular cells of the kidneys that can lead to acute kidney failure.

Afferent arteriole   Small blood vessel in the nephron that carries blood from the renal artery to the glomerulus.

Aldosterone   Mineralocorticoid hormone secreted by the adrenal cortex that causes increased reabsorption of sodium from the glomerular filtrate.

Alkaline tide   A temporary decrease in the acidity of urine from an increase of base in the blood following the secretion of HCl into gastric juices.

Alkaptonuria   An aminoaciduria marked by the excretion of large amounts of homogentisic acid into the urine, a result of incomplete metabolism of the amino acids tyrosine and phenylalanine due to the absence of homogentisic acid oxidase.

Alloisoleucine   A pathognomonic marker for Maple Sugar Urine Disease.

Amorphous crystal   Microscopic crystal formations present in either alkaline or acid urine that have no specific crystalline shape; large amounts of these crystals may obscure other elements in the microscopic field.

Amniocentesis   A procedure for the removal of amniotic fluid.

Amnion   The membranous sac that contains the fetus and amniotic fluid.

Amniostat-FLM®-PG   This is an immunologic agglutination test for the detection of phosphatidyl glycerol. The test is useful for assessing the maturity of fetal lungs.

Amperometery   The measurement of current in an electrical circuit.

Angiotensin   A vasopressor produced when renin is released from the macula densa in the juxtaglomerular apparatus of the nephron that causes contraction of the smooth muscle of arteries and arterioles.

Angiotensin-converting enzyme (ACE)   The enzyme that converts angiotensin I to angiotensin II.

Annulus   A ring structure. In the phase contrast microscope, a ring of opaque glass or other material is placed within the substage condenser, which causes a ring-shaped beam of light to pass through the specimen into the objective.

Antidiuretic hormone   A peptide hormone from the hypothalamus that renders the walls of the distal convoluted tubules and collecting ducts permeable or impermeable to water.

Anuria   The complete cessation of urine flow as a result of damage to the kidneys or a decrease in urine formation to less than 50 mL per day.

Appearance   A general term that refers to the clarity of the urine.

Arthritis   Inflammatory process affecting a joint or joints that results in pain, swelling, and stiffness.

Arthrocentesis   Removal of fluid from synovial joints.

Ascending loop of Henle   The ascending portion of the U-shaped portion of the renal tubules lying between the proximal convoluted tubule and the distal convoluted tubule.

Ascites   The accumulation of fluid in the peritoneal cavity.

β-hydroxybutyric acid   An acid (ketone) present in the urine, especially in diabetic ketoacidosis and eating disorders, when fatty acid conversion to ketones increases.

Bence-Jones protein   A light chain portion of the immunoglobulin molecules that may be deposited in the renal tubules and excreted in urine of patients with multiple myeloma.

Benign proteinuria   An increase in protein in the urine related to dehydration, stress, inflammatory process, fever, or intense activity that is not associated with increased morbidity or mortality.

Berger's disease   Most common type of glomerulonephritis when IgA, an antibody that helps the body fight infection, is increased after mucosal infection of the respiratory, gastrointestinal, or urinary tract by bacteria or viruses.

Bilirubin   The orange or yellowish pigment in bile that is derived from hemoglobin from red blood cells that lived the normal life span and have been destroyed and ingested by the macrophages of the liver, spleen, and bone marrow.

Bilirubinuria   An increase of bilirubin in the urine.

Birefringence   The production of two light waves from a single wave by a crystal containing an uneven density of molecules. As the waves emerge from the crystal, two images are formed and may be viewed using polarizing filters placed in the microscope light path.

Bladder   A muscular, membranous distensible reservoir that holds urine, located in the pelvic cavity between the ureters leading from the kidney and the urethra.

Bloodborne pathogen   Pathogenic microorganisms that are present in human blood and can cause disease in humans.

Blood–brain barrier   Designates all of the interfaces between blood, brain, and CSF.

Bowman's capsule   Part of the nephron consisting of a visceral layer of podocytes closely applied to the glomerulus and an outer parietal layer.

Brightfield microscopy   The utilization of incandescent light focused from beneath the specimen that illuminates the field to produce a dark or colored visible image on a bright background.

Bronchoalveolar lavage   A bronchoscopy procedure that uses a flexible bronchoscope designed for retrieving cells and soluble substances from the lining fluid of the distal airways and alveolar units that contain immunologic components of the lungs.

Calibration   A procedure designed to substantiate the continued accuracy of the test system throughout the laboratory reportable range of the test results for the test system.

Carcinogen   A substance that is foreign to the body, which results in the production of a cancer-producing tumor.

Casts   A molded formation in the shape of the renal tubule made of Tamm-Horsfall protein and containing various elements such as epithelial casts, red cells, white cells, bacteria, or crystals. Casts are formed in the distal convoluted tubule or the collecting duct.

Catheterized specimen   A specimen obtained by inserting a catheter or sterile tube into the bladder to obtain a specimen that is not contaminated by vaginal fluids or menstruation.

Cellular transport mechanisms   Includes both active and passive transport mechanisms which serves to filter fluids and electrolytes in the glomerulus.

Cerebrospinal fluid (CSF)   A water cushion protecting the brain and spinal cord from physical impact.

Cerumen   A substance secreted by glands at the outer third of the ear canal; may be present in the first decade of a child's life.

Chemical hygiene plan   A plan designed to provide laboratory staff with information necessary to properly store and handle chemicals.

CFTR protein   A protein that serves as a chloride channel controlling the salt content in the fluid that covers the surface of the nose and lungs.

Choroid plexus   A network of nerves, blood, and lymphatic vessels located in the floor of the ventricles of the brain and is the primary site of CSF formation.

Chromatic aberration   Different wavelengths of white light are focused by the lens at different focal points and will produce a colored halo around the specimen, causing distortion of the image.

Chronic diarrhea   Diarrhea marked by slow progression.

Chronic glomerulonephritis   The end stage of persistent glomerular damage associated with irreversible loss of renal tissue and chronic renal failure.

Chronic kidney disease   The gradual and usually permanent loss of kidney function over time, slowly, usually months to years.

Chronic pyelonephritis   Characterized by renal inflammation and fibrosis caused by recurrent and persistent renal infections, vesicourethral reflux, kidney stones, or other causes of urinary tract obstruction.

Chylous effusion   Escape of fluid from a lymphatic duct (e.g., the thoracic duct) due to an obstruction, malignancy, or traumatic disruption. The fluid typically contains lipids such as triglycerides and chylomicrons.

Chymotrypsin   A digestive enzyme produced by the pancreas and functioning in the small intestines to hydrolyze proteins.

Clarity   The quality or state of being clear or easily seen through.

Classical distal renal tubular acidosis   Tubular acidosis that occurs when the defect is in the distal tubule and may be inherited as a primary disorder or secondary to a systemic disease that affects many parts of the body.

Clean-catch specimen   A procedure for obtaining urine specimens that exposes the sample to minimal contamination.

Clean-catch urines   A procedure for obtaining a urine specimen that exposes the sample to minimal contamination.

Clinitest   A confirmatory test for glucose that relies on the ability of glucose and other nonglucose-reducing substances to reduce cupric ions to cuprous ions in the presence of heat and alkali.

Clue cells   Vaginal squamous epithelial cells that are colonized or coated with the bacteria *Gardnerella vaginalis*. These vaginal cells contaminate urine collections when clean-catch methods are not used.

Codes of Federal Regulation   A numerical system established by the federal government to identify standards used by industry and laboratories.

Coefficient of variation   100 times the standard deviation divided by the mean.

Collecting duct   Part of the nephron where the final concentration of the urine takes place under the influence of antidiuretic hormone.

Compound microscope   A combination of objective and ocular lenses of different magnifications are placed at a distance from each other to achieve a greater magnification than can be obtained by a single lens system.

Condenser   A lens system placed beneath the microscope stage responsible for concentration of light to achieve the proper illumination of the specimen. The numerical aperture of the condenser should correspond to that of the objective in use to produce the best-quality image.

Condenser diaphragm   An adjustable opening beneath the condenser to manage the amount of light entering the condenser and the proper illumination of the specimen.

Conjugated bilirubin   Bilirubin conjugated by UDP-glucuronyl transferase in the liver to form bilirubin diglucuronide, which is water soluble and excreted in the urine.

Constipation   Bowel habits characterized by a decrease in frequency and/or passage of hard, dry stools.

Contrast   The greater the difference in the brightness of the object (specimen) compared to the darker background of the field of view allows the observer to see greater detail in the object.

Cortex   The outer layer of the kidney between the renal capsule and medulla where ultrafiltration occurs.

Coulometric titration   The generation of silver ions using an electrochemical technique that creates a flow of electrons (current).

Countercurrent mechanism   The passive exchange by the diffusion of reabsorbed solutes and water from the nephron's medullary interstitium into the blood of its vascular blood supply.

Creatinine clearance (CrCl)   Test that estimates the glomerular filtration rate by comparing the creatinine levels in serum and urine, taking into consideration the patient's body surface area and urine volume. A decrease in CrCl indicates renal insufficiency.

Crescentic (rapidly progressive) glomerulonephritis   Any glomerular disease in which there is a rapid loss of renal function, usually with crescent-shaped lesions in more than 50% of the glomeruli.

Creutzfeldt-Jakob disease   One of a group of fatal neurodegenerative diseases referred to as human transmissible spongiform encephalopathy, which features an accumulation of pathological prion proteins (PrP) in the CNS.

Cumulative trauma disorder   Disorders associated with overloading of particular muscle groups from repeated use or maintaining a constrained posture.

Crystalluria   The presence of crystals in urine.

Cystatin C   A single chain, non-glycosylated, low molecular weight protein synthesized by all nucleated cells; a cysteine protein inhibitor found in elevated concentrations in patients with impaired renal function.

Cystic fibrosis   A single-gene defect manifesting in multiple body systems as chronic obstructive pulmonary disease, pancreatic exocrine deficiency, urogenital dysfunction, and abnormally high electrolyte concentration in the sweat.

Cystitis   Inflammation of the bladder usually occurring as a lower urinary tract infection that may be caused by bacterial infection, drugs, or other irritants.

Depth of Field   The focusing distance between the farthest and closest point of the specimen to the objective lens. One can change the plane of focus between these two points by using the fine adjustment on the microscope.

Descending loop of Henle   The descending portion of the U-shaped portion of the renal tubules lying between the proximal convoluted tubule and the distal convoluted tubule.

Descriptive statistics   A set of statistics used to disclose some characteristic of a sample data set and include the mean, median, mode, range, and variance.

Diabetic nephropathy   A clinical syndrome characterized by (1) persistent albuminuria (>300 mg/dL) that is confirmed on at least two occasions 3–6 months apart, (2) progressive decline in the glomerular filtration rate (GFR), (3) and hypertension.

Diarrhea   The passage of abnormally liquid or unformed stools at an increased frequency.

Diazo reaction   Bilirubin is coupled with a diazonium salt, e.g., 2,4 dichloraninline diazonium salt, in an acid medium to form azobilirubin, a pink to violet-colored compound.

Diffraction   The scattering of light waves as they come in contact with the edge of an opaque object. This occurs when the diaphragm, specimen, or molecules in the surrounding medium bends light waves, for example.

Direct bilirubin   Bilirubin conjugated by UDP-glucuronly transferase in the liver to form bilirubin diglucuronide, which is water soluble and excreted in the urine.

Distal convoluted tubule   Part of the nephron between the ascending loop of Henle and the collecting duct where the final concentration of urine begins.

Down syndrome   Is a serious disorder of autosomal chromosomes, occurring in 1 in 800 live births. The genetic origin is an extra copy of the long arm region q22.1 to q22.3 of chromosome 21.

Dysmorphic   Abnormal structure in the morphology of an element, such as red blood cells, seen in glomerulonephritis.

Dysmotility   A term that describes altered movement of feces.

Ectopia lentis   Subluxation of the ocular lens.

Efferent arteriole   Small blood vessel that carries blood away from the glomerulus to the peritubular capillaries.

Effusion   The escape of fluid into a body part, for example, the pleural (lung) cavity.

eGFR   Estimating or prediction equation to determine glomerular filtration rate from the serum creatinine.

Ehrlich's reaction   Reaction in which p-dimethylaminobenzaldehyde turns a cherry red color in the presence of urobilinogen.

Elastase-1   Belongs to the family of serine proteinase produced in the acinar cells of the pancreas.

Engineered controls   Safety equipment that isolates or removes bloodborne pathogen hazards from the workplace; represents the preferred method for controlling hazards.

Ergonomic   The study of problems related to people adjusting to their environment.

Erythroblastosis fetalis   A hemolytic disease of the newborn marked by anemia, jaundice, enlargement of the liver and spleen, and generalized edema.

Essential amino acid   An acid that cannot be synthesized by the body thus must be consumed in the diet.

Exudates   Serous fluid that contains a high concentration of protein or cells that accumulates in a body cavity because of increased capillary permeability.

Exposure control plan   A plan designed to help prevent accidental exposure of laboratory personnel to bloodborne pathogens.

Failure to thrive   A condition in which infants and children fail to gain weight and in some cases may lose it.

False positive   A test that is positive when the disease/condition or analyte is not present. This may result from an interfering substance in the specimen being tested.

False negative   A test that is negative when the disease/condition or analyte is present.

Fanconi syndrome   One of several diseases characterized by aminoaciduria associated with failure of the proximal convoluted tubules. Symptoms include rickets, polyuria, osteomalacia, and growth failure.

Fecal osmotic gap   The difference between the theoretical normal osmolality (290 mOsm/kg) and the contribution of sodium and potassium.

Fenestrated endothelium   Endothelial cells in the glomerular membrane that have pores or openings.

Fibronectin   An adhesive glycoprotein produced by fetal membranes and found in the choriodecidual junction and amniotic fluid.

First morning specimen   The sample of choice when concentrated urine is recommended. It increases the likelihood that chemicals and formed elements that may not be found in dilute, random specimens are detected.

Focal length   The measured distance traveled by light rays from the center of a lens and the focal point of the lens.

Focal point   The center point at which light rays intersect after passing through a lens.

Gestational diabetes mellitus   Any degree of glucose intolerance with onset or first recognition during pregnancy regardless of whether the condition persisted after pregnancy and not excluding the possibility that unrecognized glucose intolerance may have begun antedated or began concomitantly with the pregnancy.

Glitter cells   A term used to describe white cells that take up fluid from the surrounding medium and swell. These swollen cells exhibit a "glittering" state due to "Brownian" motion which is described as random moving of particles, of the cytoplasmic granules.

Glomerular filtration   The process of removing larger proteins when the plasma filtrate passes through the glomerular membrane and into the proximal convoluted tubule.

Glomerulonephritis   Inflammatory process that affects the glomerulus or a group of nephrotic conditions characterized by damage and inflammation of the glomeruli.

Glomerulus   A coil of approximately 40 capillary loops that is part of the renal corpuscles in the nephron of the kidney. Each is surrounded by a Bowman's capsule where the blood filtrate becomes the ultrafiltrate.

Glycorrhachia   Glucose in spinal fluid.

Gout   A type of arthritis characterized by deposition of monosodium urate crystals in joints and other tissues.

Granular casts   As casts containing cells or other elements remain in the nephron for long periods, the elements degrade over time to become coarse or fine granular casts.

Greiss reaction   A test for the presence of nitrite that involves the diazotization of nitrite with an aromatic amine to form a diazonium salt, which results in any shade of pink.

Haptoglobin   Protein carrier of hemoglobin from lysed red blood cells in the bloodstream.

Harmonic Oscillation Densitometry   A method for determining the specific gravity of urine in which the urine is placed in a glass tube with an electromagnetic coil at one end. An electric current is applied to the coil, which causes a sonic oscillation to pass through the sample. The oscillation detected is proportional to the density of the urine.

Hazard identification system   The labeling system used to categorizes chemicals into nine classes of hazardous materials.

Hemocytometer   A device for counting cells in a specific volume of fluid.

Hemarthrosis   Bleeding into joint spaces.

Hematuria   The presence of blood present in the form of intact RBCs in the urine.

Hemoglobinuria   The presence of hemoglobin from hemolyzed RBCs in the urine.

Hemosiderin   The insoluble form of iron oxide resulting from the breakdown of hemoglobin in red blood cells. Hemosiderin may be found in urinary casts after significant destruction of red cells has occurred.

Hepatic jaundice   Condition characterized by yellow staining of the skin due to increased bilirubin associated with liver damage and is an early warning sign of liver disease, e.g., hepatitis, cirrhosis.

High-resolution electrophoresis   Describes the modification of an electrophoresis procedure, which results in the separation and detection of analytes found in low concentration.

Homocystinuria An inherited disease caused by the absence of the enzyme essential to the metabolism of homocysteine. Clinical features include failure to thrive, mental retardation, cataracts, increased thrombosis risk, and death.

Hyaline cast A urinary cast containing Tamm-Horsfall protein. These casts are visually similar to the surrounding medium in a wet mount preparation and may be hard to see using brightfield microscopy.

Hyaluronan An anionic, non-sulfated glycosaminoglycan dispersed in many body tissues (e.g., connective, epithelial, and neural).

Hydramnios A condition characterized by an abnormal accumulation (typically ~2,000 mL) of amniotic fluid at term.

Hyperkalemic renal tubular acidosis A generalized transport abnormality of the distal tubules that affects the transport of electrolytes in the distal tubules. It is the most common cause of RTA and can be caused by an inherited disorder or certain drugs or medications.

Hypersthenuric Urine with a specific gravity over 1.010.

Hyperuricemia Elevated levels of uric acid in serum.

Hyposthenuric Urine with a specific gravity below 1.010.

Ictotest A tablet test for bilirubin that yields a more sharply colored diazo reaction than the reagent strip. It consists of a mat and tablet containing p-nitrobenzene-diazonium-p-toluenesulfonate, sulfosalicylic acid, sodium carbonate, and boric acid.

IgA nephropathy Most common type of glomerulonephritis when IgA, an antibody that helps the body fight infection, is increased after a mucosal infection of the respiratory, gastrointestinal, or urinary tract by bacteria or viruses.

Inborn error of metabolism Inherited disorder that results in disruption of a specific enzyme function caused by failure to inherit the gene to produce a particular enzyme.

Incident command system Is a standardized on-scene incident management concept designed specifically to allow responders to adopt an integrated organizational structure equal to the complexity and demands of any single incident or multiple incidents without being hindered by jurisdictional boundaries.

Indirect bilirubin The bilirubin formed by the degradation of hemoglobin that binds to albumin and is carried to the liver. It is not soluble in water and cannot be excreted in the urine.

Inferential statistics Statistics that make estimates of population parameters and used to make decisions concerning those parameters.

Inflammasome A multiprotein oligomer that is part of the body's innate immune system. It is responsible for activation of the inflammatory response.

Inflammatory diarrhea A form of diarrhea characterized by pain, fever, bleeding, or other signs and symptoms of inflammation.

Inhibin One of two hormones secreted by the gonads in both males and females that inhibit the production of the follicle-stimulating hormone by the pituitary gland.

Intracranial pressure The pressure inside the skull.

Intrathecal Literally means "within the sheath."

Inulin clearance Inulin, a naturally occurring polysaccharide of fructose found in artichokes, is the gold standard for measuring glomerular filtration rate.

Iontophoresis The movement of small ions in an electric field.

Iris diaphragm An adjustable opening found directly below the light source to change the amount of light entering the condenser diaphragm.

Isosthenuric A uniform specific gravity of 1.010 that is the specific gravity of plasma. This means the urine is neither concentrated nor diluted and indicates impaired renal tubular function.

Jaundice A condition marked by yellow discoloration of the body tissue and fluids caused by excessive amounts of bilirubin in the blood. It is a symptom of an array of conditions, e.g., obstruction of the bile duct by gallstones, inflammatory conditions, hepatitis, and cirrhosis.

Juxtaglomerular apparatus Comprised of the juxtaglomerular cells of the afferent arteriole and the macula densa of the distal tubule that initiates the renin-angiotensin mechanism to elevate blood pressure and increase sodium retention.

Kimmelstiel-Wilson disease A syndrome associated with diabetes mellitus, hypertension, glomerulonephrosis, edema, and retinal lesions.

Köhler illumination A method of light adjustment used to achieve the correct illumination of the substage condenser in order to focus light on the specimen plane.

Lecithin/sphingomyelin (L/S) ratio A laboratory test used to assess fetal pulmonary status. This test estimates the ratio of the amount of lecithin to sphingomyelin in amniotic fluid.

Linearity The quality or state of being linear (i.e., a straight line).

Lumbar puncture A puncture made by inserting an aspiration needle into the subarachnoid space of the spinal cord to extract spinal fluid.

Ketonemia An increase in ketones (intermediate products of fat metabolism formed during the catabolism or breakdown of fatty acids) in the blood.

Ketones Intermediate products of fat metabolism (acetone, acetoacetic acid (diacetic acid), and β-hydroxybutyric acid) formed during the catabolism or breakdown of fatty acids.

Ketonuria Increase in urinary ketones and an early indicator of diabetes mellitus.

Ketosis A condition characterized by increased ketones in the blood and urine.

Lamellar bodies Are the storage form of surfactant released into amniotic fluid by fetal breathing movements.

Legal's test Reaction of acetoacetic acid with nitroprusside/nitroferricyanide modified in the reagent strip test for ketones.

Leukocyte esterase An enzyme found in the primary granules of polymorphonuclear neutrophils, which are the most common leukocytes found in response to a bacterial infection. The presence of LE is the screening test for leukocytes used on reagent strips.

Leukocyturia   The presence of white blood cells in the urine, which often indicates the presence of an infection in the upper or lower urinary tract.

Macula densa   A group of cells in the wall of the distal convoluted tubule, next to the juxtaglomerular cells, that are sensitive to changes in salt concentration of the filtrate in the tubule.

Malabsorption   Inadequate or defective absorption of nutrients from the GI tract.

Maldigestion   A disorder of digestion which results from an intraluminal defect that leads to the incomplete breakdown of nutrients into their absorbable substrates.

Maltese cross formation   A cross of four arms with broadened ends; the formation appears in polarized specimens containing lipids in a microscopic wet preparation.

Maple syrup urine disease   Also referred to as branched chain α-ketoacid (BCKA) deficiency, MSUD is an autosomal recessive disease caused by a deficiency in a subunit of the branched-chain alpha ketoacid dehydrogenase complex.

Material Safety Data Sheets: (*See* Safety Data Sheet)

Maximal reabsorptive capacity (T_m):   The highest rate in mg/dL at which tubules can transfer a substance either from the tubules to the interstitial fluid or vice versa.

Mean   The average of a set of data.

Median   The middle value or the 50th percentile value of a sample set when the data are rank ordered by magnitude.

Medulla   The inner or central portion of the kidney.

Membranoproliferative glomerulonephritis   Inflammation of the glomeruli caused by an abnormal immune response characterized by subendothelial deposits and proliferating mesangial cells in the glomerulus.

Meningitis   An inflammation of the meninges around the brain and/or spinal cord.

Minimal change disease   Form of nephrotic syndrome most often seen in children in whom the cellular structure of the glomeruli is not altered to any significant extent.

Mode   The data point that occurs most frequently in a set of data.

Mucus   A gelatinous protein secreted by membranes in the urinary tract; increased amounts seen can be caused by bacterial infection, urinary calculi, or other irritants.

Myoglobin   An iron containing protein found in muscle cells which function to store oxygen for use in cell respiration.

Nephrolithiasis   The presence of calculi (stones) in the kidney.

Nephrotic syndrome   A condition characterized by increased glomerular permeability to proteins, resulting in marked proteinuria, edema, hypoalbuminemia, and hyperlipidemia.

Nephron   The structural and functional unit of the kidney. There are approximately 1 to 1.5 million nephrons in each kidney.

Neubauer hemocytometer   An example of a specific hemocytometer counting chamber.

Nitrite   Produced by the reduction of nitrate by the enzyme nitrate reductase produced by Gram-negative bacteria. It is the reagent strip reaction screening test for the presence of nitrate-reducing bacteria.

Nocturia   An increase in urine excretion at night.

Noninfectious glomerulonephritis   Acute glomerulonephritis associated with multisystem diseases: vasculitis collagen-vascular disease (systemic lupus erythematosus [SLE]), diabetic nephropathy, Henoch-Schlein purpura, IgA, nephropathy, and Goodpasture syndrome.

Non-ionizing radiation   Electromagnetic radiation ranging from extremely low frequency (ELF) to ultraviolet (UV).

Non-streptococcal glomerulonephritis   Glomerulonephritis caused by bacteria other than Group A beta streptococci (e.g., diplococci, other streptococci, staphylococci, and mycobacteria). Viruses have also been associated with this type of glomerulonephritis.

Numerical Aperture (NA)   A measure of the amount of light accepted by the objective lens. This affects the resolution, the contrast, and the magnification of the specimen.

Occupational and Safety Health Administration   A federal agency within the Department of Labor that was created by Congress through Public Law 91-596 in 1970 that provides federally mandated policies and procedures to ensure safety in the workplace, including laboratories and healthcare facilities.

Ochronosis   A rare condition marked by dark pigmentation of the ligaments, cartilage, fibrous tissues, skin, and urine.

Occult blood   Blood that is present in minute quantitie not seen by the naked eye.

Oligoclonal proteins   A group of specific proteins, likely to be IgG, commonly found in the spinal fluid of patients with multiple sclerosis.

Oliguria   A decrease in urine volume to < 400 mL/day.

Optical tube length   The distance between the rear focal plane of the objective and the forward focal plane of the ocular objective.

Orthostatic proteinuria   A condition where protein is found in the urine when the patient has been standing but not while reclining (supine). Proteinuria disappears when a patient is in a reclining position.

Osmotic diarrhea   Occurs when ingested, semi-absorbed, osmotically active solutes (e.g., sodium, potassium, and glucose) attract enough fluid into the lumen to exceed the reabsorptive capacity of the colon. The result is an increase in fecal water output proportional to the solute load.

Oval fat bodies   Lipids, or fat globules, can be taken up from the surrounding medium by degrading renal tubular epithelial cells. These cells are highly refractile and will exhibit a Maltese cross formation under polarizing microscopy.

p-aminohippurate: Substance used to measure tubular secretory capacity with 90% cleared by the renal tubules in a single passage through the kidney.

Paracentesis   The removal of ascites fluid from the abdominal cavity.

Parfocal The ability to achieve visualization of the specimen without major focus adjustment when switching between objectives of different magnification.

"Pass through" phenomenon Occurs in the Clinitest reaction when large amounts of glucose or other reducing substances are present in the urine and the reaction goes through the entire color range very quickly and back to dark greenish brown.

Passive transport Movement of molecules across a membrane as a result of differences in their concentration or electrical potential on opposite sides of the membrane.

Pathognomonic Indicative of a disease, especially its characteristic symptoms.

Pericardial sac A space that lies between the visceral and parietal pericardium.

Pericardiocentesis Removal or aspiration of pericardial fluid using a sterile syringe.

Pericardium The fibro serous sac enclosing the heart and the roots of the great vessels.

Peritoneal cavity A closed sac formed the lining of the abdominal cavity by the parietal peritoneum.

Peritoneum A serous membrane that is comprised of the parietal peritoneum and visceral peritoneum.

Peritubular capillaries The capillaries surrounding the renal tubules.

Personal Protective Equipment Specialized clothing or equipment worn by employees for protection against hazards (e.g., chemicals and biological organisms).

pH A measure of the hydrogen ion concentration of a solution. The negative logarithm of the hydrogen ion concentration; degree of acidity or alkalinity is expressed in pH units.

Phase contrast illumination Method of altering the phase of different light wavelengths in order to increase the visualization of elements in a microscopic specimen that have the same refractive index as the surrounding medium.

Phenylketonuria A recessive hereditary disease caused by the body's failure to oxidize phenylalanine to tyrosine due to the defective enzyme phenylalanine hydroxylase.

PLAN A plan objective is one designed to produce flatness of the field of focus and is flat on one side.

Pleural space A closed space (similar to the inside of a balloon) within which the lung has grown.

Polarizing microscopy A technique used to view objects under a microscope which utilizes light polarization to make objects appear as unique colors

Polyuria An increase in daily urine volume to over 2000 mL/day.

Population The universe of values or attributes, such as all of the fasting serum cholesterol levels of all apparently healthy males in the United States.

Porphyrias A group of inherited and acquired disorders of heme biosynthesis caused by deficiencies of specific enzymes in the biosynthetic pathway. The result is an excess production and increased excretion of precursors formed in the steps before the enzyme defect.

Posthepatic jaundice Jaundice caused by bile duct obstruction, e.g., gallstones or cancer.

Postrenal proteinuria Increase in proteins in the urine produced by the urinary or genital tract due to inflammation, malignancy, or injury.

Precision The ability to produce the same value for replicate measurements of the same sample.

Preeclampsia A complication of pregnancy manifested by increased hypertension, proteinuria, and edema.

Precipitation test Cold precipitation of proteins using sulfosalicylic acid (SSA), 3% to 7% w/v, used to confirm a positive reagent strip protein.

Prehepatic jaundice Jaundice caused by increased RBC destruction or hemolysis, e.g., hemolytic anemia.

Prerenal glucosuria Increase in urine glucose because of increased plasma glucose as a result of hormonal disorders, the most common condition is diabetes mellitus.

Prerenal proteinuria Proteinuria that occurs before the kidney and not due to renal disease. Overflow proteinuria due to increased levels of low molecular weight proteins.

Preservative An additive that protects the urine against bacterial growth and metabolism and minimizes changes in the urine.

Primary glomerulonephritis Glomerulonephritis that specifically affects the kidney.

Prion protein A protein that is capable of folding into an unusual shape and may also have the ability to cause other proteins to change their shape as well.

Protein error of indicators At a constant pH, some indicators are one color when protein is absent and another color when protein is present. It is used in reagent strips as a screening test for proteinuria.

Proteinuria An increase in the loss of protein in the urine often associated with early renal disease.

Proximal convoluted tubule The renal tubule closest to the glomerulus where the largest percentage of reabsorption of essential substances takes place.

Proximal renal tubular acidosis Very rare and occurs as a result of impairment of reabsorption of HCO_3^- in the proximal tubules, producing a urine pH >7 if plasma HCO_3^- concentration is normal, and a urine pH <5.5 if plasma HCO_3^- is already depleted. The most common cause of proximal RTA in children is Fanconi's syndrome.

Pseudocasts The appearance of cast-like elements in urine wet mounts created by collections of amorphous crystals formed by the action of the cover slip on the slide.

Pseudochylous effusion Fluid that is formed gradually through the breakdown of cellular lipid in long-standing effusion such as tuberculosis or rheumatoid pleuritis.

Pseudogout Chronic recurrent arthritis clinically similar to gout. Crystals of calcium pyrophosphate dihydrate are commonly found in the synovial fluid.

Pyelonephritis Inflammation and bacterial infection of the kidneys usually caused by a lower urinary tract infection.

Pyuria Presence of white blood cells in the urine that often indicates the presence of an infection in the upper or lower urinary tract.

Quad screen A group of four laboratory tests including uE_3, β-hCG, dimeric inhibin A and AFP usually performed at 16–18 weeks gestation to assess patients for possible Down's syndrome.

Quality control The procedures for monitoring and evaluating the quality of the analytical testing process of each method to ensure the accuracy and reliability of patient test results.

Ragocytes A granulocytes containing phagocytized immune complexes often found in patients with active rheumatoid arthritis.

Random urines A urine specimen that is collected at any time—no specified time, but the time collected should be noted on the container.

Range A measure of spread or variation in a set of data.

Reagent strip Plastic strips with chemical-impregnated absorbent pads for each test/analyte. When the pad comes in contact with urine that contains the analyte a color is produced depending on the concentration of the analyte. It is used to detect various urine analytes.

Refractive Index The comparison of the velocity of light in air with the velocity of light in a solution, in this case urine.

Refractometer Device that measures the concentration of dissolved particles by measuring the refractive index. Clinical refractometers make use of principles of light by measuring the velocity and angle at which light passes through a solution enters a prism and mathematically converts this angle (refractive index) to specific gravity.

Renal artery A branch of the abdominal aorta that supplies blood to the kidney.

Renal calyces A cuplike extension of the renal pelvis.

Renal clearance The rate at which the kidneys remove a substance from the plasma or blood or a quantitative expression of the rate at which a substance is excreted by the kidneys in relation to the concentration of the same substance in the plasma usually expressed as mL cleared per minute.

Renal glucosuria Increased levels of glucose in the urine caused by conditions that affect tubular reabsorption, e.g., Fanconi's syndrome.

Renal lithiasis Kidney stone formation.

Renal proteinuria Increase in urine protein associated with glomerular membrane damage by toxic substances or renal infections, e.g., pyelonephritis.

Renal threshold The plasma concentration at which active transport stops that allows for complete reabsorption of the substance when its plasma concentration is within normal limits. The renal threshold for glucose is 160 to 180 mg/dL.

Renal tubular acidosis Class of disorders in which excretion of hydrogen ions or reabsorption of filtered bicarbonate (HCO_3^-) is impaired leading to a chronic metabolic acidosis.

Renal tubular cells Those epithelial cells that line the proximal and distal convoluted renal tubule of the kidney.

Renal tubular disease Disorder that results from injury and damage to the tubules; it can also be caused by metabolic disorders, e.g., Fanconi's syndrome, that damage the tubules.

Renal vein The blood vessel which returns essential substances to the body.

Renin An enzyme produced in the kidney by the cells of the juxtaglomerular apparatus when (1) blood pressure declines (renal artery hypotension), (2) a decrease in blood volume is sensed, or (3) a decrease in sodium is detected in the distal tubules of the kidney.

Renin-angiotensin system Regulates flow of blood to and within the kidneys by responding to changes in blood pressure and plasma sodium content.

Renovascular disease Pertains to diseases(es) associated with blood vessels associated with the kidneys.

Resolution The ability of a lens system to distinguish two points in the field as separate and distinct.

Resolving power The shortest distance between two points that can be distinguished as separate and distinct.

Reticle A micrometer measure engraved on a glass slide and placed within the ocular lens in order to measure specimens in the field of view.

Rhabdomyolysis An acute disease characterized by destruction of skeletal muscle..

Rheostat The mechanical adjustment of light intensity found on the outside of the microscope base.

Safety Data Sheet A document that consist of 16 sections (e.g., identification, composition, hazards, first aid, firefighting concerns, and safe handling) that are relevant to chemicals being used in the laboratory.

Sample A portion or subset of a population, such as the serum cholesterol levels of all males in the laboratory.

Second-tier testing A confirmatory test that is performed when primary-screening tests, either by tandem mass spectrometry or another method, yield an equivocal result.

Secretory diarrhea A type of diarrhea caused by derangement in fluid and electrolytes transport across intestinal mucosa. There is an increase in secretion of water and electrolytes that overwhelms the reabsorptive ability of the large intestine.

Secondary glomerulonephritis Glomerulonephritis that principally involves other organs and the kidney secondarily.

Serous fluid Fluid formed as a plasma ultrafiltrate that provides lubrication between the parietal and visceral serous membranes.

Skewness A measure of the degree of asymmetry of a distribution.

Sperm motility Refers to the movement of sperm and is reported as the percentage of sperm that move.

Spherical aberration Distortion of the image caused by differential focal points of light waves passing through the outer edge and center of a lens. This causes the outer edges of the specimen to be less focused than that at the center.

Spinal tap   Also, lumbar puncture is commonly preferred method of extracting spinal fluid.

Standard deviation   A measure of the dispersion of a group of values around a mean.

Steatorrhea   Describes the presence of excess fat in stools. In quantitative terms, it represents an amount of stool fat that exceeds 7 g/day.

Sternheimer-Malbin stain   A stain composed of a crystal violet and Safranin combination used to stain urine sediment for the visualization of white blood cells, epithelial cells, and casts.

Subarachnoid hemorrhage   Bleeding into the subarachnoid space that lies between the pia mater and the arachnoid mater.

Suprapubic aspiration   A procedure for draining the bladder when it is not possible to use a catheter.

Suprapubic collection   Urine collection using direct needle aspiration through the abdominal wall into the bladder.

Surfactant   A surface-active substance that lowers surface tension.

Synovial fluid   Clear lubricating fluid of the joint, bursae, and tendon sheaths secreted by the synovial membrane of a joint. The fluid is an ultrafiltrate that contains hyaluronic acid.

Synovial joint   Joint in which the articulating surfaces are separated by synovial fluid.

Synoviocyte   Cells in the synovial membrane that secrete hyaluronic acid.

Tamm-Horsfall protein   A glycoprotein produced by the thick ascending limb of the Loop of Henle and distal convoluted tubule. It is found in normal urine and is a major component of casts.

Tandem mass spectrometry   A spectrometry technique that uses two mass spectrometers in unison to detect minute quantities of analytes in samples.

Tau protein   A unique protein that is increased in Alzheimer disease and reflects neurofibrillary tangles but the increase overlaps with a wide number of other neurological diseases.

Teratogen   A substance that acts preferentially on an embryo at precise stages of its development, thereby leading to possible anomalies and malformations.

Three-glass collection   Procedure used to determine prostatic infection in males. All portions of the urine—beginning, middle, and end—are collected in three separate containers.

Thoracentesis   A technique that uses a needle and syringe to remove pleural fluid from the thoracic cavity.

Tophus   A deposit of sodium biurate in tissues near a joint and in the ear.

Timed specimen   Specimen required when measuring the exact concentration of a urine chemical is required and not the semiquantitative (trace, small, moderate, or large) presence or absence of the analyte. Urine is collected within a specified number of hours at a specific time.

Transthyretin   Also prealbumin, is an alpha-globulin secreted by the liver that transports retinal-binding protein and thyroxine in blood and spinal fluid.

Transudate   When serous fluid passes through a membrane, especially a capillary wall, and accumulates in a body cavity.

Traumatic tap   A term used to signify trauma from the needle causing bleeding into the lumbar space.

Trichomonas vaginalis   A single cell protozoan with a flagella for propulsion. Urinary tract infection may occur in both males and females and is usually transmitted through sexual contact.

Triple test   A group of three laboratory tests including uE_3, β-hCG, and AFP usually performed at 16–18 weeks gestation to assess patients for possible Down's syndrome.

Tubular reabsorption   Process by which substances moved from the filtrate into the blood through active or passive transport.

Tubular secretion   The passage of substances from the blood in the peritubular capillaries to the tubular filtrate.

Tubulointerstitial nephritis   A heterogeneous group of disorders that share similar features of tubular and interstitial (space or gap in the kidney outside of the structure of the nephron) injury due to a toxic agent, e.g., drug or chemical.

Turbidity   Opacity due to the suspension of flaky or granular particles in a normally clear liquid, e.g., urine.

Tyrosinemia   A disease of tyrosine metabolism caused by a deficiency of the enzyme tyrosine aminotransferase.

Ultrafiltrate   The portions of a solution where the dispersed particles but not the liquid are held back.

Unconjugated bilirubin   The bilirubin formed by the degradation of hemoglobin, which binds to albumin and is carried to the liver. It is not soluble in water and cannot be excreted in the urine.

Unconjugated estriol   Estriol that circulates in blood not bound to protein.

Universal precautions   Is a practice described by National Institute for Occupational Safety and Health (NIOSH) in which every clinical laboratory should treat all human blood and other potentially infectious material as if they were known to contain infectious agents such a HBV, HIV, and other bloodborne pathogens.

Ureter   The tube that carries urine from the kidney to the bladder.

Urethra   The tube for the excretion of urine extending from the bladder to the outside.

Urethritis   Inflammation of the urethra.

Urinometer   A device, a type of hydrometer, that consists of a weighted float that has a scale calibrated in terms of specific gravity from 1.000–1.040 and is used to measure specific gravity.

Urobilin   A brown pigment formed by the oxidation of urobilinogen, a decomposition product of urobilinogen.

Urobilinogen   A bile pigment that is formed from the degradation of hemoglobin produced in the intestine from the reduction of bilirubin by the intestinal bacteria.

Urochrome   The chief pigment in urine that is the product of endogenous metabolism and under normal conditions is produced at a constant rate.

Uromodulin   An immunosuppressive protein produced in the kidney that is identical to Tamm-Horsfall protein.

Urothelial nonsquamous epithelial   Found in the lining of the bladder and urethra. The structural entity is neither cuboidal nor squamous and is called transitional epithelium. These cells have the unique ability to expand and contract, which explains the modified structure.

Vesicourethral reflux   The reflux of urine from the bladder back into the ureters, the most common anatomic cause of acute pyelonephritis.

Visceral epithelial podocytes   The third layer of the glomerular membrane consisting of cells containing podo (foot) processes that restrict large molecules, e.g., larger proteins, from passing through the glomerular membrane.

Working distance   The free space between the lower end of the objective and the upper surface of the specimen (glass slide or cover slip).

Xanthochromia   Describes the yellow color in the supernatant of centrifuged CSF.

Xenobiotic   A substance that is foreign to a living organism and is usually harmful.

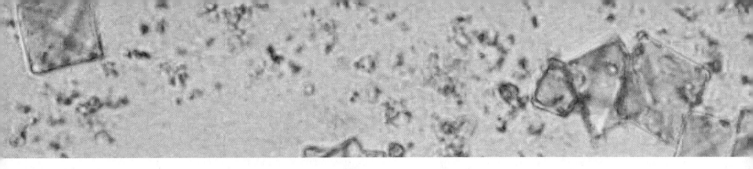

Index

Note: Page numbers with *b, f, n, or t* indicate boxes, figures, footnotes, or tables respectively.